Adult Telephone Protocols

Office Version | 3rd Edition

David A. Thompson, MD, FACEP

American Academy of Pediatrics

DEDICATED TO THE HEALTH OF ALL CHILDREN™

AAP Department of Marketing and Publications Staff

Maureen DeRosa, MPA, Director, Department of Marketing and Publications
Sandi King, MS, Director, Division of Publishing and Production Services
Jason Crase, Editorial Specialist
Shannan Martin, Publishing and Production Services Specialist
Linda Diamond, Manager, Art Direction and Production
Julia Lee, Director, Division of Marketing and Sales
Marirose Russo, Manager, Practice Services Marketing

Cover design by Wild Onion Design, Inc.

ISBN 978-1-58110-743-2
Library of Congress Control Number: Pending
MA0635

Adult Telephone Protocols: Office Version

User's Responsibility: Author and Publisher Disclaimer Notice

- These protocols are clinical guidelines that must be used in conjunction with critical thinking and clinical judgment. Therefore, these protocols are most suitable for use by physicians, nurse practitioners, or physician assistants. Nurses should receive special training before using these protocols (see Training in User's Guide). Non-licensed and non-health professionals (eg, secretaries) should not use these protocols.
- These protocols should not be used unless they have been reviewed, amended as necessary, and approved by a supervising physician or medical director responsible for overseeing their use.
- These protocols are as up-to-date as possible at the time of publication and revision. However, it is the responsibility of the supervising physician or medical director to keep these protocols current based on changes in the medical literature and medical practice. The most up-to-date versions of the protocols are available at www.stcc-triage.com/download/aap.html.
- The contents of these protocols have been carefully reviewed and tested for accuracy, but they are not, and cannot be, perfect. Therefore, the author and publisher disclaim responsibility for any harmful consequence, loss, injury, or damage associated with the use and application of information or advice contained in these protocols.
- The author and publisher do not warrant or guarantee the accuracy, safety, efficacy, or completeness of any of these protocols.
- Any person, institution, or organization using these protocols assumes full responsibility for acts or omissions arising out of their use or misuse. The user assumes all risks associated with using these protocols.
- Using this product means the user has read and accepts the Disclaimer Notice.

Urgent updates available at www.stcc-triage.com/download/aap.html

Adult Telephone Protocols: Office Version

Alphabetic Listing

Anatomic Listing

Bites/Stings

Skin, Localized Symptoms

Skin, Widespread Symptoms

Fever Symptoms

Mental and Behavioral Health Symptoms

Miscellaneous (Other)

Adult Telephone Protocols: Office Version

Category Listing

Allergies

Behavior, Psychosocial

Bites/Stings

Disease/Diagnosis (Infections)

Disease/Diagnosis (Not Infections)

Emergencies

Follow-up Calls

Foreign Body

Exposure

Medical Device, Procedure, or Surgery

Medication (Drug)

Pain

Symptoms

Trauma/Injury

Adult Telephone Protocols: Office Version

Appendix Table of Contents

ABDOMINAL PAIN (FEMALE)

DEFINITION

- Pain or discomfort located between the bottom of the rib cage and the groin crease
- Female

Pain Severity Is Defined As:

- **Mild (1-3):** Doesn't interfere with normal activities, abdomen soft and not tender to touch
- **Moderate (4-7):** Interferes with normal activities or awakens from sleep, tender to touch
- **Severe (8-10):** Excruciating pain, doubled over, unable to do any normal activities

TRIAGE ASSESSMENT QUESTIONS

Call EMS 911 Now

- Passed out (i.e., fainted, collapsed and was not responding)
  R/O: shock
  FIRST AID: Lie down with the feet elevated.
- Shock suspected (e.g., cold/pale/clammy skin, too weak to stand)
  R/O: shock
  FIRST AID: Lie down with the feet elevated.
- Sounds like a life-threatening emergency to the triager

See More Appropriate Protocol

- Chest pain
  Go to Protocol: Chest Pain (on page 48) first; then use appropriate Abdominal Pain Protocol
- Pain is mainly in upper abdomen (if needed, ask: "Is it mainly above the belly button?")
  Go to Protocol: Abdominal Pain (Upper) on page 6

Go to ED Now

- SEVERE abdominal pain (e.g., excruciating)
  R/O: acute abdomen
- Vomiting red blood or black (coffee ground) material
  R/O: gastritis, peptic ulcer disease
- Bloody, black, or tarry bowel movements
  R/O: GI bleed

Go to ED Now (or to Office With PCP Approval)

- Constant abdominal pain lasting > 2 hours
  R/O: acute abdomen
- Vomiting bile (green color)
  R/O: intestinal obstruction
- Patient sounds very sick or weak to the triager

Go to Office Now

- Vomiting and abdomen looks much more swollen than usual
- White of the eyes have turned yellow (i.e., jaundice)
  R/O: cholelithiasis, hepatitis
- Blood in urine (red, pink, or tea-colored)
  R/O: kidney stone
- Fever > 103° F (39.4° C)
- Fever > 100.5° F (38.1° C) and over 60 years of age
- Fever > 100.5° F (38.1° C) and has diabetes mellitus or a weakened immune system (e.g., HIV positive, cancer chemotherapy, organ transplant, splenectomy, chronic steroids)
- Fever > 100.5° F (38.1° C) and bedridden (e.g., nursing home patient, stroke, chronic illness, recovering from surgery)
  R/O: bacterial infection
  Note: may need ambulance transport to ED.
- Pregnant or could be pregnant (i.e., missed last menstrual period)
  R/O: spontaneous abortion or ectopic pregnancy

See Today in Office

- MODERATE OR MILD pain that comes and goes (cramps) lasts > 24 hours
- Age > 60 years
  Reason: higher risk of serious cause of abdominal pain
- Unusual vaginal discharge
  R/O: vaginitis, PID
- Patient wants to be seen

See Within 2 Weeks in Office

- Abdominal pain is a chronic symptom (recurrent or ongoing AND lasting > 4 weeks)
- Pain with sexual intercourse (dyspareunia)

Home Care

- Mild abdominal pain

HOME CARE ADVICE FOR MILD ABDOMINAL PAIN

1. **Reassurance:** A mild stomachache can be caused by indigestion, gas pains, or overeating. Sometimes a stomachache signals the onset of a vomiting illness due to a viral gastroenteritis ("stomach flu").
2. **Rest:** Lie down and rest until you feel better.
3. **Fluids:** Sip clear fluids only (e.g., water, flat soft drinks, or ½-strength fruit juice) until the pain has been gone for over 2 hours. Then slowly return to a regular diet.
4. **Diet:**
   - Slowly advance diet from clear liquids to a bland diet.
   - Avoid alcohol or caffeinated beverages.
   - Avoid greasy or fatty foods.
5. **Pass a BM:** Sit on the toilet and try to pass a bowel movement (BM). Do not strain. This may relieve the pain if it is due to constipation or impending diarrhea.
6. **Avoid NSAIDs and Aspirin:** Avoid any drug that can irritate the stomach lining and make the pain worse (especially aspirin and NSAIDs like ibuprofen).
7. **Expected Course:** With harmless causes, the pain is usually better or goes away within 2 hours. With viral gastroenteritis ("stomach flu"), belly cramps may precede each bout of vomiting or diarrhea and may last 2-3 days. With serious causes (such as appendicitis) the pain becomes constant and more severe.
8. **Pregnancy Test, When in Doubt:**
   - If there is any possibility of pregnancy, obtain and use a urine pregnancy test from the local drugstore.
   - Follow the instructions included in the package.
9. **Call Back If:**
   - Abdominal pain is constant and present for more than 2 hours.
   - Abdominal pains come and go and are present for more than 24 hours.
   - You are pregnant.
   - You become worse.

FIRST AID

First Aid Advice for Shock:

Lie down with the feet elevated.

BACKGROUND INFORMATION

General Information

- Abdominal pain is a very common symptom. Sometimes it may be a symptom of a benign gastrointestinal disorder like gas, overeating, or gastroenteritis. At times abdominal pain is a symptom of a moderately serious problem like appendicitis or biliary colic (gallstones).
- Abdominal pain may also be the warning symptom of life-threatening conditions like perforated peptic ulcer disease, mesenteric ischemia, and ruptured abdominal aortic aneurysm.
- There are multiple causes of abdominal pain in women. In women, the range of diagnoses needs to be broadened to include problems related to pregnancy and the female genitourinary organs.
- Pain in the elderly carries with it a higher risk of serious illness. In one study of elderly patients presenting to an emergency department with abdominal pain, 40% had surgical illness.

Top Causes of Abdominal Pain in Women Under 50 Years of Age

- Appendicitis
- Ectopic pregnancy
- Endometriosis
- Gallbladder disease
- Nonspecific abdominal pain
- Ovarian cyst
- Pelvic inflammatory disease
- Peptic ulcer disease
- Spontaneous abortion

Top Causes of Abdominal Pain in Women Over 50 Years of Age

- Appendicitis
- Bowel obstruction
- Diverticulitis
- Gallbladder disease
- Pancreatitis
- Peptic ulcer disease

Location of Pain and Possible Etiologies

- **RUQ:** Liver and gallbladder
- **Epigastric:** Heart, stomach, duodenum, esophagus
- **LUQ:** Spleen, stomach
- **Periumbilical:** Pancreas, early appendicitis, small bowel
- **RLQ:** Ileum, appendix, ovary, kidney
- **Suprapubic:** Uterus, bladder, rectum
- **LLQ:** Sigmoid colon, ovary, kidney

ABDOMINAL PAIN (MALE)

DEFINITION

- Pain or discomfort located between the bottom of the rib cage and the groin crease
- Male

Pain Severity Is Defined As:

- **Mild (1-3):** Doesn't interfere with normal activities, abdomen soft and not tender to touch
- **Moderate (4-7):** Interferes with normal activities or awakens from sleep, tender to touch
- **Severe (8-10):** Excruciating pain, doubled over, unable to do any normal activities

TRIAGE ASSESSMENT QUESTIONS

Call EMS 911 Now

- Passed out (i.e., fainted, collapsed and was not responding)
  R/O: shock
  FIRST AID: Lie down with the feet elevated.
- Shock suspected (e.g., cold/pale/clammy skin, too weak to stand)
  R/O: shock
  FIRST AID: Lie down with the feet elevated.
- Sounds like a life-threatening emergency to the triager

See More Appropriate Protocol

- Chest pain
  Go to Protocol: Chest Pain on page 48 first; then use appropriate Abdominal Pain Protocol
- Pain is mainly in upper abdomen (if needed, ask: "Is it mainly above the belly button?")
  Go to Protocol: Abdominal Pain (Upper) on page 6

Go to ED Now

- SEVERE abdominal pain (e.g., excruciating)
  R/O: acute abdomen
- Vomiting red blood or black (coffee ground) material
  R/O: gastritis, peptic ulcer disease
- Bloody, black, or tarry bowel movements
  R/O: GI bleed
- Unable to urinate (or only a few drops) and bladder feels very full
  R/O: urinary retention
- Pain in scrotum persists > 1 hour
  R/O: kidney stone

Go to ED Now (or to Office With PCP Approval)

- Constant abdominal pain lasting > 2 hours
  R/O: acute abdomen
- Vomiting bile (green color)
  R/O: intestinal obstruction
- Patient sounds very sick or weak to the triager

Go to Office Now

- Vomiting and abdomen looks much more swollen than usual
- White of the eyes have turned yellow (i.e., jaundice)
  R/O: cholelithiasis, hepatitis
- Blood in urine (red, pink, or tea-colored)
  R/O: kidney stone
- Fever > 103° F (39.4° C)
- Fever > 100.5° F (38.1° C) and over 60 years of age
- Fever > 100.5° F (38.1° C) and has diabetes mellitus or a weakened immune system (e.g., HIV positive, cancer chemotherapy, organ transplant, splenectomy, chronic steroids)
- Fever > 100.5° F (38.1° C) and bedridden (e.g., nursing home patient, stroke, chronic illness, recovering from surgery)
  R/O: bacterial infection
  Note: may need ambulance transport to ED.

See Today in Office

- MILD pain that comes and goes (cramps) lasts > 24 hours
- Age > 60 years
  Reason: higher risk of serious cause of abdominal pain
- Patient wants to be seen

See Within 2 Weeks in Office

- Abdominal pain is a chronic symptom (recurrent or ongoing AND lasting > 4 weeks)

Home Care

- Mild abdominal pain

HOME CARE ADVICE FOR MILD ABDOMINAL PAIN

1. **Reassurance:** A mild stomachache can be caused by indigestion, gas pains, or overeating. Sometimes a stomachache signals the onset of a vomiting illness due to a viral gastroenteritis ("stomach flu").
2. **Rest:** Lie down and rest until you feel better.
3. **Fluids:** Sip clear fluids only (e.g., water, flat soft drinks, or ½-strength fruit juice) until the pain has been gone for over 2 hours. Then slowly return to a regular diet.
4. **Diet:**
   - Slowly advance diet from clear liquids to a bland diet.
   - Avoid alcohol or caffeinated beverages.
   - Avoid greasy or fatty foods.
5. **Pass a BM:** Sit on the toilet and try to pass a bowel movement (BM). Do not strain. This may relieve pain if it is due to constipation or impending diarrhea.
6. **Avoid NSAIDs and Aspirin:** Avoid any drug that can irritate the stomach lining and make the pain worse (especially aspirin and NSAIDs like ibuprofen).
7. **Expected Course:** With harmless causes, the pain is usually better or goes away within 2 hours. With viral gastroenteritis ("stomach flu"), belly cramps may precede each bout of vomiting or diarrhea and may last 2-3 days. With serious causes (such as appendicitis) the pain becomes constant and more severe.
8. **Call Back If:**
   - Abdominal pain is constant and present for more than 2 hours.
   - Abdominal pains come and go and are present for more than 24 hours.
   - You become worse.

FIRST AID

First Aid Advice for Shock:
Lie down with the feet elevated.

BACKGROUND INFORMATION

General Information

- Abdominal pain is a very common symptom. Sometimes it may be a symptom of a benign gastrointestinal disorder like gas, overeating, or gastroenteritis. At times abdominal pain is a symptom of a moderately serious problem like appendicitis or biliary colic (gallstones). Abdominal pain may also be the warning symptom of life-threatening conditions like perforated peptic ulcer disease, mesenteric ischemia, and ruptured abdominal aortic aneurysm.
- Abdominal pain in the elderly carries with it a higher risk of serious illness.

Top Causes of Abdominal Pain in Men Under 50 Years of Age

- Appendicitis
- Gallbladder disease
- Nonspecific abdominal pain
- Peptic ulcer disease

Top Causes of Abdominal Pain in Men Over 50 Years of Age

- Appendicitis
- Bowel obstruction
- Diverticulitis
- Gallbladder disease
- Pancreatitis
- Peptic ulcer disease

Location of Pain and Possible Etiologies

- **RUQ:** Liver and gallbladder
- **Epigastric:** Heart, stomach, duodenum, esophagus, gallbladder, pancreas
- **LUQ:** Spleen, stomach
- **Periumbilical:** Pancreas, early appendicitis, small bowel
- **RLQ:** Ileum, appendix, kidney
- **Suprapubic:** Bladder, rectum, colon
- **LLQ:** Sigmoid colon, kidney

ABDOMINAL PAIN (UPPER)

DEFINITION

- Pain is primarily centered in the upper abdomen (if needed, ask: "Is it just below rib cage and above belly button?")
- Pain may radiate into chest, back, or other location.

Pain Severity Is Defined As:

- **Mild (1-3):** Doesn't interfere with normal activities, abdomen soft and not tender to touch
- **Moderate (4-7):** Interferes with normal activities or awakens from sleep, tender to touch
- **Severe (8-10):** Excruciating pain, doubled over, unable to do any normal activities

TRIAGE ASSESSMENT QUESTIONS

Call EMS 911 Now

- Passed out (i.e., fainted, collapsed and was not responding)
  R/O: shock
  FIRST AID: Lie down with the feet elevated.
- Shock suspected (e.g., cold/pale/clammy skin, too weak to stand)
  R/O: shock
  FIRST AID: Lie down with the feet elevated.
- Visible sweat on face or sweat is dripping down

See More Appropriate Protocol

- Chest pain
  Go to Protocol: Chest Pain on page 48

Go to ED Now

- SEVERE abdominal pain (e.g., excruciating)
  R/O: acute abdomen
- Pain lasting > 10 minutes and over 50 years old
  Reason: higher risk of cardiac ischemia or surgical cause of abdominal pain
- Pain lasting > 10 minutes and over 40 years old and associated chest, arm, neck, upper back, or jaw pain
  Reason: higher risk of cardiac ischemia as cause of pain
- Pain lasting > 10 minutes and over 35 years old and at least one cardiac risk factor
- Risks include: hypertension, diabetes, high cholesterol, obesity, family history of heart disease, smoking
- Pain lasting > 10 minutes and history of heart disease (i.e., heart attack, bypass surgery, angina, angioplasty, CHF)
  Reason: higher risk of cardiac ischemia as cause of pain
- Recent injury to the abdomen
- Vomiting red blood or black (coffee ground) material
  R/O: gastritis, peptic ulcer disease
- Blood in bowel movements (black/tarry or red)

Go to ED Now (or to Office With PCP Approval)

- Constant abdominal pain lasting > 2 hours
  R/O: acute abdomen
- Vomiting bile (green color)
  R/O: intestinal obstruction
- Patient sounds very sick or weak to the triager

Go to Office Now

- Vomiting and abdomen looks much more swollen than usual
- White of the eyes have turned yellow (i.e., jaundice)
  R/O: cholelithiasis, hepatitis
- Fever > 103° F (39.4° C)
- Fever > 100.5° F (38.1° C) and over 60 years of age
- Fever > 100.5° F (38.1° C) and has diabetes mellitus or a weakened immune system (e.g., HIV positive, cancer chemotherapy, organ transplant, splenectomy, chronic steroids)
- Fever > 100.5° F (38.1° C) and bedridden (e.g., nursing home patient, stroke, chronic illness, recovering from surgery)
  R/O: bacterial infection
  Note: may need ambulance transport to ED.
- Pregnant > 24 weeks
  R/O: preeclampsia

See Today in Office

- Age > 60 years
  Reason: risk of serious cause
- Patient wants to be seen

See Today or Tomorrow in Office

- MILD pain that comes and goes (cramps) lasts > 24 hours
- Alcohol abuse known or suspected

See Within 2 Weeks in Office

- Abdominal pain is a chronic symptom (recurrent or ongoing AND lasting > 4 weeks)
- Intermittent burning pains radiating into chest or sour taste in mouth
  R/O: possible reflux esophagitis

Home Care

- Mild abdominal pain

HOME CARE ADVICE FOR MILD UPPER ABDOMINAL PAIN

1. **Reassurance:** A mild stomachache can be from indigestion, stomach irritation, or overeating. Sometimes a stomachache signals the onset of a vomiting illness from a viral infection.
2. **Fluids:** Sip clear fluids only (e.g., water, flat soft drinks, or ½-strength fruit juice) until the pain is gone for 2 hours. Then slowly return to a regular diet.
3. **Diet:**
   - Slowly advance diet from clear liquids to a bland diet.
   - Avoid alcohol or caffeinated beverages.
   - Avoid greasy or fatty foods.
4. **Antacid:** If having pain now, try taking an antacid (e.g., Mylanta, Maalox). Dose: 2 tablespoons (30 mL) of liquid by mouth.
5. **Avoid NSAIDs and Aspirin:** Avoid any drug that can irritate the stomach lining and make the pain worse (especially aspirin and NSAIDs like ibuprofen).
6. **Stop Smoking:** Smoking can aggravate heartburn and stomach problems.
7. **Reducing Reflux Symptoms (GERD):** Eat smaller meals and avoid snacks for 2 hours before sleeping. Avoid the following foods, which tend to aggravate heartburn and stomach problems: fatty/greasy foods, spicy foods, caffeinated beverages, mints, and chocolate.
8. **Expected Course:** With harmless causes, the pain usually lessens or is resolved in 2 hours. With gastroenteritis, stomach cramps may precede each bout of vomiting or diarrhea. With serious causes (such as appendicitis), the pain becomes constant and severe.
9. **Call Back If:**
   - Abdominal pain is constant and present for more than 2 hours.
   - You become worse.

FIRST AID

First Aid Advice For Shock:

Lie down with the feet elevated.

BACKGROUND INFORMATION

General Information

- There are multiple causes of upper abdominal pain.
- Gastritis and peptic ulcer disease are common and typically cause pain in the upper abdomen (epigastrium), sometimes accompanied by vomiting.
- Gastroesophageal reflux disease (GERD) causes a burning pain that radiates into chest. Lying down aggravates symptoms. May get a sour or bitter taste in mouth.
- Abdominal pain in the elderly carries with it a higher risk of serious illness.

Top Causes of Upper Abdominal Pain in Individuals Under 50 Years of Age

- Appendicitis
- Gallbladder disease
- Nonspecific abdominal pain
- Peptic ulcer disease

Top Causes of Upper Abdominal Pain in Individuals Over 50 Years of Age

- Appendicitis
- Bowel obstruction
- Diverticulitis
- Gallbladder disease
- Pancreatitis
- Peptic ulcer disease

Other Causes

- Angina and heart attack
- Abdominal aortic aneurysm
- Hepatitis
- Herpes zoster
- Pneumonia

Caution—Cardiac Ischemia

- The most life-threatening cause of acute upper abdominal pain is cardiac ischemia.
- Rarely, patients may present with upper abdominal pain as the sole symptom of a myocardial infarction. Usually there will be other associated symptoms of cardiac ischemia: chest pain, shortness of breath, nausea, and/or diaphoresis.
- Cardiac ischemia should be suspected in any patients with risk factors for cardiac disease. These include: hypertension, smoking, diabetes, hyperlipidemia, a strong family history of heart disease, and age greater than 50.
- Consider cardiac ischemia in patients who complain of "indigestion."

ALCOHOL USE AND ABUSE AND DEPENDENCE

DEFINITION

- Known or suspected alcohol abuse
- Questions or concerns related to alcohol intoxication, withdrawal, dependence, or abuse

TRIAGE ASSESSMENT QUESTIONS

Call EMS 911 Now

- Coma (e.g., not moving, not talking, not responding to stimuli)
  R/O: severe alcohol intoxication, overdose, occult head trauma, hepatic encephalopathy, hypoglycemia
- Difficult to awaken or acting confused (e.g., disoriented, slurred speech)
  R/O: DTs, severe alcohol intoxication, overdose, occult head trauma, hepatic encephalopathy, hypoglycemia
- Seeing, hearing, or feeling things that are not there (i.e., visual, auditory, or tactile hallucinations)
  R/O: alcohol withdrawal, alcoholic hallucinosis
- Slow, shallow, and weak breathing
  R/O: impending respiratory arrest
- Seizure
  R/O: alcohol withdrawal seizure
- Violent behavior or threatening to kill someone
  R/O: alcohol intoxication, DTs, homicidal ideation
- Patient attempted suicide
  R/O: physical injury or overdosage
- Threatening suicide
  Reason: suicidal ideation
- Sounds like a life-threatening emergency to the triager

See More Appropriate Protocol

- Substance abuse or dependence: question or problem related to
  Go to Protocol: Substance Abuse and Dependence on page 255

Go to ED Now

- Severe abdominal pain
  R/O: pancreatitis or other acute abdomen
- Constant abdominal pain lasting > 2 hours
  R/O: pancreatitis or other acute abdomen
- Blood in bowel movements (e.g., black, tarry or red blood)
  Exception: Blood on surface of BM with constipation
  R/O: gastritis, peptic ulcer disease, esophageal varices, lower GI bleed
- Vomiting red blood or black (coffee ground) material
  R/O: gastritis, esophageal varices, Mallory-Weiss tear
- Multiple episodes of vomiting and lasting more than 2 hours
  R/O: alcoholic ketoacidosis
- Feeling very shaky (i.e., visible tremors of hands)
  R/O: alcohol dependence, alcohol withdrawal

Go to ED Now (or to Office With PCP Approval)

- Drinks alcohol daily and prior alcohol withdrawal seizures
  REASON: higher risk of alcohol withdrawal
  R/O: alcohol dependence
- Drinks alcohol daily and prior DTs
  Reason: higher risk of alcohol withdrawal
  R/O: alcohol dependence
- Patient sounds very sick or weak to the triager

See Today in Office

- White of the eyes have turned yellow (i.e., jaundice)
  R/O: alcoholic hepatitis, cirrhosis of the liver
- Fever > 101.5° F (38.6° C)
  R/O: bacterial illness

See Today or Tomorrow in Office

- Patient wants to be seen

Callback by PCP Today

- Pregnant and intoxicated or admits to drinking problem
  Reason: risk to fetus (fetal alcohol syndrome)

Call Local Agency Today

- Alcohol or drug abuse, known or suspected
  Note: The CAGE questionnaire is a simple screening tool for alcohol abuse and dependence. See Background Information.
- Requesting admission for alcohol abuse
- Requesting to talk with a counselor (mental health worker, psychiatrist, etc.)
- Alcohol use interferes with work or school
- Male and 14 or more drinks/week, or more than 4 drinks on single occasion
  Reason: at-risk drinking, further evaluation and counseling needed
- Female or elderly and 7 or more drinks/week, or more than 3 drinks on single occasion
  Reason: at-risk drinking, further evaluation and counseling needed

Home Care

- ○ Alcohol use, abuse, and dependence, questions about
- ○ Blood alcohol level, question about
- ○ Sobering up from alcohol intoxication, questions about
  Reason: caller wants to know "how to help a friend/ family member sober up"
- ○ Pregnancy and alcohol, questions about

HOME CARE ADVICE

General Information

1. **Do Not Drink and Drive.** Pick a designated driver if you and your friends are drinking alcohol.
2. **Do Not Drink Alcohol During Pregnancy:**
   - Drinking alcohol during pregnancy can harm the baby and may cause birth defects (fetal alcohol syndrome).
   - Drinking small amounts (1 drink) occasionally may be OK as research has not yet shown this to cause harm to the baby.
   - The SAFEST thing for the baby is to NOT DRINK any alcohol during pregnancy.
3. **Caring for the Intoxicated (Drunk) Adult:**
   - No medicines speed up the sobering process (i.e., drinking coffee does not help).
   - Taking a cold shower may temporarily make someone more alert, but it will not speed up the sobering process.
   - Keep alcohol away from the patient (e.g., take patient away from bar/party, remove any nearby alcohol).
   - Watch and protect the patient from harm (e.g., avoid dangerous activities, driving).
   - Lay the patient on his/her side (in case of vomiting).
   - **Call 911 If:** Difficult to awaken, difficulty with breathing, or violent behavior.
4. **What Is the Effect of Drinking Alcohol on the Blood Alcohol Level?**
   - For an average-sized person, each of the following will raise the blood alcohol level approximately 25 mg/dL: 1 oz (one shot; 30 mL) of alcohol, 4 oz (half cup; 120 mL) of wine, or 12 oz (one can; 360 mL) of beer.
   - An average adult will break down (metabolize) alcohol at a rate of 15-25 mg/dL per hour.
   - **Example:** Drinking 3-4 beers will raise your alcohol level from 0 to 100 mg/dL and it will take 4-7 hours before your alcohol level is back to zero.
5. **At What Blood Alcohol Level Are You Considered Legally Drunk?**
   - The normal blood alcohol level is 0 (zero).
   - There are various different terminologies for reporting a blood alcohol level. Each of the following has the same meaning: 80 milligrams/dL, 80 grams per cent, 80 mg/100 mL, or 0.08.
   - Drinking 3-4 drinks is sufficient to make an average-sized person legally drunk.
   - In the U.S. the legal definition of alcohol intoxication varies from state to state: 80 mg/dL–100 mg/dL.
   - In Canada it is a criminal offense to drive a car while having a blood alcohol level greater than 80 mg/dL (0.08). Some Canadian provinces have sanctions (suspensions) for levels greater than 50 mg/dL (0.05).
6. **Local Alcohol Treatment Program:**
   - If available, local alcohol treatment program: xxx-xxx-xxxx.
   - If available, local psychiatric crisis service at ________________hospital: xxx-xxx-xxxx.
7. **Call Back If:**
   - You have more questions about alcohol or alcohol abuse.
   - You become worse.

Additional Resources

1. **Alcoholics Anonymous (AA):**
   - The Alcoholics Anonymous organization is a "fellowship of men and women who share their experience, strength and hope with each other that they may solve their common problem and help others to recover from alcoholism. The only requirement for membership is a desire to stop drinking."
   - If available, local phone number: xxx-xxx-xxxx.
   - National phone number: 212-870-3400.
   - Web site: www.aa.org.
2. **Al-Anon/Alateen:**
   - The goal of Al-Anon is "to help families and friends of alcoholics recover from the effects of living with the problem drinking of a relative or friend."
   - If available, local phone number: xxx-xxx-xxxx.
   - National phone number: 888-425-2666.
   - Web site: www.al-anon.org.
   - Web site: www.al-anon.org/for-alateen.
3. **Canada—Internet Resources**
   - **Canadian Network of Substance Abuse and Allied Professionals:** This Web site lists treatment agencies for each of the provinces in Canada. Available at: www.cnsaap.ca/Eng/CanadianLandscape/Pages/default.aspx.
   - **New Brunswick:** Department of Health and Wellness Addiction Services (www.gnb.ca/0378/addiction-e.asp). Services offered by region.
   - **Newfoundland and Labrador:** Newfoundland and Labrador Addictions Services (www.health.gov.nl.ca/health/addictions/services.html). Services offered by region.
   - **Northwest Territories:** Nats`ejée K`éh Treatment Centre (www.natsejeekeh.org). The phone number is 867-874-6699.
   - **Ontario—Drug and Alcohol Registry of Treatment (DART):** This is an online database of treatment programs offered in Ontario. It is searchable by name, municipality, Local Health Integration Network (LHIN), provincial service category, and/or specific population group. Available at: www.drugandalcoholhelpline.ca. The phone number for the helpline is 800-565-8603.
4. **United States—Substance Abuse and Mental Health Services Administration (SAMHSA):**
   - This governmental agency works to improve the quality and availability of substance abuse prevention, alcohol and drug addiction treatment, and mental health services.
   - More information available at: www.samhsa.gov.
5. **United States—SAMHSA Treatment Referral Line:**
   - SAMHSA Treatment Referral Routing Service (http://samhsa.gov/treatment) is a "confidential, free, 24-hour-a-day, 365-day-a-year, information service, in English and Spanish, for individuals and family members facing substance abuse and mental health issues. This service provides referrals to local treatment facilities, support groups, and community-based organizations. Callers can also order free publications and other information in print on substance abuse and mental health issues."
   - The phone number is 800-662-HELP (4357).
6. **United States—SAMHSA Substance Abuse Treatment Facility Locator:**
   - SAMHSA has a Web tool for finding local drug abuse treatment programs.
   - This locator is available at: http://findtreatment.samhsa.gov.

BACKGROUND INFORMATION

General Information

- Approximately 6% of the population in the United States and Canada meets diagnostic criteria for alcohol abuse or dependence.
- Women and the elderly will have a higher blood alcohol level in comparison with men for the same amount of alcohol consumption.

Definitions and Patterns of Alcohol Use

- **A Drink:** 1.5 oz hard liquor (one shot or jigger; 45 mL), 5 oz wine (small glass; 150 mL), 12 oz beer (one can; 360 mL)
- **Moderate Drinking (Social Drinking):** Men who have 2 or less drinks per day. Women/elderly who have 1 or less drinks per day.

- **At-Risk Drinking:** Individuals have no apparent medical, social, or legal problems related to alcohol but drink excessively. Men who have more than 14 drinks per week or more than 4 drinks on occasion. Women/elderly who have more than 7 drinks per week or more than 3 drinks on occasion.
- Drinking alcohol during pregnancy.
- **Alcohol Abuse (Problem Drinking, Harmful Drinking):** Individuals with alcohol abuse have patterns of alcohol drinking that lead to health, occupational, legal, or social problems. This can range from minor problems like waking up with a hangover to more serious consequences such as motor vehicle accidents and missing work.
- **Alcohol Dependence (Alcoholism):** Alcoholism is a disease. Alcoholics are physically addicted to alcohol and demonstrate withdrawal symptoms when they stop drinking. Alcoholics also develop tolerance, which means that they have to drink more alcohol to achieve the same level of intoxication.
- Alcoholics feel compelled to drink and continue to drink in the face of adverse consequences.

CAGE Questionnaire:

These 4 questions are a simple way to screen for alcohol abuse and dependence. One or 2 positive answers suggest at-risk alcohol drinking and the individual should see their doctor for further evaluation. Three or 4 positive answers indicate a high likelihood of alcohol abuse and/or dependency.

- Have you ever felt you should CUT down on your drinking?
- Have people ever ANNOYED you by criticizing your drinking?
- Have you ever felt bad or GUILTY about your drinking?
- Have you ever had a drink first thing in the morning to steady your nerves or to get rid of a hangover (EYE-OPENER)?

Conversion of Alcohol Level to SI Units

- mg/dL ethanol X 0.2171 = mmol/L
- mmol/L ethanol X 4.61 = mg/dL

Caution: Always Consider the Following Associated Conditions in Individuals With Alcohol-Related Problems:

- Depression and other psychiatric illnesses
- **Gastrointestinal Complications:** Pancreatitis, gastritis, gastrointestinal bleeding
- **Liver Disease:** Hepatitis, cirrhosis
- **Infectious Diseases:** Tuberculosis, pneumonia
- **Injury:** From fights, accidents
- Malnutrition and vitamin deficiency
- **Neurologic Complications:** Seizures
- Polydrug abuse
- Suicidal ideation and attempt

ANIMAL BITE

DEFINITION

- Bite or claw wound from a pet, farm, or wild animal
- Includes follow-up calls about receiving an antibiotic for an animal bite infection

Wild Animals at Risk for RABIES:

- Bat, skunk, raccoon, fox, coyote
- Any other large wild animal

Pet Animals at Risk for RABIES:

- Outdoor pets who are stray, sick, or unvaccinated AND living in communities where rabies occurs in pets. Triagers should check with the local public health department about the risk for rabies in their community.
- Dogs and cats in developing countries.
- Unprovoked bite.

TRIAGE ASSESSMENT QUESTIONS

Call EMS 911 Now

- Major bleeding (actively dripping or spurting) that can't be stopped
  FIRST AID: Apply direct pressure to the entire wound with a clean cloth.
- Sounds like a life-threatening emergency to the triager

Go to ED Now

- Any break in skin (e.g., cut, puncture, or scratch) and wild animal at RISK for RABIES (e.g., bat, raccoon, fox, skunk, coyote, other carnivores)
  Reason: needs irrigation AND may need rabies vaccine and rabies immunoglobulin
- Any break in skin (e.g., cut, puncture, or scratch) and dog, cat, or ferret at RISK for RABIES (e.g., sick, stray, unprovoked bite, developing country)
  Reason: needs irrigation AND may need rabies vaccine and rabies immunoglobulin
- Any break in skin (e.g., cut, puncture, or scratch) and monkey
  Reason: needs irrigation and evaluation for possible herpesvirus simiae exposure

Go to ED Now (or to Office With PCP Approval)

- Cut (length > 1/8 inch or 3 mm) or skin tear and any animal
  Reason: cuts may need irrigation; larger cuts may need sutures
- Bleeding won't stop after 10 minutes of direct pressure (using correct technique)
- Sounds like a serious bite injury to the triager

Go to Office Now

- Severe pain
- No bite mark and suspicious bat exposure (e.g., bat found in same room as sleeping adult)
  Reason: postexposure rabies prophylaxis may be indicated
- Non-bite body fluid contact (e.g., saliva, brain) and animal at high-risk for RABIES (e.g., bat, raccoon, skunk, fox, coyote, and other carnivores)
  Reason: postexposure rabies prophylaxis may be indicated
- Puncture wound (holes through the skin) from cat (teeth or claws)
  Reason: 50% risk of wound infection. Antibiotics are often indicated.
- Puncture wound or small cut on face
  Reason: cosmetic risk and may need prophylactic antibiotics
- Puncture wound or small cut on hands or genitals
  Reason: increased infection risk and may need prophylactic antibiotics
  Exception: puncture from small pet (e.g., gerbil, mouse, hamster, puppy)
- Bite looks infected (e.g., red area, red streak, pus, or fever)
  R/O: cellulitis, lymphangitis

See Today in Office

- Wound and no tetanus booster in > 5 years (All animal bites are dirty)
- Patient wants to be seen

Home Care

- ○ Minor animal bite or claw wound, too small to irrigate
- ○ Small puncture wound (e.g., from gerbil, mouse, hamster, puppy)
- ○ Superficial scratch (didn't go through the dermis)
- ○ Bite that didn't break the skin
  R/O: bruise

HOME CARE ADVICE FOR MINOR ANIMAL BITE

Minor Cuts and Scratches and Puncture Wounds

1. **Bleeding:** For any bleeding, apply continuous pressure for 10 minutes.
2. **Cleaning:**
   - Wash all wounds immediately with soap and water for 5 minutes. Scrub the wound enough to make it rebleed a little.
   - Also, flush vigorously under a faucet for a few minutes.
   - Cleaning the wound helps prevent infection.
3. **Antibiotic Ointment:** Apply an antibiotic ointment (e.g., Neosporin, Bacitracin) to the bite 3 times a day for 3 days.
4. **Expected Course:** Most scratches, scrapes, and other minor bites heal up fine in 3 to 5 days
5. **Call Back If:**
   - Wound begins to look infected (redness, swelling, warmth, tender to touch, or red streaks).
   - You become worse.

Minor Bruises

1. **Treating Bruises:**
   - **Cold Pack for First 48 Hours:** For bruises or swelling, apply a cold pack or an ice bag (wrapped in a moist towel) to the area for 20 minutes. Repeat in 1 hour, then as needed for the first 48 hours after the injury (Reason: to reduce the bruising, swelling, and pain).
   - **Local Heat After 48 Hours:** After 48 hours apply a warm, moist washcloth or heating pad for 10 minutes 3 times a day to help absorb the blood.
2. **Pain Medicines:**
   - For pain relief, take acetaminophen, ibuprofen, or naproxen.

   Acetaminophen (e.g., Tylenol):
   - Take 650 mg by mouth every 4-6 hours as needed. Each Regular Strength Tylenol pill has 325 mg of acetaminophen. The most you should take each day is 3,250 mg (10 pills a day).
   - Another choice is to take 1,000 mg every 8 hours. Each Extra Strength Tylenol pill has 500 mg of acetaminophen. The most you should take each day is 3,000 mg (6 pills a day).

   Ibuprofen (e.g., Motrin, Advil):
   - Take 400 mg by mouth every 6 hours.
   - Another choice is to take 600 mg by mouth every 8 hours.

   Naproxen (e.g., Aleve):
   - Take 250-500 mg by mouth every 12 hours.

   Extra Notes:
   - Acetaminophen is thought to be safer than ibuprofen or naproxen in people over 65 years old. Acetaminophen is in many OTC and prescription medicines. It might be in more than one medicine that you are taking. You need to be careful and not take an overdose. An acetaminophen overdose can hurt the liver.
   - **Caution:** Do not take acetaminophen if you have liver disease.
   - **Caution:** Do not take ibuprofen if you have stomach problems, kidney disease, are pregnant, or have been told by your doctor to avoid this type of anti-inflammatory drug. Do not take ibuprofen for more than 7 days without consulting your doctor.
   - Use the lowest amount of medicine that makes your pain feel better.
   - Before taking any medicine, read all the instructions on the package.
3. **Expected Course:** Bruises should fade away over 7-14 days.

Who Should Call Animal Control

1. **United States—Contacting Animal Control:**
   - For patients referred in for evaluation, the ED or PCP will call the animal control center.
   - For patients not referred in, the patient should call the animal control center in the county where the bite occurred if a rabies-prone wild animal or stray pet animal attempted to bite an adult but was unsuccessful (i.e., the adult does not need to be seen). The animal control center will initiate a search for the animal. If located, any rabies-prone animals will be observed 10 days for rabies or sacrificed and tested for rabies. Dangerous strays will be taken to the local animal shelter.
2. **Canada—Contacting the Public Health Department:**
   - For adults referred into ED, the ED will call the local public health department.
   - For adults not referred into ED, the triager needs to instruct the caller to report the bite by contacting the local public health department in the area where the bite occurred (provide service referral).
   - Public health should be notified of any animal bite (or other animal contact) that might result in rabies.

Reporting Wild Animals and Strays

1. **Canada:** You can report the animal to the local medical officer of health and to the nearest CFIA veterinarian.
2. **United States:** You can report the animal to the animal control center for your county.

FIRST AID

First Aid Advice for Bleeding:

Apply direct pressure to the entire wound with a clean cloth.

First Aid Advice for All Bites and Scratches:

Wash all bite wounds and scratches with soap and warm water.

BACKGROUND INFORMATION

General

- Animal bites usually need to be seen by a physician because all bites are contaminated with saliva and are prone to wound infection.
- Bites on the hands are at increased risk of complications.
- **Wound Infection:** Any redness (regardless of size) that develops at the site of an animal bite that happened 24-96 hours previously—most likely (high specificity) indicates the onset of infection (e.g., cellulitis, lymphangitis).

Types of Wounds

- **Bruising:** There is no break in the skin. No risk of infection.
- **Abrasion or Scratch:** These are superficial wounds that don't go all the way through the skin. The risk of infection is low. Prophylactic antibiotic therapy is not indicated.
- **Laceration or Cut:** These are wounds that go through the skin (dermis) into the fat or muscle tissue. There is an intermediate risk of infection. Wound cleansing and irrigation can help prevent infection by washing out the bacteria from the wound. Sometimes debridement of the wound edges is needed. Prophylactic antibiotic therapy may be required.
- **Puncture Wound:** Intermediate risk of infection. Puncture wounds from cat bites are especially prone to getting infected; many physicians will prescribe prophylactic antibiotics for cat bites.

Rabies

- Rabies is very rare in humans but is nearly always fatal.
- **Exposure:** Bites or scratches from a bat, skunk, raccoon, fox, coyote, or other carnivores are more likely to transmit rabies than pets or other animals. These animals can transmit rabies even if they have no symptoms. Bats have transmitted rabies without a detectable bite mark. In the United States, approximately 90% of cases of rabies in humans are attributed to bats.

- **Postexposure Treatment:** Postexposure prophylaxis consists of an injection of one dose of immune globulin and 4 injections of rabies vaccine over a 14-day period. Rabies immune globulin and the first dose of rabies vaccine should be given as soon as possible after an exposure. The subsequent injections of rabies vaccine should be given on days 3, 7, and 14 after the first vaccination.
- **Incubation Period:** The incubation period for rabies in humans can be days, months, and even possibly longer than a year. Therefore, if there has been a definite or likely exposure then postexposure prophylaxis (e.g., rabies vaccine, rabies IG) should be given regardless of the interval since the exposure.
- **Risk of Transmission—Type of Animal Bite:** The risk of transmission depends on the type of animal bite. See the next section.
- **Risk of Transmission—Type of Body Fluid:** The rabies virus is transmitted through saliva and brain/nervous system tissue from infected animals. Only these specific body fluids and tissues can transmit the rabies virus. The CDC recommends that other contact such as touching an animal or contact with blood, urine, or feces is not considered an exposure; no postexposure prophylaxis is needed in these situations.

Types of Animal Bites

- **Puppy Teeth and Puncture Wounds:** This guideline does not refer in the tiny puncture wounds from puppy teeth for prophylactic antibiotics. The reason is that they barely puncture the skin (if at all) and can't be irrigated. Puppy teeth are tiny and sharp. They cause shallow punctures that look like "a dot." They occur commonly in the majority of children and adults who care for a puppy.
- **Small Indoor Pet Animal Bites:** Small indoor pets (gerbils, hamsters, guinea pigs, white mice, rats, etc.) are at no risk for rabies. Puncture wounds from these small animals also don't need to be seen. There is only a small risk for developing a wound infection (Reason: the wound infection rate is low because the bites often don't penetrate the dermis).
- **Large Pet Animal Bites:** Most bites from pets are from dogs or cats. Bites from domestic animals such as horses can be handled using these guidelines. The main risk from pet bites is serious wound infection. Cat bites become infected more often than dog bites. Claw wounds from cats are treated the same as bite wounds, since the claws may be contaminated with saliva. Bites from pet pigs or primates also have a high rate of wound infection. Bites on the hands or feet have a higher risk of infection than bites to other parts of the body.
- **Small Wild Animal Bites:** Rabbits and small rodents (such as squirrels, mice, rats, and chipmunks) rarely become infected with rabies and have not been known to transmit it to humans.These bites can sometimes get infected.
- **Bites From Rabies-Prone Wild Animals:** Bites or scratches from a bat, skunk, raccoon, fox, coyote, or other carnivores are more dangerous than other animals. These animals can transmit rabies even if they have no symptoms. There are cases where bats have transmitted rabies without a detectable bite mark *(MMWR Recomm Rep*. 2008;57[RR-3]:1–28).

Dogs and Cats and the Risk of Rabies

- **Indoor Versus Outdoor Pets:** Dogs and cats that are never allowed to roam freely outdoors are considered free of rabies. Outdoor pets who are [1] stray, sick, or unvaccinated AND [2] living in communities where rabies occurs in pets are considered at risk for rabies in the United States and Canada.
- **Metropolitan Versus Rural Location:** Dogs and cats in most metropolitan areas in the United States and Canada are free of rabies (Exception: lower Texas, Northwest Territories). Dogs and cats in rural areas have a higher risk of rabies.
- **Provoked Versus Unprovoked Bite:** An unprovoked attack by a domestic animal increases the likelihood that an animal is rabid. Note that bites inflicted while a person is attempting to feed or handle a healthy animal are considered provoked.
- **Developing Countries Versus United States and Canada:**
  Dogs and cats in developing countries have a higher risk of rabies; rabies postexposure prophylaxis is indicated if a bite occurs in a developing country.
- Nurses and physicians must check with the local public health department about the risk for rabies in their community.

Bat Bites and Rabies

- All bat bites are considered rabies-prone. During the past 2 decades, nearly all cases of human rabies in the United States and Canada were caused by bats.
- Bat bites are painless and difficult to see. A bat bite is equivalent to a puncture wound from a 27-gauge needle.
- Rabies postexposure prophylaxis should be considered when direct contact between a human and a bat has occurred, unless the exposed person can be certain a bite, scratch, or mucous membrane exposure did not occur (ACIP 1999). Exposure that occurs during sleep, involving unattended preverbal children, or involving mentally disabled individuals is included.
- Rabies postexposure prophylaxis should also be considered for persons who were in the same room as the bat and who might be unaware that a bite or direct contact had occurred (e.g., a sleeping person awakens to find a bat in the room) (ACIP 1999).
- State or provincial health departments can test bats for rabies only if human contact has occurred.

Coyote Bites and Rabies

- All coyote bites are considered rabies-prone.
- Coyotes are found throughout the United States and Canada. Parents who see a coyote often worry about the safety of their children. Parents can be reassured that in general coyotes are afraid of humans.
- Coyote bites occur less than 10 times per year in the United States. Most of them are in children less than 5 years old while unattended. The last recorded death due to a coyote attack in the United States was in 1980 in California.

Wound Irrigation—Why It's Important

- Careful wound irrigation and debridement in the ED or office are more effective at preventing infection than prophylactic antibiotics.
- The following wounds need vigorous irrigation: cuts deep enough to see fat or bloody tissue inside or cuts longer than 1/8 inch (3 mm). Puncture wounds can't be irrigated and superficial scratches don't need to be irrigated.
- All bites should be washed at home immediately for 3 minutes under running water before going in to the ED or office.

ARM PAIN

DEFINITION

- Pain in the arm.
- Not due to a traumatic injury.
- Minor muscle strain and overuse are covered in this guideline.

Pain Severity Is Defined As:

- **Mild (1-3):** Doesn't interfere with normal activities
- **Moderate (4-7):** Interferes with normal activities (e.g., work or school) or awakens from sleep
- **Severe (8-10):** Excruciating pain, unable to do any normal activities, unable to hold a cup of water

TRIAGE ASSESSMENT QUESTIONS

Call EMS 911 Now

- Shock suspected (e.g., cold/pale/clammy skin, too weak to stand)
  R/O: shock
- Similar pain previously and it was from "heart attack"
  R/O: cardiac ischemia, myocardial infarction
- Similar pain previously from "angina" and not relieved by nitroglycerin
  R/O: cardiac ischemia
- Sounds like a life-threatening emergency to the triager

See More Appropriate Protocol

- Followed a shoulder injury
  Go to Protocol: Trauma, Shoulder on page 307
- Followed a hand or wrist injury
  Go to Protocol: Trauma, Hand and Wrist on page 287
- Chest pain
  Go to Protocol: Chest Pain on page 48
- Wound looks infected
  Go to Protocol: Wound Infection on page 344
- Elbow pain is main symptom
  Go to Protocol: Elbow Pain on page 104
- Hand or wrist pain is main symptom
  Go to Protocol: Hand and Wrist Pain on page 132

Go to ED Now

- Difficulty breathing or unusual sweating (e.g., sweating without exertion)
  R/O: cardiac ischemia
- Chest pain lasting longer than 5 minutes
  R/O: cardiac ischemia
- Age > 40 and no obvious cause for pain, pain still present even when not moving the arm
  R/O: cardiac ischemia

Go to ED Now (or to Office With PCP Approval)

- Fever and red area (area very tender to touch)
  R/O: cellulitis, lymphangitis
- Fever and swollen joint
  R/O: septic arthritis
- Entire arm is swollen
  R/O: DVT of upper extremity
- Patient sounds very sick or weak to the triager

Go to Office Now

- SEVERE pain (e.g., excruciating, unable to do any normal activities)
  Reason: inadequate analgesia
  R/O: herniated cervival disk
- Red area or streak and large (> 2 in or 5 cm)
  R/O: cellulitis, erysipelas, lymphangitis
  Note: It may be difficult to determine the rash color in people with darker-colored skin.
- Cast on wrist or arm and now increasing pain
  R/O: swelling (cast may need to be bivalved)
- Weakness (i.e., loss of strength) in hand or fingers
  R/O: herniated cervical disk
- Arm pains with exertion (e.g., occurs with walking; goes away on resting)
  R/O: angina

See Today in Office

- Painful rash with multiple small blisters grouped together (i.e., dermatomal distribution or "band" or "stripe")
  R/O: herpes zoster
- Looks like a boil, infected sore, deep ulcer, or other infected rash (spreading redness, pus)
  R/O: abscess, cellulitis
- Localized rash is very painful and no fever
  R/O: cellulitis, spider bite, bee sting, herpes zoster

See Today or Tomorrow in Office

- Numbness (i.e., loss of sensation) in hand or fingers
  R/O: neuropathy, cervical radiculopathy, herniated cervical disk, carpal tunnel syndrome
- Localized pain, redness, or hard lump along vein
  R/O: superficial thrombophlebitis
- Patient wants to be seen

See Within 3 Days in Office

- MODERATE pain (e.g. interferes with normal activities) and present > 3 days
  R/O: arthritis, tendonitis, carpal tunnel syndrome
- Pain is worsened or caused by bending the neck
  R/O: cervical radiculopathy

See Within 2 Weeks in Office

- MILD pain and present > 7 days
- Arm pain is a chronic symptom (recurrent or ongoing AND lasting > 4 weeks)

Home Care

- ○ Caused by strained muscle
  R/O: muscle strain (pulled muscle)
- ○ Caused by overuse injury from recent vigorous activity (e.g., sports, lifting, physical work)
  R/O: overuse injury
- ○ Arm pain
  R/O: muscle strain, arthritis

HOME CARE ADVICE FOR ARM PAIN

Muscle Strain or Overuse

1. **Reassurance—Muscle Strain:**
   - **Definition:** A muscle strain occurs from over-stretching or tearing a muscle. People often call this a "pulled muscle." This muscle injury can occur while exercising, while lifting something, or sometimes during normal activities.
   - **Symptoms:** People often describe a sharp pain or popping when the muscle strain occurs. The muscle pain worsens with movement of the arm.
2. **Reassurance—Overuse:**
   - **Definition:** Sore muscles are common following vigorous activity (overuse injury), especially when your body is not used to this amount of activity (e.g., sports, weight lifting, moving furniture).
   - **Symptoms:** People often describe a diffuse soreness and aching in the over-used muscles.
3. **Local Cold for First 48 Hours:**
   - Apply a cold pack or an ice bag (wrapped in a moist towel) to the area for 20 minutes. Repeat in 1 hour, then every 4 hours while awake.
   - Continue this for the first 48 hours after an injury (Reason: to reduce the swelling and pain).
4. **Local Heat:**
   - Beginning 48 hours after an injury, apply a warm washcloth or heating pad for 10 minutes 3 times a day.
   - This will help increase circulation and improve healing.
   - **Local Heat (Shower Option):** If stiffness persists more than 48 hours, relax in a hot shower twice a day and gently exercise the involved part under the falling water water.
   - **Rest:** Avoid any exercise activity which causes this pain for the next 3 days.
5. **Pain Medicines:**
   - For pain relief, take acetaminophen, ibuprofen, or naproxen.

Acetaminophen (e.g., Tylenol):

- Take 650 mg by mouth every 4-6 hours as needed. Each Regular Strength Tylenol pill has 325 mg of acetaminophen. The most you should take each day is 3,250 mg (10 pills a day).
- Another choice is to take 1,000 mg every 8 hours. Each Extra Strength Tylenol pill has 500 mg of acetaminophen. The most you should take each day is 3,000 mg (6 pills a day).

Ibuprofen (e.g., Motrin, Advil):

- Take 400 mg by mouth every 6 hours.
- Another choice is to take 600 mg by mouth every 8 hours.

Naproxen (e.g., Aleve):

- Take 250-500 mg by mouth every 12 hours.

Extra Notes:

- Acetaminophen is thought to be safer than ibuprofen or naproxen in people over 65 years old.
- Acetaminophen is in many OTC and prescription medicines. It might be in more than one medicine that you are taking. You need to be careful and not take an overdose. An acetaminophen overdose can hurt the liver.

- **Caution:** Do not take acetaminophen if you have liver disease.
- **Caution:** Do not take ibuprofen if you have stomach problems, kidney disease, are pregnant, or have been told by your doctor to avoid this type of anti-inflammatory drug. Do not take ibuprofen for more than 7 days without consulting your doctor.
- Use the lowest amount of medicine that makes your pain feel better.
- Before taking any medicine, read all the instructions on the package

6. **Expected Course:**
   - **Muscle Strain:** A minor muscle strain usually hurts for 2-3 days. The pain often peaks on day 2. A more severe muscle strain can hurt for 2-4 weeks.
   - **Muscle Overuse:** Sore muscles from overuse usually hurts for 2-4 days. The pain often peaks on day 2.
7. **Call Back If:**
   - Moderate pain (e.g., interferes with normal activities) lasts more than 3 days.
   - Mild pain lasts more than 7 days.
   - You become worse.

Arm Pain—General Care Advice

1. **Pain Medicines:**
   - For pain relief, take acetaminophen, ibuprofen, or naproxen.

   Acetaminophen (e.g., Tylenol):
   - Take 650 mg by mouth every 4-6 hours as needed. Each Regular Strength Tylenol pill has 325 mg of acetaminophen. The most you should take each day is 3,250 mg (10 pills a day).
   - Another choice is to take 1,000 mg every 8 hours. Each Extra Strength Tylenol pill has 500 mg of acetaminophen. The most you should take each day is 3,000 mg (6 pills a day).

   Ibuprofen (e.g., Motrin, Advil):
   - Take 400 mg by mouth every 6 hours.
   - Another choice is to take 600 mg by mouth every 8 hours.

   Naproxen (e.g., Aleve):
   - Take 250-500 mg by mouth every 12 hours.

   Extra Notes:
   - Acetaminophen is thought to be safer than ibuprofen or naproxen in people over 65 years old. Acetaminophen is in many OTC and prescription medicines. It might be in more than one medicine that you are taking. You need to be careful and not take an overdose. An acetaminophen overdose can hurt the liver.
   - **Caution:** Do not take acetaminophen if you have liver disease.
   - **Caution:** Do not take ibuprofen if you have stomach problems, kidney disease, are pregnant, or have been told by your doctor to avoid this type of anti-inflammatory drug. Do not take ibuprofen for more than 7 days without consulting your doctor.
   - Use the lowest amount of medicine that makes your pain feel better.
   - Before taking any medicine, read all the instructions on the package
2. **Call Back If:**
   - Moderate pain (e.g., interferes with normal activities) lasts more than 3 days.
   - Mild pain lasts more than 7 days.
   - Arm swelling occurs.
   - Signs of infection occur (e.g., spreading redness, warmth, fever).
   - You become worse.

FIRST AID

First Aid Advice for Shock:

Lie down with the feet elevated.

BACKGROUND INFORMATION

Causes of Arm Pain

- **Deep Vein Thrombosis (DVT):** DVT of the arm is rare. Symptoms include arm pain and swelling.
- **Muscle Cramps:** Brief pains (1 to 15 minutes) may be due to muscle spasms. The pain should resolve completely after an episode of muscle spasm.
- **Muscle Strain (Pulled Muscle):** A muscle strain occurs from overstretching or tearing a muscle. This muscle injury can occur while exercising, while lifting something, and sometimes during normal activities. This is also referred to as a "pulled muscle."

- **Muscle Strain (Sore Muscles From Overuse):** Continuous acute pains (hours to 3 days) are often due to over-strenuous activities or forgotten muscle injuries from recent exercise or work-related activities.
- **Cervical Radiculopathy:** This is caused by pressure on the spinal nerve roots from a herniated disk or from spinal arthritis.
- **Viral Illness:** Mild bilateral diffuse muscle aches also occur with many viral illnesses.
- **Other Causes:** Unwitnessed fracture, arthritis, skin infection (cellulitis, erysipelas), bursitis.

Serious Signs and Symptoms

- Severe pain
- Red area with streak
  (R/O: cellulitis with lymphangitis; common)
- Joint swelling with fever
  (R/O: septic arthritis; rare)
- Entire arm is swollen
  (R/O: deep vein thrombosis of upper extremity; rare)

Caution: Cardiac Ischemia

- Rarely, patients may present with arm pain as the sole symptom of a myocardial infarction. Usually there will be other associated symptoms of cardiac ischemia: chest pain, shortness of breath, nausea, and/or diaphoresis.
- Cardiac ischemia should be suspected in any patients with risk factors for cardiac disease. These include: hypertension, smoking, diabetes, hyperlipidemia, a strong family history of heart disease, and age > 50.

ASTHMA ATTACK

DEFINITION

- Adult is having an asthma attack.
- Previously diagnosed as having asthma, asthmatic bronchitis, or reactive airway disease by a physician, or treated in the past with asthma medications by inhaler or nebulizer.
- Use this guideline only if the patient has symptoms that match Asthma Attack.

Symptoms of an Asthma Attack Include:

- Recurring episodes of wheezing, cough, chest tightness, and difficulty breathing.
- Wheezing is a high-pitched or whistling sound heard on expiration.

Asthma Attack Severity Is Defined As:

- **Mild:** No SOB at rest, mild SOB with walking, speaks normally in sentences, can lay down, no retractions, pulse < 100 (GREEN Zone: PEFR 80-100%)
- **Moderate:** SOB at rest, SOB with exertion and prefers to sit, cannot lie down flat, speaks in phrases, mild retractions, audible wheezing, pulse 100-120 (YELLOW Zone: PEFR 50-80%)
- **Severe:** Very SOB at rest, speaks in single words, agitated, sitting hunched forward, cannot lie down flat, retractions, usually loud wheezing, sometimes minimal wheezing because of decreased air movement, pulse >120 (RED Zone: PEFR < 50%)
- **Respiratory Arrest Imminent:** Struggling to breathe, unable to speak, drowsy, or confused

TRIAGE ASSESSMENT QUESTIONS

Call EMS 911 Now

- Severe difficulty breathing (e.g., struggling for each breath, unable to speak, or speaking in single words)
  FIRST AID: Take 4 puffs from your quick-relief inhaler (e.g., albuterol)
- Bluish lips, tongue, or face
  FIRST AID: Take 4 puffs from your quick-relief inhaler (e.g., albuterol)
- Wheezing started suddenly after medicine, an allergic food, or bee sting
  R/O: anaphylaxis
  FIRST AID: Take 4 puffs from your quick-relief inhaler (e.g., albuterol)
- Passed out (i.e., fainted, collapsed and was not responding)
- Sounds like a life-threatening emergency to the triager

Go to ED Now

- SEVERE asthma attack (e.g., very SOB at rest, speaks in single words, loud wheezes)
  FIRST AID: Take 4 puffs from your quick-relief inhaler (e.g., albuterol)

Go to ED Now (or to Office With PCP Approval)

- Peak flow rate less than 50% of baseline level (RED zone)
- Severe wheezing or coughing and doesn't have nebulizer or inhaler available
  Reason: needs immediate nebulizer or inhaler
- Chest pain
  R/O: pneumothorax
- Hospitalized before with asthma; now feels same
- Patient sounds very sick or weak to the triager

Go to Office Now

- MODERATE asthma attack (e.g., SOB at rest, speaks in phrases, audible wheezes) and not resolved after 2 nebulizer or inhaler treatments given 20 minutes apart
  Reason: may need oral corticosteroid burst
- Peak flow rate 50-80% of baseline level (YELLOW zone) after using 2 nebulizer or inhaler treatments given 20 minutes apart

See Today in Office

- Fever > 103° F (39.4° C)
  R/O: bacterial pneumonia
- Fever > 100.5° F (38.1° C) and over 60 years of age
- Coughing continuously (nonstop) that keeps from working or sleeping, and not improved after inhaler or nebulizer
  Reason: may need oral corticosteroid burst

- Asthma medicine (nebulizer or inhaler) is needed more frequently than q 4 hours
- Fever present > 3 days (72 hours)
- Patient wants to be seen

See Today or Tomorrow in Office

- MILD asthma attack (e.g., no SOB at rest, mild SOB with walking, speaks normally in sentences, mild wheezing) and persists > 24 hours on appropriate treatment
  Reason: may need oral corticosteroid burst
- Intermittent mild wheezing persists > 5 days
- Nasal discharge present > 10 days
- Sinus pain (around cheekbone or eye)

Discuss With PCP and Callback by Nurse Today

- Influenza prevalent in community (or household) and has flu symptoms (e.g., cough WITH fever, etc) with onset < 48 hours ago
  Reason: antiviral treatment may be indicated

See Within 2 Weeks in Office

- No asthma checkup in > 6 months
  Reason: review treatment program
- Missing > 1 day of work or school per month because of asthma

Home Care

- ○ MILD asthma attack (e.g., no SOB at rest, mild SOB with walking, speaks normally in sentences, mild whezing)

HOME CARE ADVICE FOR MILD ASTHMA ATTACK

1. **Quick-Relief Asthma Medicine:**
   - Start your quick-relief medicine (e.g., albuterol, salbutamol) at the first sign of any coughing or shortness of breath (don't wait for wheezing). Use your inhaler (2 puffs each time) or nebulizer every 4 hours. Continue the quick-relief medicine until you have not wheezed or coughed for 48 hours.
   - The best "cough medicine" for an adult with asthma is always the asthma medicine (Note: Don't use cough suppressants, but cough drops may help a tickly cough).
2. **Long-term–Control Asthma Medicine:** If you are using a controller medicine (e.g., inhaled steroids or cromolyn), continue to take it as directed.
3. **Drinking Liquids:** Try to drink normal amount of liquids (e.g., water). Being adequately hydrated makes it easier to cough up the sticky lung mucus.
4. **Humidifier:** If the air is dry, use a cool mist humidifier to prevent drying of the upper airway.
5. **Hay Fever:** If you have nasal symptoms from hay fever, it's OK to take antihistamines (Reason: poor control of allergic rhinitis makes asthma worse whereas antihistamines don't make asthma worse).
6. **Remove Allergens:** Take a shower to remove pollens, animal dander, or other allergens from the body and hair.
7. **Avoid Triggers:** Avoid known triggers of asthma attacks (e.g., tobacco smoke, cats, other pets, feather pillows, exercise).
8. **Work With Your Doctor:** There is no cure for asthma, but you can take charge and learn to control it. The best way to take charge of asthma is to work with your doctor (over many months) to find the right controller (preventive) medicine so your asthma is under control. If you keep having asthma attacks, then the asthma is not under control. People can die from asthma if they do not take it seriously and work with a doctor to control it.
9. **Expected Course:** If treatment is started early, most asthma attacks are quickly brought under control. All wheezing should be gone by 5 days.
10. **Call Back If:**
    - Inhaled asthma medicine (nebulizer or inhaler) is needed more often than every 4 hours.
    - Wheezing has not completely cleared after 5 days.
    - You become worse.

How to Use an Inhaler or Spacer

1. **How to Use a Metered Dose Inhaler (MDI):**
   - **Step 1:** Remove the cap and shake the inhaler.
   - **Step 2:** Hold the inhaler about 1-2 inches (2-5 cm) in front of the mouth. Breathe out—completely.
   - **Step 3:** Press down on the inhaler to release the medicine as you start to breathe in slowly.
   - **Step 4:** Breathe in slowly for 3 to 5 seconds.
   - **Step 5:** Hold your breath for 10 seconds to allow the medicine to reach deeply into your lungs.
   - If your doctor has prescribed 2 puffs, wait 1 minute and then repeat steps 2-5.
2. **How to Use an MDI With a Spacer:**
   - **Step 1:** Shake the inhaler and then attach it to the spacer or holding chamber.
   - **Step 2:** Breathe out completely.
   - **Step 3:** Place the mouthpiece of the spacer in your mouth.
   - **Step 4:** Press down on the inhaler. This will put one puff of the medicine in the holding chamber or spacer.
   - **Step 5:** Breathe in slowly for 5 seconds.
   - **Step 6:** Hold your breath for 10 seconds and then exhale.
   - If your doctor has prescribed 2 or more puffs, wait 1 minute between each puff and then repeat steps 2-6.
3. **How to Use a Dry Powder Inhaler:**
   - **Step 1:** Remove the cap and follow manufacturer's instructions to load a dose of medicine.
   - **Step 2:** Breathe out completely.
   - **Step 3:** Put the mouthpiece of the inhaler in the mouth.
   - **Step 4:** Breathe in quickly and deeply.
   - **Step 5:** Hold your breath for 10 seconds to allow the medicine to reach deeply into your lungs.
   - If your doctor has prescribed 2 or more inhalations, wait 1 minute and then repeat steps 2-5.
4. **Float Test—How to Tell if Your Inhaler (MDI) Is Empty:**
   - An empty MDI is sometimes the cause of an unresponsive asthma attack.
   - Most MDIs hold 120 puffs of albuterol or other medicine. It should say on the side of the inhaler.
   - Shaking the inhaler and hearing fluid in it is not helpful. When the medicine is gone, extra propellant still remains.
   - **The Float Test:** Place the inhaler in a bowl of water and if it floats, assume it's empty. A new and completely full inhaler will sink. The float test is not 100% reliable.

Your Peak Flow Meter

1. **Peak Flow Meter:**
   - Every adult asthmatic should have a peak flow meter.
   - A peak flow meter is a device that measures how well air moves out of your lungs.
   - The number that is obtained is called the peak expiratory flow rate (PEFR).
   - The "personal best" value is the highest PEFR number that a person obtains when they are feeling well.
2. **How to Use a Peak Flow Meter:**
   - **Step 1:** Move the indicator to the bottom of the numbered scale. Stand up.
   - **Step 2:** Take a deep breath, filling your lungs completely.
   - **Step 3:** Place the mouthpiece in your mouth and close your lips around it. Do not put your tongue inside the hole.
   - **Step 4:** Blow out as hard and fast as you can.
   - **Step 5:** Repeat the process 2 more times.
   - **Step 6:** Write down the highest of the 3 numbers.
3. **Using a Peak Flow Meter to Determine the Severity of an Asthma Attack:**
   - **GREEN Zone—MILD Attack:** PEFR 80-100% of personal best
   - **YELLOW Zone—MODERATE Attack:** PEFR 50-80%
   - **RED Zone—SEVERE Attack:** PEFR less than 50%

FIRST AID

First Aid Advice for Asthma Attack:

Take 4 puffs on your quick-relief inhaler (e.g., albuterol, salbutamol, Xopenex) right now.

BACKGROUND INFORMATION

Asthma Triggers

Different things can cause an asthma attack. These are called asthma triggers.

- Allergens (pollen, house dust, mold, animals)
- Irritants (cigarette smoke, dirt, pollution)
- Exercise
- Respiratory infections (cold or flu)
- Sudden changes in the weather (generally cold weather)

Asthma Medications

There are 2 main types of asthma medications, long-term and quick-relief:

- **A long-term–control** (preventative, controller) medicine keeps asthma attacks from starting.
- It works slowly over many weeks to stop the swelling in the airways. Adults must take it every day even when they feel fine and can breathe well. Examples of preventive medicines include inhaled steroids (e.g., AeroBid, Azmacort, Beclovent, Flovent, Pulmicort, Vanceril) and cromolyn.
- **A quick-relief** (rescue, reliever) medicine helps stop an asthma attack that has already started.
- It can keep the attack from getting serious. It works fast to stop the tightness and opens the airways in the lungs during an asthma attack. An adult should take it at the first sign of a wheeze, cough, or drop in peak flow measurement. Sometimes doctors will tell an adult to take it every day for a week or two after an asthma attack, but quick-relief medicines are not meant to be used to stop attacks every day for weeks and weeks. Examples of quick-relief medicines include inhaled or nebulized beta-agonists (e.g., Proventil, Alupent, albuterol, Ventolin, salbutamol).

Albuterol (Salbutamol) Quick-Relief Treatments for Asthma Attacks and the NAEPP Guidelines

- **Quick-Relief (Rescue) Treatment:** Bronchodilator treatment with albuterol is indicated for asthma attack symptoms. The patient should take up to 2 treatments 20 minutes apart using an inhaler (2-6 puffs) or a nebulizer.
- **Response to Treatment if PEFR < 50%:** Adults having an asthma attack with a PEFR < 50% should start oral steroid and either go to ED or call EMS 911.
- **Response to Treatment if PEFR 50-80%:** Adults with an asthma attack who have an incomplete response (PEFR 50-80%) to quick-relief treatment need to be started on a steroid burst. If they do not have access to prednisone through their on-call PCP, they need to be seen in the emergency department
- **Reference:** NAEPP Expert Panel Report 3: Guidelines for the Diagnosis and Management of Asthma—Summary Report 2007. This report is available online at: www.nhlbi.nih.gov/guidelines/asthma/asthgdln.htm.

Levalbuterol (Xopenex)

- Levalbuterol is a newer bronchodilator that is related chemically to albuterol (it is the L stereoisomer of albuterol).
- Levalbuterol costs more than albuterol.
- Generally, patients will not be using both of these medications together.

Peak Flow Meters

Peak flow meters measure how fast an adult can move air out of the lungs. Every adult asthmatic should have a peak flow meter. These measurements are very useful for grading the severity of an asthma attack. The normal peak expiratory flow rate (PEFR) for a healthy adult female is 400-500 and the normal value is 500-650 for a healthy adult male. Peak flow rates decrease during an asthma attack. In general, medications should be increased when the PEFR is less than 80% of baseline and an adult should be seen immediately in the emergency department if the PEFR is less than 50%.

- **MILD Attack:** PEFR 80-100% of baseline (personal best/GREEN zone)
- **MODERATE Attack:** PEFR 50-80% (YELLOW zone)
- **SEVERE Attack:** PEFR less than 50% (RED zone)

Using a Spacer (Holding Chamber) With an MDI

- Many individuals can benefit from using a spacer (holding chamber), especially individuals who have difficulty coordinating taking a breath and activating the MDI. For such individuals, adding a spacer to their inhaler may double the delivery of albuterol to the lungs.
- Metered-dose inhalers with a spacer work as well as a nebulizer treatment.

CAUTION: Asthma patients are at risk for asthma-related death; risk factors include:

- Current use of, or recent withdrawal from, systemic corticosteroids
- Prior intubation for asthma or admission to an intensive care unit
- Hospitalizations or multiple emergency visits for asthma within the past year
- History of psychosocial problems or denial of asthma or its severity
- History of noncompliance with asthma medication plan

ATHLETE'S FOOT

DEFINITION

- Fungus infection of the feet.
- Causes itchy rash between the toes.
- Use this guideline only if the patient has symptoms that match Athlete's Foot.

Symptoms of Athlete's Foot Include:

- Rash with redness, maceration, and fissuring between the toes, especially in the web space between the third/fourth and fourth/fifth toes.
- Often involves the insteps of the feet.
- The rash itches and burns.

TRIAGE ASSESSMENT QUESTIONS

See More Appropriate Protocol

● Doesn't match the SYMPTOMS for athlete's foot
Go to Protocol: Rash or Redness, Localized and Cause Unknown on page 216

Go to ED Now (or to Office With PCP Approval)

● Patient sounds very sick or weak to the triager

Go to Office Now

● Fever and bright red area or streak
R/O: cellulitis, lymphangitis

See Today in Office

● Rash looks infected (e.g., spreading redness, pus)
R/O: cellulitis

● Rash is very painful
R/O: cellulitis

● Diabetes
Reason: diabetic foot care

See Today or Tomorrow in Office

● After week on treatment and rash continues to spread
R/O: wrong diagnosis

● Rash has spread beyond the instep and toes
R/O: contact dermatitis from sneakers, "moccasin-type" tinea pedis

● Patient wants to be seen

See Within 3 Days in Office

● After 4 weeks on treatment and rash has not cleared completely
R/O: wrong diagnosis

Home Care

○ Athlete's foot with no complications

HOME CARE ADVICE

General Care Advice for Athlete's Foot

1. **Antifungal Cream:** Apply the antifungal cream 2 times a day to the affected areas of the feet. Continue the cream for at least 7 days after the rash is cleared.
   - Available over-the-counter in the United States as terbinafine (Lamisil AT), clotrimazole (Lotrimin AF), or miconazole (Micatin, Monistat-Derm).
   - Available over-the-counter in Canada as clotrimazole (clotrimazole cream, Canesten, Clotrimaderm) or miconazole (Micatin Cream, Micozole, Monistat-Derm).
   - Terbinafine (Lamisil AT) is most recommended but is not available in Canada.
   - Read the package instructions thoroughly on all medications that you use.
2. **Keep the Feet Clean and Dry:** Wash the feet 2 times every day. Dry the feet completely, especially between the toes. Then apply the cream. Wear clean socks and change them twice daily.
3. **Avoid Scratching:** Scratching infected feet will delay healing. Rinse the itchy feet in cool water for relief.
4. **Contagiousness:**
   - The condition is not very contagious.
   - The fungus can't grow on dry, normal skin.
   - Adults with athlete's foot do not need to miss any school or work. You can continue to play sports.
   - The socks can be washed with regular laundry. They don't need to be boiled.
5. **Expected Course:** With proper treatment, athlete's aoot should decrease substantially within 1 week and disappear within 2 weeks.

6. **Call Back If:**
    - Rash looks infected (e.g., spreading redness, streaks, pus).
    - Rash continues to spread after 1 week of treatment.
    - Rash has not cleared after 2 weeks of treatment.
    - You become worse.

Prevention

1. **Avoid being barefoot in public areas** (e.g., showers, bathrooms, swimming pools). You can get athlete's foot from walking barefoot in these areas. Wear sandals.
2. **Keep the Feet Clean and Dry:** Wash your feet with warm soapy water once a day. Rinse the feet and dry thoroughly, especially between the toes. Wear clean cotton socks and change daily.

BACKGROUND INFORMATION

General Information

- Athlete's foot is an infection caused by a fungus that grows best on the warm, damp skin of the foot and toes. It is also referred to as tinea pedis.
- It is a common malady, with up to 70% of the adult population having it at some point in their lives.
- There are both topical and oral medications that work well in treating this infection. Most healthy individuals will be able to treat athlete's foot effectively using a topical agent.

BACK PAIN

DEFINITION

- Complains of upper, mid, or lower back pain that occurs mainly in the midline.
- Not due to a traumatic injury.
- Minor muscle strain and overuse are covered in this guideline. Sciatic pain is also covered.

Pain Severity Is Defined As:

- **Mild (1-3):** Doesn't interfere with normal activities
- **Moderate (4-7):** Interferes with normal activities or awakens from sleep
- **Severe (8-10):** Excruciating pain, unable to do any normal activities

TRIAGE ASSESSMENT QUESTIONS

Call EMS 911 Now

- Passed out (i.e., fainted, collapsed and was not responding)
  R/O: AAA
  FIRST AID: Lie down with feet elevated.
- Shock suspected (e.g., cold/pale/clammy skin, too weak to stand)
  R/O: AAA
  FIRST AID: Lie down with feet elevated.
- Sounds like a life-threatening emergency to the triager

See More Appropriate Protocol

- Pain in the upper back over the ribs (rib cage) that radiates (travels) into the chest
  Go to Protocol: Chest Pain on page 48
- Pain in the upper back over the ribs (rib cage) and worsened by coughing (or clearly increases with breathing)
  Go to Protocol: Chest Pain on page 48

Go to ED Now

- Unable to urinate (or only a few drops) and bladder feels very full
  R/O: urinary retention, cauda equina syndrome
- Numbness (loss of sensation) in groin or rectal area
- Severe abdominal pain
- Abdominal pain and age > 60
  R/O: compression fracture, aortic aneurysm

Go to ED Now (or to Office With PCP Approval)

- Sudden onset of severe back pain and age > 60
  R/O: compression fracture, aortic aneurysm
- Pain radiates into groin, scrotum
  R/O: kidney stones
- Blood in urine (red, pink, or tea-colored)
- Vomiting and pain over lower ribs of back (i.e., flank-kidney area)
- Weakness of a leg or foot (e.g., unable to bear weight, dragging foot)
  R/O: nerve root impingement or cord compression
- Patient sounds very sick or weak to the triager

Go to Office Now

- Severe back pain
- Fever > 100.5° F (38.1° C) and flank pain
  R/O: pyelonephritis
- Pain or burning with urination
  R/O: pyelonephritis

See Today in Office

- Can't walk or can barely walk
  R/O: severe back strain, cord compression
- Tingling or numbness in the legs or feet
  R/O: severe back strain, cord compression
- High-risk adult (e.g., history of cancer, history of HIV, or history of IV drug abuse)
  R/O: metastasis, epidural abscess
- Rash in same area as pain (may be described as "small blisters")
  R/O: herpes zoster
- Pain radiates into the thigh or further down the leg, and in both legs
  Reason: bilateral sciatica carries higher risk

See Today or Tomorrow in Office

- Pain radiates into the thigh or further down the leg
  R/O: sciatica
- Age > 50 and no history of prior similar back pain
  Reason: higher risk of serious medical cause
- Patient wants to be seen

See Within 2 Weeks in Office

- Back pain persists > 2 weeks
- Back pain is a chronic symptom (recurrent or ongoing AND lasting > 4 weeks)

Home Care

- ○ Back pain

HOME CARE ADVICE FOR MILD BACK PAIN

1. **Reassurance:** Heavy lifting or excessive twisting can cause lower back pain. With treatment, the pain usually goes away in 1 to 2 weeks.
2. **Local Cold or Heat:** During the first 2 days after a mild injury, apply a cold pack or ice bag (wrapped in a moist towel) to the sore muscles for 20 minutes 4 times a day. Wrap the cold pack in a towel to prevent frostbite. After 2 days, apply a heating pad or hot water bottle to the most painful area for 20 minutes whenever the pain flares up. Wrap hot water bottles or heating pads in a towel to avoid burns.
3. **Sleep:** Sleep on your side with a pillow between your knees. If you sleep on your back, place a pillow under your knees to reduce stress on your lower back. Avoid sleeping on your abdomen. The mattress should be firm or reinforced with a board. Avoid water beds.
4. **Activity:** Continue ordinary activities as much as your pain permits. Continued activity is more healing for the back than rest. Avoid any activities that significantly increase the pain. Avoid heavy lifting, twisting, and strenuous exercise until completely well (Note: complete bed rest is unnecessary).
5. **Pain Medicines:**
   - For pain relief, take acetaminophen, ibuprofen, or naproxen.

   Acetaminophen (e.g., Tylenol):
   - Take 650 mg by mouth every 4-6 hours as needed. Each Regular Strength Tylenol pill has 325 mg of acetaminophen. The most you should take each day is 3,250 mg (10 pills a day).
   - Another choice is to take 1,000 mg every 8 hours. Each Extra Strength Tylenol pill has 500 mg of acetaminophen. The most you should take each day is 3,000 mg (6 pills a day).

   Ibuprofen (e.g., Motrin, Advil):
   - Take 400 mg by mouth every 6 hours.
   - Another choice is to take 600 mg by mouth every 8 hours.

   Naproxen (e.g., Aleve):
   - Take 250-500 mg by mouth every 12 hours.

   Extra Notes:
   - Acetaminophen is thought to be safer than ibuprofen or naproxen in people over 65 years old. Acetaminophen is in many OTC and prescription medicines. It might be in more than one medicine that you are taking. You need to be careful and not take an overdose. An acetaminophen overdose can hurt the liver.
   - **Caution:** Do not take acetaminophen if you have liver disease.
   - **Caution:** Do not take ibuprofen if you have stomach problems, kidney disease, are pregnant, or have been told by your doctor to avoid this type of anti-inflammatory drug. Do not take ibuprofen for more than 7 days without consulting your doctor.
   - Use the lowest amount of medicine that makes your pain feel better.
   - Before taking any medicine, read all the instructions on the package
6. **Prevention:**
   - The only way to prevent future backaches is to keep your back muscles in excellent physical condition.
   - A sedentary lifestyle (lack of exercise) is a risk factor for developing back pain.
   - Walking, stationary biking, and swimming provide good aerobic conditioning as well as exercise for your back.
   - Being overweight puts more weight on the spine and thus increases the risk of back pain. If you are overweight, work with your doctor to develop a weight-loss program.
7. **Good Body Mechanics:**
   - **Lifting:** Stand close to the object to be lifted. Keep your back straight and lift by bending your legs. Ask for lifting help if needed.
   - **Sleeping:** Sleep on a firm mattress.
   - **Sitting:** Avoid sitting for long periods of time without a break. Avoid slouching. Place a pillow or towel behind your lower back for support.
   - **Posture:** Maintain good posture.

8. **Strengthening Exercises:**
   - During the first couple days after an injury, strengthening exercises should be avoided.
   - The following exercises can help strengthen the back. Perform the following exercises 3-10 times each day, for 5-10 seconds each time.
   - **Bent Knee Sit-ups:** Lay on back, curl forward lifting shoulders about 6 inches (15 cm) off the floor.
   - **Leg Lifts:** Lay on back, lift foot 6 inches (15 cm) off floor (one leg at a time).
   - **Pelvic Tilt:** Lay on back with knees bent, push lower back against floor.
   - **Chest Lift:** Lie face down on ground, place arms by your sides, lift shoulders off the floor.
9. **Call Back If:**
   - Numbness or weakness occurs.
   - Bowel/bladder problems occur.
   - Pain persists for more than 2 weeks.
   - You become worse.

FIRST AID

First Aid Advice for Shock:

Lie down with the feet elevated.

BACKGROUND INFORMATION

General

- Lower back pain is a cause of countless visits to physicians' offices and emergency departments. It is the second most common cause of lost workdays, after cold and flu symptoms. Over 80% of people at some point in their lives have lower back pain.
- However, there is some good news. In most cases, the back pain is not serious and it has a self-limited course. Pain subsides within 4-6 weeks in 90% of individuals experiencing acute low back pain.

Four Categories of Back Pain

- **Potentially Serious:** Examples include abdominal aortic aneurysm, neoplasm, osteomyelitis, epidural abscess, vertebral fracture, and neurologic emergencies (e.g., cauda equina syndrome).
- **Sciatica (Back Pain With Neurologic Symptoms):** There is radiation of the back pain into a lower extremity suggesting lumbosacral nerve root compression. There may be associated leg weakness, numbness, or paresthesias.
- **Nonspecific Back Pain:** No neurologic symptoms. Examples include lumbar strain/sprain, degenerative osteoarthritis, lumbar disc disease, and fibromyalgia.
- **Referred Back Pain:** There are gastrointestinal causes like pancreatitis, biliary colic, and posterior-gastric ulcer; genitourinary causes like renal colic, pyelonephritis, endometriosis, and ovarian cyst.

Lumbar Strain

- Acute lower back pain in the 18- to 50-year-old age group is usually a symptom of strain of some of the 200 muscles in the back that allow us to stand upright.
- Often the triggering event is carrying something too heavy, lifting from an awkward position, bending too far backward or sideways, or overuse.
- Individuals with strained back muscles often note that the pain is increased by bending or twisting movements, relieved by assuming certain positions, and that the back muscles are tender.

Degenerative Osteoarthititis

- Degenerative osteoarthritis is a common cause of back pain in the elderly population.
- In uncomplicated osteoarthritis, individuals will complain of chronic midline back discomfort.
- Frequently, there is morning stiffness that improves as the day progresses.

Bed Rest and Overtreatment

- Complete bed rest is inconvenient and unnecessary in the majority of patients, including those who need to be examined by the physician. Complete bed rest should never be recommended over the telephone.
- Research has demonstrated that continuing ordinary activities within the limits permitted by pain results in a speedier recovery than rest (Malmivaara).

BEE STING

DEFINITION

- Stung by a honeybee, bumblebee, hornet, wasp, or yellow jacket

Three Types of Reactions

- **Local Reaction:** Localized pain, swelling, itching and mild redness at stinger site.
- **Toxic Reaction:** History of multiple stings; larger venom dose; systemic symptoms include light-headedness, vomiting, diarrhea.
- **Anaphylactic Reaction:** Severe life-threatening allergic reaction to sting.

TRIAGE ASSESSMENT QUESTIONS

Call EMS 911 Now

- Passed out (i.e., fainted, collapsed and was not responding)
  R/O: anaphylaxis
  Use FIRST AID ADVICE for anaphylaxis.
- Wheezing or difficulty breathing
  R/O: anaphylaxis
  Use FIRST AID ADVICE for anaphylaxis.
- Hoarseness, cough, or tightness in the throat or chest
  R/O: anaphylaxis
  Use FIRST AID ADVICE for anaphylaxis.
- Swollen tongue or difficulty swallowing
  Use FIRST AID ADVICE for anaphylaxis.
- Life-threatening reaction in past to sting (anaphylaxis) and < 2 hours since sting
  Note: Anaphylaxis usually starts within 20 minutes and always by 2 hours following a sting.
- Sounds like a life-threatening emergency to the triager

See More Appropriate Protocol

- Not a bee, wasp, hornet, or yellow jacket sting
  Go to Protocol: Insect Bite on page 166

Go to ED Now (or to Office With PCP Approval)

- Widespread hives, itching, or facial swelling and started within 2 hours of sting
  R/O: allergic reaction
  Note: No history of life-threatening reaction and no current anaphylactic symptoms
- Vomiting or abdominal cramps and started within 2 hours of sting
  R/O: allergic reaction
  Note: No history of life-threatening reaction and no current anaphylactic symptoms
- Patient sounds very sick or weak to the triager

Go to Office Now

- Sting inside the mouth
  R/O: swelling of the airway
- Sting on eyeball (e.g., cornea)
  R/O: corneal scar
- More than 50 stings
  Reason: risk for systemic toxic reaction from a large dose of venom
- Fever and area is red
  R/O: cellulitis, lymphangitis
  Reason: fever and looks infected
- Fever and area is very tender to touch
  R/O: cellulitis, lymphangitis
  Reason: fever and looks infected
  Note: Infection after a sting is uncommon.
- Red streak or red line and length > 2 inches (5 cm)
  R/O: lymphangitis
  Note: Lymphangitis looks like a red streak or line originating at the wound and ascending up the arm or leg toward the heart. Uncommon after a sting.

See Today in Office

- Red or very tender (to touch) area, and started over 24 hours after the sting
  R/O: cellulitis
  Note: Cellulitis is uncommon after a sting. Any redness starting in the first 24 hours is just due to the sting venom.
- Red or very tender (to touch) area, getting larger over 48 hours after the sting
  R/O: cellulitis, but probably due to venom
  NOTE: Skin infection is uncommon after a sting.

- Swelling is huge (e.g., > 4 inches or 10 cm, spreads beyond wrist or ankle)
  R/O: cellulitis, but more likely is large local reaction to venom
- Patient wants to be seen

See Within 3 Days in Office

- Widespread hives, itching, or facial swelling and started > 2 hours after sting
  R/O: allergic reaction
  Note: No history of life-threatening reaction and no anaphylactic symptoms
- Scab drains pus or increases in size, and not improved after applying antibiotic ointment for 2 days
  R/O: infected sore, impetigo

Home Care

- ○ Normal local reaction to bee, wasp, or yellow jacket sting
- ○ Scab drains pus or increases in size
  R/O: infected sore, impetigo

HOME CARE ADVICE

General Care Advice for Bee, Wasp, or Yellow Jacket Sting

1. **Try to Remove the Stinger (if Present):**
   - The stinger looks like a tiny black dot in the sting.
   - There are several different methods of removal. Removing the stinger quickly is more important than how you remove it.
   - Use a fingernail, credit card edge, or knife-edge to scrape it off. Don't pull it out (Reason: squeezes out more venom). If the stinger is below the skin surface, leave it alone. It will be shed with normal skin healing.
   - In many cases no stinger will be present. Only bees leave their stingers. Wasps, yellow jackets, and hornets do not.
2. **Local Cold for Pain—Cold Pack Method:**
   - Wrap a bag of ice in a towel (or use a bag of frozen vegetables such as peas).
   - Apply this cold pack to the area of the sting for 10-20 minutes.
   - You may repeat this as needed, to relieve symptoms of pain and swelling.
3. **Pain Medicines:**
   - For pain relief, take acetaminophen, ibuprofen, or naproxen.

   Acetaminophen (e.g., Tylenol):
   - Take 650 mg by mouth every 4-6 hours as needed. Each Regular Strength Tylenol pill has 325 mg of acetaminophen. The most you should take each day is 3,250 mg (10 pills a day).
   - Another choice is to take 1,000 mg every 8 hours. Each Extra Strength Tylenol pill has 500 mg of acetaminophen. The most you should take each day is 3,000 mg (6 pills a day).

   Ibuprofen (e.g., Motrin, Advil):
   - Take 400 mg by mouth every 6 hours.
   - Another choice is to take 600 mg by mouth every 8 hours.

   Naproxen (e.g., Aleve):
   Take 250-500 mg by mouth every 12 hours.

   Extra Notes:
   - Acetaminophen is thought to be safer than ibuprofen or naproxen in people over 65 years old. Acetaminophen is in many OTC and prescription medicines. It might be in more than one medicine that you are taking. You need to be careful and not take an overdose. An acetaminophen overdose can hurt the liver.
   - **Caution:** Do not take acetaminophen if you have liver disease.
   - **Caution:** Do not take ibuprofen if you have stomach problems, kidney disease, are pregnant, or have been told by your doctor to avoid this type of anti-inflammatory drug. Do not take ibuprofen for more than 7 days without consulting your doctor.
   - Use the lowest amount of medicine that makes your pain feel better.
   - Before taking any medicine, read all the instructions on the package
4. **Hydrocortisone Cream for Itching:**
   - Hydrocortisone cream applied to the sting area 4 times a day can also help reduce itching. Use it for a couple days until the itch is mild.
   - Available over-the-counter in United States as 0.5% and 1% cream.
   - Available over-the-counter in Canada as 0.5% cream.

5. **Antihistamine Medication for Itching:**
   If the sting becomes very itchy, take diphenhydramine (e.g., Benadryl; adult dosage 25-50 mg) by mouth.
   - Do not take diphenhydramine if you have prostate problems.
   - Antihistamines may cause sleepiness. Do not drink, drive, or operate dangerous machinery while taking antihistamines.
   - An over-the-counter antihistamine that causes less sleepiness is loratadine (e.g., Alavert or Claritin).
   - Read the package instructions thoroughly on all medications that you take.
6. **Expected Course:**
   - **Pain:** Severe pain or burning at the site lasts 1 to 2 hours. Pain after this period is usually minimal. Itching often follows the pain.
   - **Redness and Swelling:** Normal redness and swelling from the venom can increase for 24 hours following the sting. Redness at the sting site is normal. It doesn't mean that it is infected.
   - The redness can last 3 days and the swelling 7 days.
   - Stings only rarely get infected.
7. **Call Back If:**
   - Difficulty breathing or swallowing (generally develops within the first 2 hours after the sting; call 911).
   - Swelling becomes huge.
   - Sting begins to look infected.
   - You become worse.

Preventing Stings

1. **Some Outdoor Activity Tips**
   - Wear long-sleeved shirts, long pants, and shoes when you are in grassy areas or outdoors and exposed to stinging insects.
   - Avoid using perfumes and hair sprays; these attract insects.
   - Wear dark or drab-colored clothes rather than bright colors.
   - Take special care when eating or preparing food outdoors. These odors can attract insects (especially yellow jackets).

Tetanus Vaccination and Stings

1. **Getting a Tetanus Booster:**
   - Tetanus vaccination (booster) after a bee sting is not necessary.
   - However, if it has been more than 10 years since your last tetanus vaccination, it is appropriate from a preventive health care standpoint to obtain a vaccination (i.e., Td or Tdap) sometime in the next couple weeks.

Infected Sore or Scab

1. **Reassurance:**
   - Sometimes a small infected sore can develop at the site of a cut, scratch, insect bite, or sting.
   - The typical appearance is a sore smaller than 1 inch (2.5 cm) in diameter. It is often covered by a soft, honey-yellow or yellow-brown crust or scab. Sometimes the scab may drain a tiny amount pus or yellow fluid. Usually there is minimal to no pain.
   - Small infected sores usually get better with regular cleansing and use of an antibiotic ointment
2. **Cleaning:**
   - Wash the area 2-3 times daily with an antibacterial soap and warm water.
   - Gently remove any scab. The bacteria live underneath the scab. You may need to soak the scab off by placing a warm, wet washcloth (or gauze) on the sore for 10 minutes.
3. **Antbiotic Ointment:**
   - Apply an antibiotic ointment 3 times per day.
   - Cover the sore with a Band-Aid to prevent scratching and spread.
   - Use Bacitracin ointment (OTC in United States) or Polysporin ointment (OTC in Canada) or one that you already have.
4. **Avoid Picking:** Avoid scratching and picking. This can worsen and spread a skin infection.
5. **Contagiousness:**
   - Infected sores can be contagious by skin-to-skin contact.
   - Wash your hands frequently and avoid touching the sore.
   - **Work and School:** You can attend school or work if it is covered.

- **Contact Sports:** Generally, you need to receive antibiotic treatment for 3 days before you can return to the sport. There can be no pus or drainage. You should check with your trainer, if there is one for your sports team.

6. **Expected Course:**
   - The sore should stop growing in 1-2 days and it should begin improving within 2-3 days.
   - The sore should be completely healed in 7-10 days.
7. **Call Back If:**
   - Fever occurs.
   - Spreading redness or a red streak occurs.
   - Sore increases in size.
   - Sore not improving after 2 days using antibiotic ointment.
   - Sore not completely healed in 7 days (1 week).
   - New sore appears.
   - You become worse.

FIRST AID

First Aid Advice for Minor Bee Sting (Localized Symptoms Only):

- Apply a cold pack to the area of the sting for 10-20 minutes.

First Aid Advice for Anaphylaxis—Epinephrine (Pending EMS Arrival):

- If the patient has an epinephrine autoinjector, the patient should use it now.
- Use the autoinjector on the upper outer thigh. You may give it through clothing if necessary.
- Epinephrine is available in autoinjectors under trade names: EpiPen, EpiPen Jr, and Twinject. EpiPen is a single injection. Twinject has a second injection that can be used if there is no improvement after 5 minutes.

First Aid Advice for Anaphylaxis—Benadryl (Pending EMS Arrival):

- Give antihistamine orally NOW if able to swallow.
- Use Benadryl (diphenhydramine; adult dose 50 mg) or any other available antihistamine.

First Aid Advice for Anaphylactic Shock (Pending EMS Arrival):

- Lie down with feet elevated.

BACKGROUND INFORMATION

General

- *Hymenoptera* is the scientific name for the class/order of venomous insects which include: bees, wasps, hornets, yellow jackets.
- Over 95% of stings are from honey bees or yellow jackets.
- Tetanus vaccination after a bee sting is not necessary.

Local Reaction

- The stinger injects venom into the skin; it is the venom that causes the pain and other symptoms.
- The main symptoms are localized pain, swelling, itching, and mild redness at the sting site.
- **Pain:** Severe pain or burning at the site lasts 1 to 2 hours. Itching often follows the pain.
- **Swelling:** Normal swelling can increase for 24 hours following the sting. Stings of the upper face can cause marked swelling around the eye, but this is harmless.
- **Redness:** Bee stings can normally become red. That doesn't mean they are infected. Infections rarely occur in stings.
- **Expected Course:** The redness can last 3 days and the swelling 7 days.

Toxic Reaction—From a Large Number of Stings

- Nonallergic systemic reactions occur with a minimum of 50 stings in adults. Betten 2005 recommends that any adult with > 50 stings be observed in a medical setting for 24 hours for signs of delayed venom toxicity. He suggests a rule of 1 sting per kg for children.
- Symptoms of a large number of stings include vomiting and diarrhea developing within 8 hours of the stings. This venom reaction can progress over 24 hours to hemolysis, rhabdomyolysis (muscle breakdown), and renal failure.
- Death from massive envenomation occurs mainly in adults with > 500 stings. It has been estimated that the median lethal dose of honeybee venom is 500 to 1,400 stings in an adult (who is not allergic to bee stings).

Anaphylactic Reaction

- Anaphylactic reactions to *Hymenoptera* stings occur in 0.4% of patients.
- Generally, the shorter the interval between the sting and the first onset of systemic symptom, the more serious the reaction will be. Anaphylaxis usually starts within 20 minutes and almost always by 2 hours. If no symptoms occur by 2 hours, the risk for anaphylaxis is minimal.
- Systemic symptoms include: wheezing, hypotension, shock, generalized urticaria, and abdominal cramping.

Removing the Stinger

- The stingers on wasps, hornets, and yellow jackets do not detach, and thus they are able to sting multiple times.
- Honeybees are capable of stinging only once because they have tiny barbs on their stingers that gets embedded in the skin. After stinging, the stinger apparatus detaches from the bee's body and the bee dies. Therefore, it is only with honeybee stings that there is a stinger that sometimes needs to be removed.
- There are several different methods of removal. Removing the stinger quickly is more important than the type of removal used (Visscher). The patient can grab it with his fingers, scrape it out with a credit card, or use Scotch tape.

BREATHING DIFFICULTY

DEFINITION

- Difficult or labored breathing
- Also known as respiratory distress or shortness of breath (SOB)

Severity Is Defined As:

- **Mild:** Speaks normally in sentences, minimal SOB at rest and mild SOB with walking, can lay down, no retractions, pulse < 100
- **Moderate:** Speaks in phrases, difficulty breathing even at rest, SOB worsens with exertion and prefers to sit, mild retractions, audible wheezing, pulse 100-120
- **Severe:** Speaks in single words, struggling to breathe, sitting hunched forward, retractions, pulse >120

Excluded:

- Difficulty breathing because of a stuffy nose should be triaged using the COLDS protocol on page 53 or the SINUS PAIN AND CONGESTION protocol on page 231.

TRIAGE ASSESSMENT QUESTIONS

Call EMS 911 Now

- Breathing stopped and hasn't returned
  FIRST AID: Begin mouth-to-mouth breathing
- Choking on something
  FIRST AID: If breathing stopped, quickly discuss the abdominal thrust maneuver (Heimlich)
- SEVERE difficulty breathing (e.g., struggling for each breath, speaks in single words, pulse > 120)
  R/O: severe respiratory distress
- Bluish lips, tongue, or face now
  R/O: cyanosis and need for oxygen
- Difficult to awaken or acting confused (e.g., disoriented, slurred speech)
  R/O: hypoxia, hypercapnea
- Passed out (i.e., fainted, collapsed and was not responding)
  R/O: anaphylaxis, severe hypoxia, or cough syncope
- Wheezing started suddenly after medicine, an allergic food, or bee sting
  R/O: anaphylaxis
- Stridor
  R/O: upper airway obstruction
- Slow, shallow, and weak breathing
  R/O: impending respiratory arrest
- Sounds like a life-threatening emergency to the triager

See More Appropriate Protocol

- Chest pain
  Go to Protocol: Chest Pain on page 48
- Wheezing (high-pitched whistling sound) and previous asthma attacks or use of asthma medicines
  Go to Protocol: Asthma Attack on page 22
- Difficulty breathing and only present when coughing
  Go to Protocol: Cough on page 66
- Difficulty breathing and only from stuffy or runny nose
  Go to Protocol: Colds on page 53

Go to ED Now

- MODERATE difficulty breathing (e.g., speaks in phrases, SOB even at rest, pulse 100-120)
- Wheezing can be heard across the room
- Drooling or spitting out saliva (because can't swallow)
  R/O: epiglottitis, severe tonsillopharyngitis
- Any history of prior "blood clot" in leg or lungs
  Note: a "blood clot" typically would have required treatment with heparin or coumadin.
  Reason: increased risk of thromboembolism
  R/O: deep vein thrombosis
- Recent illness requiring prolonged bed rest (i.e., immobilization)
  R/O: pulmonary embolus
- Hip or leg fracture in past 2 months (e.g, or had cast on leg or ankle)
  R/O: pulmonary embolus
- Major surgery in the past month
  R/O: pulmonary embolus
- Recent long-distance travel with prolonged time in car, bus, plane, or train (i.e., hours sitting in one spot)
  Reason: immobilization during prolonged travel increases risk of pulmonary embolus

- Extra heart beats OR irregular heart beating (i.e., "palpitations")
  R/O: dysrrhythmia

Go to ED Now (or to Office With PCP Approval)

- Fever > 103° F (39.4° C)
  R/O: pneumonia
- Fever > 100.5° F (38.1° C) and over 60 years of age
  R/O: pneumonia
- Fever > 100.5° F (38.1° C) and bedridden (e.g., nursing home patient, stroke, chronic illness, recovering from surgery)
  R/O: pneumonia
- Fever > 100.5° F (38.1° C) and diabetes mellitus or immunocompromised (e.g., HIV positive, cancer chemotherapy, splenectomy, organ transplant, chronic steroids)
  R/O: pneumonia
- Periods where breathing stops and then resumes normally and bedridden (e.g., nursing home patient, CVA)
  R/O: Cheyne-Stokes
- Pregnant or postpartum (< 1 month since delivery)
  R/O: pulmonary embolus
- Patient sounds very sick or weak to the triager

Go to Office Now

- MILD difficulty breathing (e.g., minimal/no SOB at rest, SOB with walking, pulse < 100)
- Worsening difficulty breathing and not responding to usual therapy
  R/O: worsening CHF or COPD
- Continuous (nonstop) coughing
- Patient wants to be seen

HOME CARE ADVICE FOR BREATHING DIFFICULTY (Pending Office Visit)

1. **Fever Medicines:**
   - For fevers above 101° F (38.3° C) take acetaminophen or ibuprofen.
   - The goal of fever therapy is to bring the fever down to a comfortable level. Remember that fever medicine usually lowers fever 2 degrees F (1 - 1 1/2 degrees C).

   Acetaminophen (e.g., Tylenol):
   - Take 650 mg by mouth every 4-6 hours. Each Regular Strength Tylenol pill has 325 mg of acetaminophen.
   - Another choice is to take 1,000 mg every 8 hours. Each Extra Strength Tylenol pill has 500 mg of acetaminophen.
   - The most you should take each day is 3,000 mg.

   Ibuprofen (e.g., Motrin, Advil):
   - Take 400 mg by mouth every 6 hours.
   - Another choice is to take 600 mg by mouth every 8 hours.
   - Use the lowest amount that makes your pain feel better.

   Extra Notes:
   - Acetaminophen is thought to be safer than ibuprofen in people over 65 years old. Acetaminophen is in many OTC and prescription medicines. It might be in more than one medicine that you are taking. You need to be careful and not take an overdose. An acetaminophen overdose can hurt the liver.
   - **Caution:** Do not take acetaminophen if you have liver disease.
   - **Caution:** Do not take ibuprofen if you have stomach problems, kidney disease, are pregnant, or have been told by your doctor to avoid this type of anti-inflammatory drug. Do not take ibuprofen for more than 7 days without consulting your doctor.
   - Before taking any medicine, read all the instructions on the package.
2. **Call Back If:**
   - You become worse.

FIRST AID

First Aid Advice—If Not Breathing:

- If you know CPR, you should do this while waiting for the paramedics to arrive.
- Begin chest compressions and mouth-to-mouth breathing (30 compressions:2 breaths cycle). Do 100 chest compressions per minute (approximately 6 breaths).

First Aid Advice for Anaphylaxis—Epinephrine (Pending EMS Arrival):

- If the patient has an epinephrine autoinjector, the patient should use it now.
- Use the autoinjector on the upper outer thigh. You may give it through clothing if necessary.
- Epinephrine is available in autoinjectors under trade names: EpiPen, EpiPen Jr, and Twinject. EpiPen is a single injection. Twinject has a second injection that can be used if there is no improvement after 5 minutes.

First Aid Advice for Anaphylaxis—Benadryl (Pending EMS Arrival)

- Give antihistamine orally NOW if able to swallow.
- Use Benadryl (diphenhydramine; adult dose 50 mg) or any other available antihistamine.

First Aid Advice for Choking

- IF COUGHING AND BREATHING, encourage coughing.
- As long as the adult is breathing and coughing, just encourage him to cough the material up by himself (Reason: the cough reflex can usually clear the windpipe).
- Don't offer anything to drink (Reason: fluids take up space needed for air passage).

If Breathing Stops, Perform Abdominal Thrust (Heimlich) Maneuver

- If the adult can't breathe, cough, or make a sound, proceed with high abdominal thrusts.
- Grasp the adult from behind, just below the lower ribs but above the navel, in bear-hug fashion.
- Make a fist with one hand and fold the other hand over it.
- Give a sudden upward and backward jerk (at a 45° angle) to try to squeeze all the air out of the chest and pop the lodged object out of the windpipe.
- Repeat this upward abdominal thrust 10 times in rapid succession, until the object comes out.
- If the adult is too heavy for you to suspend from your arms, lay him on his back on the floor. Put your hands on both sides of the abdomen, just below the ribs, and apply sudden, strong bursts of upward pressure.

If the Adult Passes Out, Give Mouth-to-Mouth Breathing

- Quickly open the mouth and look inside to see if there is any object that can be removed with a sweep of your finger (usually there is not). Avoid "blind" sweeps.
- Then begin resuscitation. Air can usually be forced past the foreign object temporarily until help arrives.
- If mouth-to-mouth breathing doesn't move the chest, repeat the abdominal thrusts or chest compressions.

BACKGROUND INFORMATION

General

- Some adults with long-standing cardiopulmonary disorders have chronic dyspnea. Such patients generally can be evaluated in the office setting on a nonurgent basis, if current symptoms are unchanged from their baseline.
- Patients with new onset or worsening shortness of breath require more urgent follow-up.

Causes

- Anaphylaxis
- Anemia
- Anxiety states, hyperventilation syndrome
- Asthma—bronchospasm
- Congestive heart failure
- Chronic obstructive pulmonary disease
- Diabetic ketoacidosis
- Pneumonia
- Pulmonary embolism
- Spontaneous pneumothorax
- Upper respiratory infection, acute bronchitis

BURNS

DEFINITION

- Thermal burns are skin injuries from heat.
- Thermal burns include explosions, fireworks.

TRIAGE ASSESSMENT QUESTIONS

Call EMS 911 Now

- Difficulty breathing after exposure to fire, smoke, or fumes
  R/O: inhalation injury
- Difficult to awaken or acting confused (e.g., disoriented, slurred speech)
  R/O: inhalation injury, carbon monoxide poisoning
  FIRST AID: Move to fresh air
- Burn area larger than 10 palms of hand (> 10% BSA) with blisters
  Reason: large second-degree burn; risk of shock
- Sounds like a life-threatening emergency to the triager

See More Appropriate Protocol

- Chemical gets into the eye from fingers, contaminated object, spray, or splash
  Go to Protocol: Eye, Chemical In on page 108
- Sunburn
  Go to Protocol: Sunburn on page 262

Go to ED Now

- Burn area larger than 4 palms of hand (> 4% BSA)
- Burn completely circles an arm or leg
  Reason: circumferential burn
- Caused by explosion or gunpowder
  R/O: other injuries and need for debridement
- Headache or nausea after exposure to fire and smoke
  R/O: smoke inhalation, carbon monoxide poisoning

Go to ED Now (or to Office With PCP Approval)

- Hoarseness or cough after exposure to fire and smoke
  R/O: smoke inhalation
- Blister (intact or ruptured) and larger than 2 inches (5 cm)
  Reason: may need debridement
- Blister (intact or ruptured) on the hand and larger than 1 inch (2.5 cm)
  R/O: risk of contracture
- Blisters (intact or ruptured) on the face, neck, or genitals
  Reason: cosmetic concerns, possible partner abuse
- Caused by very hot substance and center of burn is white (or charred)
  R/O: full thickness third-degree burn
- Sounds like a serious burn to the triager

Go to Office Now

- SEVERE pain
  R/O: need for narcotic analgesia
- Acid or alkali (lye) burn
- Chemical on skin that causes a blister
- Looks infected (e.g., fever, red streaks, spreading red area, pus)
  R/O: cellulitis

See Today in Office

- Broken (ruptured) blister and caller doesn't want to trim the dead skin
- Suspicious history for the burn
  R/O: domestic violence or elder abuse
- Patient wants to be seen

See Within 3 Days in Office

- After 10 days and burn isn't healed
- Diabetic and minor burn of lower leg or foot
  Reason: diabetic neuropathy and decreased resistance to infection
- Minor burn and last tetanus shot > 10 years ago
  Reason: minor thermal burn, needs a tetanus booster

Home Care

- Minor thermal or chemical burn
- Mouth or lip pain from hot food or drink

HOME CARE ADVICE

First-Degree Burns or Small Blisters

1. **Reassurance:** A minor thermal or chemical burn can be treated at home.
2. **Cleaning:** Wash the area gently with an anti-bacterial liquid soap and water once a day.
3. **Ruptured (Broken or Open) Blisters:**
   - You should remove the dead blister skin for any ruptured blisters.
   - **Method 1:** The easiest way to do this is gently wipe away the dead skin with some wet gauze or a wet washcloth.
   - **Method 2:** If that fails, trim off the dead skin with a fine scissors.
4. **Antibiotic Ointment for Ruptured Blisters:**
   - Apply an antibiotic ointment (e.g., OTC bacitracin) directly to a Band-Aid or dressing (Reason: prevent unnecessary pain of applying it directly to burn).
   - Then apply the Band-Aid or dressing over the burn.
   - Change the dressing every other day. Use warm water and 1 or 2 wipes with a wet washcloth to remove any surface debris.
   - Be gentle with burns.
5. **Intact (Closed) Blisters:**
   - **First 7 Days After a Burn:** Leave intact blisters alone.
   - **After 7 Days:** You can gently remove the blisters. The easiest way to do this is gently wipe away the dead skin with some wet gauze or a wet washcloth.
6. **Expected Course:**
   - Burns usually hurt for 2-3 days.
   - **First-Degree Burns:** Usually peel like a sunburn in about a week. The skin should look nearly normal after 2 weeks.
   - **Second-Degree Burns:** Blisters usually rupture within 7 days. Second-degree burns take 14-21 days to heal (longer than first-degree burns). Sometimes the skin looks a little darker or lighter than before after it has healed.
   - **Scarring:** Fortunately, first- and second-degree burns don't leave scars.
7. **Pain Medicines:**
   - For pain relief, take acetaminophen, ibuprofen, or naproxen.

   Acetaminophen (e.g., Tylenol):
   - Take 650 mg by mouth every 4-6 hours as needed. Each Regular Strength Tylenol pill has 325 mg of acetaminophen. The most you should take each day is 3,250 mg (10 pills a day).
   - Another choice is to take 1,000 mg every 8 hours. Each Extra Strength Tylenol pill has 500 mg of acetaminophen. The most you should take each day is 3,000 mg (6 pills a day).

   Ibuprofen (e.g., Motrin, Advil):
   - Take 400 mg by mouth every 6 hours.
   - Another choice is to take 600 mg by mouth every 8 hours.

   Naproxen (e.g., Aleve):
   - Take 250-500 mg by mouth every 12 hours.

   Extra Notes:
   - Acetaminophen is thought to be safer than ibuprofen or naproxen in people over 65 years old. Acetaminophen is in many OTC and prescription medicines. It might be in more than one medicine that you are taking. You need to be careful and not take an overdose. An acetaminophen overdose can hurt the liver.
   - **Caution:** Do not take acetaminophen if you have liver disease.
   - **Caution:** Do not take ibuprofen if you have stomach problems, kidney disease, are pregnant, or have been told by your doctor to avoid this type of anti-inflammatory drug. Do not take ibuprofen for more than 7 days without consulting your doctor.
   - Use the lowest amount of medicine that makes your pain feel better.
   - Before taking any medicine, read all the instructions on the package
8. **Call Back If:**
   - Severe pain persists more than 2 hours after taking pain medicine.
   - Burn starts to look infected (pus, red streaks, increased tenderness).
   - You become worse.

Mouth or Lip Pain From Hot Food or Drink

1. **Reassurance:**
   - Minor burns of the mouth from hot food usually are painful for 2 days.
   - They heal quickly because the lining of the mouth heals twice as fast as the skin.
2. **Local Ice:**
   - Put a piece of ice in the mouth immediately for 10 minutes (Reason: reduce swelling and pain).
   - Rinse the mouth with ice water every hour for 4 hours.
3. **Expected Course:**
   - The pain usually resolves after 2 days.
   - Second-degree burns can cause some blisters that quickly turn into shallow ulcers. These take 3 or 4 days to heal. They normally have a white surface.
4. **Call Back If:**
   - Difficulty with swallowing occurs.
   - Difficulty with breathing occurs.
   - Pain becomes severe.
   - You become worse.

Preventing Tetanus

1. **Tetanus Shot:** If your last tetanus shot was more than 10 years ago, you need a booster. Call your doctor during regular office hours (within the next 3 days).

Internet Resources

1. **Canada Burn Care Facilities, Compiled by the American Burn Association:** www.ameriburn.org/CanadaFinalPub.pdf
2. **US Burn Care Facilities, Compiled by the American Burn Association:** www.ameriburn.org/BCRD2-19-09.pdf
3. **Burn Center Referral Criteria and Guidelines for Operations of Burn Centers, From the American Burn Association:** www.ameriburn.org/Chapter14.pdf

FIRST AID

First Aid Advice for Thermal Burns:

- Immediately (don't take time to remove clothing) put the burned part in cold tap water or pour cold water over it for 10 minutes.
- For burns on the face, apply a cold, wet washcloth (Reason: lessens the depth of the burn and relieves pain).

First Aid Advice for Smoke Inhalation, Chemical Fume Inhalation, or Carbon Monoxide Exposure:

- Immediately move to fresh air.
- Go outdoors (best).
- Or move to an open door/window (in extreme weather conditions).

First Aid Advice for Chemical Burns

- Immediately remove any contaminated clothing.
- Then flush the chemical off the skin with warm water for 10 minutes. For large areas, use a shower.

BACKGROUND INFORMATION

General

- The triager should first determine burn severity (i.e., first, second, third degree). Sometimes it may be a mixture.
- The triager should then estimate the size of the burn in terms of total body surface area (BSA). The victim's palm represents approximately 1% of the BSA. The Rule of Nines can also be used to estimate burn size.
- The triager should confirm that there is no inhalation injury from hot or toxic fumes. Symptoms of inhalation injury include coughing and difficulty breathing.
- The triager should also be suspicious of carbon monoxide (CO) poisoning in situations of smoke inhalation, especially in house fires. Mild symptoms of CO poisoning include headache and nausea.
- More severe poisoning can cause confusion and coma.

Causes

- **Household Burns:** Most burns are scalds from hot water or hot drinks. Others are from hot ovens, stoves, electric or kerosene space heaters, exhaust pipes, grease, hair-curling irons, clothes irons, heating grates, and cigarettes.
- **Workplace Burns:** Common sources of injury are cooking oils and hot water/steam, usually in workers involved with food preparation.

Degrees of Burns (Severity)

- **First Degree (Superficial Burns):** Reddened skin without blisters (does not need to be seen).
- **Second Degree (Partial Thickness Burns):** Reddened skin with blisters (heals from bottom up, takes 2 to 3 weeks).
  - Small intact blisters (< 2 inch; < 5 cm) can usually be left alone; initial debridement is not needed. An intact blister serves as a physiologic dressing, decreases the risk of infection, and reduces pain. However, most blisters over 1 inch (2.5 cm) will go on to rupture.
  - Large intact blisters (> 2 inch; > 5 cm) almost always rupture within a couple days of the burn. They should be debrided (remove dead blister skin). Generally, this is best done by a physician or other health care provider. All ruptured blisters need debridement (removal) of the dead skin; this can be done by the caller, a physician, or other health care provider. Most ruptured blisters are empty of fluid. A blister with a small opening and slow fluid leak can be recognized by the appearance of wrinkled skin.
- **Third Degree (Full-Thickness Burns):** Deep burns with white or charred skin. The area also loses sensation to pain and touch (i.e., numb). Usually needs a skin graft to prevent bad scarring if it is larger than a quarter (1 inch or 2.5 cm) in size. If a third-degree burn is < 1 inch (2.5 cm) in size, usually it will heal from the margins.

Rule of Nines for Estimating Burn Size:

Each part of the body contributes a predictable portion of the total BSA.

- **Head and Neck:** 9%
- **Each Arm:** 9%
- **Anterior Chest and Abdomen:** 18%
- **Entire Back:** 18%
- **Each Leg:** 18%
- **Genital Region:** 1%

Rule of Palms for Estimating Burn Size

- A person's palm (not including the fingers) represents 1% of the total BSA.
- For example, if a person had blistering of the left shoulder the size of 2 palms, the total area of blistering would be 2% of the BSA.

CAST SYMPTOMS AND QUESTIONS

DEFINITION

- Symptoms occurring in arm or leg after cast placement
- Other questions about cast care

A CAST is made of a hard material (plaster or fiberglass) and it goes all the way around the injured part (e.g., hand, arm, foot, leg).

In contrast, a SPLINT is placed on only one side of the injured part and then held in place with a soft material like a cotton gauze wrapping or an elastic bandage. Callers can use their fingers to tell the difference.

TRIAGE ASSESSMENT QUESTIONS

Go to ED Now

- Chest pain
  R/O: DVT, pulmonary embolus
- Difficulty breathing
  R/O: DVT, pulmonary embolus

Go to ED Now (or to Office With PCP Approval)

- Patient sounds very sick or weak to the triager

Go to Office Now

- SEVERE pain of fingers or toes, and not improved after pain medications and elevation
  R/O: tight cast, compartment syndrome
  Note: most follow-up cast care should be handled by doctor (e.g., orthopedist) who put on the cast.
- Numbness or tingling of fingers or toes, and not improved after elevation
  R/O: tight cast, compartment syndrome
- Blueness or pallor of fingers or toes (compared to non-injured side)
  R/O: tight cast, compartment syndrome, or simple bruising
- Increasing pain under cast and cast put on > 72 hours ago
  R/O: DVT, wound infection

See Today in Office

- Swelling of fingers or toes, and not improved after elevation
  Reason: cast check
  Note: most follow-up cast care should be handled by doctor (e.g., orthopedist) who put on the cast.
- Coolness or tingling of fingers or toes, and not improved after elevation
  Reason: cast check
- Can't wiggle fingers or toes
  Reason: cast check
- Foreign body gets stuck under the cast
- Bad odor comes from underneath the cast
  R/O: wound infection, pressure sore, poor cast hygiene
- Drainage comes through cast or out of end of cast
  R/O: wound infection, pressure sore
- Unexplained fever occurs
  R/O: wound infection, pressure sore, osteomyelitis
- Plaster cast gets wet and is soft after attempted drying
- Plaster or fiberglass cast gets wet and patient has metal pins sticking out of skin
  Reason: evaluate cast, possible replacement
- Skin becomes red or raw at edge of cast
- Cast breaks, cracks, or falls off

Discuss With PCP and Callback by Nurse Today

- SEVERE pain under the cast and not controlled with pain medications
  R/O: fracture pain
  Note: most follow-up cast care should be handled by doctor (e.g., orthopedist) who put on the cast
- Cast feels too loose
- Cast feels too tight
- Cast removal date, questions about
- Triager unable to answer question

See Within 3 Days in Office

- Patient wants to be seen

Home Care

- Pain under the cast
  Reason: expected pain from injury
- Itchy skin under the cast
- Numbness or tingling of fingers or toes and has not tried elevation
  R/O: mild swelling
- Normal cast care, questions about
- Wet cast, questions about
- Sharp edges on cast, questions about

HOME CARE ADVICE

Normal Cast Care

1. **Elevation for Arm-Wrist Cast:**
   - Elevate the arm above your heart; this will help reduce swelling and pain.
   - Elevation is especially important during the first 3 days after putting on the cast.
   - Occasional wiggling of fingers will also prevent some swelling.
2. **Elevation for Leg-Ankle Cast:**
   - Elevate the leg by propping it up on pillows. Ideally, your leg should be above your heart. This will limit the amount of swelling that occurs and reduce the pain.
   - Elevation is especially important during the first 3 days after putting on the cast.
   - Occasional wiggling of the toes will also prevent some swelling.
3. **Keep Cast Dry:**
   - Don't get the cast wet.
   - **Plaster Cast:** Wet plaster can become soft and crumble.
   - **Fiberglass:** Wet padding under a fiberglass cast can cause skin rashes.
   - **Fiberglass With Gore-Tex Liner:** Patients with this special type of water-resistant cast may have been given permission to get the cast wet. Follow the doctor's instructions.
4. **How to Bathe With a Cast:**
   - To avoid getting the cast wet, enclose it in a plastic bag for bathing. Close the upper part of the plastic with tape or an elastic strap. You can also buy a waterproof sleeve at some drugstores.
   - Use a bathtub, because it's harder to keep a cast dry in a shower. Don't submerge the cast in bathwater even though it's covered.
5. **Activities:**
   - Adults with casts can usually go to school and work (unless the doctor specifically gave patient other instructions).
   - Mild exercise of the unaffected parts of the body is fine.
   - Avoid contact or dangerous sports (Reason: fall and reinjury).
   - Avoid exercise that causes excessive sweating (Reason: cast will become damp).
   - Avoid swimming (Reason: cast will often get wet even if using a plastic bag to cover it).
6. **Walking:**
   - If the cast is on a leg, don't walk on it unless you have your physician's approval. Never walk on it the first 48 hours because it takes that long for plaster to completely dry and become strong.
   - If you were given crutches or a walker, then you should not put any body weight on the cast when walking.
7. **Call Back If:**
   - Finger or toes develop numbness, tingling, or pain.
   - Can't wiggle fingers or toes.
   - Fingers or toes become bluish or pale.
   - You become worse.

Pain and Itching

1. **Pain From Fracture(s):**
   - Fractures can be quite painful. The pain is worst the first 1-4 days after the injury and slowly decreases over the next couple weeks. A fracture takes 4-6 weeks to heal completely.
   - Many patients find that the most effective way to reduce pain is ELEVATION.
   - Patients also find that using ICE reduces pain.
   - Pain MEDICATIONS are also important.
2. **Prescription Pain Medication:**
   - The doctor who put on the cast has probably recommended or prescribed a pain medication. Take this as directed.
   - There are also over-the-counter pain medications that you can take: acetaminophen (e.g., Tylenol) and ibuprofen (e.g., Motrin)
3. **Pain Medicines:**
   - For pain relief, take acetaminophen, ibuprofen, or naproxen.

   Acetaminophen (e.g., Tylenol):
   - Take 650 mg by mouth every 4-6 hours as needed. Each Regular Strength Tylenol pill has 325 mg of acetaminophen. The most you should take each day is 3,250 mg (10 pills a day).

Another choice is to take 1,000 mg every 8 hours. Each Extra Strength Tylenol pill has 500 mg of acetaminophen. The most you should take each day is 3,000 mg (6 pills a day).

Ibuprofen (e.g., Motrin, Advil):
- Take 400 mg by mouth every 6 hours.
- Another choice is to take 600 mg by mouth every 8 hours.

Naproxen (e.g., Aleve):
- Take 250-500 mg by mouth every 12 hours.

Extra Notes:
- Acetaminophen is thought to be safer than ibuprofen or naproxen in people over 65 years old. Acetaminophen is in many OTC and prescription medicines. It might be in more than one medicine that you are taking. You need to be careful and not take an overdose. An acetaminophen overdose can hurt the liver.
- **Caution:** Do not take acetaminophen if you have liver disease.
- **Caution:** Do not take ibuprofen if you have stomach problems, kidney disease, are pregnant, or have been told by your doctor to avoid this type of anti-inflammatory drug. Do not take ibuprofen for more than 7 days without consulting your doctor.
- Use the lowest amount of medicine that makes your pain feel better.
- Before taking any medicine, read all the instructions on the package

4. **Itching:**
   - Use a hair dryer to blow some COOL air into the cast.
   - Do NOT stick anything down into the cast, such as a coat hanger or pencil, to scratch an itch. It might injure the skin and lead to infection or get stuck inside the cast.
5. **Call Back If:**
   - Pain under cast increases.
   - Pain under cast becomes severe.
   - You become worse.

Numbness and Tingling

1. **Expected Course With Elevation:**
   - Numbness and tingling can sometimes occur because of swelling and from pressure from the cast.
   - It should go away with elevation. If it does not, then you will need to be examined.
2. **Call Back If:**
   - Numbness or tingling persist after 1-2 hours of elevation.
   - You become worse.

Wet Cast

1. **Drying a Plaster Cast:**
   - A small wet spot can be blow-dried with a hair dryer. Try to dry it with the hair dryer set at a low setting (Caution: hot air can cause burns).
   - If a larger area of the cast becomes wet, you can also use a hair dryer to dry the cast.
   - Unfortunately, even if dried, a plaster cast will usually stay soft and need to be replaced.
2. **Drying a Fiberglass Cast:**
   - The outside (fiberglass portion) of a fiberglass cast is waterproof. However, the inside lining that is next to your skin is cotton and is not waterproof.
   - You usually dry the inner cotton lining with a hair dryer. Try to dry the lining with the hair dryer set at a low setting (Caution: hot air can cause burns).
   - If you can't dry it, the wet lining will cause itching or rashes under the cast.
3. **Call Back If:**
   - Cast becomes very soft.
   - Cast cracks.
   - You become worse.

Sharp Edges on Cast

1. **Sharp Edge on a Cast:**
   - If an edge is sharp you can carefully file it down with an emery board (nail file).
   - Another option is to cover the area with tape; or you can pad it with a cotton ball and some tape.
2. **Call Back If:**
   - This care advice does not help.
   - Redness or drainage occurs.
   - You become worse.

BACKGROUND INFORMATION

Casts

- A cast is a hard splint that completely encloses part of an injured arm or leg in the best position for healing.
- The purpose of a cast is to keep fractures (broken bones) from moving (immobilization) until they heal. Casts for fractures are usually applied for 4 to 6 weeks. Casts help reduce pain because when fractures move they hurt. Casts can also be used to help treat severe sprains (torn ligaments).
- The cast itself can be made out of fiberglass or plaster. Generally fiberglass is better than plaster. Fiberglass casts are lighter, less bulky, and stronger than plaster casts. Fiberglass casts are more durable, and the outside of a fiberglass cast is waterproof. Fiberglass casts are strong within 30 minutes of application. It takes plaster casts 48 hours to become completely dry and strong.
- The innermost layer of a cast is usually cotton padding to protect the skin. Gore-Tex liners are also available for use with fiberglass casts and have the advantage of being waterproof.

Common Cast Problems and Questions

- **Compartment Syndrome:** See below.
- **Pressure Sores:** A pressure sore can develop over an area of bony prominence as a result of pressure of the cast. This can usually be avoided with adequate padding at the time of casting.
- **Tight Casts:** Most questions are about tight casts. A tight cast can decrease circulation to the fingers and toes. The main symptoms are numbness, tingling, or increased pain in the fingers or toes. Other symptoms are color changes (bluish or pale) or swelling of the fingers or toes.
- **Wound Infection:** Sometimes a cast is placed over a wound. The wound can be a surgical incision from an operation or a traumatic wound from a compound fracture (bone poke through skin). These hidden wounds can become infected.

Compartment Syndrome

- **Definition:** Severely compromised capillary blood flow due to severe swelling inside a cast. This is an orthopedic emergency.
- **Complications:** Permanent muscle or nerve damage.
- **Symptoms:** Severe pain with passive stretching (flexion or extension) of fingers or toes is the most reliable sign. Other symptoms include moderate pain at rest, increasing pain, tingling, numbness, or pale fingers or toes.

CHEST PAIN

DEFINITION

- Uncomfortable pressure, fullness, squeezing, or other pain in the chest.
- This includes the area from the clavicles to the bottom of the rib cage.
- Not due to a traumatic injury.

TRIAGE ASSESSMENT QUESTIONS

Call EMS 911 Now

- Severe difficulty breathing (e.g., struggling for each breath, unable to speak).
  R/O: hypoxia, acute pulmonary edema
- Passed out (i.e., fainted, collapsed and was not responding)
  R/O: shock
- Chest pain lasting longer than 5 minutes and ANY of the following:
  - Over 50 years old
  - Over 30 years old and at least one cardiac risk factor (i.e., high blood pressure, diabetes, high cholesterol, obesity, smoker, or strong family history of heart disease)
  - Pain is crushing, pressure-like, or heavy
  - Took nitroglycerin and chest pain was not relieved
  - History of heart disease (i.e., angina, heart attack, bypass surgery, angioplasty, CHF)

  R/O: myocardial infarction, acute coronary syndrome
- Visible sweat on face or sweat dripping down face
  R/O: myocardial infarction, acute coronary syndrome
- Sounds like a life-threatening emergency to the triager

Go to ED Now

- SEVERE chest pain
- Pain also present in shoulder(s) or arm(s) or jaw
  R/O: acute coronary syndrome
- Difficulty breathing
- Cocaine use within last 3 days
  Reason: cocaine can precipitate acute coronary syndrome
- History of prior "blood clot" in leg or lungs (i.e., deep vein thrombosis, pulmonary embolism)
  Note: a "blood clot" typically would have required treatment with heparin or Coumadin.
  Reason: increased risk of thromboembolism
  R/O: deep vein thrombosis
- Recent illness requiring prolonged bed rest (i.e., immobilization)
  R/O: pulmonary embolism
- Hip or leg fracture in past 2 months (e.g., or had cast on leg or ankle)
  R/O: pulmonary embolism
- Major surgery in the past month
  R/O: pulmonary embolism
- Recent long distance travel with prolonged time in car, bus, plane, or train (i.e., within past 3 weeks; 6 or more hours' duration)
  Reason: immobilization during prolonged travel increases risk of pulmonary embolus
- Heart beating irregularly or very rapidly
  R/O: SVT, tachyarrhythmia

Go to ED Now (or to Office With PCP Approval)

- Chest pain lasting longer than 5 minutes
  Reason: chest pain is a high-risk complaint; referral for evaluation
- Intermittent chest pain and pain has been increasing in severity or frequency
  R/O: unstable angina
- Dizziness or lightheadedness
- Coughing up blood
- Patient sounds very sick or weak to the triager

See Today in Office

- Fever > 100.5° F (38.1° C)
- Intermittent chest pains persist > 3 days
- All other patients with chest pain
  Alternate Disposition: Have physician speak directly with patient
- Patient wants to be seen

Home Care

- ○ Intermittent mild chest pain lasting a few seconds each time

HOME CARE ADVICE FOR MILD CHEST PAIN

1. **Fleeting Chest Pain:** Fleeting chest pains that last only a few seconds and then go away are generally not serious. They may be from pinched muscles or nerves in your chest wall.
2. **Chest Pain Only When Coughing:** Chest pains that occur with coughing generally come from the chest wall and from irritation of the airways. They are usually not serious.
3. **Cough Medicines:**
   - **OTC Cough Syrups:** The most common cough suppressant in OTC cough medications is dextromethorphan. Often the letters DM appear in the name.
   - **OTC Cough Drops:** Cough drops can help a lot, especially for mild coughs. They reduce coughing by soothing your irritated throat and removing that tickle sensation in the back of the throat. Cough drops also have the advantage of portability—you can carry them with you.
   - **Home Remedy—Hard Candy:** Hard candy works just as well as medicine-flavored OTC cough drops. Diabetics should use sugar-free candy.
   - **Home Remedy—Honey:** An old home remedy has been shown to help decrease coughing at night. The adult dosage is 2 teaspoons (10 mL) at bedtime.
4. **Expected Course:** These mild chest pains usually disappear within 3 days.
5. **Call Back If:**
   - Severe chest pain.
   - Constant chest pain lasting longer than 5 minutes.
   - Difficulty breathing.
   - Fever.
   - You become worse.

FIRST AID

First Aid Advice for Shock:

Lie down with the feet elevated.

BACKGROUND INFORMATION

General

- Chest pain is a challenging symptom from a triage perspective as there are a number of potentially life-threatening causes of pain and no combination of symptoms that sufficiently discriminate serious from non-serious pain.
- A conservative stance in triaging these patients is recommended.

Serious Causes of Chest Pain

- **Acute Coronary Syndromes (Angina, Myocardial Infarction):** Chest pain caused by atherosclerotic blockages in the coronary arteries is the most common cause of acute coronary syndromes. This chest pain syndrome is typically seen with exertion, unless the blockage in a particular coronary artery is complete and then pain occurs at rest. Acute myocardial infarctions result from a complete loss of blood supply to the blocked coronary artery involved, often the result of an acute thrombus formation in the diseased vessel or disruption of an atherosclerotic plaque. Atherosclerotic heart disease, also referred to as ischemic heart disease, remains the leading cause of death in adults in the United States. See the Caution statement for further symptom description.
- **Pulmonary Embolus:** This potentially life-threatening process occurs when a clot, usually from a source in the lower extremities, dislodges and causes mechanical obstruction in the pulmonary arterial system of the lungs. The classic clinical picture is pleuritic chest pain, dyspnea, and hemoptysis. Some or all of these symptoms may be present. Risk factors include immobilization (e.g., bedbound, recent surgery, prolonged travel), trauma especially to the pelvis or lower extremities, and peripartum and hypercoaguable states (e.g., birth control pills, estrogen use, malignancy).
- **Pneumothorax:** Lung collapse can occur spontaneously or with trauma. The symptoms typically include pleuritic chest pain and dyspnea.

- **Thoracic Aortic Dissection:** A tear in the thoracic aorta usually presents with acute severe chest pain, often described as sharp and tearing in nature. This pain can be referred to the interscapular area. This disease entity is typically seen in the elderly.
- **Pericarditis:** Inflammation of the sac surrounding the heart or pericardium can result in positional chest pain, often pleuritic and dyspnea.

Other Less Serious Causes of Chest Pain

- **Pneumonia:** Some patients with pneumonia will complain of a sharp localized pleuritic pain. In general, any patient with pneumonia who is hypoxemic, has multilobe involvement, is unable to keep down liquids or medications, or is of advanced age or immunocompromised will require hospitalization.
- **Herpes Zoster:** Usually pain precedes the typical rash of grouped vesicles on a red base in a nerve root distribution.
- **Cholecystitis, Cholelithiasis:** The typical pain of gallstone disease is in the epigastrium and right upper quadrant, crampy in nature. Because of its location it can be confused with chest pain. Gallstone abdominal pain can radiate to the upper back in the region of the shoulder blade.
- **Costochondritis:** Caused by inflammation of the costal cartilages and/or their sternal articulations. The pain associated is typically sharp, positional, and reproducible. Costochondritis is a diagnosis of exclusion in those with risk factors for the more serious and life-threatening causes of chest pain.
- **Rib-Muscle Strain:** Typically the pain is positional, localized, intermittent, and sharp
- **Reflux Esophagitis:** Patients will often describe an acid or sour taste from the reflux of stomach contents and acid into the throat and mouth.

Myocardial Infarction—Should a Telephone Triage Nurse Recommend Aspirin?

- **Background:** Research has shown that early administration of aspirin reduces mortality from myocardial infarction. EMS 911 dispatchers sometimes instruct patients to take aspirin after an ambulance has been dispatched. Aspirin for cardiac chest pain is a standing medical order (SMO) for all EMS providers across the United States and Canada. Aspirin is also the standard of care for treating cardiac chest pain, once the patient reaches the emergency department. There is no evidence that taking aspirin at home provides any additional benefit over taking aspirin during paramedic transport or on arrival in the emergency department.
- **Telephone Triage and an EMS 911 Disposition:** Generally, these should be very short calls with the goal being to have the caller speak with the EMS 911 dispatcher as soon as possible. The triager should deliver and the caller should hear one piece of information: CALL 911 NOW. One can imagine a scenario in which the nurse triager spends too long on the phone with a caller clarifiying allergies/whether or not they already took aspirin/ explaining the difference between true aspirin and non-aspirin pain relievers (e.g., Tylenol).
- **If the Caller Asks About Aspirin:** Emphasize the importance of calling EMS 911 first. If there is no aspirin allergy, the patient may chew an aspirin (160 to 325 mg) while waiting for the paramedics to arrive.

Caution—Cardiac Ischemia

- Cardiac ischemia is the most common life-threatening cause of acute chest pain.
- Sometimes adults may present with chest pain as the sole symptom of a myocardial infarction. Often there will be other associated symptoms of cardiac ischemia: shortness of breath, nausea, and/or diaphoresis.
- Some adults can have cardiac ischemia without chest discomfort. For example, a diabetic with diaphoresis and shortness of breath.
- Women are less likely to experience chest pain and are more likely to have atypical symptoms; this can lead to delays in evaluation and treatment.
- Cardiac ischemia should be suspected in any patients with risk factors for cardiac disease. These include: hypertension, smoking, diabetes, hyperlipidemia, a strong family history of heart disease, and age over 50 years.

COLD SORES (FEVER BLISTERS OF LIP)

DEFINITION

- Recurrent sores on the outer lips caused by the herpes simplex virus.
- Use this guideline only if the patient has symptoms that match Fever Blisters.

Symptoms of Fever Blisters (Cold Sores) Include:

- Tingling or burning on the outer lip where cold sores previously occurred is an early warning sign of another episode of cold sores.
- A cold sore starts off as a cluster of painful 1-mm to 3-mm small bumps or blisters on the outer lip.
- The small blisters often rupture and form 1 big sore (i.e., cold sore).
- It is present only on one side of the mouth (i.e., doesn't cross the midline).
- Usually lasts 7-10 days.

TRIAGE ASSESSMENT QUESTIONS

Go to ED Now (or to Office With PCP Approval)

● Patient sounds very sick or weak to the triager

Go to Office Now

● Sores on the eye, eyelids, or tip of nose
R/O: herpes of the cornea

● Red streak or red area spreading from the cold sore
R/O: cellulitis

See Today in Office

● Immunocompromised (e.g., HIV positive, cancer chemotherapy, splenectomy, organ transplant, chronic steroids)
Reason: antiviral treatment indicated

● New sores occur in another area
R/O: impetigo

See Today or Tomorrow in Office

● Sores last > 2 weeks
R/O: wrong diagnosis, impetigo

● Patient wants to be seen

Callback by PCP Today

● Herpes sores are a recurrent problem, and caller wants a prescription medicine to take the next time they occur

Home Care

○ Cold sores without complications

HOME CARE ADVICE FOR COLD SORES

1. **General Information—Cold Sores**
   - Fever blisters or cold sores occur on one side of the outer lip.
   - Typically last 7-10 days.
   - Treatment with a cold sore cream can reduce the pain and shorten the course by a day or 2.
2. **Docosanol 10% Cream:**
   - Apply over-the-counter docosanol cream (trade name Abreva) to the cold sore 5 times daily until healing occurs.
   - Begin using this cream as soon as you first sense the beginning of an outbreak.
   - Docosonal is not available in Canada.
   - Read and follow the package instructions. Ask your physician's opinion.
3. **Contagiousness:**
   - Herpes from cold sores is contagious to other people. Discourage picking or rubbing the sore. Don't open the blisters. Wash your hands frequently. The cold sores are contagious until dry (approximately 5-7 days). Most cold sore sufferers note a tingling in the lip before the sore appears (prodromal phase). Patients are also contagious during this period.
   - **Eyes:** Avoid spreading the virus to someone's eye by kissing or touching; an eye infection can be serious (herpes keratitis).
   - **Mouth:** Since the blisters and mouth secretions are contagious, avoid kissing other people during this time. Avoid sharing drinking glasses, eating utensils, or razors.

- **Sex:** Avoid oral sex during this time. Herpes from sores on your mouth can spread to your partner's genital area.
- **Contact With Immunocompromised People:** Avoid contact with anyone who has eczema or a weakened immune system.

4. **Expected Course:** The pain typically subsides over 4-5 days and the sores typically heal over a 7- to 10-day period. On average, patients note recurrences 2-3 times per year.
5. **Prevention:** Since cold sores are often triggered by exposure to intense sunlight, use a lip balm containing a sunscreen (SPF 30 or higher).
6. **Recurrence:** Tingling or burning on the outer lip where cold sores previously occurred is an early sign of the new onset of recurrent cold sores.
7. **National Herpes Hotline Phone Number:** (919) 361-8488. Counselors provide information about transmission, treatment, prevention, and emotional issues. The hotline is open from 9:00 am to 7:00 pm, Eastern Time, Monday through Friday.
8. **Call Back If:**
   - Sores look infected (spreading redness).
   - Sores occur near or in the eye.
   - Sores last longer than 10 days.
   - You become worse.

BACKGROUND INFORMATION

General Information

- **Cause:** Cold sores are recurrent painful blisters on the outer lip caused by the herpes simplex virus (usually type 1).
- **Primary Herpes Simplex:** Approximately 80% of the adult population has had herpes simplex at some point in their lives. The very first episode (primary herpes simplex) of infection can present as sores on the inside of the mouth (with fever and feeling sick). More commonly, people have no symptoms at all during the first episode.
- **Recurrent Herpes Simplex Labialis (Cold Sores):** After the first episode of herpes, the herpes virus stays hidden in a facial sensory nerve. It can be reactivated by sun exposure, fever, friction, trauma, menstrual periods, stress, or physical exhaustion. Such recurrences occur in 20% of the adult population. Typically, the symptoms are confined to the lip and there is no fever. The medical term for these recurring cold sores of the lip is herpes simplex labialis. Another term that people use for this condition is fever blisters. This is a self-limiting illness that resolves without any treatment in 7-10 days.

Are There Any Over-the-Counter Treatments for Cold Sores?

- Docosanol cream (Abreva) seems to reduce severity, pain, and duration of cold sores (Sacks 2001). Docosanol is FDA approved in the United States. Ask your physician's opinion.

What Can Your Physician Prescribe for Colds Sores?

- **Topical (Cream) Prescription Treatment With Penciclovir 1%:** Use of this cream 4 times daily has been shown to reduce the severity, pain, and duration of cold sores in adults (Spruance 1997). It is more expensive than docosanol.
- **Oral (Pills) Prescription Treatment:** Available oral antiviral medications include acyclovir (Zovirax), famciclovir (Famvir), and valacyclovir (Valtrex). There may be some modest benefit obtained from using these medications; these medications may shorten symptom duration by 1 day and reduce symptoms. However, the research is not conclusive and such treatment is not standard practice (Emmert 2000). You will need to discuss this with your physician.

COLDS

DEFINITION

- Viral respiratory infection of the nose and throat.
- Use this guideline only if the patient has symptoms that match a Cold.

Symptoms of a Cold Include:

- Runny or congested (stuffy) nose is the main symptom. The nasal discharge may be clear, cloudy, yellow, or green.
- Sneezing.
- Mild fever and muscle aches, feeling tired and sleepy, headache.
- Scratchy or sore throat.
- Postnasal drip, throat clearing, cough.
- Sometimes associated with hoarseness, tearing eyes, and swollen lymph nodes in the neck.

TRIAGE ASSESSMENT QUESTIONS

Call EMS 911 Now

- ● Severe difficulty breathing (e.g., struggling for each breath, unable to speak)
- ● Very weak (e.g., can't stand)
- ● Sounds like a life-threatening emergency to the triager

See More Appropriate Protocol

- ● Runny nose is caused by pollen or other allergies
  Go to Protocol: Hay Fever (Nasal Allergies) on page 136
- ● Cough is the main symptom
  Go to Protocol: Cough on page 66
- ● Sore throat is the main symptom
  Go to Protocol: Sore Throat on page 241

Go to ED Now (or to Office With PCP Approval)

- ● Patient sounds very sick or weak to the triager
  R/O: pneumonia

Go to Office Now

- ● Fever > 103° F (39.4° C)
  R/O: pneumonia
- ● Fever > 100.5° F (38.1° C) and over 60 years of age
- ● Fever > 100.5° F (38.1° C) and has diabetes mellitus or a weakened immune system (e.g., HIV positive, cancer chemotherapy, organ transplant, splenectomy, chronic steroids)
- ● Fever > 100.5° F (38.1° C) and bedridden (e.g., nursing home patient, stroke, chronic illness, recovering from surgery)
  R/O: bacterial infection
  Note: may need ambulance transport to ED.

See Today in Office

- Fever present > 3 days (72 hours)
  R/O: bacterial sinusitis, bronchitis, pneumonia
- Fever returns after gone for over 24 hours and symptoms worse or not improved
  R/O: bacterial sinusitis, bronchitis, pneumonia
- Sinus pain (not just congestion) and fever
  R/O: bacterial sinusitis
- Earache
  R/O: otitis media

See Today or Tomorrow in Office

- Sinus congestion (pressure, fullness) present > 10 days
  R/O: bacterial sinusitis, allergic rhinitis
- Nasal discharge present > 10 days
  R/O: bacterial sinusitis, allergic rhinitis
- Using nasal washes and pain medicine > 24 hours and sinus pain (lower forehead, cheekbone, or eye) persists
  R/O: sinusitis

Strep Test Only Visit Today or Tomorrow

- Sore throat present > 5 days
  R/O: Strep pharyngitis

Home Care

- ○ Colds with no complications
- ○ Vitamin and herbal supplements for colds, questions about
- ○ Neti Pot, questions about

HOME CARE ADVICE

General Instructions for Treating a Cold

1. **Reassurance:**
   - It sounds like an uncomplicated cold that we can treat at home.
   - Colds are very common and may make you feel uncomfortable.
   - Colds are caused by viruses, and no medicine or "shot" will cure an uncomplicated cold.
   - Colds are usually not serious.
2. **For a Runny Nose With Profuse Discharge:**
   - Blow the nose.
   - Nasal mucus and discharge helps to wash viruses and bacteria out of the nose and sinuses.
   - Blowing the nose is all that is needed.
   - If the skin around your nostrils gets irritated, apply a tiny amount of petroleum ointment to the nasal openings once or twice a day.
3. **For a Stuffy Nose—Use Nasal Washes:**
   - **Introduction:** Saline (salt water) nasal irrigation is an effective and simple home remedy for treating cold symptoms and other conditions involving the nasal and sinus passages. Nasal irrigation consists of pouring, spraying, or squirting salt water into the nose and then letting it run back out.
   - **How It Helps:** The salt water rinses out excess mucus, washes out any irritants (dust, allergens) that might be present, and moisturizes the nasal cavity.
   - **Methods:** There are several ways to perform nasal irrigation. You can use a saline nasal spray bottle (available over-the-counter), a rubber ear syringe, a medical syringe without the needle, or a Neti Pot.

   Step-by-Step Instructions:
   - **Step 1:** Lean over a sink.
   - **Step 2:** Gently squirt or spray warm salt water into one of your nostrils.
   - **Step 3:** Some of the water may run into the back of your throat. Spit this out. If you swallow the salt water it will not hurt you.
   - **Step 4:** Blow your nose to clean out the water and mucus.
   - **Step 5:** Repeat steps 1-4 for the other nostril. You can do this a couple times a day if it seems to help you.

   How to Make Saline (Salt Water) Nasal Wash:
   - You can make your own saline nasal wash.
   - Add ½ tsp of table salt to 1 cup (8 oz; 240 mL) of warm water.
   - You should use sterile, distilled, or previously boiled water for nasal irrigation.
4. **Treatment for Associated Symptoms of Colds:**
   - For muscle aches, headaches, or moderate fever (more than 101° F or 38.9° C): Take acetaminophen every 4 hours.
   - **Sore Throat:** Try throat lozenges, hard candy, or warm chicken broth.
   - **Cough:** Use cough drops.
   - **Hydrate:** Drink adequate liquids.
5. **Humidifier:** If the air in your home is dry, use a cool-mist humidifier.
6. **Contagiousness:**
   - The cold virus is present in your nasal secretions.
   - Cover your nose and mouth with a tissue when you sneeze or cough.
   - Wash your hands frequently with soap and water.
   - You can return to work or school after the fever is gone and you feel well enough to participate in normal activities.
7. **Expected Course:**
   - Fever may last 2-3 days.
   - Nasal discharge 7-14 days.
   - Cough up to 2-3 weeks.
8. **Call Back If:**
   - Difficulty breathing occurs.
   - Fever lasts more than 3 days.
   - Nasal discharge lasts more than 10 days.
   - Cough lasts more than 3 weeks.
   - You become worse.

Over-the-Counter Medicines for a Cold

1. **Medicines for a Stuffy or Runny Nose:**
   - Most cold medicines that are available over-the-counter (OTC) are not helpful.
   - **Antihistamines:** Are only helpful if you also have nasal allergies.
   - If you have a very runny nose and you really think you need a medicine, you can try using a nasal decongestant for a couple days.

2. **Nasal Decongestants for a Very Stuffy or Runny Nose:**
    - If you have a very stuffy nose, nasal decongestant medicines can shrink the swollen nasal mucosa and allow for easier breathing. If you have a very runny nose, these medicines can reduce the amount of drainage. They may be taken as pills by mouth or as a nasal spray.
    - Most people do NOT need to use these medicines.
    - Pseudoephedrine (Sudafed) is available OTC in pill form. Typical adult dosage is two 30-mg tablets every 6 hours. Read package instructions.
    - Phenylephrine (Sudafed PE) is available OTC in pill form. Typical adult dosage is one 10-mg tablet every 4 hours. Read package instructions.
    - Oxymetazoline nasal drops (Afrin) are available OTC. Clean out the nose before using. Spray each nostril once, wait 1 minute for absorption, and then spray a second time. Read package instructions.
    - Phenylephrine nasal drops (Neo-Synephrine) are available OTC. Clean out the nose before using. Spray each nostril once, wait 1 minute for absorption, and then spray a second time. Read package instructions.
3. **Caution—Nasal Decongestants:**
    - Do not take these medications if you have high blood pressure, heart disease, prostate enlargement, or an overactive thyroid.
    - Do not take these medications if you are pregnant.
    - Do not take these medications if you have used an MAO inhibitor such as isocarboxazid (Marplan), phenelzine (Nardil), rasagiline (Azilect), selegiline (Eldepryl, Emsam), or tranylcypromine (Parnate) in the past 2 weeks. Life-threatening side effects can occur.
    - Do not use these medications for more than 3 days (Reason: rebound nasal congestion).
4. **Cough Medicines:**
    - **OTC Cough Syrups:** The most common cough suppressant in OTC cough medications is dextromethorphan. Often the letters DM appear in the name.
    - **OTC Cough Drops:** Cough drops can help a lot, especially for mild coughs. They reduce coughing by soothing your irritated throat and removing that tickle sensation in the back of the throat. Cough drops also have the advantage of portability—you can carry them with you.
    - **Home Remedy—Hard Candy:** Hard candy works just as well as medicine-flavored OTC cough drops. Diabetics should use sugar-free candy.
    - **Home Remedy—Honey:** An old home remedy has been shown to help decrease coughing at night. The adult dosage is 2 teaspoons (10 mL) at bedtime.
5. **OTC Cough Syrup—Dextromethorphan:**
    - Cough syrups containing the cough supppresant dextromethorphan (DM) may help decrease your cough. Cough syrups work best for coughs that keep you awake at night. They can also sometimes help in the late stages of a respiratory infection when the cough is dry and hacking. They can be used along with cough drops.
    - **Examples:** Benylin, Robitussin DM, Vicks 44 Cough Relief
    - Read the package instructions for dosage, contraindications, and other important information.
6. **Caution—Dextromethorphan:**
    - Do not try to completely suppress coughs that produce mucus and phlegm. Remember that coughing is helpful in bringing up mucus from the lungs and preventing pneumonia.
    - **Research Notes:** Dextromethorphan in some research studies has been shown to reduce the frequency and severity of cough in adults (18 years or older) without significant adverse effects. However, other studies suggest that dextromethorphan is no better than placebo at reducing a cough.
    - **Drug Abuse Potential:** It should be noted that dextromethorphan has become a drug of abuse. This problem is seen most often in adolescents. Overdose symptoms can range from giggling and euphoria to hallucinations and coma.

- **Contraindicated:** Do not take dextromethorphan if you are taking a monoamine oxidase (MAO) inhibitor now or in the past 2 weeks. Examples of MAO inhibitors include isocarboxazid (Marplan), phenelzine (Nardil), selegiline (Eldepryl, Emsam, Zelapar), and tranylcypromine (Parnate). Do not take dextromethorphan if you are taking venlafaxine (Effexor).

7. **Pain and Fever Medicines:**
   - For pain or fever relief, take acetaminophen or ibuprofen.
   - Treat fevers above 101° F (38.3° C).
   - The goal of fever therapy is to bring the fever down to a comfortable level. Remember that fever medicine usually lowers fever 2-3° F (1-1.5° C).

   Acetaminophen (e.g., Tylenol):
   - Take 650 mg by mouth every 4-6 hours as needed. Each Regular Strength Tylenol pill has 325 mg of acetaminophen. The most you should take each day is 3,250 mg (10 pills a day).
   - Another choice is to take 1,000 mg every 8 hours. Each Extra Strength Tylenol pill has 500 mg of acetaminophen. The most you should take each day is 3,000 mg (6 pills a day).

   Ibuprofen (e.g., Motrin, Advil):
   - Take 400 mg by mouth every 6 hours.
   - Another choice is to take 600 mg by mouth every 8 hours.

   Extra Notes:
   - Acetaminophen is thought to be safer than ibuprofen in people over 65 years old. Acetaminophen is in many OTC and prescription medicines. It might be in more than one medicine that you are taking. You need to be careful and not take an overdose. An acetaminophen overdose can hurt the liver.
   - **Caution:** Do not take acetaminophen if you have liver disease.
   - **Caution:** Do not take ibuprofen if you have stomach problems, kidney disease, are pregnant, or have been told by your doctor to avoid this type of anti-inflammatory drug. Do not take ibuprofen for more than 7 days without consulting your doctor.
   - Use the lowest amount of medicine that makes your pain or fever better.
   - Before taking any medicine, read all the instructions on the package.

Mineral, Vitamin, and Herbal Supplements

1. **Zinc:**
   - Some studies have reported that zinc gluconate lozenges (i.e., Cold-Eeze) may reduce the duration and severity of cold symptoms.
   - **Dosage:** Taken by mouth. You should take this with food to minimize the chance of nausea. Follow package instructions.
   - **Side Effects:** Some people complain of nausea and a bad taste in their mouth when they take zinc.
   - **Important Note About Zicam:** A zinc nasal gel (i.e., Zicam) is also available over-the-counter. There have been a number of lawsuits claiming that Zicam causes loss of smell (anosmia); it is uncertain whether this truly happens, but for now you should not use this medicine.
2. **Vitamin C:**
   - A number of experts, including Nobel Prize-winner Linus Pauling, have promoted taking high doses of this vitamin as a treatment for the common cold.
   - Research to date shows that vitamin C has minimal (if any) effect on the duration or degree of cold symptoms. Thus, it cannot be recommended as a treatment.
   - Vitamin C is probably harmless in standard doses (< 2 g daily).
3. **Echinacea:** There is no proven benefit of using this herbal remedy in treating or preventing the common cold. In fact, current research suggests that it does not help.
4. Read the package instructions thoroughly on all supplements that you take.

Neti Pot for Sinus Symptoms

1. **Neti Pot**
   - The Neti Pot is a small ceramic or plastic pot with a narrow spout. It looks like a small tea pot. Two manufacturers of the Neti Pot are the Himalayan Institute in Pennsylvania and SinuCleanse in Wisconsin.

- **How It Helps:** The Neti Pot performs nasal washing (also called nasal irrigation or "jala neti"). The salt water rinses out excess mucus, washes out any irritants (dust, allergens) that might be present, and moisturizes the nasal cavity.
- **Indications:** The Neti Pot is widely used as a home remedy to relieve conditions such as colds, sinus infections, and hay fever (nasal allergies).
- **Adverse reactions:** None. Though, not everyone likes the sensation of pouring water into their nose.
- **YouTube Instructional Video:** There are instructional videos on how to use a Neti Pot both on manufacturers' Web sites and also on YouTube.

2. **Neti Pot Step-by-Step Instructions:**
   - **Step 1:** Follow the directions on the salt package to make warm salt walter.
   - **Step 2:** Lean forward and turn your head to one side over the sink. Keep your forehead slightly higher than your chin.
   - **Step 3:** Gently insert the spout of the Neti Pot into the higher nostril. Put it far enough so that it forms a comfortable seal.
   - **Step 4:** Raise the Neti Pot gradually so the salt water flows in through your higher nostril and out of the lower nostril. Breathe through your mouth.
   - **Step 5:** When the Neti Pot is empty, blow your nose to clean out the water and mucus.
   - **Step 6:** Some of the water may run into the back of your throat. Spit this out. If you swallow the salt water it will not hurt you.
   - **Step 7:** Refill the Neti Pot and repeat on the other side. Again, exhale vigorously to clear the nasal passages.

How to Make Saline (Salt Water) Nasal Wash:

- You can make your own saline nasal wash.
- Add ½ tsp of table salt to 1 cup (8 oz; 240 mL) of warm water.
- You should use sterile, distilled, or previously boiled water for nasal irrigation.

BACKGROUND INFORMATION

General Information

- Colds are very common. The average adult experiences 3-4 colds each year.
- Viruses cause colds, and no medicine or "shot" will cure an uncomplicated cold.
- Colds are usually not serious. Most patients with colds do not need to be seen by a doctor.
- Rarely colds can lead to more serious illnesses such as: sinusitis, bronchitis, pneumonia, and otitis media. Elderly persons and individuals with a weakened immune system (due to chemotherapy, HIV positive, splenectomy, or the regular use of steroid medications) are at higher risk of developing these infectious complications.

Color of Nasal Discharge

- The nasal discharge normally changes color during different stages of a cold.
- It starts as a clear discharge and later becomes cloudy.
- Sometimes it becomes yellow or green colored for a few days; and this is still normal.
- Intermittent yellow or green discharge is more common with sleep, antihistamines, or low humidity (Reason: all of these events reduce the production of normal nasal secretions).
- Yellow or green nasal secretions suggest the presence of a bacterial sinusitis ONLY if they occur in combination with [1] sinus pain OR [2] the return of a fever after it has been gone for over 24 hours OR [3] nasal discharge persists > 10 days without improvement.
- Nasal secretions only become a problem when they block the nose and interfere with breathing through the nose. During a cold, if nasal breathing is noisy but the caller can't see blockage in the nose, it usually means the dried mucus is farther back. Nasal washes can remove it.
- Nasal mucus can become blood-tinged during a cold. It is just due to frequent wiping and blowing the nose.

Nasal Washes (Nasal Irrigation) for Sinus Symptoms

- **Introduction:** Saline (salt water) nasal irrigation is an effective and simple home remedy for treating cold symptoms and other conditions involving the nasal and sinus passages. Nasal irrigation consists of pouring, spraying, or squirting salt water into the nose and then letting it run back out.
- **How It Helps:** The salt water rinses out excess mucus, washes out any irritants (dust, allergens) that might be present, and moisturizes the nasal cavity.
- **Indications:** Nasal irrigation appears to be an effective treatment for chronic sinusitis. It may also help reduce sinus symptoms from acute viral upper respiratory infection (colds), irritant rhinitis (e.g., dust from the workplace), and allergic rhinitis (hay fever). Some doctors recommend it for rhinitis of pregnancy.
- **Adverse Reactions:** Nasal irrigation is safe and there are no serious adverse effects. However, not everyone likes the sensation of having water in their nose.
- **Methods:** There are several ways to perform nasal irrigation. None has been proven to be better than any other. Methods include use of a nasal spray bottle (available OTC), a rubber ear syringe, a Waterpik set on low, a 5- to 20-cc medical syringe without the needle, or a Neti Pot.
- **How to Make Salt Water for Nasal Irrigation:** Add ½ teaspoon of table salt to 1 cup (8 oz; 240 mL) of warm water.

Neti Pot for Sinus Symptoms

- The Neti Pot is a small ceramic or plastic pot with a narrow spout. It looks like a small tea pot. Two manufacturers of the Neti Pot are the Himalayan Institute in Pennsylvania and SinuCleanse in Wisconsin.
- **How It Helps:** The Neti Pot performs nasal washing (also called nasal irrigation or "jala neti"). The salt water rinses out excess mucus, washes out any irritants (dust, allergens) that might be present, and moisturizes the nasal cavity.
- **Indications:** The Neti Pot is widely used as a home remedy to relieve conditions such as colds, sinus infections, and hay fever (nasal allergies).
- **Adverse Reactions:** None. Nasal irrigation with a Neti Pot is safe and there are no serious adverse effects. However, not everyone likes the sensation of having salt water poured into their nose.

Neti Pot and Primary Amebic Meningoencephalitis (PAM)

- Primary amebic meningoencephalitis (PAM) is caused by *Naegleria fowleri*, the so-called "brain-eating ameba." This is an extremely rare infection. There were 32 cases in the United States between 2001 and 2010.
- The majority of the cases of PAM have occurred in the southern United States and were linked to swimming or bathing in freshwater lakes, rivers, and ponds containing this ameba. The ameba can also be found in hot springs, geothermal water sources, and poorly maintained swimming pools.
- In 2011 there were 2 cases of PAM in Louisiana that occurred after nasal irrigation with a Neti Pot. These 2 cases suggest—but are not definite proof—that the nasal irrigation fluid that the individuals used was somehow contaminated with the *N fowleri* ameba.
- The Centers for Disease Control and Prevention (CDC) recommends that individuals should use distilled, sterile, or previously boiled water for nasal irrigation. It's also important to rinse the irrigation device after each use and leave open to air-dry.

Dextromethorphan Cough Medicines for Cough

- The most common cough suppressant in OTC cough medications is dextromethorphan. Usually the letters DM appear in the name. An example is Robitussin DM.
- **Research:** Dextromethorphan in some research studies has been shown to reduce the frequency and severity of cough in adults (18 years or older) without significant adverse effects. However, other studies suggest that dextromethorphan is no better than placebo at reducing a cough.

- **Dextromethorphan and Adult Telephone Triage Guidelines:** The care advice in these guidelines continues to recommend DM-containing cough syrups. The rationale for this is: DM may reduce cough to some extent in adults, adult patients may benefit from the placebo effect of DM, many patients demand a recommendation for a cough syrup, there is no OTC medicine that works better than DM, and generally DM has no side effects.
- **Use Cough Drop or Hard Candy Instead:** Cough drops can often be used instead of cough syrups. While some would consider them a placebo similar to cough medicines, they may actually reduce coughing by soothing an irritated throat. In addition they have the advantage of portability. Hard candy probably works just as well as an OTC cough drop.
- **Use Honey for Nocturnal Cough:** See information in next column.
- **Dextromethorphan: A Drug of Abuse:** It is important to note that DM has become a drug of abuse. This problem is seen most commonly in the adolescent population. Overdose symptoms can range from giggling and euphoria to hallucinations or coma.

Honey for Cough

- **Recent Research Study:** A recent research study (Paul) compared honey to either dextromethorphan (DM) or no treatment for the treatment of nocturnal coughing. The study group contained 105 children age 2 to 18 years. Honey consistently scored the best for reducing cough frequency and cough severity. It also scored best for improving sleep. Dextromethorphan (DM) did not score significantly better than no treatment (showing its lack of efficacy).
- **How Might Honey Work?** One explanation for how honey works is that sweet substances naturally cause reflex salivation and increased airway secretions. These secretions may lubricate the airway and remove the trigger (or tickle) that causes a dry, nonproductive cough.
- **Adult Dosage:** 2 teaspoon (10 mL) at bedtime.

CONFUSION (DELIRIUM)

DEFINITION

- Diminished awareness and attention
- Confused thinking, talking "crazy" and acting strange
- Disorientation to person, place, or time
- **May Also Occur:** Hallucinations (usually visual or auditory), delusions (unrealistic thoughts), impaired judgment, decreased memory

Level of Consciousness Can Be Defined As:

- **Alert:** Normal state; oriented to person, place, and time.
- **Delirious (Confused):** Awake but confused talking, thinking, behavior.
- **Lethargic:** Very sleepy but can be awakened with verbal or tactile stimuli. When awakened, not alert.
- **Stuporous:** Very difficult to awaken and only responds to painful stimuli.
- **Comatose:** Persistent loss of consciousness. Doesn't awaken to painful stimuli.

Level of Consciousness Can Also Be Defined Using the AVPU Acronym:

- **A: A**wake
- **V:** Responding to **v**erbal stimuli
- **P:** Responding to **p**ainful stimuli
- **U: U**nresponsive

TRIAGE ASSESSMENT QUESTIONS

Call EMS 911 Now

- Difficult to awaken or acting confused (e.g., disoriented, slurred speech) and diabetic
  R/O: hypoglycemia
- Difficult to awaken or acting confused (e.g., disoriented, slurred speech) and new onset
  R/O: subarachnoid hemorrhage, meningitis, encephalitis, stroke
- Weakness of the face, arm, or leg on one side of the body and new onset
  R/O: stroke
- Numbness of the face, arm, or leg on one side of the body and new onset
  R/O: stroke
- Loss of speech or garbled speech and new onset
  R/O: stroke
- Difficulty breathing or bluish lips
  R/O: CNS symptoms of hypoxia
- Shock suspected (e.g., cold/pale/clammy skin, too weak to stand)
  R/O: shock
  FIRST AID: Lie down with the feet elevated.
- Seeing, hearing, or feeling things that are not there (i.e., visual, auditory, or tactile hallucinations)
  R/O: psychosis, substance abuse, alcohol withdrawal, alcoholic hallucinosis
- Followed a head injury
  R/O: concussion, cerebral contusion, epidural hematoma
- Drug overdose suspected
- Sounds like a life-threatening emergency to the triager

See More Appropriate Protocol

- Alcohol use, abuse, or dependence: question or problem related to
  Go to Protocol: Alcohol Use and Abuse and Dependence on page 9
- Drug abuse or dependence: question or problem related to
  Go to Protocol: Substance Abuse and Dependence on page 255

Go to ED Now

- Headache or vomiting
  R/O: meningitis, encephalitis, increased ICP, CO poisoning
- Stiff neck (can't touch chin to chest)
  R/O: meningitis
- Bizarre or paranoid behavior
  R/O: drug-induced psychosis, schizophrenia, bipolar disorder

Go to ED Now (or to Office With PCP Approval)

- Fever > 100.5° F (38.1° C)
  R/O: bacterial infection
- Patient sounds very sick or weak to the triager
  R/O: delirium due to hypoxia, shock, or sepsis

See Today in Office

- Transient confusion (i.e., completely resolved)
  Reason: course of delirium can fluctuate
- Patient wants to be seen (or caregiver requests)

See Today or Tomorrow in Office

- Long-standing confusion (e.g., dementia, stroke) and worsening
  R/O: infection, dehydration, metabolic abnormality

See Within 2 Weeks in Office

- Long-standing confusion (e.g., dementia, stroke) and NO worsening

Home Care

- Sundowning, questions about

HOME CARE ADVICE FOR CONFUSION (DELIRIUM) (Pending Office Visit)

Fever

1. **Fever Medicines:**
   - For fevers above 101° F (38.3° C) take acetaminophen or ibuprofen.
   - The goal of fever therapy is to bring the fever down to a comfortable level. Remember that fever medicine usually lowers fever 2 degrees F (1 - 1½ degrees C).

   Acetaminophen (e.g., Tylenol):
   - Take 650 mg by mouth every 4-6 hours. Each Regular Strength Tylenol pill has 325 mg of acetaminophen.
   - Another choice is to take 1,000 mg every 8 hours. Each Extra Strength Tylenol pill has 500 mg of acetaminophen.
   - The most you should take each day is 3,000 mg.

   Ibuprofen (e.g., Motrin, Advil):
   - Take 400 mg by mouth every 6 hours.
   - Another choice is to take 600 mg by mouth every 8 hours.
   - Use the lowest amount that makes your pain feel better.

   Extra Notes:
   - Acetaminophen is thought to be safer than ibuprofen in people over 65 years old. Acetaminophen is in many OTC and prescription medicines. It might be in more than one medicine that you are taking. You need to be careful and not take an overdose. An acetaminophen overdose can hurt the liver.
   - **Caution:** Do not take acetaminophen if you have liver disease.
   - **Caution:** Do not take ibuprofen if you have stomach problems, kidney disease, are pregnant, or have been told by your doctor to avoid this type of anti-inflammatory drug. Do not take ibuprofen for more than 7 days without consulting your doctor.
   - Before taking any medicine, read all the instructions on the package.
2. **Call Back If:**
   - You (i.e., patient, family member) become worse.

Questions About Sundowning

1. **Sundowning:**
   - **Definition:** Sundowning or "sundown syndrome" refers to the increased confusion that is sometimes seen in the late afternoon and evening in individuals with Alzheimer dementia and certain other brain conditions.
   - **Symptoms:** In addition to increased confusion there may be agitation, paranoia, hallucinations, and wandering (i.e., leaving house and getting lost).
2. **Sundowning—General Care Advice:**
   - Arrange for support from family, friends, and other caregivers.
   - Ensure adequate room lighting when awake. Consider a small night-light for use during the night.
   - Promote orientation by having an easily visible clock and calendar in the room.
   - Provide a structured daily routine and a familiar environment (photos of family, favorite possessions).
3. **Call Back If:**
   - You have more questions.
   - You (i.e., patient, family member) become worse.

FIRST AID

First Aid Advice for Hypoglycemia—Glucose

IF BLOOD GLUCOSE < 70 mg/dL (3.9 mmol/L) or UNKNOWN (pending EMS arrival) for conscious patients:

- Give sugar (10-15 grams glucose) by mouth IF able to swallow.
- Each of the following is equivalent to 10 g of glucose: milk (1 cup; 240 mL); orange juice (½ cup; 120 mL); prepackaged juice box (1 box); table sugar or honey (3 teaspoons; 15 mL); glucose tablets (3 tablets); glucose paste (10-15 grams).

First Aid Advice for Hypoglycemia—Glucagon

IF BLOOD GLUCOSE < 70 mg/dL (3.9 mmol/L) or UNKNOWN (pending EMS arrival):

- If family has glucagon for hypoglycemic emergencies AND the caller knows how to use it, encourage the caller to give the glucagon now.
- Inject it IM into the upper outer thigh.
- Adult dosage is 1 mg.

BACKGROUND INFORMATION

Delirium

- **Definition:** The term delirium is used to describe an alteration in level of consciousness that develops over hours to days.
- **Symptoms:** Symptoms may include disorientation, decreased attention, trouble with speech and understanding, and hallucinations. Symptoms often fluctuate.
- **Disposition:** Most adults with delirium need to be evaluated emergently.

Causes of Delirium

- Numerous acute and chronic medical conditions
- **Medications:** Especially benzodiazepines, narcotics, anticholinergics
- Substance abuse and alcohol intoxication
- Substance withdrawal (e.g., delirium tremens from alcohol withdrawal)

Conditions That Mimic Delirium

- **Depression:** Depressive symptoms, but oriented times 3
- **Dementia:** Long-standing confusion worsening over months to years
- **Psychosis:** History of psychiatric illness, paranoid thoughts

CONSTIPATION

DEFINITION

- Difficulty passing bowel movements: straining, hard stools, or rectal pressure.
- Patient feels like bowel movements do not occur frequently enough.

TRIAGE ASSESSMENT QUESTIONS

See More Appropriate Protocol

- Abdominal pain is the main symptom and adult male
  Go to Protocol: Abdominal Pain (Male) on page 4
- Abdominal pain is the main symptom and adult female
  Go to Protocol: Abdominal Pain (Female) on page 1
- Rectal bleeding or blood in stool is main symptom
  Go to Protocol: Rectal Bleeding on page 219

Go to ED Now (or to Office With PCP Approval)

- Patient sounds very sick or weak to the triager

Go to Office Now

- Constant abdominal pain lasting > 2 hours
  R/O: acute abdomen
- Vomiting bile (green color)
  R/O: intestinal obstruction
- Vomiting and abdomen looks much more swollen than usual
  R/O: intestinal obstruction

See Today in Office

- Intermittent mild abdominal pain and fever
  R/O: diverticulitis
- Abdomen is more swollen than usual
  R/O: fecal impaction
- Severe rectal pain not relieved by sitz bath or glycerine suppository
  R/O: impaction, abscess, fissure
- Last bowel movement (BM) > 4 days ago
  R/O: fecal impaction
- Leaking stool
  R/O: fecal impaction

See Within 3 Days in Office

- Constipation persists > 1 week while using care advice
- Unable to have a bowel movement (BM) without using a laxative, suppository, or enema
- Pencil-like, narrow stools
  R/O: malignancy
- Weight loss greater than 10 pounds (5 kg) and not dieting
  R/O: malignancy
- Patient wants to be seen

See Within 2 Weeks in Office

- Uses enema or laxative (e.g., lactulose, milk of magnesia) more than once a month
- Constipation is a chronic symptom (recurrent or ongoing AND lasting > 4 weeks)
  Note: for example, less than 3 BMs/week or straining greater than 25% of the time
- Minor bleeding from rectum (e.g., blood just on toilet paper, few drops, streaks on surface of normal formed BM) occurs more than twice
  R/O: anal fissure, hemorrhoids, malignancy

Home Care

- Mild constipation

HOME CARE ADVICE FOR MILD CONSTIPATION

1. **General Constipation Instructions:**
   - Eat a high-fiber diet.
   - Drink adequate liquids.
   - Exercise regularly (even a daily 15-minute walk!).
   - Get into a rhythm—try to have a BM at the same time each day.
   - Don't ignore your body's signals to have a BM.
   - Avoid enemas and stimulant laxatives.

2. **High-Fiber Diet:** A high-fiber diet will help improve your intestinal function and soften your BMs. The fiber works by holding more water in your stools.
   - Try to eat fresh fruit and vegetables at each meal (peas, prunes, citrus, apples, beans, corn).
   - Eat more grain foods (bran flakes, bran muffins, graham crackers, oatmeal, brown rice, and whole wheat bread). Popcorn is a source of fiber.
3. **Liquids:** Adequate liquid intake is important to keep your BMs soft.
   - Drink 6-8 glasses of water a day (Caution: certain medical conditions require fluid restriction).
   - Prune juice is a natural laxative.
   - Avoid alcohol.
4. **Get Into a Rhythm:**
   - Try to have a BM at the same time every day. The best time is about 30-60 minutes after breakfast or another meal (Reason: natural increased intestinal activity).
   - Do not ignore your body's signals to have a BM.
5. **Bulk Laxatives:**
   - **Metamucil (Psyllium Fiber):** One teaspoon (5 cc) in a glass of water twice daily.
   - Bulk-forming agents work like fiber to help soften the stools and improve your intestinal function. Long-term use of this type of laxative is generally safe.
   - **Side Effects:** Mild gas or a bloating sensation may occur.
   - Read the package instructions thoroughly on all medications that you use.
6. **Osmotic Laxatives:**
   - **Miralax (Polyethylene Glycol 3350):** Miralax is an osmotic agent, which means that it binds water and causes water to be retained within the stool. You can use this laxative to treat occasional constipation. Do not use for more than 2 weeks without approval from your doctor. Generally, Miralax produces a bowel movement in 1 to 3 days. Side effects include diarrhea (especially at higher doses). If you are pregnant, discuss with your doctor before using. Available in the United States.
   - **Milk of Magnesia (Magnesium Hydroxide):** This is a mild and generally safe laxative. You can use milk of magnesia for short-term treatment of constipation. (Research suggests that Miralax may be more effective.) Dosage is 2 tablespoons (30 mL) PO. Do not use if you have kidney disease.
   - Read the package instructions thoroughly on all medications that you use.
7. **Sitz Bath for Rectal Pain Due to Constipation:**
   - Take a 20-minute sitz bath. Sitting in the warm water may help relax the anal sphincter and release the bowel movement.
   - You can make a sitz bath by adding 2 ounces (60 grams) of baking soda to a bathtub containing warm water.
8. **Enemas:** Should be used rarely and only after other measures have not worked.
9. **Call Back If:**
   - Constipation continues (i.e., less than 3 BMs/week or straining more than 25% of the time) after following care advice for constipation for 2 weeks.
   - You become worse.

BACKGROUND INFORMATION

General Information

- Normal bowel movement (BM) frequency varies from 3 times a day to 3 times a week.
- Passage of a large bowel movement is not constipation, since the size of the bowel movement relates to the amount of food an individual eats and the bowel movement frequency. Large eaters have larger stools.
- The passage of small, dry, rabbit-pellet–like stools is not constipation and instead reflects the desiccation (drying-out) mechanism and insufficient fluid intake.

Lifestyle Causes

- **Inadequate Fiber in Diet:** Inadequate dietary fiber reduces intestinal motility and makes BMs hard and more difficult to pass. Fiber works by helping stools to retain water. Good sources of dietary fiber are fresh fruits and vegetables, beans, and bran. Fiber can also be taken via supplements (e.g., Metamucil).
- **Insufficient Liquids:** Insufficient liquid intake cause stools to be dry and harder to pass. Adults should drink 6-8 glasses of water daily.
- **Lack of Exercise:** Inactivity reduces bowel function, whereas exercise helps stimulate the bowels and improve regularity. Patients who are bedridden have increased problems with constipation and may develop fecal impaction.
- **Postponing Bowel Movements (BMs):** Some individuals ignore their body's signals for having a BM. This can lead to chronic problems with constipation.
- **Recent Travel:** Travel can cause constipation because it interferes with your diet and normal daily cycle.

Other Causes

- **Irritable Bowel Syndrome:** Patients with this syndrome may report abdominal pain and bloating relieved with passage of BMs. This is diagnosed clinically as there is no test that diagnoses irritable bowel syndrome.
- **Malignant Neoplasm of Colon:** Colon cancer can present initially as constipation. Suspect this in elderly patients with new onset or worsening constipation.
- **Medications:** There are a number of prescription and OTC medications that can cause or aggravate constipation. Examples include narcotic pain relievers (e.g., codeine), NSAIDs, antidepressants, calcium channel blockers (e.g., verapamil), and iron.
- **Metabolic and Endocrine:** Examples include hypercalcemia, hypokalemia, diabetes mellitus, hypothyroidism.
- **Neurologic Disease:** Constipation can occur in patients with multiple sclerosis, Parkinson disease, and spinal cord injury.
- **Pregnancy:** Constipation is common in pregnancy, especially during the third trimester.
- **Rectal Problems:** Anal fissures and hemorrhoids cause localized pain and slight bleeding. Hard BMs cause tears in the skin (anal fissure) with passage. Chronic constipation can lead to straining at BMs, which cause enlargement of the rectal veins (hemorrhoids). The pain from these 2 disorders may cause a patient to avoid having a BM, thus aggravating the constipation further.

COUGH

DEFINITION

- Cough is nonproductive (dry cough) if there is minimal clear-white or no phlegm (sputum).
- Cough is productive (wet cough) if there is yellow, green, or brown phlegm (sputum).

TRIAGE ASSESSMENT QUESTIONS

Call EMS 911 Now

- Lips or face are bluish
  R/O: hypoxia and need for oxygen
- Severe difficulty breathing (e.g., struggling for each breath, speaks in single words)
- Rapid onset of cough and has hives
  R/O: anaphylaxis
- Coughing started suddenly after medicine, an allergic food, or bee sting
  R/O: anaphylaxis
- Difficulty breathing after exposure to flames, smoke, or fumes
  R/O: inhalation injury
- Sounds like a life-threatening emergency to the triager

See More Appropriate Protocol

- Previous asthma attacks and this feels like asthma attack
  Go to Protocol: Asthma Attack on page 22

Go to ED Now

- Chest pain present when not coughing
  R/O: pneumonia, pneumothorax, pulmonary embolism
- Difficulty breathing
  R/O: pneumonia
- Passed out (i.e., fainted, collapsed and was not responding)
  R/O: hypoxia, cough syncope, pulmonary embolism

Go to ED Now (or to Office With PCP Approval)

- Patient sounds very sick or weak to the triager

Go to Office Now

- Coughed up > 1 tablespoon blood
  Exception: blood-tinged sputum
  Reason: significant hemoptysis
- Fever > 103° F (39.4° C)
  R/O: pneumonia
- Fever > 100.5° F (38.1° C) and over 60 years of age
  R/O: pneumonia
- Fever > 100.5° F (38.1° C) and has diabetes mellitus or a weakened immune system (e.g., HIV positive, cancer chemotherapy, organ transplant, splenectomy, chronic steroids)
  R/O: pneumonia
- Fever > 100.5° F (38.1° C) and bedridden (e.g., nursing home patient, stroke, chronic illness, recovering from surgery)
  R/O: pneumonia
  Note: may need ambulance transport to ED.
- Increasing ankle swelling
  R/O: congestive heart failure
- Wheezing is present
  R/O: asthma, bronchitis

See Today in Office

- SEVERE coughing spells (e.g., whooping sound after coughing, vomiting after coughing)
  R/O: whooping cough (pertussis)
- Coughing up rusty-colored (reddish-brown) or blood-tinged sputum
  R/O: pneumonia
- Fever present > 3 days (72 hours)
  R/O: bacterial sinusitis, bronchitis, pneumonia
- Fever returns after gone for over 24 hours and symptoms worse or not improved
  R/O: bacterial sinusitis, bronchitis, pneumonia
- Sinus pain persists after using nasal washes and pain medicine > 24 hours
  R/O: bacterial sinusitis
- Known COPD or other severe lung disease (i.e., bronchiectasis, cystic fibrosis, lung surgery) and worsening symptoms (i.e., increased sputum purulence or amount, increased breathing difficulty)
  R/O: exacerbation
  Reason: may need antibiotic therapy

See Today or Tomorrow in Office

- Continuous (nonstop) coughing interferes with work or school and no improvement using cough treatment per care advice
  Reason: may need codeine or asthma medication
- Patient wants to be seen

See Within 3 Days in Office

- Cough has been present for > 10 days
  R/O: bacterial sinusitis, bronchitis
- Allergy symptoms are also present (e.g., itchy eyes, clear nasal discharge, postnasal drip)
  R/O: asthmatic cough
- Nasal discharge present > 10 days
  R/O: bacterial sinusitis
- Exposure to TB (tuberculosis)
- Taking an ACE inhibitor medication (e.g., benazepril/Lotensin, captopril/Capoten, enalapril/Vasotec, lisinopril/Zestril)
  R/O: ACE inhibitor as cause. See list in Background Information.

Home Care

- Cough with no complications
  R/O: viral URI
- Cough with cold symptoms (e.g., runny nose, postnasal drip, throat clearing)
  R/O: postnasal drip syndrome (upper airway cough syndrome)

HOME CARE ADVICE

General Care Advice for Mild to Moderate Cough

1. **Reassurance:**
   - Coughing is the way that our lungs remove irritants and mucus. It helps protect our lungs from getting pneumonia.
   - You can get a dry hacking cough after a chest cold. Sometimes this type of cough can last 1-3 weeks and be worse at night.
   - You can also get a cough after being exposed to irritating substances like smoke, strong perfumes, and dust.
2. **Cough Medicines:**
   - **OTC Cough Syrups:** The most common cough suppressant in OTC cough medications is dextromethorphan. Often the letters DM appear in the name.
   - **OTC Cough Drops:** Cough drops can help a lot, especially for mild coughs. They reduce coughing by soothing your irritated throat and removing that tickle sensation in the back of the throat. Cough drops also have the advantage of portability—you can carry them with you.
   - **Home Remedy—Hard Candy:** Hard candy works just as well as medicine-flavored OTC cough drops. Diabetics should use sugar-free candy.
   - **Home Remedy—Honey:** This old home remedy has been shown to help decrease coughing at night. The adult dosage is 2 teaspoons (10 mL) at bedtime. Honey should not be given to infants under 1 year of age.
3. **OTC Cough Syrup—Dextromethorphan:**
   - Cough syrups containing the cough supppresant dextromethorphan (DM) may help decrease your cough. Cough syrups work best for coughs that keep you awake at night. They can also sometimes help in the late stages of a respiratory infection when the cough is dry and hacking.
   - They can be used along with cough drops.
   - **Examples:** Benylin, Robitussin DM, Vicks 44 Cough Relief
   - Read the package instructions for dosage, contraindications, and other important information.
4. **Caution—Dextromethorphan:**
   - Do not try to completely suppress coughs that produce mucus and phlegm. Remember that coughing is helpful in bringing up mucus from the lungs and preventing pneumonia.
   - **Research Notes:** Dextromethorphan in some research studies has been shown to reduce the frequency and severity of cough in adults (18 years or older) without significant adverse effects. However, other studies suggest that dextromethorphan is no better than placebo at reducing a cough.
   - **Drug Abuse Potential:** It should be noted that dextromethorphan has become a drug of abuse. This problem is seen most often in adolescents. Overdose symptoms can range from giggling and euphoria to hallucinations and coma.

- **Contraindicated:** Do not take dextromethorphan if you are taking a monoamine oxidase (MAO) inhibitor now or in the past 2 weeks. Examples of MAO inhibitors include isocarboxazid (Marplan), phenelzine (Nardil), selegiline (Eldepryl, Emsam, Zelapar), and tranylcypromine (Parnate). Do not take dextromethorphan if you are taking venlafaxine (Effexor).

5. **Coughing Spasms:**
   - Drink warm fluids. Inhale warm mist (Reason: both relax the airway and loosen up the phlegm).
   - Suck on cough drops or hard candy to coat the irritated throat.
6. **Prevent Dehydration:**
   - Drink adequate liquids.
   - This will help soothe an irritated or dry throat and loosen up the phlegm.
7. **Avoid Tobacco Smoke:** Smoking or being exposed to smoke makes coughs much worse.
8. **Fever Medicines:**
   - For fevers above 101° F (38.3° C) take acetaminophen or ibuprofen.
   - The goal of fever therapy is to bring the fever down to a comfortable level. Remember that fever medicine usually lowers fever 2 degrees F (1 - 1½ degrees C).

   Acetaminophen (e.g., Tylenol):
   - Take 650 mg by mouth every 4-6 hours. Each Regular Strength Tylenol pill has 325 mg of acetaminophen.
   - Another choice is to take 1,000 mg every 8 hours. Each Extra Strength Tylenol pill has 500 mg of acetaminophen.
   - The most you should take each day is 3,000 mg.

   Ibuprofen (e.g., Motrin, Advil):
   - Take 400 mg by mouth every 6 hours.
   - Another choice is to take 600 mg by mouth every 8 hours.
   - Use the lowest amount that makes your pain feel better.

   Extra Notes:
   - Acetaminophen is thought to be safer than ibuprofen in people over 65 years old. Acetaminophen is in many OTC and prescription medicines. It might be in more than one medicine that you are taking. You need to be careful and not take an overdose. An acetaminophen overdose can hurt the liver.
   - **Caution:** Do not take acetaminophen if you have liver disease.
   - **Caution:** Do not take ibuprofen if you have stomach problems, kidney disease, are pregnant, or have been told by your doctor to avoid this type of anti-inflammatory drug. Do not take ibuprofen for more than 7 days without consulting your doctor.
   - Before taking any medicine, read all the instructions on the package.
9. **Expected Course:**
   - The expected course depends on what is causing the cough.
   - Viral bronchitis (chest cold) causes a cough that lasts 1 to 3 weeks. Sometimes you may cough up lots of phlegm (sputum, mucus). The mucus can normally be white, gray, yellow, or green.
10. **Call Back If:**
    - Difficulty breathing.
    - Cough lasts more than 3 weeks.
    - Fever lasts more than 3 days.
    - You become worse.

Cough With Cold Symptoms

1. **Reassurance:**
   - It sounds like an uncomplicated cold that we can treat at home.
   - Colds are very common and may make you feel uncomfortable.
   - Colds are caused by viruses, and no medicine or "shot" will cure an uncomplicated cold.
   - Colds are usually not serious.
2. **For a Runny Nose With Profuse Discharge: Blow the Nose:**
   - Nasal mucus and discharge help to wash viruses and bacteria out of the nose and sinuses.
   - Blowing the nose is all that is needed.
   - If the skin around your nostrils gets irritated, apply a tiny amount of petroleum ointment to the nasal openings once or twice a day.
3. **For a Stuffy Nose—Use Nasal Washes:**
   - **Introduction:** Saline (salt water) nasal irrigation is an effective and simple home remedy for treating cold symptoms and other conditions involving the nasal and sinus passages. Nasal irrigation consists of pouring, spraying, or squirting salt water into the nose and then letting it run back out.

- **How It Helps:** The salt water rinses out excess mucus, washes out any irritants (dust, allergens) that might be present, and moisturizes the nasal cavity.
- **Methods:** There are several ways to perform nasal irrigation. You can use a saline nasal spray bottle (available over-the-counter), a rubber ear syringe, a medical syringe without the needle, or a Neti Pot.

Step-by-Step Instructions:

- **Step 1:** Lean over a sink.
- **Step 2:** Gently squirt or spray warm salt water into one of your nostrils.
- **Step 3:** Some of the water may run into the back of your throat. Spit this out. If you swallow the salt water it will not hurt you.
- **Step 4:** Blow your nose to clean out the water and mucus.
- **Step 5:** Repeat steps 1-4 for the other nostril. You can do this a couple times a day if it seems to help you.

How to Make Saline (Salt Water) Nasal Wash:

- You can make your own saline nasal wash.
- Add ½ tsp of table salt to 1 cup (8 oz; 240 mL) of warm water.
- You should use sterile, distilled, or previously boiled water for nasal irrigation.

4. **Medicines for a Stuffy or Runny Nose:**
   - Most cold medicines that are available over-the-counter (OTC) are not helpful.
   - **Antihistamines:** Are only helpful if you also have nasal allergies.
   - If you have a very runny nose and you really think you need a medicine, you can try using a nasal decongestant for a couple days.
5. **Nasal Decongestants for a Very Stuffy or Runny Nose:**
   - If you have a very stuffy nose, nasal decongestant medicines can shrink the swollen nasal mucosa and allow for easier breathing. If you have a very runny nose, these medicines can reduce the amount of drainage. They may be taken as pills by mouth or as a nasal spray.
   - Most people do NOT need to use these medicines.
   - Pseudoephedrine (Sudafed) is available OTC in pill form. Typical adult dosage is two 30-mg tablets every 6 hours. Read package instructions.
   - Phenylephrine (Sudafed PE) is available OTC in pill form. Typical adult dosage is one 10-mg tablet every 4 hours. Read package instructions.
   - Oxymetazoline nasal drops (Afrin) are available OTC. Clean out the nose before using. Spray each nostril once, wait 1 minute for absorption, and then spray a second time. Read package instructions.
   - Phenylephrine nasal drops (Neo-Synephrine) are available OTC. Clean out the nose before using. Spray each nostril once, wait 1 minute for absorption, and then spray a second time. Read package instructions.
6. **Caution—Nasal Decongestants:**
   - Do not take these medications if you have high blood pressure, heart disease, prostate enlargement, or an overactive thyroid.
   - Do not take these medications if you are pregnant.
   - Do not take these medications if you have used an MAO inhibitor such as isocarboxazid (Marplan), phenelzine (Nardil), rasagiline (Azilect), selegiline (Eldepryl, Emsam), or tranylcypromine (Parnate) in the past 2 weeks. Life-threatening side effects can occur.
   - Do not use these medications for more than 3 days (Reason: rebound nasal congestion).
7. **Pain and Fever Medicines:**
   - For pain or fever relief, take acetaminophen or ibuprofen.
   - Treat fevers above 101° F (38.3° C).
   - The goal of fever therapy is to bring the fever down to a comfortable level. Remember that fever medicine usually lowers fever 2-3° F (1-1.5° C).

Acetaminophen (e.g., Tylenol):

- Take 650 mg by mouth every 4-6 hours as needed. Each Regular Strength Tylenol pill has 325 mg of acetaminophen. The most you should take each day is 3,250 mg (10 pills a day).
- Another choice is to take 1,000 mg every 8 hours. Each Extra Strength Tylenol pill has 500 mg of acetaminophen. The most you should take each day is 3,000 mg (6 pills a day).

Ibuprofen (e.g., Motrin, Advil):

- Take 400 mg by mouth every 6 hours.
- Another choice is to take 600 mg by mouth every 8 hours.

Extra Notes:

- Acetaminophen is thought to be safer than ibuprofen in people over 65 years old.
- Acetaminophen is in many OTC and prescription medicines. It might be in more than one medicine that you are taking. You need to be careful and not take an overdose. An acetaminophen overdose can hurt the liver.
- **Caution:** Do not take acetaminophen if you have liver disease.
- **Caution:** Do not take ibuprofen if you have stomach problems, kidney disease, are pregnant, or have been told by your doctor to avoid this type of anti-inflammatory drug. Do not take ibuprofen for more than 7 days without consulting your doctor.
- Use the lowest amount of medicine that makes your pain or fever better.
- Before taking any medicine, read all the instructions on the package.

8. **Contagiousness:**
   - The cold virus is present in your nasal secretions.
   - Cover your nose and mouth with a tissue when you sneeze or cough.
   - Wash your hands frequently with soap and water.
   - You can return to work or school after the fever is gone and you feel well enough to participate in normal activities.
9. **Expected Course:**
   - Fever may last 2-3 days.
   - Nasal discharge 7-14 days.
   - Cough up to 2-3 weeks.
10. **Call Back If:**
    - Difficulty breathing occurs.
    - Fever lasts more than 3 days.
    - Nasal discharge lasts more than 10 days.
    - Cough lasts more than 3 weeks.
    - You become worse.

BACKGROUND INFORMATION

General Information

- A cough is the sound made when the cough reflex suddenly expels air and secretions from the lungs.
- Cough is one of the most common symptoms that patients experience. It is the fifth most common reason for visits to physicians.
- The common cold is the single most common cause of acute cough (i.e., cough < 3 weeks in duration).
- Smokers may have a chronic cough, especially in the morning.

Why We Cough—A Cough Has 2 Important Functions:

- Serves to clear the airways of infection, mucus, foreign bodies, and other irritants.
- Protects against aspiration of oral and stomach contents.

Causes of Coughing

- **Most Common Causes:** Postnasal drip syndrome from a cold, allergic rhinitis, and sinusitis
- **Other Common Causes:** Asthma, bronchitis, pneumonia, gastroesophageal reflux, and smoking
- **Less Common Causes:** Lung cancer, congestive heart failure, pulmonary embolism, TB, whooping cough, and ACE inhibitor drugs

Angiotensin-Converting Enzyme (ACE) Inhibitors Can Cause a Dry Chronic Cough.

Generic and trade name listing:

- Benazepril—Lotensin
- Captopril—Capoten
- Cilazapril—Inhibace
- Enalapril, Enalaprilat—Vasotec
- Fosinopril—Monopril
- Lisinopril—Zestril
- Moexipril—Univasc
- Perindopril—Aceon, Coversyl
- Quinapril—Accupril
- Ramipril—Altace
- Trandolapril—Mavik

Sputum or Phlegm

- The presence of purulent sputum is a poor predictor of whether an infection is caused by a viral or bacterial respiratory infection.
- Yellow or green phlegm is a normal part of the healing process of viral tracheitis or bronchitis. This means the lining of the trachea was damaged by the viral infection and is being coughed up as new mucosa replaces it.
- Bacteria are not a common cause of tracheitis or bronchitis in healthy people. Antibiotics are not indicated for the viral bronchitis seen with colds.
- The main treatment of a productive cough is to facilitate it with good fluid intake, a humidifier (if the air is dry), and warm chicken broth or tea for coughing spasms.
- Only in COPD or other severe chronic lung disease (e.g., bronchiectasis, cystic fibrosis, lung surgery) is the amount or purulence of sputum important.

Antibiotics for Cough

- **Acute Bronchitis:** Routine antbiotic therapy provides no meaningful benefit in the treatment of acute bronchitis. There is no effect on duration of illness, severity of symptoms, or return to work.
- **Common Cold:** Colds are caused by viruses, and no medicine, "shot," or antibiotic will cure an uncomplicated cold.
- **Pneumonia:** Pneumonia is often caused by bacteria; antibiotic therapy is usually needed.
- **Whooping Cough (Pertussis):** Whooping cough is caused by a bacteria *(Bordetella pertussis)*. Treatment with antibiotics is indicated when whooping cough is diagnosed or strongly suspected.

Dextromethorphan Cough Medicines for Cough

- The most common cough suppressant in OTC cough medications is dextromethorphan. Usually the letters DM appear in the name. An example is Robitussin DM.
- **Research:** Dextromethorphan in some research studies has been shown to reduce the frequency and severity of cough in adults (18 years or older) without significant adverse effects. However, other studies suggest that dextromethorphan is no better than placebo at reducing a cough.
- **Dextromethorphan and Adult Telephone Triage Guidelines:** The care advice in these guidelines continues to recommend DM-containing cough syrups. The rationale for this is: DM may reduce cough to some extent in adults, adult patients may benefit from the placebo effect of DM, many patients demand a recommendation for a cough syrup, there is no OTC medicine that works better than DM, and generally DM has no side effects.
- **Use Cough Drop or Hard Candy Instead:** Cough drops can often be used instead of cough syrups. While some would consider them a placebo similar to cough medicines, they may actually reduce coughing by soothing an irritated throat. In addition they have the advantage of portability. Hard candy probably works just as well as an OTC cough drop.
- **Use Honey for Nocturnal Cough:** See information below.
- **Dextromethorphan—A Drug of Abuse:** It is important to note that DM has become a drug of abuse. This problem is seen most commonly in the adolescent population. Overdose symptoms can range from giggling and euphoria to hallucinations or coma.

Honey for Cough

- **Recent Research Study:** A recent research study (Paul) compared honey to either dextrometho-rphan (DM) or no treatment for the treatment of nocturnal coughing. The study group contained 105 children age 2 to 18 years. Honey consistently scored the best for reducing cough frequency and cough severity. It also scored best for improving sleep. Dextromethorphan (DM) did not score significantly better than no treatment (showing its lack of efficacy).
- **How Might Honey Work?** One explanation for how honey works is that sweet substances naturally cause reflex salivation and increased airway secretions. These secretions may lubricate the airway and remove the trigger (or tickle) that causes a dry, nonproductive cough.
- **Adult Dosage:** 2 teaspoon (10 mL) at bedtime.

DENTAL PROCEDURE ANTIBIOTIC PROPHYLAXIS

DEFINITION

- Patient is requesting antibiotic prophylaxis prior to a dental procedure.

TRIAGE ASSESSMENT QUESTIONS

Go to ED Now (or to Office With PCP Approval)

- Patient sounds very sick or weak to the triager

Discuss With PCP and Callback by Nurse Today

- Has both SPECIFIED CARDIAC CONDITION and SPECIFIED DENTAL PROCEDURE, and NO standing order to call in prescription for antibiotic
  Reason: antibiotic prescription needed
  Note: see relevant definitions in Background Information
- Has both SPECIFIED CARDIAC CONDITION and SPECIFIED DENTAL PROCEDURE, and already taking antibiotics for something else
  Reason: current antibiotic may or may not be effective
- Joint replacement surgery in past 2 years
  Reason: antibiotic prescription may be needed
  Note: see CDA November 2007 statement in Background Information
- Triager unable to answer question

See Within 3 Days in Office

- Patient wants to be seen

Home Care

- Has both SPECIFIED CARDIAC CONDITION and SPECIFIED DENTAL PROCEDURE, and standing order to call in prescription for antibiotic
  Reason: antibiotic prescription needed
  Note: see relevant definitions in Background Information
- Does not have SPECIFIED CARDIAC CONDITION
  Reason: antibiotic prophylaxis is not indicated
- Does not have SPECIFIED DENTAL PROCEDURE
  Reason: antibiotic prophylaxis is not indicated

HOME CARE ADVICE

Antibiotic Prohylaxis Is Indicated

1. **You Should Take Antibiotics Before the Dental Procedure:**
   - Given what you have told me about your heart condition and the planned dental work, it sounds like you should take antibiotics before the procedure.
   - Take the antibiotic 1 hour before the start of the dental procedure.
2. **Recommended Antibiotic—Follow Call Center Policy and the Physician's Practice Rules:**
   Call in prescription for one of the following antibiotics:
   - Amoxicillin 2 grams PO
   - **Unable to Take Medications by Mouth:** Ampicillin 2 grams IM (intramuscular shot) or IV (intravenous) or cefazolin 1 gram IM or IV.
   - **Allergic to Penicillins:** Clindamycin 600 mg PO, IM, IV, or azithromycin (Zithromax) 500 mg PO.
3. **Caution—Antibiotics:**
   - Ask patient about allergies.
   - Intramuscular antibiotics generally should not be used in patients taking Coumadin or who have a coagulopathy.
4. **Call Back If:**
   - You have more questions.

Antibiotic Prohylaxis Is Not Indicated

1. **You Do Not Need to Take Antibiotics Before This Dental Procedure:** Given what you have told me about your heart condition and the planned dental work, it sounds like you do NOT need to take antibiotics before the procedure.
2. **Disclaimer:**
   - These are guidelines for general practice. Occasionally, antibiotic prophylaxis may still be advised for an individual patient. If you have any type of heart condition, you should ask your cardiologist about this.
   - The full text of the American Heart Association (AHA) guideline for prevention of infective endocarditis is available online at: http://circ.ahajournals.org/cgi/reprint/CIRCULATIONAHA.106.183095.

- There are some cardiac conditions that have an increased lifetime risk of endocarditis, yet the AHA has deemed that anitibiotic prophyaxis is not indicated. If you develop symptoms of endocarditis, such as unexplained fever, talk with your doctor right away.

3. **Call Back If:**
   - You have more questions.

Additional Resources

1. **The American Heart Association** has created a wallet card that physicians can give to their patients. It is available online at: www.heart.org/idc/groups/heart-public/@wcm/@hcm/documents/downloadable/ucm_307644.pdf.
2. **The wallet card is also available in Spanish:** www.heart.org/idc/groups/heart-public/@wcm/@hcm/documents/downloadable/ucm_311663.pdf.

BACKGROUND INFORMATION

General

- In 2007 the American Heart Association (AHA) released new guidelines regarding antibiotic prophylaxis prior to procedures for the purpose of preventing infective endocarditis.
- There are substantive changes in these new 2007 guidelinies; antibiotic prophylaxis is now indicated in fewer patients than previously. Antibiotic prophylaxis is indicated in patients who have both a SPECIFIED CARDIAC CONDITION and a SPECIFIED DENTAL PROCEDURE (see paragraphs below).
- The full text of the AHA guideline for prevention of infective endocarditis is available online at: http://circ.ahajournals.org/cgi/reprint/CIRCULATIONAHA.106.183095
- Canadian Dental Association (CDA) released a statement in November 2007 that disagreed with a part of the AHA 2007 antibiotic prophylaxis guidelines. Specifically, the CDA recommended that prophylactic antibiotics should be considered for all patient types undergoing dental procedures during the first 2 years following joint replacement.

Specified Cardiac Conditions

Antibiotic prophylaxis prior to specified dental procedures is recommended for the following cardiac conditions (AHA 2007):

- Prosthetic cardiac valve (artificial valve)
- Previous infective endocarditis
- Congenital heart disease (CHD), specifically:
  - Unrepaired cyanotic CHD, including palliative shunts and conduits.
  - Completely repaired congenital heart defect with prosthetic material or device, whether placed by surgery or by catheter intervention, during the first 6 months after the procedure.
  - Repaired CHD with residual defects at the site or adjacent to the site of a prosthetic patch or prosthetic device (which inhibit endothelialization).
  - Or cardiac transplantation recipients who develop cardiac valvulopathy.
  - Note: Except for the conditions listed above, antibiotic prophylaxis is no longer recommended for any other form of CHD. Antibiotic prophylaxis is no longer recommended for mitral valve prolapse (MVP).

Specified Dental Procedures

- Antibiotic prophylaxis is recommended for patients with the above specified cardiac conditions for all dental procedures that involve manipulation of gingival tissue or the periapical region of teeth, or perforation of the oral mucosa (AHA 2007). Examples include:
  - Teeth cleaning
  - Dental extraction (tooth removal)
  - Biopsies
  - Dental implant placement and reimplantation of avulsed teeth
  - Endodontic surgery (e.g., root canal)
  - Periodontal procedures (e.g., surgery, scaling, root planing)
  - Placement of orthodontic bands
  - Suture removal

  Note: The following dental procedures do not need antibiotic prophylaxis: routine anesthetic injections through noninfected tissue, taking dental radiographs, placement of removable prosthodontic or orthodontic appliances, adjustment of orthodontic appliances, placement of orthodontic brackets, shedding of primary teeth, and bleeding from trauma to the lips or oral mucosa.

DEPRESSION

DEFINITION

- Patient/caller states that he or she has depression.
- Feelings of sadness or hopelessness.
- Decreased pleasure or interest in daily activities.

TRIAGE ASSESSMENT QUESTIONS

Call EMS 911 Now

- Sounds like a life-threatening emergency to the triager

See More Appropriate Protocol

- Questions or concerns about suicide thoughts, threats, and attempts
  Go to Protocol: Suicide Concerns on page 259

Go to ED Now (or to Office With PCP Approval)

- Bizarre or confused behavior
  R/O: psychosis, bipolar disorder

Call Local Agency Now

- Recurrent thoughts of death (e.g., "life is not worth living") but not threatening suicide
  R/O: major depression
- Patient sounds very upset or severely depressed (e.g., multiple symptoms of depression)
  R/O: major depression, anxiety

Discuss With PCP and Callback by Nurse Today

- Started on antidepressant medications > 2 weeks ago and not feeling any better
  Reason: antidepressant medications require 2-4 weeks to work
- Pregnant

Call Local Agency Today

- Symptoms interfere with work or school
  R/O: major depression
- Symptoms persisting > 2 weeks
  R/O: major depression
- Requesting to talk with a counselor (mental health worker, psychiatrist, etc.)

See Within 3 Days in Office

- History of manic-depression (bipolar disorder)
- Significant weight loss > 10 pounds (5 kg) and not dieting
  R/O: depression, organic pathology
- Known or suspected alcohol or drug abuse
  R/O: substance abuse as cause or contributing factor for depression
- Patient wants to be seen

See Within 2 Weeks in Office

- Feels depressed only on days just before menstrual period
  R/O: premenstrual syndrome (PMS)

Home Care

- Mild depression
- Recent death of a loved one
  Reason: bereavement, grieving
- Referral phone numbers for depression, questions about

HOME CARE ADVICE FOR DEPRESSION

General

1. **Reassurance:**
   - People with depression do get through this—even people who feel as badly as you feel now.
   - You can be helped.
   - Encourage the caller to talk about his/her problems and feelings.
   - Offer hope.
2. **Phrases to Use or Avoid:**
   - **Use:** Tell me more about how you are doing, I'm sorry, what is the hardest part of your day?
   - **Avoid:** I understand how you feel, he is in the Lord's hands, it is for the best.
3. **Suggestions for Healthy Living:**
   There are things that you can do to make yourself feel better:
   - **Eat Healthy:** Eat a well-balanced diet.
   - **Get More Sleep:** Most people need 7-8 hours of sleep each night. Being well-rested improves your attitude and your sense of physical well-being.

- **Communicate:** Share how you are feeling with someone in your life who is a good listener.
- Make certain that your spouse, family, or friends know how you are feeling.
- **Exercise Regularly:** Take a daily walk.
- **Avoid Alcohol.**

4. **Stay Active—Staying Active Can Also Make You Feel Better:**
   - Get out of of your house or apartment periodically. Go on an outing with a family member or a friend. Go to the store. Go to a movie.
   - Become involved in community activities (e.g., church, school, clubs, parent-teacher associations).
   - Start a new hobby.
   - Take a daily walk.
5. **Call Back If:**
   - Sadness or depression symptoms persist more than 2 weeks.
   - You want to talk with a counselor.
   - You feel like harming yourself.
   - You become worse.

Special Situations

1. **Death of a Loved One:**
   - Sadness and depression symptoms are common and normal after the death of a loved one.
   - Encourage the caller to talk about his/her troubles.
   - Let the caller know that taking time to grieve is important, and it is part of the healing process.
   - **Suggest:** Review a photo album or share your favorite memories with a friend or family member.
   - Support of family and friends is important.
2. **Premenstrual Syndrome:**
   - Some women experience depression symptoms and irritability during the couple days prior to their menstrual period. This is because of fluctuations in female hormone levels as the menstrual period approaches.
   - Your doctor can help you with this.

Referral Phone Numbers for Depression and Additional Resources

1. **Local Mental Health Program Phone Numbers:**
   - If available, local mental health program: xxx-xxx-xxxx.
   - If available, local psychiatric crisis service at ________ hospital: xxx-xxx-xxxx.
2. **United States Hotline and Helplines—NAMI Information Helpline:**
   - National Alliance on Mental Illness.
   - "NAMI is dedicated to the eradication of mental illnesses and to the improvement of the quality of life of all whose lives are affected by these diseases." "The National Alliance for the Mentally Ill (NAMI) is a network of local support groups for the mentally ill and their families."
   - The NAMI Helpline is an information and referral source for locating community mental health programs. National toll-free phone number: 800-950-NAMI (6264), Monday through Friday, 10:00 am–6:00 pm, Eastern time.
   - www.nami.org
3. **United States—Substance Abuse and Mental Health Services Administration (SAMHSA) Treatment Referral Line:**
   - SAMHSA Treatment Referral Routing Service (http://samhsa.gov/treatment) is a "confidential, free, 24-hour-a-day, 365-day-a-year, information service, in English and Spanish, for individuals and family members facing substance abuse and mental health issues. This service provides referrals to local treatment facilities, support groups, and community-based organizations. Callers can also order free publications and other information in print on substance abuse and mental health issues."
   - The phone number is 800-662-HELP (4357).
4. **United States—Mood Disorders Organizations:**
   - Anxiety and Depression Association of America (ADAA).
   - There is a "Find a Therapist" link on the home page.
   - www.adaa.org.
   - Telephone: 240-485-1001.

5. **Canada—Internet Resources**
   - **Canadian Network of Substance Abuse and Allied Professionals:** This Web site lists treatment agencies for each of the provinces in Canada. Available at: www.cnsaap.ca/Eng/CanadianLandscape/Pages/default.aspx.
   - **New Brunswick:** Department of Health and Wellness Addiction Services (www.gnb.ca/0378/addiction-e.asp). Services offered by region.
   - **Newfoundland and Labrador:** Newfoundland and Labrador Addictions Services (www.health.gov.nl.ca/health/addictions/services.html). Services offered by region.
   - **Northwest Territories:** Nats`ejée K`éh Treatment Centre (www.natsejeekeh.org). The phone number is 867-874-6699.
   - **Ontario—Drug and Alcohol Registry of Treatment (DART):** This is an online database of treatment programs offered in Ontario. It is searchable by name, municipality, Local Health Integration Network (LHIN), provincial service category, and/or specific population group. Available at: www.drugandalcoholhelpline.ca/. The phone number for the helpline is 800-565-8603.
6. **Canada—Mood Disorder Organization:**
   - **Ontario:** Mood Disorders Association of Ontario (MDAO)—888-486-8236.
   - www.mooddisorders.ca

BACKGROUND INFORMATION

General Information

- Depression is common, with 1 in 20 Americans getting depressed each year. Women are affected twice as often as men.
- Depression is treatable.

Symptoms

Patients with depression describe persisting symptoms of depressed mood and/or markedly decreased pleasure or interest in daily activities (anhedonia). They may also have one or more of the following symptoms:

- Significant weight loss (or gain) and not dieting
- Inability to sleep (insomnia) or increased sleeping (hypersomnia)
- Observed or reported psychomotor agitation or retardation
- Loss of energy
- Feelings of guilt or worthlessness
- Diminished ability to concentrate
- Recurrent thoughts of death; suicidal ideation, gestures, or attempts

Causes

Depression seems to be caused by a chemical imbalance in the brain. Stresses in life can sometimes trigger a new episode of depression or worsen existing depression. Causes can include:

- Death of a loved one
- Divorce, separation, or other relationship problems
- Loss of a job, stress from money problems
- Going off to college
- Certain medications
- Severe or long-standing medical illness

Treatment

- Depression can be treated with psychiatric counseling or medications. Sometimes both are necessary.
- Healthy living habits can improve one's sense of well-being. Good habits for healthy living include eating healthy, getting enough sleep, and exercising regularly.

Caution—Suicidal Ideation—Intent and Plan

- **Intent:** It is appropriate to directly ask patients about their intent to harm themselves or end their own life. Such questions will not provoke a suicide attempt and may instead give the patient a chance to unburden themselves. Any patient who is threatening self-harm now needs to be seen immediately for evaluation.
- **Plan:** This refers to the extent to which the patient has prepared for a suicide attempt. Does the patient have a specific method in mind (e.g., gun, knife, overdose)? Does the patient have access to the verbalized method (e.g., hoarded pills, firearm in house)? Access to lethal methods increases the risk of suicide attempt and death. Generally, a patient with a specific plan is considered at higher suicide risk than a patient who is threatening suicide but has no plan.

DIABETES, HIGH BLOOD SUGAR

DEFINITION

- Patient with known diabetes mellitus
- Has a high blood sugar (hyperglycemia), defined as a blood glucose > 200 mg/dL (11 mmol/L)
- Has symptoms of high blood sugar
- Has questions regarding high blood sugar

Symptoms of High Blood Sugar (Hyperglycemia) Include:

- **Mild Hyperglycemia:** Most often patient will have no symptoms.
- **Moderate Hyperglycemia:** Polyuria, polydipsia, fatigue, blurred vision.
- **Severe Hyperglycemia:** Confusion and coma.
- **Diabetic Hetoacidosis (DKA):** Fruity odor on breath, vomiting, rapid breathing, weakness, confusion, and coma.

TRIAGE ASSESSMENT QUESTIONS

Call EMS 911 Now

- Unconscious or difficult to awaken
  R/O: diabetic ketoacidosis (DKA), severe hyperglycemia, profound hypoglycemia
- Acting confused (e.g., disoriented, slurred speech)
  R/O: DKA, severe hyperglycemia, hypoglycemia
- Very weak (e.g., can't stand)
  R/O: DKA, severe hyperglycemia, hypoglycemia
- Sounds like a life-threatening emergency to the triager

Go to ED Now

- Vomiting and signs of dehydration (e.g., very dry mouth, light-headed, etc.)
  Reason: may need IV hydration, possible DKA
- Blood glucose > 240 mg/dL (13 mmol/L) and rapid breathing
  R/O: DKA

Go to ED Now (or to Office With PCP Approval)

- Blood glucose > 500 mg/dL (27.5 mmol/L)
- Blood glucose > 240 mg/dL (13 mmol/L) AND urine ketones moderate-large (or more than 1+)
  R/O: DKA
- Blood glucose > 240 mg/dL (13 mmol/L) and vomiting and unable to check urine ketones
  R/O: DKA
- Vomiting lasting > 4 hours
  R/O: DKA, dehydration
- Patient sounds very sick or weak to the triager
  R/O: severe dehydration, DKA, hyperglycemia, hypoglycemia, possible bacterial infection

Go to Office Now

- Fever > 100.5° F (38.1° C)
  Reason: diabetics are immunocompromised, consider possibility of bacterial infection

Call Transferred to PCP Now

- Caller has urgent medication question about med that PCP prescribed and triager unable to answer question

Discuss With PCP and Callback by Nurse Within 1 Hour

- Blood glucose > 400 mg/dL (22 mmol/L)
  Reason: significant hyperglycemia
- Blood glucose > 300 mg/dL (16.5 mmol/L) AND 2 or more times in a row
  Reason: obtain PCP input regarding medication adjustment and diet
- Urine ketones moderate-large
  Reason: obtain PCP input regarding medication adjustment and diet

See Today in Office

- New-onset diabetes suspected (e.g., frequent urination, weak, weight loss)
- Symptoms of high blood sugar (e.g., frequent urination, weak, weight loss) and not able to test blood glucose
- Patient wants to be seen

Discuss With PCP and Callback by Nurse Today

- Caller has nonurgent medication question about med that PCP prescribed and triager unable to answer question

Home Care

- ○ Blood glucose > 240 mg/dL (13 mmol/L)
  Reason: hyperglycemia
- ○ Blood glucose 60-240 mg/dL (3.5 -13 mmol/L)
- ○ Sick-day rules for diabetes mellitus, questions about

HOME CARE ADVICE

Treating High Blood Sugar (Hyperglycemia)

1. **General**
   - **Definition of Hyperglycemia:** Fasting blood glucose more than 140 mg/dL (7.5 mmol/L) or random blood glucose more than 200 mg/dL (11 mmol/L).
   - **Symptoms of Mild Hyperglycemia:** Frequent urination, increased thirst, fatigue, blurred vision.
   - **Symptoms of Severe Hyperglycemia:** Weakness, progressing to confusion and coma.
2. **Treatment—Liquids:**
   - Drink at least 1 glass (8 oz or 240 mL) of water per hour for the next 4 hours (Reason: adequate hydration will reduce hyperglycemia).
   - Generally, you should try to drink 6-8 glasses of water each day.
3. **Treatment—Insulin:**
   - Continue to take your insulin, as prescribed by your doctor.
   - **Sliding Scale Insulin:** IF your doctor has given you instructions to take extra rapid-acting (e.g., lispro, aspart) or short-acting (regular) insulin when your blood sugar is high, give yourself the insulin dose your doctor has recommended.
4. **Treatment—Diabetes Medications:**
   Continue taking your diabetes pills.
5. **Measure and Record Your Blood Glucose:**
   - Every day you should measure your blood glucose before breakfast and before going to bed.
   - Record the results and show them to your doctor at your next office visit.
6. **Daily Blood Glucose Goals:**
   You and your doctor should decide on what your blood glucose goals should be. Typical goals for many people who perform daily finger-stick blood testing at home are:
   - **Preprandial (Before Meal):** 70-130 mg/dL (3.9-7.2 mmol/L)
   - **Postprandial (2-3 Hours After a Meal):** Less than 180 mg/dL (10 mmol/L)
7. **Expected Course:**
   You should call back in 3-5 days if:
   - Your blood sugar continues to get above 240 mg/dL (13 mmol/L).
   - Your blood sugar continues to be higher than your daily glucose goals (set by you and your doctor).
   - It has been longer than 6 months since you had an hemoglobin A1C test.
8. **Call Back If:**
   - Blood glucose more than 300 mg/dL (16.5 mmol/L), 2 or more times in a row.
   - Urine ketones become moderate or large.
   - Vomiting lasting more than 4 hours or unable to drink any liquids.
   - Rapid breathing occurs
   - You become worse.

Sick-Day Rules

1. **General:**
   - Do not stop taking your insulin. During illness the blood sugar often rises.
   - Check your blood glucose every 2-4 hours. Write down the results.
   - Check for ketones in your urine. Ketones can be a sign of dehydration or poorly controlled diabetes.
   - Drink liquids. It is important to prevent dehydration. Drink small amounts frequently.
   - Avoid hypoglycemia. If your appetite is bad, you are not eating solid food, and your blood glucose is less than 200 mg/dL (11 mmol/L), then you should be drinking sugar-containing liquids. Examples are soda, clear juices, sports drinks.

2. **Insulin—Do Not Stop Taking It:**
   - If you are supposed to be using insulin, do not stop taking it.
   - The reason is that during an illness you may need even more insulin than usual.
3. **Insulin—Supplemental Insulin for Hyperglycemia:**
   - **Note to Triager:** Supplemental rapid-acting (e.g., lispro, aspart) or short-acting (regular) insulin is sometimes needed in addition to usual insulin doses for treating hyperglycemia. Most patients should already have been given sick-day rules education by their doctor and instructions on when to use supplemental insulin. THE TRIAGE NURSE MUST DISCUSS ALL INSULIN DOSING WITH THE DOCTOR BEFORE GIVING RECOMMENDATIONS TO THE PATIENT. In most cases it is best if the doctor talks directly with the patient.
   - **Total Daily Dose (TDD):** The total daily dose is calculated by adding up ALL insulin administered during a USUAL day.
   - **Typical Sick-Day Insulin Supplementation:** Urine ketones negative or trace: If glucose is 80-240 mg/dL (4.5-13 mmol/L), give usual dose. If glucose is 250-400 mg/dL (14-22 mmol/L), supplemental insulin dosage is 10% of TDD. If glucose is over 400 mg/dL (22 mol/L), supplemental insulin dosage is 20% of TDD.
   - **Typical Sick-Day Insulin Supplementation:** Urine ketones moderate: If glucose is 80-240 mg/dL (4.5-13 mmol/L), give usual dose. If glucose is 250-400 mg/dL (14-22 mmol/L), supplemental insulin dosage is 20% of TDD. If glucose is over 400 mg/dL (22 mol/L), supplemental insulin dosage is 20% of TDD.
4. **Insulin—Decreased Insulin for Hypoglycemia:**
   - **Note to Triager:** Decreased insulin dosing is sometimes needed in patients with a blood glucose < 80 mg/dL (4.5 mmol/L), especially if there is decreased oral intake. THE TRIAGE NURSE MUST DISCUSS ALL INSULIN DOSING WITH THE DOCTOR BEFORE GIVING RECOMMENDATIONS TO THE PATIENT. In most cases it is best if the doctor talks directly with the patient.
   - **Typical Sick-Day Insulin Reduction:** For blood glucose < 80 mg/dL (4.5 mmol/L) and there is decreased oral intake: Do not give rapid-acting (e.g., lispro, aspart) or short-acting (regular) insulin. Reduce intermediate-acting insulin (e.g., NPH, lente, 70/30) by 20%.
5. **Diet:**
   - **Appetite OK, Minimal Nausea:** Continue your normal diabetic meal plan. Avoid spicy or greasy foods.
   - **Appetite Fair, Moderate Nausea:** Eat a bland diet. Try small amounts of food 6-8 times a day. Take ½ to 1 cup (120-240 mL) of food or liquids every 1-2 hours.
   - **Appetite Poor, Severe Nausea, Can't Eat Solid Food:** Drink plenty of liquids. Try to drink 4-8 oz (120-240 mL) per hour. If glucose more than 240 mg/dL (13 mmol/L), drink sugar-free liquids (e.g., water, broth). If glucose less than 200 mg/dL (11 mmol/L), drink sugar-containing liquids (e.g., sports drinks, juice, soda).
   - Advance diet as you improve.
6. **Liquids:**
   - Drink more fluids, at least 8-10 glasses daily (8 oz or 240 mL each glass).
   - Even more liquids are needed if there is fever, vomiting, or diarrhea.
7. **Check Blood Glucose:**
   - When you are ill, you should measure your blood glucose every 2-4 hours.
   - Write down the results.
8. **Check Urine for Ketones:**
   - Check your urine for ketones whenever you are ill or if your blood glucose is more than 240 mg/dL (13 mmol/L).
   - You can buy a testing kit at your local pharmacy.
9. **Call Back If:**
   - Blood glucose more than 300 mg/dL (16.5 mmol/L), 2 or more times in a row.
   - Urine ketones become moderate or large.
   - Vomiting lasting more than 4 hours.
   - Rapid breathing occurs.
   - You become worse or have more questions.

Additional Resources

1. **American Diabetes Association (ADA):**
   - Telephone number: 1-800-DIABETES (342-2383)
   - Web site: www.diabetes.org
2. **US National Diabetes Education Program:**
   - Telephone number: 301/496-3583
   - Web site: http://ndep.nih.gov
3. **Canadian Diabetes Association:**
   - Telephone number: 1-800-226-8464
   - Web site: www.diabetes.ca

FIRST AID

First Aid Advice for Hypoglycemia—Glucose

IF BLOOD GLUCOSE < 70 mg/dL (3.9 mmol/L) or UNKNOWN (pending EMS arrival) for conscious patients:

- Give sugar (10-15 grams glucose) by mouth IF able to swallow.
- Each of the following is equivalent to 10 g of glucose: milk (1 cup; 240 mL); orange juice (½ cup; 120 mL); prepackaged juice box (1 box); table sugar or honey (3 teaspoons; 15 mL); glucose tablets (3 tablets); glucose paste (10-15 grams).

First Aid Advice for Hypoglycemia—Glucagon

IF BLOOD GLUCOSE < 70 mg/dL (3.9 mmol/L) or UNKNOWN (pending EMS arrival):

- If family has glucagon for hypoglycemic emergencies AND the caller knows how to use it, encourage the caller to give the glucagon now.
- Inject it IM into the upper outer thigh.
- Adult dosage is 1 mg

BACKGROUND INFORMATION

Causes of High Blood Sugar (Hyperglycemia)

- Noncompliance with taking insulin or other diabetes medicines. Omission of insulin is the most common cause. Malfunction of insulin pumps also occurs.
- Noncompliance with diabetes diet.
- Infections, bacterial or viral, increase insulin requirements.
- Combination of these factors.

Diabetes Mellitus

- **Definition:** Diabetes mellitus is an endocrine condition in which patients have elevated blood glucose levels (hyperglycemia). The classic symptoms of untreated or undertreated diabetes are: frequent urination (polyuria), polydipsia (excessive thirst), and involuntary weight loss.
- **The Role of Insulin:** Insulin is a hormone produced by the pancreas to help process food. Eating food makes the blood glucose rise and insulin makes the blood glucose fall.
- **Classification of Diabetes Mellitus:** There are 4 different classes of diabetes mellitus: type 1 diabetes, type 2 diabetes, gestational diabetes mellitus, and other.

Type 1 Diabetes

- **Other Names:** Insulin-dependent diabetes mellitus (IDDM), juvenile-onset diabetes.
- **Physiology:** There is no production of insulin by the body.
- **Ketosis-prone:** Patients with this type of diabetes are ketosis-prone, which means that if they do not receive daily insulin shots their bodies break down fats and produce ketones. The ketones spill into the urine and can be measured. Patients with type 1 diabetes are susceptible to developing diabetic ketoacidosis (DKA), a life-threatening condition.
- **Onset:** It most commonly first appears in childhood or adolescence. Approximately 10% of diabetics are type 1.
- **Treatment:** Insulin therapy is always required and needs to be given subcutaneously at least once daily. Patients striving for tighter control of their blood glucose will take insulin more often than once a day. Recommended therapy for type 1 diabetes includes: 1) use of multiple-dose insulin injections (3–4 injections per day) and 2) matching of mealtime (prandial) insulin to carbohydrate intake, premeal blood glucose, and anticipated activity.

Type 2 Diabetes

- **Other names:** Non–insulin-dependent diabetes mellitus (NIDDM), adult-onset diabetes.
- **Physiology:** In type 2 diabetes, there is decreased insulin production and decreased sensitivity to insulin.

- **Not Ketosis-prone:** These patients are not prone to ketosis. DKA rarely occurs.
- **Onset:** It more commonly develops in elderly and overweight adults.
- **Treatment:** The initial and most important treatments are exercise and weight loss. When these measures fail, there are pills that can be prescribed to help the body make more insulin or use the insulin more effectively. Occasionally patients require insulin therapy.

Diabetic Ketoacidosis (DKA)

- **Definition:** Blood glucose > 250 mg/dL (12 mmole/L) with acidosis and ketosis (urine ketones moderate to large)
- **Symptoms of DKA:** In addition to symptoms of hyperglycemia, fruity odor on breath, vomiting, rapid/deep breathing, confusion, and coma
- **Causes:** Noncompliance with using insulin in type 1 diabetes, infection

Five Types of Insulin for Diabetes

- **Rapid-acting (Humalog/Lispro, NovoLog/ Aspart):** Onset 5-15 minutes; peaks 30-90 minutes; effective duration 5 hours
- **Short-acting (Regular, Humulin R, Novolin R):** Onset 30-60 minutes; peaks 2-3 hours; effective duration 5-8 hours
- **Intermediate-acting (NPH, Lente, Humulin N, Humulin L, Novolin N, Novolin L):** Onset 2-4 hours; peaks 4-12 hours; effective duration 10-18 hours
- **Long-acting (Lantus/Glargine, Detemir, Levemir):** Onset 2-4 hours; no true peak; effecive duration 18-24 hours
- **Premixed (Humulin 70/30, Humulin 50/50, Humalog Mix, NovoLog Mix):** 2 peaks; effective duration 10-16 hours; depends on mixture

Insulin Administration—Different Dosing Regimens

- **Sliding Insulin Scale:** Generally only used in the hospital.
- **Insulin Algorithm:** The patient checks his/her blood glucose before each meal and then adjusts insulin dosing based upon BOTH the blood glucose and an estimated caloric count for the meal. This is considered prandial insulin because it is given with (just before) meals. Rapid-acting (Humalog/lispro or NovoLog/aspart) or short-acting (regular) are used for prandial insulin dosing.
- **Once-daily Insulin:** This is not considered physiologic insulin dosing as it only provides the basal insulin and does not provide the needed prandial increases. However, it may be an effective addition for some type 2 diabetic patients on oral medications as their need for insulin is low. Intermediate-acting insulin (NPH) or long-acting insulin (Lantus/glargine) are used.
- **Twice-daily Insulin:** Intermediate-acting insulin (NPH) or long-acting insulin (Lantus/glargine) can be used in twice-daily regimens. Twice-daily insulin dosing may be sufficient for type 2 diabetic patients because they still make sufficient insulin on their own to handle prandial (mealtime) insulin needs.
- **Flexible Insulin Regimens:** In this type of regimen both an intermediate-acting insulin (for basal insulin needs) AND a rapid or ultrashort-acting insulin (for prandial insulin needs) are used.

Exubera—Inhaled Form of Insulin—No Longer Available

- Exubera is the first-ever inhaled insulin. It comes in a dry powder inhaler.
- It was approved by the FDA in January 2006 for the treatment of type 1 and type 2 diabetes mellitus
- On October 18, 2007, Pfizer announced that it would no longer be making Exubera.

Five Types of Oral Medications for Diabetes

- **Sulfonylureas:** Examples include glyburide (Micronase, Diabeta), glipizide (Glucotrol, Glucotrol XL), and glimepiride (Amaryl).
- **Biguanides:** Examples include metformin (Glucophage, Fortamet).
- **Thiazolidinediones:** Examples include rosiglitazone (Avanida) and pioglitazone (Actos).
- **Alplha-glucosidase Inhibitors:** Examples include acarbose (Precose) and miglitol (Glyset).
- **Meglitinides:** Examples include repaglinide (Prandin) and nateglinide (Starlix).

Goals for Diabetes Management

- **HbA1c:** The HbA1c is the primary goal for diabetes management. Depending on the patient, it should be measured 2-4 times a year. The American Diabetes Association (ADA) recommends a goal of less than 7.0% for nonpregnant adults.
- **Blood Glucose:** Depending on the patient, the blood glucose should be measured 1-3 times per day. The ADA recommends the following blood glucose goals: Preprandial (before meal): 70-130 mg/dL (3.9-7.2 mmol/L); postprandial (2-3 hours after a meal): Less than 180 mg/dL (10 mmol/L).
- **Goals Should Be Individualized Based Upon:** Age/life expectancy, duration of diabetes, comorbid conditions, hypoglycemic unawareness, history of severe hypoglycemic reactions, and other individual considerations.
- **Internet Resource:** ADA Standards of Medical Care in Diabetes 2012

Glycosylated Hemoglobin (HbA1c)

- The HbA1c provides a good estimate of how well a patient has managed his/her diabetes during the past 2-3 months. With good diabetes management the HbA1c goes down and with poor management it goes up. In general, the higher the HbA1c, the greater the risk of the long-term diabetic complications.
- **Goal:** The American Association of Clinical Endocrinologists (AACE) and the American College of Endocrinology (ACE) recommend a target glycosylated hemoglobin level (HbA1c) of less than 6.5%. The American Diabetes Association (ADA) recommends a goal of less than 7.0% for nonpregnant adults. The Canadian Diabetes Associations also recommends a goal of less than 7.0%

Long-term Complications of Diabetes Mellitus

- **Eye Disease (e.g., Retinopathy):** Diabetes is the leading cause of blindness.
- Heart disease (e.g., coronary heart disease, myocardial infarction)
- Kidney disease (e.g., renal failure, proteinuria)
- Nerve disease (e.g., peripheral and autonomic neuropathy)
- Stroke

Converting Glucose Levels: mg/dL and mmol/L

- In the United State glucose is typically measured using the units mg/dL. Nearly every country in the world (including Canada) measures glucose levels using the units mmol/L.
- To convert mmol/L of glucose to mg/dL, multiply by 18.
- To convert mg/dL of glucose to mmol/L, divide by 18 or multiply by 0.055.

DIABETES, LOW BLOOD SUGAR

DEFINITION

- Patient with known diabetes mellitus
- Has a low blood sugar (hypoglycemia), defined as a a blood glucose < 70 mg/dL (3.9 mmol/L)
- Has symptoms of low blood sugar
- Has questions regarding low blood sugar

Symptoms of Low Blood Sugar (Hypoglycemia) Include:

- **Mild Hypoglycemia:** Dizziness, shakiness, weakness, trembling, sweating, headache, nervousness, and hunger. Some patients with mild hypoglycemia experience no symptoms.
- **Severe Hypoglycemia:** Unable to speak, confusion, seizures, and coma.
- **Hypoglycemic Unawareness:** Some diabetics have no symptoms of hypoglycemia and can lose consciousness without ever knowing their blood glucose levels were dropping. This condition is mainly seen in adults with long-standing diabetes. These patients need more frequent checks of their blood glucose level.

TRIAGE ASSESSMENT QUESTIONS

Call EMS 911 Now

- Unconscious or difficult to awaken
  R/O: severe hypoglycemia, insulin coma
- Seizure occurs
  R/O: severe hypoglycemia
- Acting confused (e.g., disoriented, slurred speech)
  R/O: severe hypoglycemia
- Very weak (e.g., can't stand)
  R/O: symptomatic hypoglycemia
- Sounds like a life-threatening emergency to the triager

Go to ED Now

- Vomiting and signs of dehydration (e.g., no urine > 12 hours, very dry mouth, dark urine, etc.)
  Reason: may need IV hydration

Go to ED Now (or to Office With PCP Approval)

- Low blood sugar symptoms persist > 15 minutes and using low blood sugar care advice
- Low blood glucose (< 70 mg/dL or 3.9 mmol/L) persists > 15 minutes and using low blood sugar care advice
- Patient sounds very sick or weak to the triager
  R/O: severe dehydration, hypoglycemia, possible bacterial infection

Call Transferred to PCP Now

- Diabetes medication overdose (e.g., insulin error) and triager unable to answer question
  Note: Triager should consider medication, dose, and whether patient is alone. An upgrade to EMS 911 may be indicated in some circumstances.
- Caller has urgent medication question about med that PCP prescribed and triager unable to answer question

Discuss With PCP and Callback by Nurse Within 1 Hour

- Low blood sugar symptoms with no other adult present AND hasn't tried care advice
  Note: Obtain contact information. Recruit family or friend to help. Consider upgrade to EMS 911 based on social support and ability to recontact.
- Low blood glucose (< 70 mg/dL or 3.9 mmol/L) with no other adult present AND hasn't tried care advice
  Note: Obtain contact information and make a call back in 15 minutes. Recruit family or friend to help. Consider upgrade to EMS 911 based on social support and ability to recontact.
- Blood glucose < 70 mg/dL (3.9 mmol/L) or symptomatic AND cause unknown
  Reason: unexplained hypoglycemia
  Note: Causes can include extra insulin, delayed meal or insufficient food, strenuous exercise.

See Today in Office

- Patient wants to be seen

Discuss With PCP and Callback by Nurse Today

- Morning (before breakfast) blood glucose < 80 mg/dL (4.5 mmol/L) and more than once in past week
  Reason: obtain PCP input regarding medication adjustment and diet
- Evening (after bedtime snack) blood glucose < 100 mg/dL (5.6 mmol/L) and more than once in past week
  Reason: obtain PCP input regarding medication adjustment and diet
- Caller has nonurgent medication question about med that PCP prescribed and triager unable to answer question

Home Care

- ○ Blood glucose < 70 mg/dL (3.9 mmol/L) or symptomatic AND has other adult present
  Reason: cause known, another adult is present
- ○ Low blood sugar prevention, questions about
- ○ Sick-day rules for diabetes mellitus, questions about

HOME CARE ADVICE

Treating Low Blood Sugar (Hypoglycemia)

1. **Reassurance:**
   - It sounds like an episode of low blood sugar (hypoglycemia) that we can treat at home.
   - Low blood sugar can result from taking too much diabetes medication, delayed meals, strenuous exercise, or a combination of these factors.
2. **Definition**
   - Low blood sugar (hypoglycemia) is defined as a blood glucose less than 70 mg/dL (3.9 mmol/L).
   - **Symptoms of Mild Hypoglycemia:** Shakiness, weakness, not thinking clearly, headache, trembling, sweating, dizziness, palpitations, and hunger.
   - **Symptoms of Severe Hypoglycemia:** Unable to speak, confusion, seizures, and coma.
   - **Contributing Factors:** Too much insulin, delayed meal, insufficient food, strenuous exercise, alcohol.
3. **Treatment: Eat Some (10-15 g) Sugar Now.**
   Each of the following is equivalent to 10 g of glucose:
   - Milk (1 cup; 240 mL)
   - Orange juice (½ cup; 120 mL)
   - Prepackaged juice box (1 box)
   - Table sugar or honey (3 teaspoons; 15 mL)
   - Glucose tablets (3 tablets)
4. **Treatment—If Patient Is Taking Precose (Acarbose):**
   - In this case low blood sugar must be treated with commercial glucose tablets. Take 3 glucose tablets now. If glucose tablets are not available, milk may work.
   - **Special Note:** Juice, candies, and table sugar are not effective because of the mechanism of action of this diabetic pill.
   - **Expected Course:** The symptoms of hypoglycemia should resolve in 10-15 minutes. After the symptoms resolve, eat a small snack to prevent this from recurring. Examples include: cheese and crackers, a glass of milk, or half a sandwich. If the symptoms of hypoglycemia are not better in 15 minutes, eat some more glucose (10 g).
5. **Call Back If:**
   - There is no improvement within 30 minutes.
   - Sleepiness or confusion occur.
   - You become worse.

Preventing Low Blood Sugar

1. **Prevention**
   - **Meals:** Do not skip or delay meals. Try to eat meals and snacks at the same time every day.
   - **Glucose:** Keep some type of sugar (e.g., glucose tablets or gels, honey, juice box) with you at all times. Do you have them available at work, at school, during exercise, and in your car?
   - **Dieting:** Talk with your doctor before starting a weight-loss program.
2. **Inform Your Friends and Family:**
   - If you take insulin or any other diabetic medication, you are at risk of having a hypoglycemic spell. Inform your family, close friends, and coworkers that you have diabetes and what to do if you have hypoglycemia.
   - Wear a medical alert bracelet that identifies that you have diabetes.

3. **Daily Blood Glucose Goals**
   You and your doctor should decide on what your blood glucose goals should be. Typical goals for many people who perform daily finger-stick blood testing at home are:
   - **Preprandial (Before Meal):** 70-130 mg/dL (3.9-7.2 mmol/L)
   - **Postprandial (2-3 Hours After a Meal):** Less than 180 mg/dL (10 mmol/L)
4. **Daily Records:**
   - Measure your blood glucose before breakfast and before going to bed.
   - Record the results and show them to your doctor at your next office visit.
5. **Call Back If:**
   - Morning blood glucose < 80 mg/dL (4.5 mmol/L) more than once in a week.
   - Bedtime blood < 100 mg/dL (5.5 mmol/L) more than once in a week.
   - You have more questions.
   - You become worse.

Sick-Day Rules

1. **General:**
   - Do not stop taking your insulin. During illness the blood sugar often rises.
   - Check your blood glucose every 2-4 hours. Write down the results.
   - Check for ketones in your urine. Ketones can be a sign of dehydration or poorly controlled diabetes.
   - Drink liquids. It is important to prevent dehydration. Drink small amounts frequently.
   - Avoid hypoglycemia. If your appetite is bad, you are not eating solid food, and your blood glucose is less than 200 mg/dL (11 mmol/L), then you should be drinking sugar-containing liquids. Examples are soda, clear juices, sports drinks.
2. **Insulin—Do Not Stop Taking It:**
   - If you are supposed to be using insulin, do not stop taking it.
   - The reason is that during an illness, you may need even more insulin than usual.
3. **Insulin—Supplemental Insulin for Hyperglycemia**
   - **Note to Triager:** Supplemental rapid-acting (e.g., lispro, aspart) or short-acting (regular) insulin is sometimes needed in addition to usual insulin doses for treating hyperglycemia. Most patients should already have been given sick-day rules education by their doctor and instructions on when to use supplemental insulin. THE TRIAGE NURSE MUST DISCUSS ALL INSULIN DOSING WITH THE DOCTOR BEFORE GIVING RECOMMENDATIONS TO THE PATIENT. In most cases it is best if the doctor talks directly with the patient.
   - **Total Daily Dose (TDD):** The total daily dose is calculated by adding up ALL insulin administered during a USUAL day.
   - **Typical Sick-Day Insulin Supplementation:** Urine ketones negative or trace: If glucose is 80-240 mg/dL (4.5-13 mmol/L), give usual dose. If glucose is 250-400 mg/dL (14-22 mmol/L), supplemental insulin dosage is 10% of TDD. If glucose is over 400 mg/dL (22 mol/L), supplemental insulin dosage is 20% of TDD.
   - **Typical Sick-Day Insulin Supplementation:** Urine ketones moderate: If glucose is 80-240 mg/dL (4.5-13 mmol/L), give usual dose. If glucose is 250-400 mg/dL (14-22 mmol/L), supplemental insulin dosage is 20% of TDD. If glucose is over 400 mg/dL (22 mol/L), supplemental insulin dosage is 20% of TDD.
4. **Insulin—Decreased Insulin for Hypoglycemia:**
   - **Note To Triager:** Decreased insulin dosing is sometimes needed in patients with a blood glucose < 80 mg/dL (4.5 mmol/L), especially if there is decreased oral intake. THE TRIAGE NURSE MUST DISCUSS ALL INSULIN DOSING WITH THE DOCTOR BEFORE GIVING RECOMMENDATIONS TO THE PATIENT. In most cases it is best if the doctor talks directly with the patient.
   - **Typical Sick-Day Insulin Reduction:** For blood glucose < 80 mg/dL (4.5 mmol/L) and there is decreased oral intake: Do not give rapid-acting (e.g., lispro, aspart) or short-acting (regular) insulin. Reduce intermediate acting insulin (e.g., NPH, lente, 70/30) by 20%.

5. **Diet:**
   - **Appetite OK, Minimal Nausea:** Continue your normal diabetic meal plan. Avoid spicy or greasy foods.
   - **Appetite Fair, Moderate Nausea:** Eat a bland diet. Try small amounts of food 6-8 times a day. Take ½ to 1 cup (120-240 mL) of food or liquids every 1-2 hours.
   - **Appetite Poor, Severe Nausea, Can't Eat Solid Food:** Drink plenty of liquids. Try to drink 4-8 oz (120-240 mL) per hour. If glucose more than 240 mg/dL (13 mmol/L), drink sugar-free liquids (e.g., water, broth). If glucose less than 200 mg/dL (11 mmol/L), drink sugar-containing liquids (e.g., sports drinks, juice, soda).
   - Advance diet as you improve.
6. **Liquids:**
   - Drink more fluids, at least 8-10 glasses daily (8 oz or 240 mL each glass).
   - Even more liquids are needed if there is fever, vomiting, or diarrhea.
7. **Check Blood Glucose:**
   - When you are ill, you should measure your blood glucose every 2-4 hours.
   - Write down the results.
8. **Check Urine for Ketones:**
   - Check your urine for ketones whenever you are ill or if your blood glucose is more than 240 mg/dL (13 mmol/L).
   - You can buy a testing kit at your local pharmacy.
9. **Call Back If:**
   - Blood glucose more than 300 mg/dL (16.5 mmol/L), 2 or more times in a row.
   - Urine ketones become moderate or large.
   - Vomiting lasting more than 4 hours.
   - Rapid breathing occurs.
   - You become worse or have more questions.

Additional Resources

1. **American Diabetes Association (Ada):**
   - Telephone number: 1-800-DIABETES (342-2383)
   - Web site: www.diabetes.org
2. **US National Diabetes Education Program:**
   - Telephone number: 301/496-3583
   - Web site: http://ndep.nih.gov
3. **Canadian Diabetes Association:**
   - Telephone number: 1-800-226-8464
   - Web site: www.diabetes.ca

FIRST AID

First Aid Advice for Hypoglycemia—Glucose

IF BLOOD GLUCOSE < 70 mg/dL (3.9 mmol/L) or UNKNOWN (pending EMS arrival) for conscious patients:

- Give sugar (10-15 grams glucose) by mouth IF able to swallow.
- Each of the following is equivalent to 10 g of glucose: milk (1 cup; 240 mL); orange juice (½ cup; 120 mL); prepackaged juice box (1 box); table sugar or honey (3 teaspoons; 15 mL); glucose tablets (3 tablets); glucose paste (10-15 grams).

First Aid Advice for Hypoglycemia—Glucagon

IF BLOOD GLUCOSE < 70 mg/dL (3.9 mmol/L) or UNKNOWN (pending EMS arrival):

- If family has glucagon for hypoglycemic emergencies AND the caller knows how to use it, encourage the caller to give the glucagon now.
- Inject it IM into the upper outer thigh.
- Adult dosage is 1 mg

BACKGROUND INFORMATION

Causes and Risk Factors for Low Blood Sugar (Hypoglycemia)

- **Aggressive Diabetes Control:** Intensive glycemic control reduces the long-term complications of diabetes. Unfortunately, it also increases the frequency of hypoglycemia.
- Alcohol ingestion
- History of other recent episodes of hypoglycemia
- Prolonged or vigorous exercise
- Renal failure
- Too much diabetes medication (e.g., insulin, pills) or too little food
- Combination of these factors

Diabetes Mellitus

- **Definition:** Diabetes mellitus is an endocrine condition in which patients have elevated blood glucose levels (hyperglycemia). The classic symptoms of untreated or undertreated diabetes are: frequent urination (polyuria), polydipsia (excessive thirst), and involuntary weight loss.

- **The Role of Insulin:** Insulin is a hormone produced by the pancreas to help process food. Eating food makes the blood glucose rise and insulin makes the blood glucose fall.
- **Classification of Diabetes Mellitus:** There are 4 different classes of diabetes mellitus: type 1 diabetes, type 2 diabetes, gestational diabetes mellitus, and other.

Type 1 Diabetes

- **Other Names:** Insulin-dependent diabetes mellitus (IDDM), juvenile-onset diabetes.
- **Physiology:** There is no production of insulin by the body.
- **Ketosis-prone:** Patients with this type of diabetes are ketosis-prone, which means that if they do not receive daily insulin shots their bodies break down fats and produce ketones. The ketones spill into the urine and can be measured. Patients with type 1 diabetes are susceptible to developing diabetic ketoacidosis (DKA), a life-threatening condition.
- **Onset:** It most commonly first appears in childhood or adolescence. Approximately 10% of diabetics are type 1.
- **Treatment:** Insulin therapy is always required and needs to be given subcutaneously at least once daily. Patients striving for tighter control of their blood glucose will take insulin more often than once a day. Recommended therapy for type 1 diabetes includes: 1) use of multiple-dose insulin injections (3–4 injections per day) and 2) matching of mealtime (prandial) insulin to carbohydrate intake, premeal blood glucose, and anticipated activity.

Type 2 Diabetes

- **Other Names:** Non–insulin-dependent diabetes mellitus (NIDDM), adult-onset diabetes.
- **Physiology:** In type 2 diabetes, there is decreased insulin production and decreased sensitivity to insulin.
- **Not Ketosis-prone:** These patients are not prone to ketosis. DKA rarely occurs.
- **Onset:** It more commonly develops in elderly and overweight adults.
- **Treatment:** The initial and most important treatments are exercise and weight loss. When these measures fail, there are pills that can be prescribed to help the body make more insulin or use the insulin more effectively. Occasionally patients require insulin therapy.

Diabetic Ketoacidosis (DKA)

- **Definition:** Blood glucose > 250 mg/dL (12 mmole/L) with acidosis and ketosis (urine ketones moderate to large)
- **Symptoms of DKA:** In addition to symptoms of hyperglycemia, fruity odor on breath, vomiting, rapid/deep breathing, confusion, and coma
- **Causes:** Noncompliance with using insulin in type 1 diabetes, infection

Five Types of Insulin for Diabetes

- **Rapid-acting (Humalog/Lispro, NovoLog/Aspart):** Onset 5-15 minutes; peaks 30-90 minutes; effective duration 5 hours
- **Short-acting (Regular, Humulin R, Novolin R):** Onset 30-60 minutes; peaks 2-3 hours; effective duration 5-8 hours
- **Intermediate-acting (NPH, Lente, Humulin N, Humulin L, Novolin N, Novolin L):** Onset 2-4 hours; peaks 4-12 hours; effective duration 10-18 hours
- **Long-acting (Lantus/Glargine, Detemir, Levemir):** Onset 2-4 hours; no true peak; effecive duration 18-24 hours
- **Premixed (Humulin 70/30, Humulin 50/50, Humalog Mix, NovoLog Mix):** 2 peaks; effective duration 10-16 hours; depends on mixture

Insulin Administration—Different Dosing Regimens

- **Sliding Insulin Scale:** Generally only used in the hospital.
- **Insulin Algorithm:** The patient checks his/her blood glucose before each meal and then adjusts insulin dosing based upon BOTH the blood glucose and an estimated caloric count for the meal. This is considered prandial insulin because it is given with (just before) meals. Rapid-acting (Humalog/lispro or NovoLog/aspart) or short-acting (regular) are used for prandial insulin dosing.

- **Once-daily Insulin:** This is not considered physiologic insulin dosing as it only provides the basal insulin and does not provide the needed prandial increases. However, it may be an effective addition for some type 2 diabetic patients on oral medications as their need for insulin is low. Intermediate-acting insulin (NPH) or long-acting insulin (Lantus/glargine) are used.
- **Twice-daily Insulin:** Intermediate-acting insulin (NPH) or long-acting insulin (Lantus/glargine) can be used in twice-daily regimens. Twice-daily insulin dosing may be sufficient for type 2 diabetic patients because they still make sufficient insulin on their own to handle prandial (mealtime) insulin needs.
- **Flexible Insulin Regimens:** In this type of regimen both an intermediate-acting insulin (for basal insulin needs) AND a rapid or ultrashort-acting insulin (for prandial insulin needs) are used.

Exubera—Inhaled Form of Insulin—No Longer Available

- Exubera is the first-ever inhaled insulin. It comes in a dry powder inhaler.
- It was approved by the FDA in January 2006 for the treatment of type 1 and type 2 diabetes mellitus
- On October 18, 2007, Pfizer announced that it would no longer be making Exubera.

Five Types of Oral Medications for Diabetes

- **Sulfonylureas:** Examples include glyburide (Micronase, Diabeta), glipizide (Glucotrol, Glucotrol XL), and glimepiride (Amaryl).
- **Biguanides:** Examples include metformin (Glucophage, Fortamet).
- **Thiazolidinediones:** Examples include rosiglitazone (Avanida) and pioglitazone (Actos).
- **Alplha-glucosidase Inhibitors:** Examples include acarbose (Precose) and miglitol (Glyset).
- **Meglitinides:** Examples include repaglinide (Prandin) and nateglinide (Starlix).

Goals for Diabetes Management

- **HbA1c:** The HbA1c is the primary goal for diabetes management. Depending on the patient, it should be measured 2-4 times a year. The American Diabetes Association (ADA) recommends a goal of less than 7.0% for nonpregnant adults.
- **Blood Glucose:** Depending on the patient, the blood glucose should be measured 1-3 times per day. The ADA recommends the following blood glucose goals: Preprandial (before meal): 70-130 mg/dL (3.9-7.2 mmol/L); postprandial (2-3 hours after a meal): Less than 180 mg/dL (10 mmol/L).
- **Goals Should Be Individualized Based Upon:** Age/life expectancy, duration of diabetes, comorbid conditions, hypoglycemic unawareness, history of severe hypoglycemic reactions, and other individual considerations.
- **Internet Resource:** ADA Standards of Medical Care in Diabetes 2012

Glycosylated Hemoglobin (HbA1c)

- The HbA1c provides a good estimate of how well a patient has managed his/her diabetes during the past 2-3 months. With good diabetes management the HbA1c goes down and with poor management it goes up. In general, the higher the HbA1c, the greater the risk of the long-term diabetic complications.
- **Goal:** The American Association of Clinical Endocrinologists (AACE) and the American College of Endocrinology (ACE) recommend a target glycosylated hemoglobin level (HbA1c) of less than 6.5%. The American Diabetes Association (ADA) recommends a goal of less than 7.0% for nonpregnant adults. The Canadian Diabetes Associations also recommends a goal of less than 7.0%

Long-term Complications of Diabetes Mellitus

- **Eye Disease (e.g., Retinopathy):** Diabetes is the leading cause of blindness.
- Heart disease (e.g., coronary heart disease, myocardial infarction)
- Kidney disease (e.g., renal failure, proteinuria)
- Nerve disease (e.g., peripheral and autonomic neuropathy)
- Stroke

Converting Glucose Levels: mg/dL and mmol/L

- In the United State glucose is typically measured using the units mg/dL. Nearly every country in the world (including Canada) measures glucose levels using the units mmol/L.
- To convert mmol/L of glucose to mg/dL, multiply by 18.
- To convert mg/dL of glucose to mmol/L, divide by 18 or multiply by 0.055.

DIARRHEA

DEFINITION

- Diarrhea is the sudden increase in the frequency and looseness of BMs (bowel movements, stools).

Diarrhea Severity Is Defined As:

- **Mild:** Mild diarrhea is the passage of a few loose or mushy BMs.
- **Severe:** Severe diarrhea is the passage of many (e.g., more than 15) watery BMs.

TRIAGE ASSESSMENT QUESTIONS

Call EMS 911 Now

- ● Shock suspected (e.g., cold/pale/clammy skin, too weak to stand)
  R/O: shock
  FIRST AID: Lie down with the feet elevated.
- ● Difficult to awaken or acting confused (e.g., disoriented, slurred speech)
- ● Sounds like a life-threatening emergency to the triager

See More Appropriate Protocol

- ● Vomiting also present and worse than the diarrhea
  Go to Protocol: Vomiting on page 335
- ● Blood in stool and without diarrhea
  Go to Protocol: Rectal Bleeding on page 219

Go to ED Now (or to Office With PCP Approval)

- ● Severe abdominal pain
  R/O: acute abdomen
- ● Black bowel movements
  R/O: peptic ulcer disease
  Note: Pepto-Bismol can cause darkening of the stool.
- ● Drinking very little and has signs of dehydration (e.g., no urine > 12 hours, very dry mouth, very light-headed)
  Reason: may need IV hydration
- ● Patient sounds very sick or weak to the triager

Go to Office Now

- ● Constant abdominal pain lasting > 2 hours
  R/O: acute abdomen
- ● Age < 60 years and has had > 15 diarrhea stools in past 24 hours
  Reason: severe diarrhea, higher risk of dehydration
- ● Age > 60 years and has had > 6 diarrhea stools in past 24 hours
  Reason: high risk for dehydration

See Today in Office

- Abdominal pain
  Exception: pain clears completely with each passage of diarrhea stool
- Fever > 101° F (38.3° C)
  R/O: bacterial diarrhea
- Blood in the stool
  R/O: bacterial diarrhea
- Mucus or pus in stool has been present > 2 days and diarrhea is more than mild
- Immunocompromised (e.g., HIV positive, cancer chemotherapy, splenectomy, organ transplant, chronic steroids)
  Reason: broader range of causes

Callback by PCP Today

- Travel to a foreign country in past month
  Reason: antibiotic therapy may be indicated for traveler's diarrhea
- Recent antibiotic therapy (i.e., within last 2 months)
  R/O: C difficile *diarrhea, antibiotic side effect*
- Tube feedings (e.g., nasogastric, g-tube, j-tube)
  R/O: osmotic diarrhea
- Age > 70 years
  Reason: higher morbidity

See Within 3 Days in Office

- Diarrhea persists > 7 days
- Patient wants to be seen

See Within 2 Weeks in Office

- Diarrhea is a chronic symptom (recurrent or ongoing AND lasting > 4 weeks)

Home Care

- ○ Mild diarrhea
  Reason: probable viral gastroenteritis

HOME CARE ADVICE FOR MILD DIARRHEA

1. **Reassurance:** In healthy adults, new-onset diarrhea is usually caused by a viral infection of the intestines, which you can treat at home. Diarrhea is the body's way of getting rid of the infection. Here are some tips on how to keep ahead of the fluid losses.
2. **Fluids:**
   - Drink more fluids, at least 8-10 glasses (8 oz or 240 mL) daily.
   - **Example:** Sports drinks, diluted fruit juices, soft drinks.
   - Supplement this with saltine crackers or soups to make certain that you are getting sufficient fluid and salt to meet your body's needs.
   - Avoid caffeinated beverages (Reason: caffeine is mildly dehydrating).
3. **Nutrition:**
   - Maintaining some food intake during episodes of diarrhea is important.
   - Ideal initial foods include boiled starches/cereals (e.g., potatoes, rice, noodles, wheat, oats) with a small amount of salt to taste.
   - Other acceptable foods include: bananas, yogurt, crackers, soup.
   - As your stools return to normal consistency, resume a normal diet.
4. **Diarrhea Medication—Bismuth Subsalicylate (e.g., Kaopectate, Pepto-Bismol):**
   - Helps reduce diarrhea, vomiting, and abdominal cramping.
   - **Adult Dosage:** 2 tablets or 2 tablespoons (30 mL) by mouth every hour if diarrhea continues to a maximum of 8 doses in a 24-hour period.
   - Do not use for more than 2 days.
   - This medication can make the stools look dark or even black (but not red or tarry).
5. **Diarrhea Medication—Imodium A-D:**
   - Helps reduce diarrhea.
   - **Adult Dosage:** 2 caplets or 4 teaspoonfuls (20 mL) initially by mouth. May take an additional caplet or 2 teaspoonfuls with each subsequent loose BM. Maximum of 4 caplets or 8 teaspoonfuls (40 mL) each day.
   - Do not use if there is a fever greater than 100.5° F (38.1° C) or if there is blood or mucus in the stools.
   - Do not use for more than 2 days.
   - Read and follow the package instructions carefully.
6. **Expected Course:** Viral diarrhea lasts 4-7 days. Always worse on days 1 and 2.
7. **Call Back If:**
   - Signs of dehydration occur (e.g., no urine for more than 12 hours, very dry mouth, lightheaded, etc.).
   - Diarrhea persists over 7 days.
   - You become worse.

FIRST AID

First Aid Advice for Shock:
Lie down with the feet elevated.

BACKGROUND INFORMATION

General

- The majority of adults with acute diarrhea (less than 14 days' duration) have an infectious etiology for their diarrhea, and in most cases the infection is a virus. Other common causes of acute diarrhea are food poisoning and medications.
- Maintaining hydration is the cornerstone of treatment of adults with acute diarrhea.
- In general, an adult who is alert, feels well, and who is not thirsty or dizzy is NOT dehydrated. A couple loose or runny stools do not cause dehydration. Frequent, watery stools can cause dehydration
- Antibiotic therapy is only rarely required in the treatment of acute diarrhea. Two types of acute diarrhea that require antibiotic therapy are *C difficile* diarrhea and (sometimes) traveler's diarrhea.

Traveler's Diarrhea

- Traveler's diarrhea typically begins within 2 weeks of traveling to a foreign country. There are bacteria in the water and food that the body is not used to and a diarrheal infection is the result. Traveler's diarrhea is also called "mummy tummy," "Montezuma's revenge," and "turista."

- **Symptoms:** Passage of at least 3 loose stools a day; accompanying symptoms may include nausea, vomiting, abdominal cramping, fecal urgency, and fever.
- **Region and Risk:** Travelers to the following developing areas have a HIGH RISK (40%) of getting traveler's diarrhea: Latin America, Africa, Southern Asia. There is an INTERMEDIATE RISK (15%) with travel to: Northern Mediterranean countries, Middle East, China, and Russia. Travelers to the United States, Western Europe, Canada, and Japan have a LOW RISK (2-4%) of getting traveler's diarrhea.
- **Prevention—Diet:** Avoid uncooked foods (salad). Cooked foods (served steaming hot) are usually safe as are dry foods (e.g., bread). Avoid ice cubes and tap water. Drink steaming beverages (e.g., coffee, tea) or carbonated drinks (e.g., bottled soft drinks, beer). Fruits that can be pealed are usually safe (oranges, bananas, apples).
- **Prevention—Bismuth Subsalicylate:** Bismuth (Pepto-Bismol 8 tablets daily PO) is approximately 65% effective at preventing traveler's diarrhea.
- **Prevention—Antibiotics:** Antibiotic chemoprophylaxis (prevention) during travel may be indicated in certain circumstances. Rifaximin (200 mg PO BID with meals) is approximately 70-80% effective at preventing traveler's diarrhea.
- **Treatment—Antidiarrheal Agents:** Bismuth subsalicylate (Pepto-Bismol) and loperamide (Imodium A-D) are both effective at reducing the diarrhea symptoms.
- **Treatment—Antibiotics:** Antibiotic therapy is sometimes recommended to treat this type of diarrhea, especially if the symptoms are more than mild. There are a number of antibiotics that are effective including ciprofloxacin (Cipro), azithromycin (Zithromax), and rifaximin (Xifaxan 200 mg PO TID for 3 days).

Causes

- Antibiotic side effect (e.g., temporary diarrhea from Augmentin/amoxicillin clavulanic acid)
- Bacterial gastroenteritis (i.e., *Campylobacter, Salmonella, Shigella*)
- Cathartics, excessive use of (e.g., magnesium citrate, milk of magnesia)
- Food poisoning
- Giardiasis
- Inflammatory bowel disease
- Irritable bowel syndrome
- Traveler's diarrhea
- Pseudomembranous colitis. Pseudomembranous colitis is an inflammation in the colon that occurs in some people from taking antibiotics. It is usually caused by an overgrowth of a specific type bacteria called *Clostridium difficile (C difficile)*. Other names that are used to describe this illness include antibiotic-associated diarrhea and *C difficile* colitis.
- Viral gastroenteritis.

Dehydration—Estimation by Telephone

Mild Dehydration

- **Urine Production:** Slightly decreased.
- **Mucous Membranes:** Normal.
- Heart rate < 100 beats/minute.
- Slightly thirsty.
- **Capillary Refill:** < 2 seconds.
- **Treatment:** Can usually treat at home.

Moderate Dehydration

- **Urine Production:** Minimal or absent.
- **Mucous Membranes:** Dry inside of mouth.
- Heart rate 100-130 beats/minute.
- Thirsty, light-headed when standing.
- **Capillary Refill:** > 2 seconds.
- **Treatment:** Must be seen; Go to ED NOW (or PCP Triage).

Severe Dehydration

- **Urine Production:** None > 12 hours.
- **Mucous Membranes:** Very dry inside of mouth.
- Heart rate > 130 beats/minute.
- Very thirsty, very weak, and light-headed; fainting may occur.
- **Capillary Refill:** > 2-4 seconds.
- **Treatment:** Must be seen immediately; Go to ED Now or CALL EMS 911 NOW.

Signs of Shock

- Confused, difficult to awaken, or unresponsive.
- Heart rate (pulse) is rapid and weak.
- Extremities (especially hands and feet) are bluish or gray, and cold.
- Too weak to stand or very dizzy when tries to stand.
- **Capillary Refill:** > 4 seconds.
- **Treatment:** Lie down with the feet elevated; CALL EMS 911 NOW.

DIZZINESS

DEFINITION

- Patient complains of dizziness, light-headedness, or feeling woozy.
- Patient feels like he/she might faint, but has not.
- Transient blurring of vision may be associated.

Dizziness Severity Is Defined As:

- **Mild:** Walking normally
- **Moderate:** Interferes with normal activities (e.g., work, school)
- **Severe:** Unable to stand, requires support to walk, feels like passing out now

TRIAGE ASSESSMENT QUESTIONS

Call EMS 911 Now

- Shock suspected (e.g., cold/pale/clammy skin, too weak to stand)
  R/O: shock
  FIRST AID: Lie down with the feet elevated.
- Difficult to awaken or acting confused (e.g., disoriented, slurred speech)
- Fainted, and still feels dizzy afterwards
  R/O: arrhythmia, shock
- Severe difficulty breathing
  R/O: hypoxia
- Overdose (accidental or intentional) of medications
- New neurologic deficit that is present now
- Weakness of the face, arm, or leg on one side of the body
- Numbness of the face, arm, or leg on one side of the body
- Loss of speech or garbled speech
  R/O: stroke
- Heart beating < 50 beats per minute OR > 140 beats per minute
  Reason: symptomatic bradycardia-tachycardia
- Sounds like a life-threatening emergency to the triager

See More Appropriate Protocol

- Chest pain
  Go to Protocol: Chest Pain on page 48
- Rectal bleeding, bloody stool, or tarry-black stool
  Go to Protocol: Rectal Bleeding on page 219
- Vomiting is main symptom
  Go to Protocol: Vomiting on page 335
- Diarrhea is main symptom
  Go to Protocol: Diarrhea on page 89
- Headache is main symptom
  Go to Protocol: Headache on page 140

Go to ED Now (or to Office With PCP Approval)

- SEVERE dizziness (e.g., unable to stand, requires support to walk, feels like passing out now)
  R/O: severe labyrinthitis, CVA
- Severe headache
  R/O: migraine, aneurysm
- Extra heart beats OR irregular heart beating (i.e., "palpitations")
  R/O: dysrrhythmia
- Difficulty breathing
  R/O: hypoxia
- Drinking very little and has signs of dehydration (e.g., no urine > 12 hours, very dry mouth, very light-headed)
  Reason: IV hydration needed
- Follows bleeding (e.g., stomach, rectum, vagina)
  Exception: became dizzy from sight of small amount of blood
  R/O: hypovolemic shock from major blood loss
- Patient sounds very sick or weak to the triager

Go to Office Now

- Light-headedness (dizziness) present now, after 2 hours of rest and fluids
- Spinning or tilting sensation (vertigo) present now
- Fever > 103° F (39.4° C)
- Fever > 100.5° F (38.1° C) and has diabetes mellitus or a weakened immune system (e.g., HIV positive, cancer chemotherapy, organ transplant, splenectomy, chronic steroids)

See Today in Office

- Vomiting occurs with dizziness
- Patient wants to be seen

Discuss With PCP and Callback by Nurse Today

- Taking a medicine that could cause dizziness (e.g., blood pressure medications, diuretics)
- Diabetes
  Note: Patient should check his/her glucose level when feeling dizzy

See Within 2 Weeks in Office

- Dizziness not present now but is a chronic symptom (recurrent or ongoing AND lasting > 4 weeks)

Home Care

- ○ Poor fluid intake probably causing dizziness
- ○ Recent heat exposure probably causing dizziness
- ○ Sudden or prolonged standing probably causing dizziness

HOME CARE ADVICE FOR DIZZINESS

1. **Temporary dizziness** is usually a harmless symptom. It can be caused by not drinking enough water during sports or hot weather. It can also be caused by skipping a meal, too much sun exposure, standing up suddenly, standing too long in one place, or even a viral illness.
2. **Some Causes of Temporary Dizziness:**
   - **Poor Fluid Intake:** Not drinking enough fluids and being a little dehydrated is a common cause of temporary dizziness. This is always worse during hot weather.
   - **Standing Up Suddenly:** Standing up suddenly (especially getting out of bed) or prolonged standing in one place are common causes of temporary dizziness. Not drinking enough fluids always makes it worse. Certain medications can cause or increase this type of dizziness (e.g., blood pressure medications).
   - **Heat Exposure:** Hot weather, hot tubs, or too much sun exposure are common causes of temporary dizziness. Not drinking enough fluids always makes it worse.
3. **Drink Fluids:** Drink several glasses of fruit juice, other clear fluids, or water. This will improve hydration and blood glucose. If you have a fever or have had heat exposure, make sure the fluids are cold.
4. **Cool Off:** If the weather is hot, apply a cold compress to the forehead or take a cool shower or bath.
5. **Rest for 1-2 Hours:** Lie down with feet elevated for 1 hour. This will improve circulation and increase blood flow to the brain.
6. **Stand Up Slowly:**
   - In the mornings, sit up for a few minutes before you stand up. That will help your circulation make the adjustment.
   - If you have to stand up for long periods of time, contract and relax your leg muscles to help pump the blood back to the heart.
   - Sit down or lie down if you feel dizzy.
7. **Call Back If:**
   - Still feel dizzy after 2 hours of rest and fluids.
   - Passes out (faints).
   - You become worse.

FIRST AID

First Aid Advice for Shock:

Lie down with the feet elevated.

First Aid Advice for Anaphylaxis—Epinephrine (Pending EMS Arrival):

- If the patient has an epinephrine autoinjector, the patient should use it now.
- Use the autoinjector on the upper outer thigh. You may give it through clothing if necessary.
- Epinephrine is available in autoinjectors under trade names: EpiPen, EpiPen Jr, and Twinject. EpiPen is a single injection. Twinject has a second injection that can be used if there is no improvement after 5 minutes.

First Aid Advice for Anaphylaxis—Benadryl (Pending EMS Arrival):

- Give antihistamine orally NOW if able to swallow.
- Use Benadryl (diphenhydramine; adult dose 50 mg) or any other available antihistamine.

BACKGROUND INFORMATION

There Are 2 Main Types of Dizziness: Light-headedness and Vertigo

- **Light-headedness:** This type of dizziness results from decreased blood flow to the brain. Equivalent terms that patients may use include feeling faint, spacey, weak, giddy, or woozy. Light-headedness is often aggravated by standing up and relieved by lying down.
- **Vertigo:** Patients with vertigo have the sensation that they or their environment are spinning. They may complain that the floor seems to be tilting. As a result, patients with vertigo often report difficulty with walking and standing because they feel like they are going to fall down. Vertigo typically has a neurologic etiology, resulting from some condition affecting the ear or the brain. Vertigo is usually aggravated by changes in head position.

Causes of Light-headedness

- Anyone can develop temporary dizziness or light-headedness from standing up suddenly, standing too long in one place, skipping a meal, dehydration, too much sun or hot tub exposure, or overexertion.
- Acute blood loss (e.g., gastrointestinal bleeding, vaginal bleeding).
- Cardiac disorders with decreased cardiac output (e.g., arrhythmias, valvular heart disease, cardiomyopathies).
- Fever.
- Heat exhaustion.
- Medication side effect.
- Metabolic (e.g., hypoglycemia).
- Orthostatic hypotension (e.g., anti-hypertensive medications).
- Panic disorder and hyperventilation.
- **Viral Syndrome:** Patients with viral illnesses (e.g., colds, flu) often report some dizziness along with all the other symptoms that they are experiencing.
- **Volume Depletion and Dehydration:** From vomiting, diarrhea, sweating.

EAR, SWIMMER'S (OTITIS EXTERNA)

DEFINITION

- An infection or irritation of the skin that lines the ear canal.
- Typically, the patient has been swimming recently or uses Q-tips frequently.
- Use this guideline only if the patient has symptoms that match Swimmer's Ear.

Symptoms of Swimmer's Ear Include:

- Itchy or painful ear canal.
- Discomfort when the earlobe is moved up and down (always present).
- The ear feels plugged or full.
- Sometimes a discharge; may be clear, white, or yellow.
- Fever is unusual; its presence suggests a more serious infection.

TRIAGE ASSESSMENT QUESTIONS

See More Appropriate Protocol

- Symptoms do not match swimmer's ear
  Go to Protocol: Earache on page 102

Go to ED Now (or to Office With PCP Approval)

- Pink or red swelling behind the ear
  R/O: mastoiditis
- Stiff neck (can't touch chin to chest)
  R/O: meningitis, cervical lymphadenitis
- Patient sounds very sick or weak to the triager
  Reason: feeling unwell is not typical of otitis externa

Go to Office Now

- Diabetes mellitus or a weakened immune system (e.g., HIV positive, cancer chemotherapy, transplant patient)
  Reason: higher risk for malignant otitis externa, should be examined
- Outer ear (earlobe) is red and/or swollen
  R/O: cellulitis
- Fever > 100.5° F (38.1° C)
  Reason: fever is uncommon in otitis externa

See Today in Office

- SEVERE earache pain
- Yellow or green discharge from ear canal
  R/O: otitis externa or otitis media with perforation
- Decreased hearing (or another adult says that the ear canal is completely blocked with discharge)
  Reason: debris/discharge will need to be removed manually
- Swollen lymph node near ear
  R/O: lymphadenitis
- Patient wants to be seen

See Today or Tomorrow in Office

- Diagnosis is uncertain
  Reason: see physician for confirmation of diagnosis
- Ear symptoms persist after 3 days of home treatment

Home Care

- ○ Swimmer's ear with no complications
- ○ Preventing swimmer's ear, questions about

HOME CARE ADVICE

Treatment of Mild Swimmer's Ear

1. **White Vinegar Rinses:** Vinegar (acetic acid) restores the normal acid pH of the ear canal. This helps swimmer's ear to get better. Rinse the ear canals twice daily with ½-strength white vinegar (dilute it with equal parts water). Here are some instructions on how to do this:
   - Lie down with the affected ear upward. Fill the ear canal.
   - After 5 minutes, remove the fluid by tilting the head to one side and gently pulling on the ear.
   - Continue doing this twice daily until the ear canal returns to normal.
   - **Caution:** Do not do use if you have ear tubes or hole in eardrum.

2. **Pain Medicines:**
   - For pain relief, take acetaminophen, ibuprofen, or naproxen.

   Acetaminophen (e.g., Tylenol):
   - Take 650 mg by mouth every 4-6 hours as needed. Each Regular Strength Tylenol pill has 325 mg of acetaminophen. The most you should take each day is 3,250 mg (10 pills a day).
   - Another choice is to take 1,000 mg every 8 hours. Each Extra Strength Tylenol pill has 500 mg of acetaminophen. The most you should take each day is 3,000 mg (6 pills a day).

   Ibuprofen (e.g., Motrin, Advil):
   - Take 400 mg by mouth every 6 hours.
   - Another choice is to take 600 mg by mouth every 8 hours.

   Naproxen (e.g., Aleve):
   - Take 250-500 mg by mouth every 12 hours.

Extra Notes:
   - Acetaminophen is thought to be safer than ibuprofen or naproxen in people over 65 years old. Acetaminophen is in many OTC and prescription medicines. It might be in more than one medicine that you are taking. You need to be careful and not take an overdose. An acetaminophen overdose can hurt the liver.
   - **Caution:** Do not take acetaminophen if you have liver disease.
   - **Caution:** Do not take ibuprofen if you have stomach problems, kidney disease, are pregnant, or have been told by your doctor to avoid this type of anti-inflammatory drug. Do not take ibuprofen for more than 7 days without consulting your doctor.
   - Use the lowest amount of medicine that makes your pain feel better.
   - Before taking any medicine, read all the instructions on the package

3. **Local Heat:** If pain is moderate to severe, apply a heating pad (set on low) or hot water bottle (wrapped in a towel) to outer ear for 20 minutes (CAUTION: avoid burns). This will also increase drainage.
4. **Avoid Earplugs:** If pus or cloudy fluid is draining from the ear canal, wipe the pus away as it appears. Avoid plugging with cotton (Reason: retained pus causes irritation or infection of the ear canal).
5. **Avoid Swimming:** Try to avoid swimming until symptoms are gone.
6. **Contagiousness:** Swimmer's ear is not contagious.
7. **Expected Course:** With treatment, symptoms should improve in 3 days and resolve within 7 days.
8. **Call Back If:**
   - Ear symptoms last longer than 7 days with treatment.
   - You become worse.

Prevention of Swimmer's Ear

1. **Prevention—Keep Ear Canals Dry:**
   - Try to keep your ear canals dry.
   - After showers, hair washing, and swimming, help the water run out by tilting the head to one side. You can also use a hair dryer set on the lowest setting to dry out your ears.
2. **Prevention—Avoid Cotton Swabs:**
   - Avoid cotton swabs (i.e., Q-tips, cotton tip applicator).
   - These remove the protective earwax of the ear canal.
3. **Prevention—Rinse Ear Canal With Vinegar After Swimming:**
   - After swimming, place several drops of ½-strength white vinegar (dilute it with equal parts water) in your ear canals.
   - After 5 minutes, remove the fluid by tilting the head to one side and gently pulling on the ear.
   - **Reason:** Vinegar (acetic acid) restores the normal acid pH of the ear canal.
   - **Indication:** You may want to try this if you tend to get swimmer's ear frequently.
   - **Caution:** Do not use if you have ear tubes or hole in eardrum.

BACKGROUND INFORMATION

General Information About Otitis Externa (Swimmer's Ear)

- Otitis externa is an infection of the skin that lines the ear canal. It is also referred to as swimmer's ear.
- **Cause:** When water repeatedly gets trapped in the ear canal (usually from swimming), the lining becomes wet and swollen. This makes the skin of the ear canal susceptible to superficial infection (swimmer's ear). Ear canals were meant to be dry.
- **Earwax (Cerumen):** Cerumen is produced by the ear canal as a natural waterproofing agent. Thus, frequent use of cotton ear swabs depletes the wax barrier and increases the likelihood of developing otitis externa. On the other hand, excessive amounts of earwax can inhibit water drainage from the ear, leading to chronic wetness, ear canal skin maceration, and then on to otitis externa.

Treatment of Otitis Externa

- **Antibiotic Ear Drops:** Otitis externa is usually treated with antibiotic ear drops. Examples include Cortisporin Otic, Floxin Otic, and Cipro HC Otic.
- **Oral Antibiotics:** Occasionally more severe cases are treated with oral antibiotics.
- **Acetic Acid Solution:** Milder cases of otitis externa can be treated with an acetic acid solution.
- Household white vinegar contains acetic acid; instructions for use are to rinse the ear canals twice daily with ½-strength white vinegar (dilute it with equal parts water). Acetic acid is also available by prescription (e.g., Acetic Acid Otic, Vosol).
- Pain medications.

EAR PIERCING

DEFINITION

- Area around pierced earring is red, tender, or swollen.
- Earlobes can also become torn or lacerated.

TRIAGE ASSESSMENT QUESTIONS

Go to ED Now (or to Office With PCP Approval)

- ● Earring tore completely through the earlobe
  Reason: may need sutures
- ● Skin is split open or gaping (or length > ¼ inch or 6 mm)
  Reason: may need sutures
- ● Bleeding at the piercing site has not stopped after 10 minutes of direct pressure
- ● Part of jewelry (clasp) is stuck inside the earlobe
  Reason: removal of foreign body
- ● Patient sounds very sick or weak to the triager

Go to Office Now

- ● Ear pain and entire lower ear is red or swollen
  R/O: cellulitis of earlobe
- ● Ear pain and entire upper ear is red or swollen
  R/O: auricular chondritis of helix
- ● Ear pain and fever
  R/O: cellulitis, chondritis

See Today or Tomorrow in Office

- Swollen lymph node (in front of or behind earlobe)
  R/O: lymphadenitis
- Symptoms of minor pierced ear infection (e.g., localized redness just at earring site, slight discharge), and not improving 3 days following care advice (e.g., cleaning, antibiotic ointment)
  R/O: minor local infection, inadequate cleaning of area, contact dermatitis
- Small tear in earlobe from earring injury and no tetanus booster > 10 years
  Reason: need for tetanus vaccination
- Patient wants to be seen

See Within 2 Weeks in Office

- Large thick scar has developed at the earring site over the last couple months
  R/O: keloid

Home Care

- ○ Symptoms of minor pierced ear infection (e.g., localized redness just at earring site, slight discharge)
- ○ Small tear in earlobe from earring injury
- ○ Aftercare instructions for new ear piercings, questions about

HOME CARE ADVICE

Caring of Minor Infection at an Ear Piercing Site

1. **Reassurance:**
   - This sounds like a minor infection that you can treat at home.
   - The most important thing to do is to keep the piercing site clean. It's also important to apply an antibiotic ointment; it should get better. I can give you instructions on how to do both of these.
2. **General Care Advice for New Piercings (Less Than 6 Weeks Old):**
   - Leave the earring in at all times. If you take it out, the hole can close, sometimes even within a few minutes.
   - Posts should be made out of surgical steel, 14- to 18-karat gold, or some other metal (e.g., titanium) that does not cause skin allergy. However, some piercing salons recommend that gold posts should be avoided immediately after a piercing, because even higher quality gold can contain trace amounts of nickel.
   - Make certain that phones are clean.
   - Be careful when brushing your hair.
   - Change and use a clean pillowcase every 2 days.
   - AVOID playing with the earring/jewelry.
   - AVOID SMOKING DURING THE HEALING PERIOD (Reason: it prolongs healing).
   - AVOID wearing heavy/large/dangling earrings.
   - AVOID hanging any accessories from piercing until it is completely healed.

3. **General Care Advice for Established Piercings (6 Weeks and Older):**
   - Make certain that phones are clean.
   - Be careful when brushing your hair.
   - Change and use a clean pillowcase every 2 days.
   - AVOID playing with the earring/jewelry.
   - AVOID SMOKING DURING THE HEALING PERIOD (Reason: it prolongs healing).
   - AVOID wearing heavy/large/dangling earrings.
   - AVOID hanging any accessories from piercing until it is completely healed.
4. **Treatment—Cleaning Instructions:**
   - **Step 1:** Wash your hands with soap and water.
   - **Step 2:** Soak the area in warm saline (salt water) solution 3 times per day for 5-10 minutes. For ear piercings it is easiest to place a saline-soaked cotton ball directly on the piercing site.
   - **Step 3:** Wash the piercing site with 3 times a day. Use a cotton swab (Q-tip) dipped in an ear care antiseptic solution (usually contains benzalkonium chloride). If you do not have ear care antiseptic, you can use just a tiny amount of liquid antibacterial soap (e.g., Dial); be certain to rinse it off completely.
   - **Step 4:** Gently pat area dry using clean gauze or a disposable tissue.
5. **Treatment—Antibiotic Ointment:**
   - Apply a small amount of antibiotic ointment to piercing site 3 times per day.
   - Use Bacitracin ointment (OTC in United States) or Polysporin ointment (OTC in Canada) or one that you already have.
   - Rotate (turn) the earring several times to prevent the skin from sticking to the post.
6. **Expected Course:**
   - With proper care, most minor piercing site infections should clear up in a couple days.
   - You should see a doctor if it does not improve within 3 days or if it gets worse.
7. **Saline Solution—How to Make It:**
   - Place ½ teaspoon of non-iodized (iodine-free) salt into a cup (8 oz or 240 mL) of warm water. You can use sea salt to make the saline (salt) solution.
   - Stir the water until the salt dissolves.
8. **Call Back If:**
   - Not improved after 3 days.
   - Pain increases.
   - Spreading redness occurs.
   - You become worse.

Very Small Tear in Earlobe

1. **General Care Advice for Ear Piercings:**
   - Make certain that phones are clean.
   - Be careful when brushing your hair.
   - Change and use a clean pillowcase every 2 days.
   - AVOID playing with the earring/jewelry.
   - AVOID SMOKING DURING THE HEALING PERIOD (Reason: it prolongs healing).
   - AVOID wearing heavy/large/dangling earrings.
   - AVOID hanging any accessories from piercing until it is completely healed.
2. **Bleeding:**
   - Using gauze or clean cloth, apply direct pressure to the area from both sides.
   - Call back if the bleeding does not stop after 10 minutes.
3. **Tetanus Vaccine:** If your last tetanus shot was given more than 10 years ago, then you need a booster.
4. **Call Back If:**
   - Ear looks infected.
   - You become worse.

Aftercare Instructions for a New Ear Piercing

1. **General Care Advice for New Piercings (Less Than 6 Weeks Old):**
   - Leave the earring in at all times. If you take it out, the hole can close, sometimes even within a few minutes.
   - Posts should be made out of surgical steel, 14- to 18-karat gold, or some other metal (e.g., titanium) that does not cause skin allergy. However, some piercing salons recommend that gold posts should be avoided immediately after a piercing, because even higher quality gold can contain trace amounts of nickel.
   - Make certain that phones are clean.
   - Be careful when brushing your hair.
   - Change and use a clean pillowcase every 2 days.

- AVOID playing with the earring/jewelry.
- AVOID SMOKING DURING THE HEALING PERIOD (Reason: it prolongs healing).
- AVOID wearing heavy/large/dangling earrings.
- AVOID hanging any accessories from piercing until it is completely healed.

2. **Treatment—Cleaning Instructions:**
   - **Step 1:** Wash your hands with soap and water.
   - **Step 2:** Soak the area in warm saline (salt water) solution 3 times per day for 5-10 minutes. For ear piercings it is easiest to place a saline-soaked cotton ball directly on the piercing site.
   - **Step 3:** Wash the piercing site with 3 times a day. Use a cotton swab (Q-tip) dipped in an ear care antiseptic solution (usually contains benzalkonium chloride). If you do not have ear care antiseptic, you can use just a tiny amount of liquid antibacterial soap (e.g., Dial); be certain to rinse it off completely.
   - **Step 4:** Gently pat area dry using clean gauze or a disposable tissue.
3. **Saline Solution—How to Make It:**
   - Place ½ teaspoon of non-iodized (iodine-free) salt into a cup (8 oz or 240 mL) of warm water. You can use sea salt to make the saline (salt) solution.
   - Stir the water until the salt dissolves.
4. **Expected Course:**
   - **First 1-3 Days:** There might be some mild bruising, mild swelling, and mild tenderness. Rarely, there might be very slight bleeding (a couple spots of blood at piercing site).
   - **During Healing Period:** You may note some itching at the site. You also may note whitish-yellow fluid (not pus) that coats the jewelry and forms a crust when it dries.
   - **After Healing Period:** Sometimes jewelry will not move freely within the piercing tract; this is OK and you should not try to force the jewelry to move. If you forget to clean the piercing for a couple days, you may note normal but slightly smelly secretions. This should be prevented; thus, it is important to remember to clean the piercing as part of your normal daily good hygiene.
5. **Healing Period—How Long Does It Take?**
   - A piercing heals from the outside in, so it can look healed on the outside and still be fragile on the inside.
   - Reputable piercing studios provide aftercare instructions and these aftercare instructions should be followed for the duration of the healing time.
   - Healing times vary from person to person. The values below are averages.
   - **Earlobe (Soft Lower Part of Ear):** 6-8 weeks.
   - **Ear Cartilage:** 6-9 months.
6. **Call Back If:**
   - You have more questions.

BACKGROUND INFORMATION

General

- Piercing guns should not be used. Two problems with piercing guns are tissue injury and exposure to body fluids from repeated prior use. The Association of Professional Piercers (APP) recommends against using piercing guns.
- Individuals should have their ears pierced by someone who is experienced and uses sterile technique.
- Reputable piercing studios provide aftercare instructions and these instructions should be followed for the entire duration of the healing time.

Healing Times for Ear Piercings

- Healing times vary from person to person. The values below are averages.
- **Earlobe (Soft Lower Part of Ear):** 6-8 weeks.
- **Ear Helix (Folded Rim of Skin and Cartilage of the Upper Outer Ear):** 6-9 months.

Complications of Ear Piercing—Common

Minor complications occur in about 30% of people who have their ears pierced. These complications most commonly happen in the first few days or weeks after piercing.

- **Contact Dermatitis:** Contact dermatitis is fairly common and most often is the result of allergic reaction to nickel (contained in some piercing jewelry). Piercing jewelry should be made of hypoallergenic metal. Examples of metals that cause the least amount of allergy are stainless steel, titanium, platinum, palladium, and niobium. Titanium has the least risk of allergic reaction. Even gold posts should be avoided immediately after a piercing because even higher quality gold can contain trace amounts of nickel.
- **Embedded Clasp:** The backing (clasp, ball) gets stuck (embedded) under the skin. The most common cause is that the earring post is too short (the thickness of earlobes varies) or the clasp is squeezed on too tightly. A visit to the doctor is often necessary to extract the embedded clasp.
- **Local Infection:** A minor local infection at the piercing site may occur in 10-30% of individuals, even when the piercing is performed in a sterile manner by professionals. Symptoms of a local infection include yellow discharge, crusting, and mild irritation.
- **Traumatic Injury:** Tears of skin can occur because of a pulling injury on jewelry. The most common site is the earlobe and a common scenario is the earring getting hooked on an article of clothing during dressing or undressing.

Complications of Ear Piercing—Uncommon

- **Auricular Chondritis:** This is a serious infection of the ear cartilage that occurs in a piercing through the cartilage of the helix. The helix is the folded rim of skin and cartilage of the upper outer ear. This infection can begin weeks after an ear piercing and it usually requires IV antibiotics.
- **Blood-borne Infections—Hepatitis B and C:** Blood-borne infections can be transmitted by sharing earrings with other people or through use of unsanitary piercing needles. Professional piercing studios follow strict sanitation guidelines and utilize sterile single-use piercing needles.
- **Cellulitis:** Rarely a local infection at a piercing site can spread into the surrounding skin and cause cellulitis; symptoms are spreading redness and increasing pain at the site. In such cases oral antibiotic therapy is needed.
- **Blood-borne Infections:** HIV.
- **Keloid:** A keloid is the medical term for excessive scar formation at wound or surgical site. It develops over months. It occurs because some individuals are simply prone to developing excessive scar formation and not because of how the piercing was performed.

Causes of Pierced Ear Infections

- The most common causes of infection are piercing the ears with unsterile equipment, inserting unsterile posts, or frequently touching the earlobes with dirty hands.
- Another frequent cause is earrings that are too tight either because the post is too short (the thickness of earlobes varies) or the clasp is closed too tightly. Tight earrings don't allow air to enter the channel through the earlobe. Also, the pressure from tight earrings reduces blood flow to the earlobe and makes it more vulnerable to infection. Often this can be prevented by leaving the clasp at the notch on the post.
- Some inexpensive earrings have rough areas on the posts that scratch the channel and can result in infection. Heavy earrings can cause breaks in the skin lining the channel. Inserting the post at the wrong angle also can scratch the channel, so a mirror should be used until insertion becomes second nature. Posts containing nickel can also cause an itchy, allergic reaction.

EARACHE

DEFINITION

- Pain or discomfort in or around ear
- Not due to a traumatic injury

Pain Severity Is Defined As:

- **Mild (1-3):** Doesn't interfere with normal activities
- **Moderate (4-7):** Interferes with normal activities or awakens from sleep
- **Severe (8-10):** Excruciating pain, unable to do any normal activities

TRIAGE ASSESSMENT QUESTIONS

Call EMS 911 Now

- Sounds like a life-threatening emergency to the triager

See More Appropriate Protocol

- Moving the earlobe or touching the ear clearly increases the pain
  Go to Protocol: Ear, Swimmer's (Otitis Externa) on page 95

Go to ED Now (or to Office With PCP Approval)

- Pink or red swelling behind the ear
  R/O: mastoiditis
- Stiff neck (can't touch chin to chest)
  R/O: meningitis
- Patient sounds very sick or weak to the triager

Go to Office Now

- SEVERE earache pain
- Fever > 103° F (39.4° C)
- Pointed object was inserted into the ear canal (e.g., a pencil, stick, or wire)
  R/O: TM perforation

See Today in Office

- Diabetes mellitus or a weakened immune system (e.g., HIV positive, cancer chemotherapy, transplant patient)
  Reason: higher risk for malignant otitis externa, should be examined
- All other earaches
  Exceptions: earache lasting < 1 hour, and earache from air travel
  R/O: otitis media or otitis externa
- Patient wants to be seen

Home Care

- Mild earache and ear congestion (fullness) occurring during air travel
  R/O: barotitis media
- Earache < 60 minutes' duration that is now completely gone

HOME CARE ADVICE FOR EARACHE

1. **Pain Medicines:**
   - For pain relief, take acetaminophen, ibuprofen, or naproxen.

   Acetaminophen (e.g., Tylenol):
   - Take 650 mg by mouth every 4-6 hours as needed. Each Regular Strength Tylenol pill has 325 mg of acetaminophen. The most you should take each day is 3,250 mg (10 pills a day).
   - Another choice is to take 1,000 mg every 8 hours. Each Extra Strength Tylenol pill has 500 mg of acetaminophen. The most you should take each day is 3,000 mg (6 pills a day).

   Ibuprofen (e.g., Motrin, Advil):
   - Take 400 mg by mouth every 6 hours.
   - Another choice is to take 600 mg by mouth every 8 hours.

   Naproxen (e.g., Aleve):
   - Take 250-500 mg by mouth every 12 hours.

   Extra Notes:
   - Acetaminophen is thought to be safer than ibuprofen or naproxen in people over 65 years old. Acetaminophen is in many OTC and prescription medicines. It might be in more than one medicine that you are taking. You need to be careful and not take an overdose. An acetaminophen overdose can hurt the liver.

- **Caution:** Do not take acetaminophen if you have liver disease.
- **Caution:** Do not take ibuprofen if you have stomach problems, kidney disease, are pregnant, or have been told by your doctor to avoid this type of anti-inflammatory drug. Do not take ibuprofen for more than 7 days without consulting your doctor.
- Use the lowest amount of medicine that makes your pain feel better.
- Before taking any medicine, read all the instructions on the package

2. **Local Cold for Pain:** Apply a cold pack or a cold, wet washcloth to the outer ear for 20 minutes to reduce pain while the pain medicine takes effect (Note: Some individuals prefer local heat instead of cold for 20 minutes).
3. **Avoid Earplugs:** If pus or cloudy fluid is draining from the ear canal, wipe the pus away as it appears. Avoid plugging with cotton (Reason: retained pus causes irritation or infection of the ear canal).
4. **Contagiousness:** Ear infections are not contagious.
5. **Earache During Air Travel:** Ear pain and stuffiness can occur during air travel. This results from too rapid changes in air pressure.
6. **Treatment—Earache During Air Travel:** There are a number of different maneuvers that you can use to reduce the pressure and pain, including yawning, chewing gum, or swallowing. You can also try to exhale while pinching your nose and keeping your lips closed.
7. **Prevention of Earache During Air Travel:** Using a nasal decongestant approximately 1 hour before takeoff can sometimes help. Decongestants shrink the swollen nasal passages and open up the tube connecting the nose and the ear (eustacian) to help normalize ear pressure. They can be taken as pills by mouth or as a nasal spray.
   - **Pseudoephedrine (Sudafed):** Available over-the-counter in pill form. Typical adult dosage is two 30-mg tablets every 6 hours.
   - **Phenylephrine Nasal Drops (Neo-Synephrine):** Available over-the-counter. Clean out the nose before using. Spray each nostril once, wait 1 minute for absorption, and then spray a second time. Read package instructions.
   - Do not take these medications if you have high blood pressure, heart disease, or prostate enlargement. Do not use these medications for more than 3 days (Reason: excessive use can cause rebound nasal congestion).
   - Read the package instructions thoroughly on all medications that you take.
8. **Call Back If:**
   - You become worse.

BACKGROUND INFORMATION

Causes of Earache

- Ear pain can be primary or referred. Primary ear pain originates from the ear itself. Examples include otitis media and otitis externa.
- **Otitis Media:** An infection of the middle portion of the ear behind the tympanic membrane. It is very common in children but less common in adults.
- **Otitis Externa:** Also called swimmer's ear; it is an infection of the external ear canal. Swimmers and people who use Q-tips frequently are more likely to get it. Otitis externa is more common than otitis media in adults.
- **Referred Ear Pain:** Referred ear pain means that the pain originates from a disease process outside of the ear. Because of the manner in which the nerves run in the head the pain may be perceived as being in the ear. Examples of referred ear pain include dental abscess, TMJ syndrome, and tonsillitis.

ELBOW PAIN

DEFINITION

- Pain in the elbow.
- Not due to a traumatic injury.
- Minor muscle strain and overuse are covered in this guideline.

Pain Severity Is Defined As:

- **Mild (1-3):** Doesn't interfere with normal activities
- **Moderate (4-7):** Interferes with normal activities (e.g., work or school) or awakens from sleep
- **Severe (8-10):** Excruciating pain, unable to do any normal activities, unable to hold a cup of water

TRIAGE ASSESSMENT QUESTIONS

Call EMS 911 Now

- Shock suspected (e.g., cold/pale/clammy skin, too weak to stand)
  R/O: shock
- Similar pain previously and it was from "heart attack"
  R/O: cardiac ischemia, myocardial infarction
- Similar pain previously from "angina" and not relieved by nitroglycerin
  R/O: cardiac ischemia
- Sounds like a life-threatening emergency to the triager

See More Appropriate Protocol

- Chest pain
  Go to Protocol: Chest Pain on page 48
- Followed an injury
  Go to Protocol: Trauma, Elbow on page 277
- Wound looks infected
  Go to Protocol: Wound Infection on page 344

Go to ED Now

- Difficulty breathing or unusual sweating (e.g., sweating without exertion)
  R/O: cardiac ischemia
- Age > 40 and associated chest or jaw pain, and pain lasting > 5 minutes
  R/O: cardiac ischemia

Go to ED Now (or to Office With PCP Approval)

- Red area or streak, and fever
  R/O: cellulitis, lymphangitis
  Note: It may be difficult to determine the rash color in people with darker-colored skin.
- Swollen joint and fever
  R/O: septic arthritis, infected bursitis
- Entire arm is swollen
  R/O: DVT of upper extremity
- Patient sounds very sick or weak to the triager

Go to Office Now

- SEVERE pain (e.g., excruciating, unable to do any normal activities)
- Weakness (i.e., loss of strength) in hand or fingers
  Exception: not truly weak; hand feels weak because of pain
  R/O: herniated cervical disk

See Today in Office

- Swollen joint
  R/O: arthritis
- Fluid-filled sack located directly over point of elbow
  R/O: olecranon bursitis, infected bursitis.
  Note: The "point" refers to the posterior elbow and the skin area directly over the olecranon process.
- Looks like a boil, infected sore, deep ulcer, or other infected rash (spreading redness, pus)
  R/O: impetigo, abscess, cellulitis
- Painful rash with multiple small blisters grouped together (i.e., dermatomal distribution or band or stripe)
  R/O: herpes zoster
- Numbness (i.e., loss of sensation) in hand or fingers
  R/O: cervical radiculopathy, herniated cervical disk, carpal tunnel syndrome
- Can't move joint normally (bend and straighten completely)
  R/O: arthritis, unobserved injury

See Within 3 Days in Office

- MODERATE pain (e.g., interferes with normal activities) and present > 3 days
  R/O: arthritis, tendonitis, carpal tunnel syndrome
- Patient wants to be seen

See Within 2 Weeks in Office

- MILD pain (e.g., does not interfere with normal activities) and present > 7 days
- Elbow pain is a chronic symptom (recurrent or ongoing AND lasting > 4 weeks)

Home Care

- Elbow pain
- Caused by bumping elbow, with transient burning pain shooting (radiating) into hand and fingers
  R/O: "bruised funny bone"
- Caused by overuse from recent vigorous activity (e.g., vigorous activity, tennis, golf, throwing a baseball)
  R/O: overuse injury, tendinitis, strain

HOME CARE ADVICE

Elbow Pain

1. **Reassurance—Elbow Pain:**
   - Usually elbow pain is not serious. You have told me that there is no redness, numbness, or swelling.
   - Causes of elbow pain can include a strained muscle, a forgotten minor injury, and tendinitis.
2. **Pain Medicines:**
   - For pain relief, take acetaminophen, ibuprofen, or naproxen.

   Acetaminophen (e.g., Tylenol):
   - Take 650 mg by mouth every 4-6 hours as needed. Each Regular Strength Tylenol pill has 325 mg of acetaminophen. The most you should take each day is 3,250 mg (10 pills a day).
   - Another choice is to take 1,000 mg every 8 hours. Each Extra Strength Tylenol pill has 500 mg of acetaminophen. The most you should take each day is 3,000 mg (6 pills a day).

   Ibuprofen (e.g., Motrin, Advil):
   - Take 400 mg by mouth every 6 hours.
   - Another choice is to take 600 mg by mouth every 8 hours.

   Naproxen (e.g., Aleve):
   - Take 250-500 mg by mouth every 12 hours.

   Extra Notes:
   - Acetaminophen is thought to be safer than ibuprofen or naproxen in people over 65 years old. Acetaminophen is in many OTC and prescription medicines. It might be in more than one medicine that you are taking. You need to be careful and not take an overdose. An acetaminophen overdose can hurt the liver.
   - **Caution:** Do not take acetaminophen if you have liver disease.
   - **Caution:** Do not take ibuprofen if you have stomach problems, kidney disease, are pregnant, or have been told by your doctor to avoid this type of anti-inflammatory drug. Do not take ibuprofen for more than 7 days without consulting your doctor.
   - Use the lowest amount of medicine that makes your pain feel better.
   - Before taking any medicine, read all the instructions on the package
3. **Expected Course:** If this does not get better during the next week or if it recurs, then you should make an appointment with your doctor.
4. **Call Back If:**
   - Moderate pain (e.g., interferes with normal activities) lasts more than 3 days.
   - Mild pain lasts more than 7 days.
   - Swollen joint or fever occurs.
   - You become worse.

Overuse of Elbow

1. **Reassurance—Overuse:**
   - **Definition:** Activities associated with repetitive forceful use of the elbow can cause soreness, muscle strain, and tendinitis. Such activities can include tennis, throwing of a baseball, golf, and certain types of repetitive forceful motions (e.g., washing the car, scrubbing the floor).
   - **Symptoms:** Soreness and tenderness of the elbow. Pain increases with certain movements.
2. **Apply Local Cold:**
   - Apply a cold pack or an ice bag (wrapped in a moist towel) to the area for 20 minutes. Repeat in 1 hour, then every 4 hours while awake.
   - Continue this for the first 48 hours after an injury (Reason: reduce the swelling and pain).

3. **Apply Local Heat:**
    - Beginning 48 hours after an injury, apply a warm washcloth or heating pad for 10 minutes 3 times a day.
    - This will help increase circulation and improve healing.
4. **Pain Medicines:**
    - For pain relief, take acetaminophen, ibuprofen, or naproxen.

Acetaminophen (e.g., Tylenol):

- Take 650 mg by mouth every 4-6 hours as needed. Each Regular Strength Tylenol pill has 325 mg of acetaminophen. The most you should take each day is 3,250 mg (10 pills a day).
- Another choice is to take 1,000 mg every 8 hours. Each Extra Strength Tylenol pill has 500 mg of acetaminophen. The most you should take each day is 3,000 mg (6 pills a day).

Ibuprofen (e.g., Motrin, Advil):

- Take 400 mg by mouth every 6 hours.
- Another choice is to take 600 mg by mouth every 8 hours.

Naproxen (e.g., Aleve):

- Take 250-500 mg by mouth every 12 hours.

Extra Notes:

- Acetaminophen is thought to be safer than ibuprofen or naproxen in people over 65 years old. Acetaminophen is in many OTC and prescription medicines. It might be in more than one medicine that you are taking. You need to be careful and not take an overdose. An acetaminophen overdose can hurt the liver.
- **Caution:** Do not take acetaminophen if you have liver disease.
- **Caution:** Do not take ibuprofen if you have stomach problems, kidney disease, are pregnant, or have been told by your doctor to avoid this type of anti-inflammatory drug. Do not take ibuprofen for more than 7 days without consulting your doctor.
- Use the lowest amount of medicine that makes your pain feel better.
- Before taking any medicine, read all the instructions on the package

5. **Rest:** Avoid any exercise activity which causes this pain for the next 3 days.
6. **Expected Course:**
    - For minor injuries, pain should improve over a 2- to 3-day period and disappear within 7 days.
    - If this does not get better during the next week or if it recurs, then you should make an appointment with your doctor.
7. **Call Back If:**
    - Moderate pain (e.g., interferes with normal activities) lasts more than 3 days.
    - Mild pain lasts more than 7 days.
    - Swollen joint or fever occurs.
    - You become worse.

Bruised Funny Bone

1. **Reassurance—Bruised Funny Bone:**
    - It sounds like a "bruised funny bone" that we can treat at home.
    - A direct blow to the inner side of the posterior elbow can cause numbness, tingling, and burning in the hand. The involved fingers are usually the middle, ring, and little fingers.
    - Your funny bone is actually a nerve (ulnar) which wraps around the posterior part of your elbow.
2. **Expected Course:** Symptoms from "bruising your funny bone" usually last only a few minutes. If the symptoms last longer than 30 minutes or if this problem seems to happen to you frequently, then you should see your doctor for evaluation.
3. **Call Back If:** You become worse.

FIRST AID

First Aid Advice for Shock:

Lie down with the feet elevated.

BACKGROUND INFORMATION

General

- Elbow pain is a common symptom and there are a number of causes.
- Elbow pain is almost always not serious and it generally originates from the muscles or tendons of the elbow region, as a result of overuse or injury.

Causes of Elbow Pain

- Arthritis
- Cancer (rare; in a patient with known cancer metastasis)
- Cardiac ischemia (rare)
- Cellulitis
- Fracture, dislocation, contusion
- Lateral epicondylitis (tennis elbow)
- Medial epicondylitis (golfer's elbow)
- Olecranon bursitis
- Muscle strain

Serious Signs and Symptoms

- Severe pain
- Red area with streak
  R/O: cellulitis with lymphangitis; common
- Joint swelling with fever
  R/O: septic arthritis; rare
- Entire arm is swollen
  R/O: deep vein thrombosis of upper extremity; rare

Caution: Cardiac Ischemia

- Rarely patients may present with elbow pain as the sole symptom of a myocardial infarction. Usually there will be other associated symptoms of cardiac ischemia: chest pain, shortness of breath, nausea, and/or diaphoresis.
- Cardiac ischemia should be suspected in any patients with risk factors for cardiac disease. These include: hypertension, smoking, diabetes, hyperlipidemia, a strong family history of heart disease, and age > 50.

EYE, CHEMICAL IN

DEFINITION

- Chemical gets into the eye from fingers, contaminated object, spray, or splash.

TRIAGE ASSESSMENT QUESTIONS

Go to ED Now

- Acid or alkali was the chemical
  Exception: mild agents such as household bleach or ammonia—instead call Poison Center
  FIRST AID: Irrigate eye immediately before going to the ED.
  NOTE: acid and alkali defined in Background Information
- Shortness of breath
  Reason: possible bronchospasm or pulmonary involvement

Go to ED Now (or to Office With PCP Approval)

- Sounds like a serious injury to the triager
- Call Poison Center now
- Possibly harmful substance in the eye
  Exception: Mace, pepper spray, soap, sunscreen lotion, or other obviously harmless substance
  FIRST AID: Irrigate eye immediately before calling Poison Center.

Go to Office Now

- Cloudy spot or sore on the cornea (clear central part of eye)
  FIRST AID: Irrigate eye immediately after exposure to harmful substance.
- Blurred vision that persists >1 hour after irrigation
  R/O: corneal damage
- Eye pain that persists > 1 hour after irrigation
  R/O: corneal damage
- Continued tearing or blinking that persists > 1 hour after irrigation
  R/O: corneal damage

See Today in Office

- Redness persists > 24 hours
  FIRST AID: Irrigate eye immediately afterwards.
  R/O: conjunctivitis
- Patient wants to be seen

Home Care

- Mace or pepper spray was sprayed into face/eyes
  FIRST AID: Irrigate eye immediately.
- Eye irritation from harmless chemical
  FIRST AID: Irrigate eye immediately.
  Note: See harmless list.

HOME CARE ADVICE FOR HARMLESS CHEMICAL IN THE EYE

1. **Irrigate the Eye Immediately.**
2. **Eye Irrigation Method #1—Immersion:**
   - Immerse the entire face into a sink or basin filled with lukewarm tap water.
   - With the face under water, open and close the eyelids. You may need to use your fingers. Look from side to side.
3. **Eye Irrigation Method #2—Flushing:**
   - Slowly pour lukewarm water into the eye from a pitcher or glass.
   - Or place your head under a gently running faucet or shower.
   - Hold the eyelid open during this process.
4. **Duration of Irrigation for Harmless Substances:**
   - For harmless substances (e.g., household soap, sunscreen, or hair spray), irrigation only needs to be carried out for 2-3 minutes.
   - For stronger chemicals that cause more irritation and stinging (e.g., ammonia, vinegar, alcohol, or household bleach), flush the eye for 5-10 minutes.
5. **Vasoconstrictor Eyedrops:** Red eyes from irritants usually feel much better after the irritant has been washed out. If they remain uncomfortable and bloodshot, use some long-acting vasoconstrictor eyedrops (e.g., Visine). Use 1 to 2 drops. May repeat once in 8-12 hours.

6. **Contacts:** Patients with contact lenses need to switch to glasses temporarily (Reason: to prevent damage to the cornea).
7. **Expected Course:** The pain and discomfort usually pass 1 hour after irrigation.
8. **Call Back If:**
   - Pain or blurred vision lasts longer than 1 hour after irrigation.
   - Redness lasts longer than 24 hours.
   - You become worse.

FIRST AID

First Aid Advice for Chemical in the Eye:

- Immediate and thorough irrigation of the eye with tap water should be done as quickly as possible (Reason: to prevent damage to the cornea).
- If one eye is not burned, cover it (if possible) while irrigating the other.

Duration of Irrigation:

- For HARMLESS SUBSTANCES (e.g., sunscreen or hair spray), irrigation only needs to be carried out for 2-3 minutes.
- For STRONGER CHEMICALS that cause more irritation and stinging (e.g., ammonia, vinegar, alcohol, or household bleach), flush the eye for 5-10 minutes.
- For ACIDS, irrigate the eye continuously for 10 minutes.
- For ALKALIS, irrigate the eye continuously for 20 minutes.
- For any CHEMICAL PARTICLES that can't be flushed away, wipe them away with a moistened cotton swab.

Special Notes:

- Never irrigate with antidotes such as vinegar (Reason: the chemical reaction can cause more damage).
- Tell the patient to call back immediately if they are unable to carry out the irrigation (Reason: needs a topical anesthetic in the ED).

BACKGROUND INFORMATION

Causes

- **Harmless Chemicals:** These include soap, hair spray, and sunscreen. They cause no symptoms or transient irritation.
- **Harmless Chemicals That Cause More Stinging:** Examples are alcohol or hydrocarbons. They cause temporary stinging and superficial irritation (pink sclera), but no lasting damage.
- **Harmful Chemicals:** Acids (e.g., toilet bowl cleaners) and alkalis (e.g., oven cleaners) splashed into the eye can cause severe eye pain and permanently damage the cornea. Alkali burns cause more damage than acid burns.
- **Mace and Pepper Spray:** Mace and pepper spray are used in personal protection devices. Eye exposure results in marked eye pain and tearing. Usually these symptoms subside in 30 minutes and there is no lasting damage.

Harmless Chemicals

- The following liquid products are harmless to the eye: bubble bath, cosmetics, deodorant, foods (e.g., lemon juice), glow stick liquid, hair conditioner, hair spray, hand lotion, laundry detergent (liquid), medications, shampoo, shaving cream, soap, sunscreen, and toothpaste.
- The following substances are also harmless but will cause transient irritation: hydrogen peroxide, ethyl alcohol (ethanol), automobile gasoline, and vinegar. Brief irrigation of the eye is indicated.

Harmful Chemicals

- Eye contact with acids or alkalis can cause severe damage to the eye. Both need immediate irrigation followed by immediate referral to an emergency department.
- **Acids:** Acids include hydrochloric acid, nitric acid, sulfuric acid, phosphoric acid, oxalic acid, or any other product labeled as an acid. Products that are called drain cleaners, toilet bowl cleaners, metal cleaners, descalers, or battery fluid can be assumed to contain acid until proven otherwise.

- **Alakalis:** Alkalis include lime, lye, potassium hydroxide, sodium hydroxide, calcium hydroxide, and industrial-strength ammonia. Any product that is called a drain cleaner, oven cleaner, bathroom cleaner, or industrial cleaner should be assumed to contain alkali until proven otherwise.
- Two weak alkalis that usually don't cause any harm are household bleach and household ammonia. For these exposures, instruct the caller to call the Poison Center after irrigation to determine if the particular product is harmful.

Call Poison Center

- Tell the caller to call the Poison Center immediately after irrigation is completed. One exception to this would be a definitely harmless chemical. Another exception to this would be a definitely harmful chemical like an acid or alkali (since for these the victim should go immediately to the emergency department after irrigation).
- **United States:** Give them the national toll-free number: 800-222-1222.
- **Canada:** Call local poison control center.
- **If a Poison Control Center Is Unavailable:** Triager, call back the patient in 10-20 minutes after the irrigation time is up. Ask the remaining triage questions.

EYE, FOREIGN BODY

DEFINITION

- A foreign body (FB) or object becomes lodged in the eye.
- The main symptoms are irritation, pain, tearing, and blinking.
- Also includes calls about a contact stuck in the eye.

TRIAGE ASSESSMENT QUESTIONS

See More Appropriate Protocol

- Doesn't sound like FB in the eye
  Go to Protocol: Eye, Red Without Pus on page 115
- Foreign body is a chemical
  Go to Protocol: Eye, Chemical In on page 108

Go to ED Now (or to Office With PCP Approval)

- FB stuck on eyeball
  R/O: embedded foreign body
- FB hit eye at high speed (e.g., small metallic chip from hammering, lawn mower, BB gun, explosion)
  R/O: intraocular foreign body
- Cloudy spot on the cornea (clear part of the eye)
  R/O: retained FB, tiny abrasion
- Sounds like a serious injury to the triager

Go to Office Now

- Severe eye pain
- Sharp FB (even if FB was removed)
  R/O: corneal abrasion, other eye damage
- Eye has been washed out > 30 minutes ago and still feels like FB is still present
  Reason: FB can cause corneal abrasion
- Eye has been washed out > 30 minutes ago and pain persists
  Reason: FB can cause corneal abrasion
- Eye has been washed out > 30 minutes ago and tearing or blinking persists
  Reason: FB can cause corneal abrasion
- Eye has been washed out > 30 minutes ago and blurred vision persists
  Reason: FB can cause corneal abrasion

See Today in Office

- Yellow or green pus occurs
  R/O: retained FB
- Contact lens stuck in eye and unable to remove using care advice
- Patient wants to be seen

Home Care

- Minor FB in the eye (e.g., eyelash, dirt, sand)
  Reason: probably can be removed at home
- FB was successfully removed, and now no symptoms
- Contact lens stuck in eye

HOME CARE ADVICE

Removing a Foreign Body From the Eye

1. **Treatment for Numerous Particles (Such as Dirt or Sand):**
   - Clean around the eye with a wet washcloth first.
   - Try to open and close the eye repeatedly while submerging that side of the face in a pan of water.
2. **Treatment for a Particle in a Corner of the Eye:** Try to get it out with a moistened cotton swab or the corner of a moistened cloth.
3. **Treatment for a Particle Under the Lower Lid:**
   - Pull the lower lid out by pulling down on the skin over the cheekbone.
   - Touch the particle with a moistened cotton swab.
   - If that does not work, try pouring water on the speck while pulling the lower lid out.
4. **Treatment for a Particle Under the Upper Lid:**
   - If particle cannot be seen, it is probably under the upper lid, the most common hiding place.
   - Try to open and close the eye several times while it is submerged in a pan or bowl of water. Or turn your head to the side and flush the eye using the faucet.
   - If this fails, pull the upper lid out and draw it over the lower lid. This maneuver, and tears, will sometimes dislodge the particle. By doing this the lower eyelashes may sweep the particle out from under the upper eyelid.

5. **Expected Course:** The discomfort, redness, and excessive tearing usually pass 1 to 2 hours after the FB is removed.
6. **Contacts:** Patients with contact lenses need to switch to glasses temporarily (Reason: to prevent damage to the cornea).
7. **Call Back If:**
   - This approach does not remove all the foreign material from the eye (i.e., the sensation of "grittiness" or pain persists).
   - Vision does not return to normal after the eye has been irrigated.
   - Foreign object has been removed, but tearing and blinking persist.
   - You become worse.

Removing a Contact Lens

1. **Reassurance:**
   - It sounds like something you should be able to remove at home.
   - It may reassure you to know, if you did not know this already, that a contact lens cannot go behind the eyeball. A contact lens can sometimes get hidden under your upper or lower eyelid.
   - I am going to give you some instructions.
   - Your first step will be to wash your hands with soap and water.
2. **Moisten the Contact Lens:**
   - Place several drops of saline into the eye.
   - You may need to repeat this in 5 minutes (Reason: hydrates soft contacts; helps lubricate and float soft and hard contacts).
3. **Removing a Soft Contact Lens:**
   - Look upward.
   - Pull down your lower eyelid with your middle finger.
   - Touch contact lens with your index finger and slide the lens downward to the lower white part of your eye.
   - Gently pinch the contact lens between your thumb and index finger and remove it from your eye.
4. **Removing a Hard Contact Lens—Blink Method:**
   - Pull outwards on the skin at the corner of the eye (right index finger for right eye; left index finger for left eye).
   - Cup your other hand under the eye to catch the contact lens.
   - Blink several times.
5. **Removing a Hard Contact Lens—Plunger Method**
   - Use a contact lens "plunger" to remove the contact lens.
   - If you do not have one, you can get one at a local pharmacy. This is a small, flexible plastic tool that has a suction cup on it.
6. **Call Back If:**
   - Unable to remove the contact lens.
   - Pain or foreign body sensation persists more than 2 hours after removing the contact lens.
   - You become worse.

FIRST AID

First Aid Advice for Glass Fragments on the Eyelids:

- **Method 1:** Bend forward and close the eyes. Have someone blow on the closed eyelids to get the flakes of glass off the skin.
- **Method 2:** Another technique is to touch the flakes of glass with a piece of tape.
- To get off any remaining glass, splash water on the eyelids and face. Cover the eyes with a wet washcloth. Do not rub your eyes.

BACKGROUND INFORMATION

General Information

- Foreign bodies in the eye need to be removed, as they can damage the eye.
- The most common objects that get in the eye are an eyelash or a piece of dried mucus (sleep). Particulate matter such as sand, dirt, sawdust, or grit can be blown into the eyes. Tree and plant pollen can also get blown into the eyes.
- Rubbing the eye can lead to the foreign object scratching the cornea (clear part in center of eye).

EYE, PUS OR DISCHARGE

DEFINITION

- Yellow or green discharge (pus) in one or both eyes.
- Dried pus on the eyelids and eyelashes. The eyelashes are especially likely to be matted together following sleep.
- The white portions of the eye (sclera) may be pink or red (not required).
- The eyelids are usually puffy due to irritation from the infection.
- Includes calls about adults receiving antibiotic eyedrops who are not improving or may be allergic to the eyedrops.

TRIAGE ASSESSMENT QUESTIONS

See More Appropriate Protocol

- Eye exposure to chemical or fumes
  Go to Protocol: Eye, Chemical In on page 108
- Redness of white of eye (sclera), but no pus or a small amount of transient pus
  Go to Protocol: Eye, Red Without Pus on page 115

Go to ED Now (or to Office With PCP Approval)

- Severe pain
  R/O: corneal ulcer
- Patient sounds very sick or weak to the triager
  R/O: periobital cellulitis

Go to Office Now

- Blurred vision
- Cloudy spot or sore seen on the cornea (clear part of the eye)
  R/O: corneal ulcer, herpes
- Eyelids are very swollen (shut or almost)
  R/O: periorbital cellulitis or preseptal cellulitis
- Eyelid (outer) is very red and painful (or tender to touch)
- Fever > 104° F (40.0° C)
- Eye pain/discomfort that is more than mild
  R/O: corneal ulcer, herpes, hyperacute bacterial conjunctivitis

See Today in Office

- Discharge from penis
  R/O: sexually transmitted disease (STD), chlamydia conjunctivitis
- New or abnormal vaginal discharge
  R/O: sexually transmitted disease (STD), chlamydia conjunctivitis
- Using antibiotic eyedrops > 3 days but pus persists
  R/O: resistant bacteria
- Using antibiotic eyedrops and now eyes have become very itchy (especially after eyedrops are put in)
  R/O: eye allergy to antibiotic
- Lots of yellow or green nasal discharge
  R/O: concurrent sinusitis
- Immunocompromised (e.g., HIV positive, cancer chemotherapy, splenectomy, organ transplant, chronic steroids)
- Patient wants to be seen

See Today or Tomorrow in Office

- Fever present > 3 days (72 hours)
- Bleeding on white of the eye
  Reason: probably hemorrhagic conjunctivitis from adenovirus or enterovirus, but patient needs reassurance

Callback by PCP Today

- Eye with yellow/green discharge or eyelashes stick together, but NO standing order to call in antibiotic eyedrops

Home Care

- Eye with purulent discharge
  Reason: probable mild bacterial or viral conjunctivitis without complications
- Very small amount of discharge and only in corner of eye
  Reason: probable viral conjunctivitis without complications

HOME CARE ADVICE FOR PUS OR DRAINAGE FROM EYE (Pending Talking With Your Doctor)

1. **Reassurance:** Pinkeye is a common complication of a cold or it can be acquired from exposure to a child or adult who has had it recently. Pinkeye responds to treatment with antibiotic eyedrops and is not harmful to vision.
2. **Prescription Antibiotic Eyedrops—United States:**
   - Use tobramycin eyedrops—2 drops 4-6 times daily.
   - Continue using eyedrops until you have awakened 2 mornings without pus in the eyes.
   - Read the package instructions and warnings.
3. **OTC Antibiotic Eyedrops—Canada:**
   - Polysporin eyedrops are available over-the-counter (OTC). Use 2 drops 4-6 times daily.
   - Continue using the eyedrops until you have awakened 2 mornings without pus in the eyes.
   - Read the package instructions and warnings.
4. **Eyelid Cleansing:**
   - Gently wash eyelids and lashes with warm water and wet cotton balls (or cotton gauze).
   - Remove all the dried and liquid pus.
   - Do this as often as needed.
5. **Contacts:**
   - Individuals with contact lenses need to switch to glasses temporarily (Reason: to prevent damage to the cornea).
   - Disinfect the contacts before wearing them again (or discard them if disposable).
6. **Expected Course:** With treatment, the yellow discharge should clear up in 3 days. The red eyes may persist for several more days.
7. **Contagiousness:**
   - Pinkeye is contagious. Try not to touch your eyes. Wash your hands frequently. Do not share towels.
   - You may return to work or school. Avoid physical contact (e.g., shaking hands) until the symptoms have resolved.
8. **Call Back If:**
   - You become worse.

BACKGROUND INFORMATION

Causes of Ocular Discharge

- Bacterial conjunctivitis (thick white-yellow discharge; eyelashes sticky or eyes feel "glued" shut in morning)
- Viral conjunctivitis (thin, clear-white discharge)
- Allergic conjunctivitis (itching, clear-white discharge)
- Chemical conjunctivitis from exposure to chemicals, fumes (eye irritation, tearing)

Bacterial Conjunctivitis

Purulent discharge from the eye with redness is suggestive of a bacterial conjunctivitis. Bacterial conjunctivitis requires treatment with antibiotic eyedrops. It is a common complication of a cold and starts off as a viral conjunctivitis. The symptoms can occur in one or both eyes. Other symptoms that a caller might describe include:

- Mild discomfort or mild burning of the eye(s).
- Dried pus on the eyelids and eyelashes; eyelids are stuck together upon awakening; eye discharge tends to recur througout the day.
- Eyelids may be puffy due to irritation from the infection.
- Tearing.

Eye Discharge and Cause

- Red eyes without a discharge are presumed to not be bacterial. A small amount of pus (or mucus) that's only present in the corner of the eye is usually viral or due to an irritant. Even matting (sticking together) of the eyelids after a night's sleep and that doesn't recur during the day is viral, unless it progresses.
- Eye discharge that recurs throughout the day is 80% bacterial according to Weiss 1993. Note: some viruses can cause purulent conjunctivitis (e.g., adenovirus).

Caution—Eye Pain or Blurred Vision

Patients with significant eye pain or any blurred vision need to be seen within 4 hours as significant eye pain and blurred vision do not generally occur in patients with regular conjunctivitis.

EYE, RED WITHOUT PUS

DEFINITION

- Redness or pinkness of the sclera and inner eyelids
- May have increased tearing (watery eye)
- Not due to a traumatic injury

Excluded: Yellow or green pus in the eyes;
see Eye, Pus or Discharge protocol on page 113.

TRIAGE ASSESSMENT QUESTIONS

See More Appropriate Protocol

- Chemical got in the eye
  Go to Protocol: Eye, Chemical In on page 108
- Piece of something got in the eye
  Go to Protocol: Eye, Foreign Body on page 111
- Eye redness following an injury
  Go to Protocol: Trauma, Eye on page 280
- Yellow or green pus in the eyes
  Go to Protocol: Eye, Pus or Discharge on page 113

Go to ED Now (or to Office With PCP Approval)

- Severe eye pain
  R/O: acute angle-closure glaucoma
- Patient sounds very sick or weak to the triager
  R/O: periobital cellulitis

Go to Office Now

- Blurred vision
- Cloudy spot or sore seen on the cornea (clear part of the eye)
  R/O: corneal ulcer, herpes
- Eyelids are very swollen (shut or almost)
  R/O: periorbital cellulitis or preseptal cellulitis
- Eyelid (outer) is very red
  R/O: periorbital cellulitis or preseptal cellulitis
- Vomiting
  R/O: acute angle-closure glaucoma, migraine
- Foreign body sensation ("feels like something is in there")
  R/O: corneal abrasion, foreign body
- Recent eye surgery and has increasing eye pain
  R/O: endophthalmitis
- Eye pain/discomfort that is more than mild
  R/O: corneal ulcer, herpes, iritis

See Today in Office

- Patient wants to be seen
- Eye pain present > 24 hours
  R/O: forgotten corneal abrasion, occult foreign body, iritis, herpes simplex
- Bleeding on white of the eye and is taking Coumadin or known bleeding disorder (e.g., thrombocytopenia)
  Reason: need for testing of INR, prothrombin time
- Only 1 eye is red, and persists > 48 hours
  R/O: tiny foreign body

See Today or Tomorrow in Office

- Red eyes present > 7 days
- Bleeding on white of the eye
  R/O: subconjunctival hemorrhage, conjunctivitis

Home Care

- Red eye caused by sunscreen, smoke, smog, chlorine, food, soap, or other mild irritant
  Reason: probable minor chemical conjunctivitis
- Red eye caused by contact lens
  Reason: probable contact lens overuse
- Red eye and no complications
  R/O: viral conjunctivitis (pinkeye)

HOME CARE ADVICE FOR EYE, RED WITHOUT PUS

1. **Red Eye Caused by Mild Irritant** (e.g., sunscreen, smoke, smog, chlorine, food, soap, or other mild irritant):
   - **Reassurance:** Most eye irritants cause transient redness of the eyes.
   - **Face Cleansing:** Wash the face, then the eyelids, with a mild soap and water. This will remove any irritants. Also try to avoid the irritant.
   - **Eye Irrigation:** Irrigate the eye with warm water for 2-3 minutes.
   - **Vasoconstrictor Eyedrops:** If your eyes remain uncomfortable after irrigation and are still bloodshot, use some long-acting OTC vasoconstrictor eye drops (e.g., Visine). Use 1 to 2 drops. May repeat once in 8-12 hours.
   - **Remove Contacts:** Remove your contact lenses; you need to switch to glasses temporarily (Reason: to prevent damage to the cornea).

- **Expected Course:** After removal of the irritant, the eyes usually return to normal color in 1 to 2 hours.

2. **Red Eye Caused by Contacts:**
   - **Reassurance:** It is reassuring that you have no blurred vision and that there is minimal to no discomfort. Sometimes people who wear contacts can develop eye irritation, especially if they wear their contacts too long.
   - **Remove Contacts:** Remove your contact lenses; you need to switch to glasses temporarily (Reason: to prevent damage to the cornea).
   - **No Rubbing:** Do not rub your eyes (Reason: can cause a corneal abrasion or worsen an existing abrasion).
   - **Expected Course:** The pain and irritation should go away over the next 12-24 hours. If it does not, you will need an examination (Reason: possible corneal abrasion or ulcer).
3. **Red Eye Caused by Pinkeye:**
   - **Reassurance:** It is reassuring that you have no blurred vision and that there is minimal to no discomfort. One cause of minor eye redness is pinkeye (viral conjunctivitis). People with pinkeye may often note mild eye irritation and a watery discharge. Often it affects both eyes. It can occur with a cold. It generally is not serious.
   - **Remove Contacts:** Remove your contact lenses; you need to switch to glasses temporarily (Reason: to prevent damage to the cornea).
   - **No Rubbing:** Do not rub your eyes (Reason: can cause a corneal abrasion or worsen an existing abrasion).
   - **Contagiousness:** Pinkeye is extremely contagious. Try not to touch your eyes. Wash your hands frequently. Do not share towels.
   - **Expected Course:** Pinkeye with a cold usually lasts about 7 days.
4. **Call Back If:**
   - Blurred vision or increasing pain.
   - No improvement.
   - You become worse.

BACKGROUND INFORMATION

General

- The presence of either severe pain or blurring of the vision in a patient with a red eye requires urgent evaluation.
- Common causes of a red eye include blepharitis, conjunctivitis, allergy, and subconjunctival hemorrhage.

Causes

- Abrasion of cornea
- Acute angle-closure glaucoma
- Blepharitis
- Conjunctivitis—allergic
- Conjunctivitis—chemical/irritants (e.g., sunscreen, soap, chlorinated pool water, smoke, or smog)
- Conjunctivitis—viral
- Corneal foreign body
- Corneal ulcer
- Episcleritis and scleritis
- Glaucoma
- Keratitis (inflammation of the cornea)
- Subconjunctival hemorrhage
- Trauma
- Uveitis (iritis, iridoscyclitis)

Blepharitis

- **Definition:** Blockage of the oil glands along the eyelid margins results in inflammation. Crusting and flaking skin are present at the base of the eyelashes.
- **Pain:** Minimal to absent. May describe chronic irritation of eyelids and eyes.
- **Vision Loss:** None.
- **Treatment:** Gentle daily scrubbing of the eyelid margins with a dilute baby shampoo solution and frequent application of warm compresses.

Viral Conjunctivitis

- **Definition:** Viral infection of the conjunctiva of the eye. The whites of the eyes become diffusely red or pink because of blood vessel dilatation in the conjunctiva. A watery discharge is common. Mild eyelid swelling may occur. Usually both eyes are affected. It is also called pinkeye.
- **Pain:** Minimal to absent. May describe mild irritation or itching.
- **Vision Loss:** None.
- **Treatment:** Viral conjunctivitis resolves on its own. Some physicians will prescribe antibiotic drops so as to prevent bacterial superinfection. Viral conjunctivitis is contagious; the patient should not share towels, should wash hands frequently, and should avoid close contact with others for 2 weeks.

Subconjunctival Hemorrhage

- **Definition:** Localized area of bleeding into the white area (sclera) of the eye. The fragile blood vessels in this area can rupture as a result of minor and sometimes forgotten trauma or from forceful coughing or vomiting. It can also occur spontaneously. It is nearly always unilateral.
- **Pain:** None.
- **Vision Loss:** None.
- **Treatment:** No specific treatment is required. Area of hemorrhage should gradually clear in 2-3 weeks.

FAINTING

DEFINITION

- Fainting is a brief (transient) loss of consciousness (passing out) with falling down.
- Spontaneous recovery with return to full awareness usually occurs in less than 1 minute.
- Also called passing out or syncope.
- **Note:** Remaining unconscious (coma) is an emergency.

TRIAGE ASSESSMENT QUESTIONS

Call EMS 911 Now

- Still unconscious
  R/O: coma, postictal after unwitnessed seizure
- Still feels dizzy or light-headed
  R/O: hypovolemia, arrhythmia
- Difficult to awaken or acting confused (e.g., disoriented, slurred speech)
  R/O: shock, CVA, hypoglycemia, postictal
- Difficulty breathing
  R/O: hypoxia and need for oxygen
- Lips or face are bluish now
  R/O: hypoxia and need for oxygen
- Shock suspected (e.g., cold/pale/clammy skin, too weak to stand)
  R/O: shock
  FIRST AID: Lie down with the feet elevated.
- Bleeding (e.g., vomiting blood, rectal bleeding or tarry stools, severe vaginal bleeding)
- Chest pain
  R/O: AMI, PE
- Extra heartbeats or heart is beating fast (i.e., "palpitations")
  R/O: dysrhythmia
- Heart beating < 50 beats per minute OR > 140 beats per minute
- Fainted suddenly after medicine, allergic food, or bee sting
  R/O: anaphylaxis
- Sounds like a life-threatening emergency to the triager

Go to ED Now

- Fainted > 15 minutes ago and still looks pale (pale skin, pallor)
  R/O: anemia, GI bleeding
- Fainted > 15 minutes ago and still feels too weak or dizzy to stand
  R/O: hypovolemia, dehydration
- History of heart problems or congestive heart failure
  Reason: greater risk of arrhythmia as cause of syncope
- Occurred during exercise
  R/O: cardiac arrhythmia, structural heart disease
- Any head or face injury
  Reason: suggests sudden loss of consciousness (short duration of warning)

Go to ED Now (or to Office With PCP Approval)

- Age > 50 years
  Reason: higher risk for cardiac disease and other serious causes of syncope
- Drinking very little and has signs of dehydration (e.g., no urine > 12 hours, very dry mouth)
- Fainted 2 times in 1 day
- Patient sounds very sick or weak to the triager

See Today in Office

- All other patients, and now alert and feels fine
  Exception: Simple faint due to stress, pain, prolonged standing, or suddenly standing
- Patient wants to be seen

See Within 2 Weeks in Office

- Simple fainting is a chronic symptom (has occurred multiple times)

Home Care

- Sudden standing caused simple fainting, and now alert and feels fine
  R/O: simple faint
- Prolonged standing caused simple fainting, and now alert and feels fine
  R/O: simple faint
- Fear, stress, or pain caused simple fainting, and now alert and feels fine
  R/O: simple faint (vasovagal syncope)

HOME CARE ADVICE FOR SIMPLE FAINT

General Care Advice

1. **Treatment:**
   - Lie down with feet elevated for 10 minutes (Reason: simple fainting is due to temporarily decreased blood flow to the brain).
   - Drink some fruit juice, especially if you have missed a meal or have not eaten in over 6 hours.
2. **Expected Course:** Most adults with a simple faint are back to normal after lying down for 10 minutes.
3. **Warning Symptoms for Fainting:**
   - Fainting usually has early warning symptoms (e.g., dizziness, blurred vision, nausea, feeling cold or warm).
   - If you feel these warning symptoms, immediately lie down to prevent falling down. You only have 5 seconds to act (Reason: almost impossible to faint when lying down).
   - Lying down (even on the floor) is less embarrassing than fainting, no matter where you are.
   - Sitting down (with head between knees) is certainly better than staying standing up but is less effective than lying down.
4. **Pregnancy Test, When in Doubt:**
   - If there is any possibility of pregnancy, obtain and use a urine pregnancy test from the local drugstore.
   - Follow the instructions included in the package.
5. **Call Back If:**
   - You pass out again on the same day.
   - You are pregnant.
   - You become worse.

Simple Faint From Standing Up Suddenly

1. **Reassurance:**
   - Standing up suddenly after lying down can cause temporary dizziness in anyone. If you don't sit back down when this happens, fainting can sometimes occur.
   - It is caused by temporary blood pooling in the legs and not enough blood getting to the brain.
   - It is usually not serious and is preventable.
2. **Prevention:**
   - Most fainting can be prevented.
   - When getting out of bed, sit on the edge for a few minutes before standing. If you feel dizzy, sit or lie down.
   - **Water and Salt Are Key:** If you have this tendency, drink extra fluids every day. Also, add some mildy salty foods (saltine crackers, soup) to your diet.

Simple Faint From Prolonged Standing

1. **Reassurance:**
   - Standing for too long in one position is a common cause of fainting.
   - It is caused by temporary blood pooling in the legs and not enough blood getting to the brain.
   - It is usually not serious and it is preventable.
2. **Prevention:**
   - If prolonged standing is required, repeatedly contract and relax the leg muscles. This will pump the blood back to the heart.
   - Try to avoid standing in one place for too long with your knees locked.
   - **Water and Salt Are Key:** If you have this tendency, drink extra fluids every day. Also, add some mildy salty foods (saltine crackers, soup) to your diet.

Simple Faint From Fear/Stress/Pain

1. **Reassurance:**
   - Some people faint if they experience a painful, frightening, or emotional event. Examples include getting a shot, having a bloody wound, or seeing someone else bleed.
   - For some people this is a normal reaction to stress and shouldn't cause any lasting effects.
   - It is caused by temporary blood pooling in the legs and not enough blood getting to the brain.
   - It is usually not serious and it is preventable.
2. **Prevention:**
   - Preventing fainting from stressful events is not always possible. However, here are some important tips that may help.
   - If you know you are at risk for fainting under certain circumstances (such as a shot in the doctor's office), lie down in advance.
   - Try thinking about something else. Visualize yourself on the beach or with a friend.
   - You can also learn relaxation exercises (relaxing every muscle in the body).

FIRST AID

First Aid Advice for Fainting:

Lie down with the feet elevated.

First Aid Advice for Shock:

Lie down with the feet elevated.

BACKGROUND INFORMATION

General

- Fainting (syncope) is a transient loss of consciousness due to a reduction in cerebral blood flow.
- Thus, anything that temporarily reduces blood flow to the brain can cause a person to faint; if sitting the person loses postural tone and slumps over, if standing the person falls to the ground.
- There are serious and nonserious causes of syncope.

Findings Suggestive of Serious Cause for Syncope

- Age > 50
- Known cardiac disease
- Presence of head or face injury
- Persisting decreased level of alertness after syncopal event
- Occurs during exercise
- **Has Other Symptoms:** Cardiorespiratory, neurologic, GI, or genitourinary

Causes of Syncope That Require Emergent Evaluation

- Abdominal aortic aneurysm
- Arrhythmias and cardiac conduction disorders resulting in bradycardia and tachycardia
- CVA/TIA
- Ectopic pregnancy
- GI bleeding
- Myocardial infarction
- Pulmonary embolism
- Seizure (may be mistaken for syncope)
- Subarachnoid hemorrhage

Findings Suggestive of Nonserious Cause for Syncope

- Age < 50
- No injury from fainting
- Now feels normal and is fully alert
- **No Other Symptoms:** Cardiorespiratory, neurologic, GI, or genitorurinary

Simple Faints

- **Introduction:** Simple faints can occur in healthy individuals due to stress, pain, prolonged standing, or suddenly standing up. It is the most common reason for syncope; perhaps 80% of all fainting occurs in this manner. It is also called vasovagal or vasomotor syncope.
- **Physiology:** When an individual is exposed to some sort of stimulus (e.g., pain, stress, prolonged standing), a reflex controlled by the vasomotor center in the brain stem is triggered; it tells the blood vessels in the legs to dilate, causing pooling of blood in the legs; there is less blood flow to the brain; as a result fainting occurs.
- **Warning Signs (Pre-syncope):** There are a number of warning signs that occur immediately before a simple faint. These include pallor, dizziness (light-headedness), feeling cold or warm, blurred vision, nausea or vague stomach discomfort, sweating, feeling cold. These warning symptoms last for 5 to 10 seconds before passing out occurs. Fainting can sometimes be prevented by sitting down, or even better lying down.
- **Symptoms:** A brief period of warning symptoms (e.g., dizziness, nausea), followed by unconsciousness, with return to full awareness usually in less than 1 minute; afterwards feeling normal.
- **Expected Course:** There is often a feeling of tiredness or mild malaise (e.g, being "washed out") for a period of time after a vasovagal fainting episode.
- **Predisposing Factors:** Mild dehydration, fasting, hot weather, sleep deprivation, recent illness, pregnancy, change in altitude.
- **Causes:** Listed on next page.

Simple Faints—Causes

- **Prolonged Standing in One Position Prior to Fainting (Called Orthostatic Syncope):** This is a common cause of simple faints. It commonly occurs at church, graduations, weddings, school assemblies, parades, etc. It is more common if one keeps one's knees "locked"—due to pooling of blood in the legs. Anyone who stands long enough in one position will eventually faint.
- **Standing Up Suddenly (Especially After Lying Down) Prior to Fainting (Called Orthostatic Syncope):** Usually this just causes transient dizziness. It is more common in the morning after overnight fasting and relative dehydration.
- **Sudden Fearful or Disgusting Event (Emotional Pain) Prior to Fainting (Called Vasovagal Syncope):** Examples are any kind of blood-and-guts scenario such as seeing someone vomit, bleed, or pass a stool. Seeing a badly injured person or pet can precipitate syncope. It can also occur prior to an injection or public performance (e.g., a speech or musical recital).
- **Sudden Physical Pain Prior to Fainting (Called Vasovagal Syncope):** Examples are receiving an injection (e.g., postimmunization syncope), having a sliver or sutures removed, or blood draw for lab tests. The stress of the experience probably has more to do with the syncope than the pain itself.

FEVER

DEFINITION

- Fever is the only symptom.

Fever can be defined using one of the following measurements:

- Oral temperature > 100.0° F (37.8° C).
- Ear (tympanic) temperature > 100.4° F (38.0° C).
- Rectal temperature > 100.4° F (38.0° C).
- Forehead temperature strips are unreliable.

Note: If another symptom is present, see that guideline (e.g., symptoms of cough, runny nose, sore throat, earache, abdominal pain, diarrhea, vomiting).

TRIAGE ASSESSMENT QUESTIONS

Call EMS 911 Now

- Difficult to awaken or acting confused (e.g., disoriented, slurred speech)
  R/O: sepsis, shock
- Pale cold skin and very weak (can't stand)
- Difficulty breathing and has bluish lips, tongue or face
  R/O: cyanosis and need for oxygen
- Rash with purple (or blood-colored) spots or dots
  R/O: meningococcemia
- Sounds like a life-threatening emergency to the triager

See More Appropriate Protocol

- Fever onset within 24 hours of receiving vaccine
  Go to Protocol: Immunization Reactions on page 155
- Fever onset 6-12 days after measles vaccine OR 14-28 days after chickenpox vaccine
  Go to Protocol: Immunization Reactions on page 155

Go to ED Now

- Headache and stiff neck (can't touch chin to chest)
  R/O: meningitis
- Difficulty breathing
  R/O: pneumonia
- IV drug abuse
  R/O: endocarditis

Go to ED Now (or to Office With PCP Approval)

- Fever > 103° F (39.4° C)
  R/O: bacterial infection
- Fever > 100.5° F (38.1° C) and over 60 years of age
  R/O: bacterial infection
- Fever > 100.5° F (38.1° C) and diabetes mellitus or a weakened immune system (e.g., HIV positive, chemotherapy, splenectomy)
  R/O: bacterial infection
- Fever > 100.5° F (38.1° C) and bedridden (e.g., nursing home patient, stroke, chronic illness, recovering from surgery)
  R/O: bacterial infection
  Note: may need ambulance transport to ED.
- Fever > 100.5° F (38.1° C) and indwelling urinary catheter (e.g., Foley, coudé)
  R/O: bacterial infection
- Drinking very little and has signs of dehydration (e.g., no urine > 12 hours, very dry mouth, very light-headed)
- Patient sounds very sick or weak to the triager

Go to Office Now

- Fever > 100.5° F (38.1° C) and surgery in the past month
  R/O: UTI or other bacterial infection
- Transplant patient (e.g., liver, heart, lung, kidney)
  R/O: bacterial infection
- Has central line, PICC line, or peripheral intravenous line
  R/O: catheter bacteremia
- Widespread rash and cause unknown

See Today in Office

- Patient wants to be seen

See Today or Tomorrow in Office

- Fever present > 3 days (72 hours)
  Reason: unexplained fever
- Intermittent fever > 100.5° F persists > 3 weeks
- Fever > 100.5° F (38.1° C) and foreign travel to a developing country in the past month
  R/O: malaria, typhoid fever, dengue, leptospirosis, rickettsia, et.al.

Home Care

- ○ Fever without localizing symptoms

HOME CARE ADVICE FOR FEVER

1. **Reasurance:** The presence of a fever usually means that you have an infection. Most fevers are good and help the body fight infection. The goal of fever therapy is to bring the fever down to a comfortable level. Use the following definitions to help put the level of fever into proper perspective:
   - **100-102° F (37.8 - 38.9° C):** Low-grade fevers and may help body fight infection.
   - **102-104° F (38.9 - 40° C):** Moderate-grade fevers; cause discomfort.
   - **Over 104° F (over 40° C):** High fevers; cause discomfort, weakness, headache, lethargy.
   - **Over 107° F (over 41.7° C):** The fever itself can be harmful.
2. **For All Fevers:**
   - Drink cold fluids orally to prevent dehydration (Reason: good hydration replaces sweat and improves heat loss via skin). Adults should drink 6-8 glasses of water daily.
   - Dress in one layer of lightweight clothing and sleep with one light blanket.
   - For fevers 100-101° F (37.8-38.3° C) this is the only treatment and fever medicine is unnecessary.
3. **Fever Medicines:**
   - For fevers above 101° F (38.3° C) take acetaminophen or ibuprofen.
   - The goal of fever therapy is to bring the fever down to a comfortable level. Remember that
   - fever medicine usually lowers fever 2 degrees F (1 - 1½ degrees C).

   Acetaminophen (e.g., Tylenol):
   - Take 650 mg by mouth every 4-6 hours. Each Regular Strength Tylenol pill has 325 mg of acetaminophen.
   - Another choice is to take 1,000 mg every 8 hours. Each Extra Strength Tylenol pill has 500 mg of acetaminophen.
   - The most you should take each day is 3,000 mg.

   Ibuprofen (e.g., Motrin, Advil):
   - Take 400 mg by mouth every 6 hours.
   - Another choice is to take 600 mg by mouth every 8 hours.
   - Use the lowest amount that makes your pain feel better.

   Extra Notes:
   - Acetaminophen is thought to be safer than ibuprofen in people over 65 years old. Acetaminophen is in many OTC and prescription medicines. It might be in more than one medicine that you are taking. You need to be careful and not take an overdose. An acetaminophen overdose can hurt the liver.
   - **Caution:** Do not take acetaminophen if you have liver disease.
   - **Caution:** Do not take ibuprofen if you have stomach problems, kidney disease, are pregnant, or have been told by your doctor to avoid this type of anti-inflammatory drug. Do not take ibuprofen for more than 7 days without consulting your doctor.
   - Before taking any medicine, read all the instructions on the package.
4. **Lukewarm Shower for Reducing Fever:** Take the fever medicine first. Take a lukewarm shower or bath for 10 minutes. Lukewarm water should be warm enough that it does not make you shiver but cold enough that it helps cool you off and reduce your temperature. Do not sponge yourself with rubbing alcohol.
5. **Expected Course:** Most fevers from a viral illness such as a cold fluctuate between 99.5 and 103° F (37.5 - 39.5° C) and last for 2 or 3 days.
6. **Contagiousness:** You can return to work or school after the fever is gone.
7. **Call Back If:**
   - Fever lasts longer than 3 days (72 hours).
   - You become worse.

FIRST AID

First Aid Advice for Shock:

Lie down with the feet elevated.

BACKGROUND INFORMATION

General

- In most clinical situations, fever does no major harm and may actually benefit the host defense mechanism. But nonetheless, fever is an abnormal finding that can signal a serious illness, especially in the old, frail, and immunocompromised adult. The absence of fever in a significant or overwhelming infection forebodes poorly.
- Adults tend to run lower fevers than children. Fever may be further blunted or even absent in elderly patients.
- Rectal temperatures are generally about 1° F (0.6° C) above oral temperatures.

Commonly Associated Symptoms

- The fever itself can cause significant muscle aches, nausea, light-headedness, weakness, and headache.
- **Chills:** Chills can sometimes precede fever. A fever occurs because the "thermostat" in the hypothalamus gets set to a higher temperature. The hypothalamus then causes the body temperature to rise in 2 ways. First, vasoconstriction of the peripheral blood vessels occurs and blood is shunted centrally. The patient notices a cold sensation in the hands and feet ("I feel really cold") and will often seek blankets or extra warmth. Second, shivering occurs from muscular contractions ("I am shivering, I have the chills").
- **Sweats:** These occur when the hypothalamic "thermostat" gets reset downward. Body temperature falls from vasodilation and sweating ("I feel hot and sweaty").

Broad Categories—Causes of Fever

- Infections
- Neoplasms
- Collagen vascular disorders
- Drugs

Normal Body Temperature

- 98.6° F (37° C) is the temperature that most physicians, nurses, laypersons, and medical references state is the "normal" temperature. Most people forget to qualify this result by including the site at which the temperature was taken (oral, tympanic, rectal).
- However, a study (Mackowiak) showed that the correct average daily oral temperature is 98.2° F (36.8° C) in healthy adults.
- The average temperature of healthy elderly patients is the same as younger adults. Though there is some data to suggest that the average temperature in chronically ill elderly patients is lower than that of other healthy adults. Interpretation of a temperature reading in a chronically ill elderly adult must be done with some caution. Given that lower baseline temperatures are expected in this group of patients, it would be easy to miss a fever if the conventional fever standards were applied to chronically ill elderly patients.

Normal Variations of Body Temperature

- There is a normal daily awake-sleep cycle variation in temperature, with the low occurring at 6:00 am and the high occurring at 6:00 pm. The low and high temperatures vary by 0.9° F (0.6° C).
- In women, temperature increases about 0.9° F (0.6° C) at the time of ovulation.
- Temperature can go up in response to exercise and as a result of climatic factors.

Recording the Temperature During the Triage Phone Call

- Record the temperature that the patient gives you and the site at which it was taken.
- For example, "Patient reports a temperature this morning of 101.2 F (oral)."

FOOT PAIN

DEFINITION

- Pain in the foot
- Not due to a traumatic injury

Pain Severity Is Defined As:

- **Mild (1-3):** Doesn't interfere with normal activities
- **Moderate (4-7):** Interferes with normal activities (e.g., work or school) or awakens from sleep, limping
- **Severe (8-10):** Excruciating pain, unable to do any normal activities, unable to walk

TRIAGE ASSESSMENT QUESTIONS

See More Appropriate Protocol

- Followed an injury
  Go to Protocol: Trauma, Ankle and Foot on page 274

Go to ED Now

- Entire foot is cool or blue in comparison to other foot
  R/O: iliofemoral arterial occlusion (ischemic foot)
- Purple or black skin on foot or toe
  R/O: iliofemoral arterial occlusion (ischemic foot) or arterial emboli

Go to ED Now (or to Office With PCP Approval)

- Red area or streak, and fever
  R/O: cellulitis, lymphangitis.
  Note: it may be difficult to determine the rash color in people with darker-colored skin.
- Swollen foot and fever
  R/O: cellulitis
- Patient sounds very sick or weak to the triager

See Today in Office

- SEVERE pain (e.g., excruciating, unable to do any normal activities)
  R/O: forgotten trauma, ischemic foot, acute gouty arthritis
- Looks like a boil, infected sore, deep ulcer, or other infected rash (spreading redness, red streak, pus)
  R/O: abscess, cellulitis, ulcer
- Swollen foot
  Exception: localized bump from bunions, calluses, insect bite, sting
  R/O: forgotten trauma, cellulitis
- Numbness in one foot (i.e., loss of sensation)
  R/O: nerve root compression, herniated disk

See Within 3 Days in Office

- MODERATE pain (e.g., interferes with normal activities, limping) and present > 3 days
  R/O: sciatica, arthritis, stress fracture
- Numbness or tingling in feet and new or increased
  R/O: diabetic neuropathy
- Pain in the big toe joint
  R/O: acute gouty arthritis of first MTP joint
- Patient wants to be seen

See Within 2 Weeks in Office

- MILD pain (e.g., does not interfere with normal activities) and present > 7 days
  R/O: arthritis, Achilles tendonitis, plantar heel pain, bunions
- Foot pain is a chronic symptom (recurrent or ongoing AND lasting > 4 weeks)
  R/O: arthritis, Achilles tendonitis, plantar heel pain, callus
- Caused by known bunions, plantar wart, or flatfeet

Home Care

- Foot pain
- Caused by overuse from recent vigorous activity (e.g., jogging, aerobics, prolonged walking)
  R/O: overuse injury
- Caused by transient muscle cramps in the foot
  R/O: muscle cramps, nocturnal cramps

HOME CARE ADVICE

Foot Pain and Overuse

1. **Reassurance—Foot Pain:** The symptoms you describe do not sound serious. You have told me that there is no redness, swelling, or fever. You have also told me that there has been no recent major injury.
2. **Reassurance—Overuse:**
   - It sounds like an overuse injury.
   - Foot pain and soreness are very common following vigorous activity. Such activities include sports like tennis and basketball, jogging, and certain types of work (lots of walking).
3. **Aggravating Factors:** There are a number of things that can cause or aggravate foot pain:
   - **Aging:** Foot pain is more common in the elderly. During the aging process, the feet widen and flatten, and the skin becomes drier.
   - **Pregnancy:** Foot pain is more common in pregnant women. During pregnancy hormones cause the ligaments to relax, and the extra weight causes increased stress on the feet.
   - **Obesity:** Foot pain is also more common in overweight individuals. Being overweight puts excess stress on the bones and soft tissues of the feet.
   - **Overuse:** People that are in professions that require prolonged standing and walking commonly report foot pain.
   - **Shoes:** Poorly fitting or overly tight shoes are the underlying cause of many painful foot conditions. High heels are bad for feet.
4. **Pain Medicines:**
   - For pain relief, take acetaminophen, ibuprofen, or naproxen.

   Acetaminophen (e.g., Tylenol):
   - Take 650 mg by mouth every 4-6 hours as needed. Each Regular Strength Tylenol pill has 325 mg of acetaminophen. The most you should take each day is 3,250 mg (10 pills a day).
   - Another choice is to take 1,000 mg every 8 hours. Each Extra Strength Tylenol pill has 500 mg of acetaminophen. The most you should take each day is 3,000 mg (6 pills a day).

   Ibuprofen (e.g., Motrin, Advil):
   - Take 400 mg by mouth every 6 hours.
   - Another choice is to take 600 mg by mouth every 8 hours.

   Naproxen (e.g., Aleve):
   - Take 250-500 mg by mouth every 12 hours.

   Extra Notes:
   - Acetaminophen is thought to be safer than ibuprofen or naproxen in people over 65 years old. Acetaminophen is in many OTC and prescription medicines. It might be in more than one medicine that you are taking. You need to be careful and not take an overdose. An acetaminophen overdose can hurt the liver.
   - **Caution:** Do not take acetaminophen if you have liver disease.
   - **Caution:** Do not take ibuprofen if you have stomach problems, kidney disease, are pregnant, or have been told by your doctor to avoid this type of anti-inflammatory drug. Do not take ibuprofen for more than 7 days without consulting your doctor.
   - Use the lowest amount of medicine that makes your pain feel better.
   - Before taking any medicine, read all the instructions on the package
5. **Call Back If:**
   - Swelling, redness, or fever occur.
   - Severe pain not relieved by pain medication.
   - Pain persists more than 7 days.
   - You become worse.

Muscle Cramps

1. **Reassurance—Musle Cramps:**
   - Muscle cramps can occur in the feet.
   - During attacks, break the muscle spasm by stretching the muscle in the direction opposite to how it is being pulled by the cramp or spasm. For example, for a foot cramp, pull the foot and toes backward as far as they will go.
2. **Expected Course:**
   - Muscle cramps usually last 5 to 30 minutes. Once the muscle cramp stops, the muscle quickly returns to normal. The pain should go away completely.

- If you have frequent muscle cramps, then you may need to see your doctor. Sometimes the doctor can give medications to reduce the muscle cramps.

3. **Call Back If:**
   - Fever or redness occurs.
   - Foot is cool or blue in comparison to other side.
   - You become worse.

General Foot Care

1. **Keep Your Feet Healthy:**
   - Examine your feet on a regular basis. Check for sores, redness, and calluses.
   - Avoid going barefoot in warm, damp places like locker rooms.
   - Change your socks or hose daily or whenever they get damp.
   - If you are overweight, work on losing weight.
2. **Keep Your Feet Clean:**
   - Wash your feet daily using a mild soap (e.g., Dove) and lukewarm water. Rinse off all soap.
   - Dry your feet thoroughly, especially between the toes.
   - Put a small amount of lotion (unscented with lanolin) on your feet after bathing; this will help seal moisture in the skin. Do not put lotion between your toes.
3. **Wear Shoes That Fit:**
   - Shoes should have a wide toe box, so that your toes do not feel cramped.
   - The shoe's toe cap should be 0.25-0.5 inch (6-12 mm; or approximately one finger width) longer than the longest toe in the foot.
   - Buy new shoes later in the day (Reason: feet swell during the day and become larger).
   - Avoid high heels. Heels should not be taller than 2 inches.
4. **Wear the Right Shoe for the Right Activity:**
   - Wear running shoes for running
   - Wear the correct type of protective shoes for your workplace.
5. **Call Back If:**
   - You have more questions.

BACKGROUND INFORMATION

Some Common Conditions—Causing Heel Pain

- **Achilles Tendinitis:** This is an inflammation of the Achilles tendon where it attaches to the back of the heel bone. It can be caused by inadequate warming up and overuse.
- **Haglund Deformity (Pump Bump):** This is a bursitis that develops on the posterior aspect of the heel. It is caused by the pressure of the rim of the shoe rubbing up against the heel.
- **Heel Spurs:** These are bony growths on the underside of the heel bone where the plantar tendons attach. The pain is located on the front portion of the underside of the heel.
- **Plantar Fasciitis:** This is an inflammation of the band of connective tissue (fascia) that runs along the sole (plantar aspect) of the foot. This band of fascia runs from the heel to the ball of the foot.

Some Common Conditions—Causing Arch and Ball of Foot Pain

- **Bunion (Hallux Valgus):** An enlargement of the foot joint (first MTP) at the base of the big toe. The big toe angles inward and the joint protrudes outward. A bunion can be caused by poorly fitting shoes, can be inherited, or can sometimes develop without any known cause. It can be painful. Surgery by a podiatrist is sometimes needed.
- **Bunionette (Tailor Bunion):** An enlargement of the foot joint (fifth MTP) at the base of the little toe. The little toe angles inward and the joint protrudes outwards.
- **Calluses:** Are areas of thickened skin on the bottom (sole) of the foot. They can be painful or painless. Poor fitting and overly tight shoes are the most common cause of this condition. The constant rubbing is what causes the skin to thicken.
- **Flatfeet:** Flatfee (no arch) can be inherited or can develop in adulthood. When it develops in adulthood it is also called posterior tibial tendon dysfunction (PTTD).
- **Morton Neuroma:** This is a pinched nerve. The most common location is on the sole of the foot between the third and fourth metatarsals. It can be caused by wearing shoes that are too tight, that then squeeze the bones together.

- **Muscle Cramps:** Brief pains (1 to 15 minutes) may be due to muscle spasms. Foot or calf muscles are especially prone to cramps that awaken from sleep. The pain should resolve completely after an episode of muscle spasm. Muscle cramps can occur more commonly in pregnancy.
- **Plantar Fasciitis:** This is an inflammation of the band of connective tissue (fascia) that runs along the sole (plantar aspect) of the foot. This band of fascia runs from the heel to the ball of the foot.
- **Plantar Warts:** A plantar wart looks a lot like a callus on the sole of the foot. The difference is that it is caused by a viral infection. The skin is thickened, slightly raised, and may contain tiny black specks. The black specks are thrombosed capillaries.
- **Stress Fracture:** This is a hairline partial fracture of the foot. Strenuous activities like jogging, high-impact aerobics, and hiking can cause this overuse injury.

FROSTBITE

DEFINITION

- Frostbite is a cold injury to the skin.
- Use this protocol only if the patient has symptoms that match Frostbite.

Symptoms of Frostbite Include:

- Numbness, tingling, and pain of frostbitten part.
- Frostbitten hand and fingers may feel stiff or clumsy.
- Significant pain occurs during rewarming.
- True frostbite causes white, hard, completely numb skin. It can cause serious skin damage and always requires medical attention after rewarming.
- Common sites for frostbite are the toes, fingers, nose, ears, and penis.

Frostbite Severity Is Defined As:

- **Frostnip:** There is temporary numbness and tingling that goes away after rewarming. This is actually not true frostbite since there is no injury to the skin.
- **First Degree (Mild):** White and waxy (hard) while frozen; erythema and swelling persist after rewarming.
- **Second Degree:** Same as first degree, plus blisters with clear fluid that appear in 6 to 24 hours.
- **Third Degree (Severe):** Hemorrhagic blisters progressing to skin necrosis.
- **Fourth Degree:** Skin necrosis (tissue death), gangrene.

TRIAGE ASSESSMENT QUESTIONS

Call EMS 911 Now

● Unconscious
R/O: severe hypothermia
FIRST AID: Wrap adult in warm blankets.

● Slurred speech
R/O: severe hypothermia
FIRST AID: Wrap adult in warm blankets.

● Confused thinking
R/O: severe hypothermia
FIRST AID: Wrap adult in warm blankets.

● Stumbling or falling
R/O: severe hypothermia
FIRST AID: Wrap adult in warm blankets.

● Body temperature < 95° F (35° C) rectally or < 94° F (34.4° C) orally
R/O: severe hypothermia
FIRST AID: Wrap adult in warm blankets.

Go to ED Now (or to Office With PCP Approval)

● Severe shivering that persists > 10 minutes after rewarming and drying
R/O: severe hypothermia
FIRST AID: Wrap adult in warm blankets.

● Patient sounds very sick or weak to the triager

Go to Office Now

● After hour of rewarming and skin color and sensation don't return to normal
R/O: severe frostbite

● Looks infected (e.g., spreading redness, red streak, pus)
R/O: cellulitis, lymphangitis

● Unusually severe cold exposure and any other symptoms

See Today in Office

● White, hard, completely numb skin (before rewarming)
R/O: severe frostbite (especially of the fingers or toes)

● Frostbitten part develops blisters
R/O: second-degree frostbite

● Patient wants to be seen

Home Care

○ Mild frostbite symptoms
R/O: frostnip, mild frostbite

HOME CARE ADVICE FOR FROSTBITE

1. **Frostbite Treatment—Rewarming:** Rewarm the area rapidly with wet heat:
   - Move into a warm room.
   - **For Frostbite of an Extremity (e.g., Fingers, Toes):** Place the frostbitten part in very warm water. A bathtub or sink is often the quickest approach. The water should be very warm (104° to 108° F, or 40° to 42° C), but not hot enough to burn. Immersion in this warm water should continue until a pink flush signals the return of circulation to the frostbitten part (usually 30 minutes). At this point, the numbness should disappear.
   - **For Frostbite of the Face (e.g., Ears, Nose):** Apply warm, wet washcloths to frostbitten area of the face. Continue doing this until a pink flush signals the return of circulation to the frostbitten area (usually 30 minutes).
   - With more severe frostbite, the last 10 minutes of rewarming is usually quite painful.
   - If not using a tub, keep the rest of your body warm by covering yourself with plenty of blankets.
2. **Frostbite Treatment—Common Mistakes:**
   - A common error is to apply snow to the frostbitten area or to massage it. Both can cause damage to thawing tissues.
   - Do not rewarm with dry heat, such as a heat lamp or electric heater, because frostbitten skin cannot sense burning.
   - Do not rewarm if there is a high likelihood of refreezing in the next couple hours. Freezing-warming-freezing causes more damage than freezing-warming.
3. **Drink Warm Liquids:** Drink warm liquids (e.g., hot chocolate).
4. **Pain Medicines:**
   - For pain relief, take acetaminophen, ibuprofen, or naproxen.

   Acetaminophen (e.g., Tylenol):
   - Take 650 mg by mouth every 4-6 hours as needed. Each Regular Strength Tylenol pill has 325 mg of acetaminophen. The most you should take each day is 3,250 mg (10 pills a day).
   - Another choice is to take 1,000 mg every 8 hours. Each Extra Strength Tylenol pill has 500 mg of acetaminophen. The most you should take each day is 3,000 mg (6 pills a day).

   Ibuprofen (e.g., Motrin, Advil):
   - Take 400 mg by mouth every 6 hours.
   - Another choice is to take 600 mg by mouth every 8 hours.

   Naproxen (e.g., Aleve):
   - Take 250-500 mg by mouth every 12 hours.

   Extra Notes:
   - Acetaminophen is thought to be safer than ibuprofen or naproxen in people over 65 years old.
   - Acetaminophen is in many OTC and prescription medicines. It might be in more than one medicine that you are taking. You need to be careful and not take an overdose. An acetaminophen overdose can hurt the liver.
   - **Caution:** Do not take acetaminophen if you have liver disease.
   - **Caution:** Do not take ibuprofen if you have stomach problems, kidney disease, are pregnant, or have been told by your doctor to avoid this type of anti-inflammatory drug. Do not take ibuprofen for more than 7 days without consulting your doctor.
   - Use the lowest amount of medicine that makes your pain feel better.
   - Before taking any medicine, read all the instructions on the package
5. **Aloe Vera Ointment:** Apply aloe vera ointment to the area of frostbite twice daily for 5 days.
6. **Tetanus Booster for Frostbite:** If your last tetanus shot was given more than 10 years ago, then you need a booster.
7. **Call Back If:**
   - Color and sensation do not return to normal after 1 hour of rewarming.
   - Frostbitten part develops blisters.
   - You become worse.

FIRST AID

First Aid Advice for Hypothermia:

- Remove wet clothing.
- Wrap in warm blankets (or clothing, sleeping bag, even newspaper).

- Move into a warm space (e.g., home, building, car, tent).

First Aid Advice for Frostbite:

- Rewarm the frostbitten area rapidly with wet heat.
- Move into a warm room.
- **For Frostbite of an Extremity (e.g., Fingers, Toes):** Place the frostbitten part in very warm water. A bathtub or sink is often the quickest approach. The water should be very warm (104 to 108° F, or 40 to 42° C), but not hot enough to burn. Immersion in this warm water should continue until a pink flush signals the return of circulation to the frostbitten part (usually 30 minutes).
- **For Frostbite of the Face (e.g., Ears, Nose):** Apply warm, wet washcloths to frostbitten area of the face. Continue doing this until a pink flush signals the return of circulation to the frostbitten area (usually 30 minutes). Note: Do not rewarm a frostbitten area if there is a chance of refreezing.

First Aid Advice for Frostbite During Transport to a Medical Facility:

- Wrap frostbitten area in warm blanket or clean dressing.
- Protect frostbitten area from injury.
- Avoid walking on frozen feet if possible (Reason: may cause further tissue injury).

BACKGROUND INFORMATION

General

- Frostbite and hypothermia are 2 distinct and independent medical problems.
- Frostbite results from a cold injury to the skin. The body's core temperature can be normal. In frostbite, the nerves, blood vessels, and skin cells of a part of the body are temporarily frozen. The ears, nose, penis, fingers, and toes are most commonly affected.
- In contrast, hypothermia signifies a marked decrease in the body's core temperature, and frostbite may not be present. Hypothermia is defined as a body temperature < 95° F (35° C) rectally and can be fatal without intervention.

Factors Contributing to Frostbite

- **Alcohol, Mental Illness:** Impairs judgment and reduces normal self-protective actions.
- **Medical Conditions:** A number of medical conditions predispose to frostbite. Patients with diabetes, congestive heart failure, peripheral vascular condition, Raynaud disease, and previous frostbite are all at greater risk.
- **Type of Contact:** The frostbite is much worse if the skin and clothing are also wet at the time of cold exposure. Touching bare hands to cold metal and volatile products (like gasoline) stored outside during freezing weather can cause immediate frostbite.
- **Duration of Contact:** The longer the cold exposure the greater both the heat loss and the likelihood of frostbite. The wind velocity on a cold day (windchill index) also determines how quickly frostbite occurs.

Frostbite Prevention—General

- Change wet gloves or socks immediately.
- Set limits on the time spent outdoors when the windchill temperature falls below zero.
- Know the earliest warnings of frostbite. Pain, tingling, and numbness are signals from your body that you are not dressed adequately for the weather and that you need to go indoors.

Frostbite Prevention—Clothing

- **Clothing:** Dress in layers for cold weather. The first layer should be long underwear preferably made of polypropylene or polyester (wicks moisture away from skin). The middle layer(s) should be fleece or wool. The outer layer serves as a wind-breaker and also needs to be waterproof. The layers should be loose, not tight.
- **Hand Protection:** Mittens are warmer than gloves. You may wish to wear a thin glove under the mitten.
- **Footwear:** Avoid tight shoes that might interfere with circulation. Wear 1-2 pairs of socks made from wool or a wool blend. You may also wish to wear a thin liner sock made from polyester or polypropylene (wick away moisture) under the wool socks.
- **Head Wear:** Wear a hat because over 50% of heat loss occurs from the head.

HAND AND WRIST PAIN

DEFINITION

- Pain in the hand or wrist.
- Not due to a traumatic injury.
- Minor muscle strain and overuse are covered in this guideline.

Pain Severity Is Defined As:

- **Mild (1-3):** Doesn't interfere with normal activities
- **Moderate (4-7):** Interferes with normal activities (e.g., work or school) or awakens from sleep
- **Severe (8-10):** Excruciating pain, unable to use hand at all

TRIAGE ASSESSMENT QUESTIONS

Call EMS 911 Now

- Similar pain previously and it was from "heart attack"
  R/O: cardiac ischemia, myocardial infarction
- Similar pain previously from "angina" and not relieved by nitroglycerin
  R/O: cardiac ischemia
- Sounds like a life-threatening emergency to the triager

See More Appropriate Protocol

- Followed an injury
  Go to Protocol: Trauma, Hand and Wrist on page 287
- Chest pain
  Go to Protocol: Chest Pain on page 48
- Caused by an animal bite
  Go to Protocol: Animal Bite on page 13
- Wound looks infected
  Go to Protocol: Wound Infection on page 344

Go to ED Now (or to Office With PCP Approval)

- Fever and red area (or area very tender to touch)
  R/O: cellulitis, lymphangitis
- Fever and swollen joint
  R/O: septic arthritis, cellulitis
- Patient sounds very sick or weak to the triager

Go to Office Now

- SEVERE pain (e.g., excruciating, unable to use hand at all)
  R/O: un-witnessed trauma, inflammatory arthritis
- Red area or streak and large (> 2 in or 5 cm)
  R/O: cellulitis, erysipelas, lymphangitis.
  Note: It may be difficult to determine the rash color in people with darker-colored skin.

See Today in Office

- Weakness (i.e., loss of strength) of new onset in hand or fingers
  R/O: herniated cervical disk
  Exception: not truly weak, hand feels weak because of pain
  Note: This question describes a patient with both hand pain and weakness. In contrast, a stroke patient will have sudden onset of painless weakness.
- Numbness (i.e., loss of sensation) of new onset in hand or fingers
  R/O: neuropathy, cervical radiculopathy, herniated cervical disk, carpal tunnel syndrome.
  Exception: slight tingling; numbness present > 2 weeks.
  Note: This question describes a patient with both hand pain and numbness. In contrast, a stroke patient will have sudden onset of painless numbness/weakness.
- Looks like a boil, infected sore, deep ulcer, or other infected rash (spreading redness, pus)
  R/O: impetigo, abscess, cellulitis
- Localized rash is very painful (no fever)
  R/O: early cellulitis, bee sting, inflammatory arthritis

See Within 3 Days in Office

- MODERATE pain (e.g., interferes with normal activities) and present > 3 days
  R/O: arthritis, tendonitis, carpal tunnel syndrome
- Weakness or numbness in hand or fingers and present > 2 weeks
  R/O: tendonitis, carpal tunnel syndrome, cervical radiculopathy
  Reason: chronic symptoms
- Pain is worsened or caused by bending the neck
  R/O: cervical radiculopathy, herniated cervical disk

- Pain is worsened by using computer keyboard and/or mouse
  R/O: carpal tunnel syndrome
- Swollen joint of new onset
  R/O: inflammatory arthritis
- Patient wants to be seen

See Within 2 Weeks in Office

- MILD pain (e.g., does not interfere with normal activities) and present > 7 days
- Morning stiffness of hand(s) is a chronic symptom (recurrent or ongoing AND lasting > 4 weeks)
  R/O: degenerative or inflammatory arthritis
- Hand or wrist pain is a chronic symptom (recurrent or ongoing AND lasting > 4 weeks)
  R/O: arthritis, tendonitis, carpal tunnel syndrome

Home Care

- ○ Caused by bumping elbow, and had transient burning pain shooting (radiating) into hand and fingers
  R/O: "bruised funny bone"
- ○ Caused by overuse injury from recent vigorous activity (e.g., sports, repetitive motions, heavy lifting)
  R/O: overuse injury, strain
- ○ Hand or wrist pain

HOME CARE ADVICE FOR HAND AND WRIST PAIN

Muscle Strain and Overuse

1. **Reassurance:** Muscle strain and irritation are very common following: vigorous activity (e.g., throwing a ball, playing tennis), repetitive forceful motions (e.g., washing the car, scrubbing the floor), or heavy lifting.
2. **Local Cold for First 48 Hours**
   - Apply a cold pack or an ice bag (wrapped in a moist towel) to the area for 20 minutes. Repeat in 1 hour, then every 4 hours while awake.
   - Continue this for the first 48 hours after an injury (Reason: to reduce the swelling and pain).
3. **Local Heat**
   - Beginning 48 hours after an injury, apply a warm washcloth or heating pad for 10 minutes 3 times a day.
   - This will help increase circulation and improve healing.
4. **Rest:** You should try to avoid (or minimize) doing the activity that caused the pain for the next 1-2 weeks.
5. **Pain Medicines:**
   - For pain relief, take acetaminophen, ibuprofen, or naproxen.

   Acetaminophen (e.g., Tylenol):
   - Take 650 mg by mouth every 4-6 hours as needed. Each Regular Strength Tylenol pill has 325 mg of acetaminophen. The most you should take each day is 3,250 mg (10 pills a day).
   - Another choice is to take 1,000 mg every 8 hours. Each Extra Strength Tylenol pill has 500 mg of acetaminophen. The most you should take each day is 3,000 mg (6 pills a day).

   Ibuprofen (e.g., Motrin, Advil):
   - Take 400 mg by mouth every 6 hours.
   - Another choice is to take 600 mg by mouth every 8 hours.

   Naproxen (e.g., Aleve):
   - Take 250-500 mg by mouth every 12 hours.

   Extra Notes:
   - Acetaminophen is thought to be safer than ibuprofen or naproxen in people over 65 years old. Acetaminophen is in many OTC and prescription medicines. It might be in more than one medicine that you are taking. You need to be careful and not take an overdose. An acetaminophen overdose can hurt the liver.
   - **Caution:** Do not take acetaminophen if you have liver disease.
   - **Caution:** Do not take ibuprofen if you have stomach problems, kidney disease, are pregnant, or have been told by your doctor to avoid this type of anti-inflammatory drug. Do not take ibuprofen for more than 7 days without consulting your doctor.
   - Use the lowest amount of medicine that makes your pain feel better.
   - Before taking any medicine, read all the instructions on the package

6. **Expected Course:** For minor injuries, pain should improve over a 2- to 3-day period and disappear within 7 days.
7. **Call Back If**
   - MODERATE pain (e.g. interferes with normal activities) lasts more than 3 days.
   - MILD pain lasts more than 7 days.
   - Arm swelling occurs.
   - Signs of infection occur (e.g., spreading redness, warmth, fever).
   - You become worse.

Bruised Funny Bone

1. **Reassurance**
   - It sounds like a "bruised funny bone" that we can treat at home.
   - A direct blow to the inner side of the posterior elbow can cause numbess, tingling, and burning in the hand. The involved fingers are usually the middle, ring and little fingers.
   - Your funny bone is actually a nerve (ulnar) which wraps around the posterior part of your elbow.
2. **Expected Course:** Symptoms from "bruising your funny bone" usually last only a few minutes. If the symptoms last longer than 30 minutes or if this problem seems to happen to you frequently, then you should see your doctor for evaluation.
3. **Call Back If:** You become worse.

Hand and Wrist Pain—General Care Advice

1. **Reassurance:** Hand and wrist pain can be caused by strained muscles, tendonitis, and mild arthritis.
2. **Pain Medicines:**
   - For pain relief, take acetaminophen, ibuprofen, or naproxen.

   Acetaminophen (e.g., Tylenol):
   - Take 650 mg by mouth every 4-6 hours as needed. Each Regular Strength Tylenol pill has 325 mg of acetaminophen. The most you should take each day is 3,250 mg (10 pills a day).
   - Another choice is to take 1,000 mg every 8 hours. Each Extra Strength Tylenol pill has 500 mg of acetaminophen. The most you should take each day is 3,000 mg (6 pills a day).

   Ibuprofen (e.g., Motrin, Advil):
   - Take 400 mg by mouth every 6 hours.
   - Another choice is to take 600 mg by mouth every 8 hours.

   Naproxen (e.g., Aleve):
   - Take 250-500 mg by mouth every 12 hours.

   Extra Notes:
   - Acetaminophen is thought to be safer than ibuprofen or naproxen in people over 65 years old.
   - Acetaminophen is in many OTC and prescription medicines. It might be in more than one medicine that you are taking. You need to be careful and not take an overdose. An acetaminophen overdose can hurt the liver.
   - **Caution:** Do not take acetaminophen if you have liver disease.
   - **Caution:** Do not take ibuprofen if you have stomach problems, kidney disease, are pregnant, or have been told by your doctor to avoid this type of anti-inflammatory drug. Do not take ibuprofen for more than 7 days without consulting your doctor.
   - Use the lowest amount of medicine that makes your pain feel better.
   - Before taking any medicine, read all the instructions on the package
3. **Call Back If**
   - MODERATE pain (e.g. interferes with normal activities) lasts more than 3 days.
   - MILD pain lasts more than 7 days.
   - Signs of infection occur (e.g., spreading redness, warmth, fever).
   - You become worse.

BACKGROUND INFORMATION

Causes

- Arthritis (e.g., degenerative, gouty, infectious, inflammatory, traumatic).
- **Carpal Tunnel Syndrome:** Is caused by compression of the median nerve at the wrist. Numbness is typically noted in the thumb, index, and ring fingers but may be poorly localized. It is seen more commonly in diabetics, pregnancy, rheumatoid arthritis, and in individuals whose jobs require repetitive wrist movements.
- Cellulitis.
- Overuse injury (tendonitis).
- Trauma (e.g., contusion, dislocation, fracture, sprain, strain).

Serious Signs and Symptoms

- Severe pain
- Red area with streak
  (R/O: cellulitis with lymphangitis; common)
- Joint swelling with fever
  (R/O: septic arthritis; rare)
- Entire arm is swollen
  (R/O: deep vein thrombosis of upper extremity; rare)

Caution: Cardiac Ischemia

- Rarely patients may present with arm pain as the sole symptom of a myocardial infarction. Usually there will be other associated symptoms of cardiac ischemia: chest pain, shortness of breath, nausea, and/or diaphoresis.
- Cardiac ischemia should be suspected in any patients with risk factors for cardiac disease. These include: hypertension, smoking, diabetes, hyperlipidemia, a strong family history of heart disease, male gender, and age > 60.

HAY FEVER (NASAL ALLERGIES)

DEFINITION

- An allergic reaction of the nose and sinuses to an inhaled substance, for example, pollen, mold, or dust.
- An itchy nose and clear discharge are common.
- Use this guideline only if the patient has symptoms that match Hay Fever.

Symptoms of Hay Fever (Nasal Allergies) Include:

- Runny nose (clear nasal discharge)
- Stuffy nose (nasal congestion)
- Sneezing and sniffing
- Itching of nose, eyes, and roof of mouth
- Watery eyes
- Ear fullness (ear congestion)
- No fever

TRIAGE ASSESSMENT QUESTIONS

See More Appropriate Protocol

- Wheezing (high-pitched whistling sound) and previous asthma attacks or use of asthma medicines
  Go to Protocol: Asthma Attack on page 22
- Doesn't match the symptoms for nasal allergy
  Go to Protocol: Colds on page 53

Go to ED Now (or to Office With PCP Approval)

- Patient sounds very sick or weak to the triager

See Today in Office

- Lots of coughing
  R/O: associated asthma
- Lots of yellow or green discharge from nose, present > 3 days
  R/O: bacterial sinusitis

See Today or Tomorrow in Office

- Nasal discharge present > 10 days
  R/O: bacterial sinusitis
- Moderate-severe nasal allergy symptoms (i.e., interfere with sleep, school, or work) and taking antihistamines > 2 days
  R/O: poor control
- Patient wants to be seen

See Within 2 Weeks in Office

- Nasal allergies occur only certain times of year and diagnosis of hay fever has never been confirmed by a physician
  R/O: seasonal allergic rhinitis (hay fever)
- Nasal allergies occur year-round
  R/O: perennial allergic rhinitis; multiple allergies to pollens, house dust, pets, foods
- Snores most nights of month
  R/O: chronic nasal congestion, sleep apnea

Home Care

- ○ Nasal allergies occur only certain times of year
  R/O: seasonal allergic rhinitis (hay fever)

HOME CARE ADVICE

General Care Advice for Hay Fever

1. **Wash Off Pollen Daily:** Remove pollen from the body with hair washing and a shower, especially before bedtime.
2. **Avoiding Pollen:**
   - Stay indoors on windy days.
   - Keep windows closed in home, at least in bedroom; use air conditioner.
   - Use a high-efficiency house air filter (HEPA or electrostatic).
   - Keep windows closed in car, turn AC on recirculate.
   - Avoid playing with outdoor dog.
3. **For a Stuffy Nose—Use Nasal Washes:**
   - **Introduction:** Saline (salt water) nasal irrigation is an effective and simple home remedy for treating cold symptoms and other conditions involving the nasal and sinus passages. Nasal irrigation consists of pouring, spraying, or squirting salt water into the nose and then letting it run back out.
   - **How It Helps:** The salt water rinses out excess mucus, washes out any irritants (dust, allergens) that might be present, and moisturizes the nasal cavity.

- **Methods:** There are several ways to perform nasal irrigation. You can use a saline nasal spray bottle (available over-the-counter), a rubber ear syringe, a medical syringe without the needle, or a Neti Pot.

Step-by-Step Instructions:

- **Step 1:** Lean over a sink.
- **Step 2:** Gently squirt or spray warm salt water into one of your nostrils.
- **Step 3:** Some of the water may run into the back of your throat. Spit this out. If you swallow the salt water it will not hurt you.
- **Step 4:** Blow your nose to clean out the water and mucus.
- **Step 5:** Repeat steps 1-4 for the other nostril. You can do this a couple times a day if it seems to help you.

How to Make Saline (Salt Water) Nasal Wash:

- You can make your own saline nasal wash.
- Add ½ tsp of table salt to 1 cup (8 oz; 240 mL) of warm water.
- You should use sterile, distilled, or previously boiled water for nasal irrigation.

4. **Antihistamine Medications for Hay Fever:**
    - Antihistamines help reduce sneezing, itching and runny nose.
    - You may need to take antihistamines continuously during pollen season (Reason: continuously is the key to control).
    - Loratadine is a newer (second-generation) antihistamine. The dosage of loratadine (e.g., OTC Claritin, Alavert) is 10 mg once a day.
    - Cetirizine is a newer (second-generation) antihistamine. The dosage of cetirizine (e.g., OTC Zyrtec) is 10 mg once a day.
    - **Caution:** Antihistamines may cause sleepiness. Do not drink, drive, or operate dangerous machinery while taking antihistamines.
    - Loratadine and cetirizine cause less sleepiness than diphenhydramine (Benadryl) or chlorpheniramine (Chlor-Trimeton, Chlor-Tripolon).
    - Read the package instructions thoroughly on all medications that you take.
5. **Nasal Decongestant Nose Drops for Stuffy Nose:**
    - Antihistamines do not help nasal congestion (stuffiness), but decongestant nose drops do. Decongestants shrink the swollen nasal mucosa and allow for easier breathing.
    - Phenylephrine nasal drops (e.g., Neo-Synephrine) are available over-the-counter. Clean out the nose before using. Spray each nostril once, wait 1 minute for absorption, and then spray a second time.
    - **Caution:** Do not take this medication if you have high blood pressure, heart disease, or prostate enlargement. Do not take these medications if you are pregnant. Do not take these medications if you have used an MAO inhibitor such as isocarboxazid (Marplan), phenelzine (Nardil), rasagiline (Azilect), selegiline (Eldepryl, Emsam), or tranylcypromine (Parnate) in the past 2 weeks. Life-threatening side effects can occur.
    - Do not use these medications for more than 3 days (Reason: rebound nasal congestion).
    - Read the package instructions thoroughly on all medications that you use.
6. **For Eye Allergies:** For eye symptoms, wash pollen off the face and eyelids. Then apply cold, wet compresses. Oral antihistamines will usually bring all eye symptoms under control.
7. **Call Back If:**
    - Symptoms are not controlled in 2 days with continuous antihistamines.
    - You become worse.

Neti Pot for Sinus Symptoms

1. **Neti Pot**
    - The Neti Pot is a small ceramic or plastic pot with a narrow spout. It looks like a small teapot. Two manufacturers of the Neti Pot are the Himalayan Institute in Pennsylvania and SinuCleanse in Wisconsin.
    - **How It Helps:** The Neti Pot performs nasal washing (also called nasal irrigation or "jala neti"). The salt water rinses out excess mucus, washes out any irritants (dust, allergens) that might be present, and moisturizes the nasal cavity.

- **Indications:** The Neti Pot is widely used as a home remedy to relieve conditions such as colds, sinus infections, and hay fever (nasal allergies).
- **Adverse Reactions:** None. Though, not everyone likes the sensation of pouring water into their nose.
- **YouTube Instructional Video:** There are instructional videos on how to use a Neti Pot both on manufacturers' Web sites and also on YouTube.

2. **Neti Pot Step-by-Step Instructions:**
    - **Step 1:** Follow the directions on the salt package to make warm salt walter.
    - **Step 2:** Lean forward and turn your head to one side over the sink. Keep your forehead slightly higher than your chin.
    - **Step 3:** Gently insert the spout of the Neti Pot into the higher nostril. Put it far enough so that it forms a comfortable seal.
    - **Step 4:** Raise the Neti Pot gradually so the salt water flows in through your higher nostril and out of the lower nostril. Breathe through your mouth.
    - **Step 5:** When the Neti Pot is empty, blow your nose to clean out the water and mucus.
    - **Step 6:** Some of the water may run into the back of your throat. Spit this out. If you swallow the salt water it will not hurt you.
    - **Step 7:** Refill the Neti Pot and repeat on the other side. Again, exhale vigorously to clear the nasal passages.

How to Make Saline (Salt Water) Nasal Wash:

- You can make your own saline nasal wash.
- Add ½ tsp of table salt to 1 cup (8 oz; 240 mL) of warm water.
- You should use sterile, distilled, or previously boiled water for nasal irrigation.

BACKGROUND INFORMATION

General Information

- Many patients correctly self-diagnose this condition. Confirmation of this diagnosis by a physician is helpful and becomes essential if symptoms are more than mild.
- Many patients with allergic rhinitis also have symptoms of allergic conjunctivitis (watery itchy eyes).

Two Types of Allergic Rhinitis

- **Seasonal Allergic Rhinitis:** Hay fever is the non-medical term people use to describe seasonal allergic rhinitis due to pollens. Patients who suffer from hay fever note that their symptoms are worse during certain seasons of the year. Such individuals usually have an allergy to pollen, grasses, or trees. Depending on the specific allergy, the symptoms may be worse in the spring, summer, or fall. A few unfortunate individuals may experience allergic symptoms in all 3 seasons. Hay fever is not specifically an allergy to hay nor do sufferers have a fever.
- **Perennial Allergic Rhinitis:** Patients with this type of allergic rhinitis may report nasal symptoms all year long. Alternatively they may complain of sporadic symptoms throughout the year, not confined to any particular season. Such individuals often have an allergy to dust mites, mold, mildew, feathers, or animal dander.

Nasal Washes (Nasal Irrigation) for Sinus Symptoms

- **Introduction:** Saline (salt water) nasal irrigation is an effective and simple home remedy for treating cold symptoms and other conditions involving the nasal and sinus passages. Nasal irrigation consists of pouring, spraying, or squirting salt water into the nose and then letting it run back out.
- **How It Helps:** The salt water rinses out excess mucus, washes out any irritants (dust, allergens) that might be present, and moisturizes the nasal cavity.
- **Indications:** Nasal irrigation appears to be an effective treatment for chronic sinusitis. It may also help reduce sinus symptoms from acute viral upper respiratory infection (colds), irritant rhinitis (e.g., dust from the workplace), and allergic rhinitis (hay fever). Some doctors recommend it for rhinitis of pregnancy.

- **Adverse Reactions:** Nasal irrigation is safe and there are no serious adverse effects. However, not everyone likes the sensation of having water in their nose.
- **Methods:** There are several ways to perform nasal irrigation. None has been proven to be better than any other. Methods include use of a nasal spray bottle (available OTC), a rubber ear syringe, a Waterpik set on low, a 5- to 20-cc medical syringe without the needle, or a Neti Pot.
- **How to Make Salt Water for Nasal Irrigation:** Add ½ teaspoon of table salt to 1 cup (8 oz; 240 mL) of warm water.

Neti Pot for Sinus Symptoms

- The Neti Pot is a small ceramic or plastic pot with a narrow spout. It looks like a small teapot. Two manufacturers of the Neti Pot are the Himalayan Institute in Pennsylvania and SinuCleanse in Wisconsin.
- **How It Helps:** The Neti Pot performs nasal washing (also called nasal irrigation or "jala neti"). The salt water rinses out excess mucus, washes out any irritants (dust, allergens) that might be present, and moisturizes the nasal cavity.
- **Indications:** The Neti Pot is widely used as a home remedy to relieve conditions such as colds, sinus infections, and hay fever (nasal allergies).
- **Adverse Reactions:** None. Nasal irrigation with a Neti Pot is safe and there are no serious adverse effects. However, not everyone likes the sensation of having salt water poured into their nose.

Neti Pot and Primary Amebic Meningoencephalitis (PAM)

- Primary amebic meningoencephalitis (PAM) is caused by *Naegleria fowleri*, the so-called "brain-eating ameba." This is an extremely rare infection. There were 32 cases in the United States between 2001 and 2010.
- The majority of the cases of PAM have occurred in the southern United States and were linked to swimming or bathing in fresh water lakes, rivers, and ponds containing this ameba. The ameba can also be found in hot springs, geothermal water sources, and poorly maintained swimming pools.
- In 2011 there were 2 cases of PAM in Louisiana that occurred after nasal irrigation with a Neti Pot. These 2 cases suggest—but are not definite proof—that the nasal irrigation fluid that the individuals used was somehow contaminated with the *Naegleria fowleri* ameba.
- The Centers for Disease Control and Prevention (CDC) recommends that individuals should use distilled, sterile, or previously boiled water for nasal irrigation. It's also important to rinse the irrigation device after each use and leave open to air-dry.

Caution—There Are Other Illnesses That Have Nasal Symptoms Similar to Hay Fever:

- **Viral Rhinitis:** Also known as the common cold. Runny or stuffy nose is the main symptom. The nasal discharge may be clear, cloudy, yellow, or green. The patient usually has other symptoms of a cold: fever, muscle aches, sore throat, and headache.
- **Bacterial and Viral Sinusitis:** Yellow or green nasal secretions suggest the possibility of bacterial sinus infection (sinusitis) if they occur in combination with [1] sinus pain OR [2] the return of a fever after it has been gone for over 24 hours OR [3] secretions lasting longer than 10 days without improvement.
- **Rhinitis Medicamentosa:** Prolonged continuous use (longer than 5 days) of over-the-counter decongestant nose drops can lead to "rebound" congestion where the nose becomes even stuffier.
- **Occupational Exposure:** Airborne irritants in the workplace can cause nasal problems.

HEADACHE

DEFINITION

- Pain or discomfort of the head.
- The face and ears are excluded.
- Not due to a traumatic injury.

Pain Severity Is Defined As:

- **Mild (1-3):** Doesn't interfere with normal activities
- **Moderate (4-7):** Interferes with normal activities or awakens from sleep
- **Severe (8-10):** Excruciating pain, unable to do any normal activities

TRIAGE ASSESSMENT QUESTIONS

Call EMS 911 Now

- Difficult to awaken or acting confused (e.g., disoriented, slurred speech)
  R/O: subarachnoid hemorrhage, meningitis
- Weakness of the face, arm, or leg on one side of the body and new onset
  R/O: stroke
- Numbness of the face, arm, or leg on one side of the body and new onset
  R/O: stroke
- Loss of speech or garbled speech and new onset
  R/O: stroke
- Passed out (i.e., fainted, collapsed and was not responding)
- Sounds like a life-threatening emergency to the triager

See More Appropriate Protocol

- Followed a head injury within last 3 days
  Go to Protocol: Trauma, Head on page 290
- Sinus pain of forehead and yellow or green nasal discharge
  Go to Protocol: Sinus Pain and Congestion on page 231

Go to ED Now

- Unable to walk without falling
  R/O: cerebellar stroke
- Stiff neck (can't touch chin to chest)
  R/O: meningitis
- Possibility of carbon monoxide exposure
  R/O: CO poisoning

Go to ED Now (or to Office With PCP Approval)

- Severe headache, states "worst headache" of life
  R/O: migraine, CNS bleed
- Severe headache, sudden onset (i.e., reaching maximum intensity within 30 seconds)
  R/O: migraine, CNS bleed
- Severe pain in one eye
  R/O: angle-closure glaucoma
- Loss of vision or double vision
  R/O: temporal arteritis
- Patient sounds very sick or weak to the triager

Go to Office Now

- Fever > 103° F (39.4° C)
  R/O: bacterial infection
- Fever > 100.5° F (38.1° C) and has diabetes mellitus or a weakened immune system (e.g., HIV positive, cancer chemotherapy, organ transplant, splenectomy, chronic steroids)
  R/O: meningitis, encephalitis

Callback by PCP or Subspecialist Within 1 Hour

- Severe headache and has had severe headaches before
  R/O: migraine
- Severe headache and not relieved by pain meds
  R/O: new-onset migraine, CNS bleed, brain tumor
- Severe headache and vomiting
  R/O: migraine, increased ICP
- Severe headache and fever

See Today in Office

- New headache and immunocompromised (e.g., HIV positive, cancer chemotherapy, chronic steroid treatment)
  Reason: greater risk of organic pathology
- Fever present > 3 days (72 hours)
  R/O: sinusitis
- Patient wants to be seen

See Today or Tomorrow in Office

- Unexplained headache that is present > 24 hours
  R/O: sinusitis or other treatable cause
- New headache and age > 50
  Reason: greater risk of organic pathology

See Within 2 Weeks in Office

- Headache is a chronic symptom (recurrent or ongoing AND lasting > 4 weeks)
  R/O: tension headache, migraine headache

Home Care

- Mild-moderate headache
  R/O: tension headache
- Similar to previously diagnosed migraine headaches
  R/O: migraine headache
- Similar to previously diagnosed muscle-tension headaches

HOME CARE ADVICE FOR HEADACHE

1. **Reassurance—Migraine Headache:**
   - You have told me that this headache is similar to previous migraine headaches that you have had. If the pattern or severity of your headache changes, you will need to see your physician.
   - Migraine headaches are also called vascular headaches. A migraine can be anywhere from mild to severely painful. Sufferers often describe it as throbbing or pulsing. It is often just on one side. Associated symptoms include nausea and vomiting. Some individuals will have visual or other neurological warning symptoms (aura) that a migraine is coming.
   - This sounds like a painful headache that you are having, but there are pain medications you can take and other instructions I can give you to reduce the pain.
2. **Reassurance—Muscle Tension Headache:**
   - You have told me that this headache is similar to your previously diagnosed muscle tension headaches.
   - The majority of headaches are caused by muscle tension.
   - The discomfort is usually diffuse and may be described as a "tight band" around the head. It may radiate down into the neck and shoulders. The discomfort can be aggravated by emotional stress.
   - This sounds like a painful headache that you are having, but there are pain medications you can take and other instructions I can give you to reduce the pain.
3. **Pain Medicines:**
   - For pain relief, take acetaminophen, ibuprofen, or naproxen.

   Acetaminophen (e.g., Tylenol):
   - Take 650 mg by mouth every 4-6 hours as needed. Each Regular Strength Tylenol pill has 325 mg of acetaminophen. The most you should take each day is 3,250 mg (10 pills a day).
   - Another choice is to take 1,000 mg every 8 hours. Each Extra Strength Tylenol pill has 500 mg of acetaminophen. The most you should take each day is 3,000 mg (6 pills a day).

   Ibuprofen (e.g., Motrin, Advil):
   - Take 400 mg by mouth every 6 hours.
   - Another choice is to take 600 mg by mouth every 8 hours.

   Naproxen (e.g., Aleve):
   - Take 250-500 mg by mouth every 12 hours.

   Extra Notes:
   - Acetaminophen is thought to be safer than ibuprofen or naproxen in people over 65 years old. Acetaminophen is in many OTC and prescription medicines. It might be in more than one medicine that you are taking. You need to be careful and not take an overdose. An acetaminophen overdose can hurt the liver.
   - **Caution:** Do not take acetaminophen if you have liver disease.
   - **Caution:** Do not take ibuprofen if you have stomach problems, kidney disease, are pregnant, or have been told by your doctor to avoid this type of anti-inflammatory drug. Do not take ibuprofen for more than 7 days without consulting your doctor.
   - Use the lowest amount of medicine that makes your pain feel better.
   - Before taking any medicine, read all the instructions on the package.
4. **Migraine Medication:** If your doctor has prescribed specific medication for your migraine, take it as directed as soon as the migraine starts.
5. **Rest:** Lie down in a dark, quiet place and try to relax. Close your eyes and imagine your entire body relaxing.
6. **Local Cold:** Apply a cold, wet washcloth or cold pack to the forehead for 20 minutes.
7. **Stretching:** Stretch and massage any tight neck muscles.

8. **Call Back If:**
   - Headache lasts longer than 24 hours.
   - You become worse.

BACKGROUND INFORMATION

Common Causes

- During the course of a year, the majority of adults suffer headaches.
- **Migraine Headaches:** Are also referred to as vascular headaches. The headache is moderate to severe in intensity, described as throbbing or pulsing in nature, and usually unilateral. Associated symptoms include nausea and vomiting. Some individuals will have visual or other neurological warning symptoms (aura) that a migraine is coming.
- **Muscle Tension Headaches:** The majority of headaches are caused by muscle tension. The discomfort is usually diffuse and may be described as a "tight band" around the head. It may radiate down into the neck and shoulders. The discomfort can be aggravated by emotional stress.
- **Sinusitis:** Headaches occur with sinusitis. The headache is usually located in the forehead area and the individual has associated sinus symptoms (nasal discharge, congestion, postnasal drip).
- **Viral Illness:** A mild to moderate headache frequently accompanies many febrile illnesses (cold, flu, pharyngitis). Sometimes the headache is related to fever. A moderate headache that persists after the fever has resolved is a red flag that something more serious may be causing the headache.

Less Common Causes

- **Acute Glaucoma:** The affected individual will have eye pain.
- **Brain Tumor:** Approximately 60-70% of patients with a brain tumor will complain of headaches. The headache is typically described as dull, slowly but steadily worsening over weeks, worse in the morning, and frontal in location.
- **Caffeine Withdrawal:** This occurs in individuals who drink large amounts of caffeine (e.g., coffee, tea, colas) and suddenly stop. Some caffeine drinkers will note a headache upon arising that goes away after their first cup of coffee.
- **Carbon Monoxide Exposure:** Frequently there will be a group (e.g., the entire family) of people with the same symptoms.
- **Subarachnoid Hemorrhage:** Subarachnoid hemorrhage needs to be considered in any severe sudden onset headache. A typical presentation is the "worst headache ever" (79%). Other supporting symptoms of subarachnoid hemorrhage include: neck pain or stiffness (33%), vomiting (28%), and loss of consciousness (64%). Subarachnoid hemorrhage is a life-threatening problem.
- **Temporal Arteritis:** The other term for this is giant cell arteritis. Typically this presents as a unilateral headache in an individual over 55 years old. There may be tenderness of the scalp over the area of the temporal artery. Fifty percent of patients report painful chewing from jaw claudication. Other symptoms can include muscle aches, fever, and malaise. Permanent visual loss can occur in 20% of patients with temporal arteritis; any change in vision requires emergent evaluation as immediate steroid therapy is indicated.
- **Lumbar Puncture Headache:** This is a complication of lumbar puncture. Typically occurs 12-24 hours after the procedure and the headache is aggravated by sitting up or standing.
- **Meningitis, Encephalitis:** Accompanying symptoms may include fever, confusion, stiff neck.
- **Preeclampsia:** Should be considered in any patient that is more than 20 weeks pregnant and any postpartum patient in the first 4 weeks after delivery. Clinical presentation typically consists of persistent headache, visual symptoms (spots or flashing lights), epigastric pain, hand and face swelling, sudden weight gain (e.g., more than 3 lb or 1.4 kg in 1 week), proteinuria, and blood pressure over 140/90.
- **Pseudotumor Cerebri:** This is also known as benign intracranial hypertension.

HEART RATE AND HEARTBEAT QUESTIONS

DEFINITION

- Fast heart rate (> 100 beats/minute)
- Slow heart rate (< 60 beats/minute)
- Skipped or extra heartbeats (irregular heartbeat)
- Palpitations are an increased sensation (or awareness) of an unduly rapid, forceful, or irregular heartbeat.

TRIAGE ASSESSMENT QUESTIONS

Call EMS 911 Now

- Passed out (i.e., fainted, collapsed and was not responding)
  R/O: arrhythmia
- Shock suspected (e.g., cold/pale/clammy skin, too weak to stand)
  R/O: arrhythmia, shock
- Difficult to awaken or acting confused (e.g., disoriented, slurred speech)
  R/O: arrhythmia, shock
- Visible sweat on face or sweat dripping down face
  R/O: hypoglycemia, arrhythmia, serious pathology
- Unable to walk, or can only walk with assistance (e.g., requires support)
  R/O: arrhythmia, shock
- Received SHOCK from implantable cardiac defibrillator and has persisting symptoms (i.e., palpitations, light-headedness)
  R/O: recurrent ventricular tachyarrhythmia, defibrillator system failure
- Sounds like a life-threatening emergency to the triager

See More Appropriate Protocol

- Chest pain
  Go to Protocol: Chest Pain on page 48

See Today in Office

- Patient wants to be seen

Go to ED Now

- Difficulty breathing
  R/O: arrhythmia
- Dizziness, light-headedness, or weakness
- Heart beating very rapidly (e.g., > 130/minute) and present now
  Exception: during exercise
  R/O: SVT, tachyarrhythmia
- Heart beating very slowly (e.g., < 50/minute)
  Exception: athlete
  R/O: bradycardia

Go to ED Now (or to Office With PCP Approval)

- History of heart disease (i.e., heart attack, bypass surgery, angina, angioplasty)
  Reason: higher risk of serious cardiac dysrhythmias
- Age > 60 years
  Reason: higher risk of serious cardiac dysrhythmias
- New or worsened shortness of breath with activity (dyspnea on exertion)
  R/O: new-onset atrial fibrillation
- Taking water pill (i.e., diuretic) or heart medication (e.g., digoxin)
  R/O: hypokalemia, digoxin toxicity
- Patient sounds very sick or weak to the triager

Call Transferred to PCP Now

- Wearing a "Holter monitor" or "cardiac event monitor"
  Reason: notify PCP
- Received SHOCK from implantable cardiac defibrillator (and now feels well)
  Reason: notify PCP

See Today in Office

- Heart beating very rapidly (e.g., > 130/minute) and not present now
  Exception: during exercise
  R/O: SVT, tachyarrhythmia
- Skipped or extra beat(s) and increases with exercise or exertion
- Skipped or extra beat(s) and occurs 4 or more times per minute
  R/O: PVCs, PACs

See Within 3 Days in Office

- History of hyperthyroidism or taking thyroid medication
  Reason: may be causing symptoms
- Known or suspected substance abuse (e.g., cocaine, alcohol abuse)
  Reason: needs counseling
- Palpitations and no improvement after following care advice

See Within 2 Weeks in Office

- Problems with anxiety or stress
- Palpitations are a chronic symptom (recurrent or ongoing AND lasting > 4 weeks)

Home Care

- Palpitations
- Skipped or extra beat(s) and occurs < 4 times/minute

HOME CARE ADVICE FOR PALPITATIONS

1. **Reassurance:**
    - Everybody has palpitations at some point in their lives. Sometimes it is simply a heightened awareness of the heart's normal beating.
    - Occasional extra heartbeats are experienced by most everyone. Lack of sleep, stress, and caffeinated beverages can make palpitations worse.
    - Patients with anxiety or stress may describe a "rapid heartbeat" or "pounding" in their chest from their heart beating.
2. **Health Basics:**

- **Sleep:** Try to get sufficient amount of sleep. Lack of sleep can aggravate palpitations. Most people need 7-8 hours of sleep each night.
- **Exercise:** Regular exercise will improve your overall health, improve your mood, and is a simple method to reduce stress.
- **Diet:** Eat a balanced healthy diet.
- **Liquid Intake:** Drink adequate liquids, 6-8 glasses of water daily.

3. **Avoid Caffeine:**
    - Avoid caffeine-containing beverages (Reason: caffeine is a stimulant and can aggravate palpitations).
    - Examples of caffeine-containing beverages include coffee, tea, colas, Mountain Dew, Red Bull, and some energy drinks.
4. **Avoid Diet Pills:** Do not use diet pills (Reason: they act as stimulants).
5. **Limit Alcohol:** Limit your alcohol consumption to no more than 2 drinks a day. Ideally, eliminate alcohol entirely for the next 2 weeks.
6. **Limit Smoking:** Stop or reduce your smoking.
7. **Expected Course:** If your symptoms do not improve over the next couple days, then you should make an appointment to see your doctor.
8. **Call Back If:**
    - Chest pain, light-headedness, or difficulty breathing occurs.
    - Heart beating more than 130 beats/minute.
    - More than 3 extra or skipped beats/minute.
    - You become worse.

BACKGROUND INFORMATION

General

- **Normal Heart Rate:** The normal heart rate is regular and between 60 and 100 beats per minute. The heart rate increases with exercise, emotional stress, and fever. Athletes may have a resting pulse of less than 60.
- **Palpitations:** Everybody experiences palpitations at some point in their lives. In most circumstances it is simply a heightened awareness of the heart's normal beating.
- **Rapid Heart Rate:** Patients with anxiety or stress may describe a "rapid heartbeat" or "pounding" in their chest from their heart beating. If they are able to measure their own heart rate, they will relate that the heart is beating regularly at < 130 beats/minute. Patients with a heart rate greater than 130 (excluding during exercise) require evaluation.

- **Extra Heartbeats:** Occasional extra heartbeats are also experienced by almost everyone. Patients may state that their heart "jumps," "skips a beat," or "flip-flops." Lack of sleep, stress, and caffeinated beverages can aggravate this condition. If the patient states that this is occurring 4 or more times per minute on an ongoing basis, then they require physician evaluation.
- **Automatic Implantable Cardioverter Defibrillator (AICD):** This internal device analyzes the cardiac rhythm and automatically delivers a shock to the heart when needed. The patient can feel the shock. A patient with an AICD typically has a past history of either ventricular fibrillation, symptomatic ventricular tachycardia, or unexplained syncope.

Causes

- **Anxiety:** Stress, panic disorder, hyperventilation.
- **Endocrine:** Hyperthyroidism, hypoglycemia.
- **Exercise:** Exercise and physical work are the most common cause of temporary tachycardia.
- **Cardiac Disease:** Underlying cardiac disease predisposes an individual to cardiac dysrrhythmias: angina, myocardial infarction, congestive heart failure, valvular heart disease.
- **Cardiac Dysrhythmias:** PACs, PVCs, SVT, VT, atrial fibrillation, etc.
- **Dehydration:** The heart rate speeds up with volume depletion.
- **Medication:** Thyroid hormone, digoxin (Lanoxin), diet pills.
- **Stimulants:** Caffeine, cocaine, tobacco.

HEAT EXPOSURE (HEAT EXHAUSTION AND HEATSTROKE)

DEFINITION

- Symptoms following exposure to high environmental temperatures or vigorous physical activity during hot weather

TRIAGE ASSESSMENT QUESTIONS FOR HEAT INJURY

Call EMS 911 Now

- Fever > 104° F (40.0° C)
  R/O: heatstroke
- Unconscious or difficult to awaken
  R/O: heatstroke
- Acting confused (e.g., disoriented, slurred speech)
  R/O: heatstroke
- Seizure has occurred
  R/O: heatstroke
- Very weak (e.g., can't stand)
  R/O: heatstroke, severe heat exhaustion
- Has fainted (passed out)
  R/O: heat syncope
- Sounds like a life-threatening emergency to the triager

See More Appropriate Protocol

- Swelling of both ankles (i.e., pedal edema) and worsened by hot weather
  Go to Protocol: Leg Swelling and Edema on page 180

Go to ED Now

- Unable to walk or can only walk with assistance (e.g., requires support)
  R/O: heat exhaustion
  FIRST AID: for heat exhaustion
- Fever > 103° F (39.4° C)

Go to ED Now (or to Office With PCP Approval)

- Vomiting interferes with drinking fluids
  R/O: need for IV fluids
- Dizziness, fever, or muscle cramps persist after 2 hours of oral fluids and rest
  R/O: need for IV fluids
- Patient sounds very sick or weak to the triager

Go to Office Now

- Fever > 100.5° F (38.1° C) and over 60 years of age
  R/O: heat exhaustion or bacterial illness
- Fever > 100.5° F (38.1° C) and has diabetes mellitus or a weakened immune system (e.g., HIV positive, cancer chemotherapy, organ transplant, splenectomy, chronic steroids)
  R/O: heat exhaustion or bacterial illness
- Fever > 100.5° F (38.1° C) and bedridden (e.g., nursing home patient, stroke, chronic illness, recovering from surgery)
  R/O: heat exhaustion or bacterial illness

See Today in Office

- Patient wants to be seen

Home Care

- Normal muscle cramps or sore muscles from heat exposure
  R/O: heat cramps
- Normal transient (1 to 2 hours) fever (< 103° F or 39.4° C) from heat exposure
  R/O: mild heat exhaustion
- Normal hot, flushed (pink) skin from heat exposure
  R/O: mild heat exhaustion
- Normal mild dehydration suspected (e.g., dizziness, weakness, nausea) from heat exposure
  R/O: mild heat exhaustion, dehydration

HOME CARE ADVICE FOR HEAT INJURY

1. **Mild Heat Exposure Symptoms:**
   - **Heat Cramps:** Heat cramps are a common reaction to excessive heat exposure. They are not usually serious but can be a warning sign of impending heat exhaustion. Heat cramps mean that your body needs more liquids and salt.
   - **Temperature Elevation:** The body can normally become overheated from sun exposure and/or exercise. The temperature should come down to normal after lost fluids are replaced and you have been able to rest for 1 or 2 hours.

- **Facial Flushing:** Your skin can become very pink or flushed when you become overheated. The skin color should return to normal in 1 or 2 hours.
- **Dizziness:** Dizziness is usually due to mild dehydration from all the sweating that occurs with heat exposure. It should disappear in 1 to 2 hours after the lost fluids are replaced.

2. **Move to a Cool, Shady Area:**
   - Move to a cool, shady area. If possible, move into an air-conditioned place.
   - Remove excess clothing or equipment (e.g., sports gear, protective work uniforms).
   - Rest until feeling better.
3. **Drink Liquids to Rehydrate:**

   What?
   - Drink a sports-rehydration drink (e.g., Gatorade or Powerade), which contains sugar and salt.
   - Or, drink water, and eat some salty foods (e.g., potato chips or pretzels).

   How Much?
   - Approximately 1 cup (240 mL) every 15 minutes for the next 1-2 hours.
   - Your urine (pee) color can help you tell if you have drunk enough liquids. Dark-yellow urine suggests dehydration. Clear or light-yellow urine suggests that you have drunk enough liquids.
4. **Avoid:**
   - Don't take salt tablets (Reason: they may cause vomiting).
   - Don't drink carbonated beverages (Reason: bubbles fill up stomach).
   - Don't drink alcohol or caffeinated beverages (Reason: they are dehydrating).
5. **Cool Bath for Elevated Temperature:**
   - After you drink some water, take a cool bath or shower for 5 minutes (Reason: brings down the temperature more quickly).
   - **Fever Medications:** Fever medications like acetaminophen (Tylenol) are of no value in reducing a body temperature elevation from heat exposure.
6. **Call Back If:**
   - Fever rises more than 103° F (39.4° C).
   - Dizziness, fever, or muscle cramps last more than 2 hours.
   - Vomiting interferes with taking fluids.
   - You become worse.

FIRST AID

First Aid Advice for Heatstroke or Sunstroke:

- Call EMS 911 immediately.
- Move to a cool, shady area. If possible, move into an air-conditioned place.
- Remove excess clothing or equipment (e.g., sports gear, protective work uniforms).
- Sponge the entire body surface with cool water (as cool as tolerated without shivering). If available, place ice packs on the neck, armpits, and groin. Fan the patient to increase evaporation.
- Keep the feet elevated to counteract shock.
- If the patient is awake, give as much cold water or sports drink (e.g., Gatorade, Powerade) as he or she can tolerate.
- Fever medicines are of no value for heatstroke.

First Aid for Heat Exhaustion:

- Put the patient in a cool place. Lie down with the feet elevated.
- Undress patient (except for underwear) so the body surface can give off heat.
- Sponge the entire body surface continuously with cool water (as cool as tolerated without shivering).
- Fan the patient to increase evaporation.
- After 2 or 3 glasses of water, drive the patient in to be seen. During the drive, provide unlimited amounts of water.

BACKGROUND INFORMATION

Cause

- The body's temperature rises when internal heat production and external heat exposure exceeds the capacity of the body to dispel heat.
- Heat injuries generally occur as a result of exposure to high temperatures and/or high humidity.

Types of Heat Injuries

There are 5 main reactions to hot environmental temperatures:

- **Heatstroke or Sunstroke:** Hot, flushed skin; high fever > 105° F (40.5° C) rectally; the absence of sweating (in 50%); confusion or unconsciousness; and shock are present. Exertional heatstroke occurs with exertion/exercise and the onset is usually rapid. Classic heatstroke typically occurs during heat waves and the onset is usually gradual. A rectal temperature is more accurate than an oral temperature in these disorders. Heatstroke is a life-threatening emergency with a 10-70% mortality rate if not treated promptly. EMS 911 transport is required.

- **Heat Exhaustion:** Symptoms may include profuse sweating, headache, nausea, vomiting, dizziness, and weakness. The body temperature can range from normal to 104° F (40° C). The onset is usually gradual. Patients with heat exhaustion are dehydrated and depleted of electrolytes (sodium, potassium). Treatment consists of rest, fluid, and electrolyte replacement.
- **Heat Syncope:** This is an orthostatic syncope that develops from standing up too suddenly or from prolonged standing.
- **Heat Cramps:** Severe muscle cramps in the limbs (especially calf or thigh muscles) and abdomen are present. No fever. Heat tetany (manifested by carpopedal spasm) may occur. Heat cramps are caused by decreased electrolytes and fluids in the muscle tissues. Treatment consists of rest, fluid, and electrolyte replacement.
- **Heat Edema:** Many individuals experience heat edema during the first few days of hot weather or after traveling to a warmer climate. There may be mild swelling of the feet and ankles and some puffiness of the fingers. Typically, the body adjusts to the higher temperatures (acclimatizes) in a couple of days and the swelling resolves.

Preventing Heat Reactions:

- When you are working or exercising in a hot environment, you need to drink large amounts of cool liquids. This means 1 cup every 15 minutes. Water is the ideal solution for replacing lost sweat. Very little salt is lost. Special glucose-electrolyte solutions (sports drinks) offer no advantage over water unless exercising for longer than an hour.
- Take 5-minute water breaks in the shade every 25 minutes. Drink water even if you are not thirsty. Thirst is often delayed until a person is almost dehydrated. You cannot drink too much water during hot weather.
- Avoid salt tablets because they slow down stomach emptying and delay the absorption of fluids.
- Wear a single layer of lightweight clothing. Change it if it becomes wet with perspiration.
- Athletic coaches recommend that exercise sessions be shortened and less vigorous if the temperature exceeds 82° F (28° C), especially if the humidity is high.
- When using a hot tub, limit exposure to 15 minutes and have a buddy system in case a heat reaction suddenly occurs. Hot tubs and saunas should be avoided by people with a fever. Hot tubs and saunas should not be used after vigorous exercise when the body needs to release heat.
- During heat waves, spend as much time as possible in cool environments (e.g., with air-conditioning) or use an electric fan. Slow down. It takes at least a week to acclimate to a hot environment.

HIGH BLOOD PRESSURE

DEFINITION

- Systolic blood pressure > 140 or
- Diastolic blood pressure > 90 or
- Taking medications for high blood pressure

If adult is having symptoms (e.g., headache, chest pain, difficulty breathing), then go to that guideline first and use this guideline afterward.

TRIAGE ASSESSMENT QUESTIONS

Call EMS 911 Now

- Sounds like a life-threatening emergency to the triager

Go to L&D Now (or to Office With PCP Approval)

- Pregnant and new hand or face swelling
  R/O: preeclampsia
- Pregnant > 20 weeks and BP > 140/90
  R/O: preeclampsia

Go to ED Now (or to Office With PCP Approval)

- BP > 160/100 and any cardiac or neurologic symptoms (e.g., chest pain, difficulty breathing, unsteady gait, blurred vision)
  R/O: hypertensive emergency
- Patient sounds very sick or weak to the triager

Discuss With PCP and Callback by Nurse Within 1 Hour

- BP = 180/110 and missed most recent dose of blood pressure medication
  Reason: needs to take medicine and recheck blood pressure

See Today in Office

- BP > 180/110
  Reason: asymptomatic hypertension, stage 2. May need medication adjustment or initiation.
- Patient wants to be seen
  Reason: for BP check

Discuss With PCP and Callback by Nurse Today

- Ran out of BP medications
  Reason: refill
- Taking BP medications and feels is having side effects (e.g., impotence, cough, dizziness)
  Reason: may need dose adjustment or new med

See Within 2 Weeks in Office

- BP > 160/100
  Reason: asymptomatic hypertension, stage 2. May need medication adjustment or initiation.
- BP > 140/90 and is taking BP medications
  Reason: may need medication adjustment, or counseling regarding lifestyle modifications
- BP > 140/90 and is not taking BP medications
  Reason: may need medication initiation, or counseling regarding lifestyle modifications
- BP > 120/90 and no improvement after lifestyle modifications per care advice
  Reason: may need medication initiation, adjustment, or counseling regarding lifestyle modifications
- BP > 130/80 and history of heart problems, kidney disease, or diabetes
  Reason: high normal BP, but high-risk patient; may need medication adjustment or initiation

Home Care

- BP < 140/90 and taking BP medications
  Reason: hypertension, treatment goal usually < 140/90
- BP 120-139/80-89
  Reason: prehypertension, lifestyle modification recommended
- BP < 120/80
  Reason: normal blood pressure

HOME CARE ADVICE

General Care Advice for High Blood Pressure

1. **General:**
   - Untreated high blood pressure may cause damage to the heart, brain, kidneys, and eyes.
   - Treatment of high blood pressure can reduce the risk of stroke, heart attack, and heart failure.
   - The goal of blood pressure treatment for most patients with hypertension is to keep the blood pressure under 140/90.
2. **BP 120-139/80-89**
   - This is considered borderline high blood pressure, or prehypertension.
   - Sometimes, changes in your lifestyle can reduce your blood pressure without medications.
   - If your blood pressure stays elevated during the next month, you should go in to see the doctor and get your blood pressure checked.
3. **BP Less Than 120/80**
   - This is considered normal blood pressure.
4. **Lifestyle Changes**
   The following lifestyle changes can help you reduce your blood pressure:
   - Maintain a healthy weight. Lose weight if you are overweight.
   - Do 30 minutes of aerobic physical activity (e.g., brisk walking) most days of the week.
   - Eat a diet high in fresh fruits and low-fat dairy products. Limit your intake of saturated and total fat. Choose foods that are lower in salt.
   - If you smoke, you should stop.
   - If you drink alcohol, you should limit your daily alcohol drinking. Women should have no more than 1 drink per day. Men should have no more than 2 drinks per day. A drink is defined as 1.5-oz hard liquor (one shot or jigger; 45 mL), 5-oz wine (small glass; 150 mL), or 12-oz beer (one can; 360 mL).
5. **Call Back If:**
   - Headache, blurred vision, difficulty talking, or difficulty walking occurs.
   - Chest pain or difficulty breathing occurs.
   - You want to go in to the office for a blood pressure check.
   - You become worse.

Missed Dose of Blood Pressure Medication

1. **What to Do When You Miss a Dose of Your Blood Pressure Medication:**
   - Generally, you should take a missed dose as soon as you remember.
   - If it is more than 8 hours until your next dose, take the missed dose of medication now.
   - If it is less than 8 hours until your next dose, skip the missed dose and take the medicine at the next regularly scheduled time.
   - Do NOT take 2 doses of a blood pressure medication at the same time because you missed a dose.
2. **Call Back If:**
   - Headache, blurred vision, difficulty talking, or difficulty walking occurs.
   - Chest pain or difficulty breathing occurs.
   - You want to come in to the office for a blood pressure check.
   - You become worse.

Internet Resource—National High Blood Pressure Education Program

1. **Internet Resource—National High Blood Pressure Education Program**
   - My Blood Pressure Wallet Card: www.nhlbi.nih.gov/health/public/heart/hbp/hbpwallet.htm
   - Your Guide to Lowering Blood Pressure: www.nhlbi.nih.gov/health/public/heart/hbp/hbp_low/index.htm

BACKGROUND INFORMATION

General Information

- **Systolic Vs Diastolic:** The blood pressure (BP) reading is written as 2 numbers, the systolic pressure and the diastolic pressure. For example, if a person had a BP of 130/65, then 130 would be the systolic blood pressure and 65 would be the diastolic blood pressure.
- **Definition of High Blood Pressure:** An adult has hypertension (high blood pressure) if the blood pressure (BP) readings consistently show a BP greater than 140/90, that is, a systolic BP over 140 OR a diastolic BP over 90.
- Untreated hypertension may cause damage to the heart, brain, kidneys, and eyes.
- There are age-related increases in blood pressure, such that over 50% of adults over the age of 60 have hypertension.
- Automatic home BP measurement devices can sometimes be unreliable. Have patient check BP in both arms. If there is another adult in the home, consider checking his/her BP to see if the device is functioning correctly.
- Current research casts substantial doubt on the common belief that hypertension causes headaches. However, it is important to emphasize that a patient who has a severe headache which he or she describes as being the "worst headache" or having sudden onset (thunderclap) deserves an emergency evaluation.

Blood Pressure Classification In Adults

- **Normal:** Less than 120/80
- **Prehypertension:** Between 120-139/80-89
- **Hypertension—Stage 1:** Between 140-159/90-99
- **Hypertension—Stage 2:** Greater than 159/99

Benefits of Antihypertensive Medications

- Reduce incidence of stroke by 35-40%
- Reduce incidence of myocardial infarction by 20-25%
- Reduce incidence of congestive heart failure by more than 50%

HIVES

DEFINITION

- A very itchy rash made up of flat raised/swollen spots patches of skin.
- Use this guideline only if the patient has symptoms that match Hives.

Symptoms of Hives (Urticaria) Include:

- Itchy, swollen patches or bumps that appear suddenly.
- Patches change shape and location frequently; any one patch generally only lasts for a few hours then fades away.
- Sizes of patches vary from ½ inch (6 mm) to several inches across.
- In whites and individuals with lighter skin tones, hives appear pink or red in color, with a central area of paleness (welts).

Itching Severity Is Defined As:

- **Mild:** Doesn't interfere with normal activities
- **Moderate-Severe:** Interferes with work, school, sleep, or other activities

TRIAGE ASSESSMENT QUESTIONS

Call EMS 911 Now

- Difficulty breathing or wheezing now
  R/O: anaphylaxis
- Rapid onset of swollen tongue
  R/O: anaphylaxis
- Rapid onset of hoarseness or cough
  R/O: anaphylaxis
- Very weak (e.g., can't stand)
  R/O: anaphylaxis
- Difficult to awaken or acting confused (e.g., disoriented, slurred speech)
  R/O: anaphylaxis
- Life-threatening reaction (anaphylaxis) in the past to similar substance (e.g., food, insect bite/sting, chemical, etc.) and < 2 hours since exposure
  Reason: high likelihood of recurrent severe reaction
- Sounds like a life-threatening emergency to the triager

See More Appropriate Protocol

- Bee, wasp, or yellow jacket sting within last 24 hours
  Go to Protocol: Bee Sting on page 32
- Taking a new medicine now or within last 3 days
  Exception: antihistamine, decongestant or other OTC cough/cold medicines
  Go to Protocol: Rash, Widespread on Drugs (Drug Reaction) on page 212
- Doesn't match the symptoms of hives
  Go to Protocol: Rash, Widespread and Cause Unknown on page 209

Go to ED Now

- Swollen tongue
  R/O: angioedema
- Widespread hives and onset < 2 hours of exposure to high-risk allergen (e.g., peanuts, tree nuts, fish, or shellfish)

Go to ED Now (or to Office With PCP Approval)

- Patient sounds very sick or weak to the triager

See Today in Office

- MODERATE-SEVERE hives persist (i.e., hives interfere with normal activities or work) and taking antihistamine (e.g., Benadryl, Claritin) > 24 hours
- Hives have become worse and taking oral steroids (e.g., prednisone) > 24 hours
- Abdominal pain
  R/O: gastrointestinal angioedema
- Joint swelling
  R/O: serum sickness reaction
- Fever
  R/O: treatable infection as cause of hives
- Patient wants to be seen

See Today or Tomorrow in Office

- Hives persist > 1 week

See Within 3 Days in Office

- Widespread hives and onset > 2 hours of exposure to high-risk allergen (e.g., peanuts, tree nuts, fish, or shellfish)
- Hives from food reaction and diagnosis never confirmed by a physician

- Hives has occurred 3 or more times in the last year and the cause is not known
  Reason: needs diagnosis confirmed, possible further workup

Home Care

- ○ Hives from food reaction
- ○ Localized hives
- ○ Widespread hives

HOME CARE ADVICE FOR HIVES

Hives From Food Reaction

1. **Food-Related Hives:**
   - Foods can cause transient hives, especially around the mouth.
   - Some are mild food allergies; others can occur in anyone (e.g., with strawberries).
   - Hives from foods usually disappear within 6 hours.
2. **Antihistamine (e.g., Benadryl) for Hives From Food:**
   - One or two dosages of an antihistamine will accelerate the clearing of this type of hives.
   - Benadryl (diphenhydramine) is an antihistamine. The adult dose is 25-50 mg. If the hives are still present after 6 hours, repeat the Benadryl.
   - If Benadryl is not available, use any hay fever or cold medicine that contains an antihistamine. Examples of other antihistamines are chlorpheniramine (Chlor-Trimeton, Chlor-Tripolon) and loratadine (Claritin, Alavert). Loratadine is a newer (second-generation) antihistamine and it causes less sedation than diphenhydramine.
   - **Caution:** This type of medication may cause sleepiness. Do not drink alcohol, drive, or operate dangerous machinery while taking antihistamines. Do not take these medications if you have prostate enlargement.
   - Read the package instructions thoroughly on all medications that you take.
3. **Prevention:** In the future, avoid any food you think caused the hives.
4. **Call Back If:**
   - Severe hives or severe itching persist more than 24 hours despite taking an antihistamine (e.g., Benadryl).
   - You become worse.

Localized Hives

1. **Localized Hives:**
   - For localized hives, wash the allergic substance off the skin with soap and water.
   - If itchy, massage the area with a cold washcloth or ice.
   - Localized hives usually disappear in a few hours and don't need treatment with an oral antihistamine (e.g., Benadryl).
2. **Hydrocortisone Cream:**
   - For very itchy spots, apply hydrocortisone cream 4 times a day as needed.
   - Available OTC in United States as 0.5% and 1% cream.
   - Available OTC in Canada as 0.5% cream.
3. **Prevention:** Try to avoid any substance that you think caused the hives.
4. **Call Back If:**
   - Severe hives or severe itching persist more than 24 hours despite taking an antihistamine (e.g., Benadryl).
   - Hives last more than 1 week.
   - You become worse.

Widespread Hives

1. **Widespread Hives:**
   - Remove allergens. For widespread hives be certain to take a bath or shower, if triggered by pollens or animal contact. Change clothes.
   - Take a cool bath for 10 minutes to relieve itching. Rub very itchy areas with an ice cube for 10 minutes.
   - Hives normally come and go for 3 or 4 days, then disappear.
2. **Antihistamine (e.g., Claritin) for Widespread Hives:**
   - Take an antihistamine like loratadine (e.g., OTC Claritin, Alavert) for widespread hives that itch. The adult dosage of loratadine is 10 mg by mouth once each day. Continue the antihistamine until the hives have been gone for 24 hours.
   - Loratidine is a newer (second-generation) antihistamine and it causes less sedation than diphenhydramine (Benadryl) or chlorpheniramine (Chlor-Trimeton).

- **Caution:** This type of medication may cause sleepiness. Do not drink alcohol, drive, or operate dangerous machinery while taking antihistamines. Do not take these medications if you have prostate enlargement.
- Read the package instructions thoroughly on all medications that you take.

3. **Contagiousness:** Hives are not contagious. You can return to work or school if the hives do not interfere with normal activities.
4. **Prevention:** If you identify a substance that causes hives, try to avoid that substance in the future.
5. **Call Back If:**
   - Severe itching persists longer than 24 hours while taking an antihistamine.
   - Hives persist longer than 1 week.
   - You become worse.

FIRST AID

First Aid Advice for Anaphylaxis—Epinephrine (Pending EMS Arrival):

- If the patient has an epinephrine autoinjector, the patient should use it now.
- Use the autoinjector on the upper outer thigh. You may give it through clothing if necessary.

Epinephrine is available in autoinjectors under trade names: EpiPen, EpiPen Jr, and Twinject. EpiPen is a single injection. Twinject has a second injection that can be used if there is no improvement after 5 minutes.

First Aid Advice for Anaphylaxis—Benadryl (Pending EMS Arrival):

- Give antihistamine orally NOW if able to swallow.
- Use Benadryl (diphenhydramine; adult dose 50 mg) or any other available antihistamine.

First Aid Advice for Anaphylactic Shock (Pending EMS Arrival):

- Lie down with feet elevated.

BACKGROUND INFORMATION

General

- The medical term for hives is urticaria.
- Hives are sometimes an allergic skin reaction to something that the patient has eaten, touched, or in some other manner been exposed to. Hives are not contagious.
- Hives usually come and go for several days to a week. Sometimes they can reappear weeks or months later. Some individuals have chronic urticaria, and symptoms can be intermittently present for months.

Causes of Hives

- **Localized:** Localized hives are usually due to skin contact with plants, pollen, food, a chemical, or pet saliva. Dermographism is the term used to describe patients who have localized hives in response to firm stroking of the skin. Localized hives are not caused by drugs, infection, or swallowed foods. Localized hives usually resolve in less than 4 hours.
- **Widespread:** Widespread hives can be an allergic reaction to a food, cosmetic product, drug, insect bite, or other substance. Sometimes widespread hives shows up after a viral infection. Stress may bring on or aggravate hives. Often the cause is not found (idiopathic).

Definitions

- **Anaphylactic Reaction:** Anaphylaxis is a serious allergic reaction that is rapid in onset and may cause death.
- **Severe Allergic Reaction:** Any associated symptoms besides skin findings: swollen tongue, shortness of breath, syncope, abdominal pain.
- **Localized Hives:** Hives on one area of the body only.
- **Widespread Hives:** Hives on multiple (2 or more) areas of the body.

IMMUNIZATION REACTIONS

DEFINITION

- Patient believes they are having a reaction to a recent immunization.
- Reactions to anthrax, chickenpox (varicella), hepatitis A, hepatitis B, HPV (human papillomavirus), influenza, Japanese encephalitis, MMR (measles, mumps, rubella), meningococcal, pneumococcal, polio, rabies, shingles (herpes zoster), smallpox (vaccinia), Td (tetanus, diphtheria), Tdap (tetanus, diphtheria, pertussis), and yellow fever vaccines are covered.
- Use this guideline only if the patient has symptoms that match Immunization Reaction.

Symptoms of an Immunization Reaction (Vaccine Reaction) Include:

- MINOR TEMPORARY ADVERSE REACTIONS ARE COMMON. Examples include local pain and swelling at the injection site, fever, headache, muscle aches. Most local reactions at the injection site occur within 2 days. Fever with most vaccines begins within 24 hours and lasts 2-3 days. With live vaccines (MMR and chickenpox), fever and systemic reactions usually begin within 1 and 4 weeks.
- SERIOUS ADVERSE REACTIONS ARE RARE. Anaphylaxis can occur with any vaccine. Anaphylactic symptoms start within 2 hours (usually within 20 minutes) after injection.

TRIAGE ASSESSMENT QUESTIONS

Call EMS 911 Now

- ● Difficulty with breathing or swallowing starts within 2 hours after injection
  R/O: anaphylactic reaction
- ● Difficult to awaken or acting confused (e.g., disoriented, slurred speech)
  R/O: acute encephalopathy
- ● Unresponsive, passed out, or very weak
  R/O: acute encephalopathy
- ● Sounds like a life-threatening emergency to the triager

Go to ED Now (or to Office With PCP Approval)

- ● Sounds like a severe, unusual reaction to the triager
  R/O: brachial neuritis, etc.

Go to Office Now

- ● Fever > 103° F (39.4° C)
  R/O: severe reaction, bacteremia
- ● Fever > 100.5° F (38.1° C) and over 60 years of age
- ● Fever > 100.5° F (38.1° C) and has diabetes mellitus or a weakened immune system (e.g., HIV positive, cancer chemotherapy, organ transplant, splenectomy, chronic steroids)
- ● Fever > 100.5° F (38.1° C) and bedridden (e.g., nursing home patient, stroke, chronic illness, recovering from surgery)
  R/O: bacterial infection
  Note: may need ambulance transport to ED
- ● Measles vaccine and purple/blood-colored rash (onset day 6-12)
  R/O: purpura or petechiae, thrombocytopenia
- ● Redness or red streak around the injection site begins > 48 hours after shot
  R/O: cellulitis, lymphangitis

See Today in Office

- ● Fever present > 3 days (72 hours)
  R/O: bacterial superinfection
- ● Smallpox vaccine and eye pain, eye redness, or rash on eyelids
  R/O: inadvertent innoculation and resultant vaccinial keratitis

See Today or Tomorrow in Office

- ● Deep lump follows (in 2 to 8 weeks) Td or Tdap shot, and becomes tender to the touch
  R/O: secondary bacterial infection
- ● Patient wants to be seen

Home Care

- ○ Mild immunization reaction
- ○ Painless lump at tetanus-diphtheria (Td) injection site
- ○ Immunization reactions, questions about

HOME CARE ADVICE FOR IMMUNIZATION REACTIONS

General Home Care Advice

1. **Cold Pack for Local Reaction at Injection Site:**
    - Apply a cold pack or ice in a wet washcloth to the area for 20 minutes. Repeat in 1 hour.
    - Then apply as needed for the first 48 hours after the injection (Reason: reduce the pain and swelling).
2. **Pain and Fever Medicines:**
    - For pain or fever relief, take acetaminophen or ibuprofen.
    - Treat fevers above 101° F (38.3° C).
    - The goal of fever therapy is to bring the fever down to a comfortable level. Remember that fever medicine usually lowers fever 2-3° F (1-1.5° C).

    Acetaminophen (e.g., Tylenol):
    - Take 650 mg by mouth every 4-6 hours as needed. Each Regular Strength Tylenol pill has 325 mg of acetaminophen. The most you should take each day is 3,250 mg (10 pills a day).
    - Another choice is to take 1,000 mg every 8 hours. Each Extra Strength Tylenol pill has 500 mg of acetaminophen. The most you should take each day is 3,000 mg (6 pills a day).

    Ibuprofen (e.g., Motrin, Advil):
    - Take 400 mg by mouth every 6 hours.
    - Another choice is to take 600 mg by mouth every 8 hours.

    Extra Notes:
    - Acetaminophen is thought to be safer than ibuprofen in people over 65 years old. Acetaminophen is in many OTC and prescription medicines. It might be in more than one medicine that you are taking. You need to be careful and not take an overdose. An acetaminophen overdose can hurt the liver.
    - **Caution:** Do not take acetaminophen if you have liver disease.
    - **Caution:** Do not take ibuprofen if you have stomach problems, kidney disease, are pregnant, or have been told by your doctor to avoid this type of anti-inflammatory drug. Do not take ibuprofen for more than 7 days without consulting your doctor.
    - Use the lowest amount of medicine that makes your pain or fever better.
    - Before taking any medicine, read all the instructions on the package.
3. **Td or Tdap Vaccination Lump:**
    - A painless lump (or nodule) sometimes develops at the Td or Tdap injection site 1 or 2 weeks later.
    - It is harmless and usually will disappear in about 2 months.
4. **Call Back If:**
    - Fever lasts more than 3 days.
    - Pain lasts more than 3 days.
    - Injection site starts to look infected.
    - You become worse.

Common Harmless Reactions—Reassurance

1. **Anthrax Vaccine:**
    - A small lump at injection site (in 50%)
    - Local pain, redness, swelling, and itching at injection site (in 30-60%)
    - Moderate local reactions 1-5 inches (2-13 cm) wide (in 1-5%)
    - Large local reactions (in less than 1%)
    - Muscle aches and joint aches (in 20%)
    - Headaches (in 20%)
    - Fever and chills (in 5%)
2. **Chickenpox Vaccine:**
    - Local pain at injection site (in 25%).
    - Fever (in 10-15%).
    - Mild chickenpox-like rash (2-5 spots) occurring up to 1 month after vaccination (in 5%). There is minimal chance of transmission of the vaccine virus to others; only 3 cases of transmission in over 14 million vaccines. Adults with these vaccine rashes can go to work or school. Keep rash covered with clothing or Band-Aid. Avoid contact with immunocompromised individuals (e.g., HIV, cancer chemotherapy, transplant recipients).

3. **Hepatitis A (HAV) Vaccine:**
    - Local pain at injection site (in 50%)
    - Headache (in 15%)
    - Tiredness (in 7%)
    - Fever
4. **Hepatitis B (HBV) Vaccine:**
    - Local pain at injection site (in 25%)
    - Fever (in 1%)
5. **Human Papillomavirus (HPV) Vaccine:**
    - Pain and tenderness at the injection site (in 80%).
    - Mild redness and mild swelling at the injection site (in 25%)
    - Fever over 100.4° F (38.0° C) (in 10%) and fever over 102° F (38.9° C) (in 1-2%)
    - Malaise, nausea, headache, body aches.
6. **H1N1 Influenza Vaccine (Inactivated; Injected):**
    - Local pain, redness, swelling at injection site.
    - Fever.
    - Muscle aches, headache, nausea.
    - If these symptoms occur, they usually last 1-2 days.
7. **H1N1 Influenza Intranasal Vaccine:**
    - This vaccine is made from a weakened virus; it does not cause swine flu but can cause mild flu-like symptoms, including:
        - Runny nose or nasal congestion
        - Fever, chills, muscle aches, and feeling tired
        - Headache
        - Sore throat
        - Vomiting, diarrhea
8. **Influenza (TIV; Injection) Vaccine:**
    - Local pain at injection site.
    - Fever.
    - Aches.
    - If these symptoms occur, they usually last 1-2 days.
9. **Influenza (LAIV; Intranasal) Vaccine:**
    - This vaccine is made from a weakened virus; it does not cause influenza but can cause mild symptoms in people who get it:
        - Runny nose or nasal congestion
        - Fever, chills, muscle aches, and feeling tired
        - Headache
        - Sore throat
10. **Japanese Encephalitis Vaccine:**
    - Pain, redness, or tenderness at the injection site (in 20%)
    - Malaise, nausea, headache, abdominal pain, body aches (in 10%)
11. **Measles, Mumps, Rubella (MMR) Vaccine:**
    - Local pain at injection site (in 10%).
    - Fever and rash occur within 7 to 12 days following the injection (in 5%). The fever is usually between 101° F and 103° F (38.3° C and 39.5° C) and lasts 2 to 3 days. The mild pink rash is mainly on the trunk and lasts 2 to 3 days. No treatment is necessary. You are not contagious.
    - Temporary mild pain and stiffness in the joints. This typically occurs in women (in 25% of women).
    - Temporary lymph node swelling.
12. **Meningococcal Vaccine:**
    - Mild local reaction (sore injection site) is common (50-70%).
    - Headache (40%).
    - Joint pain (20%).
    - Fever (1%).
    - The vaccine does not cause meningitis.
13. **Pneumococcal Vaccine:**
    - Mild pain, tenderness, swelling, OR redness at the injection site (in 50%)
    - Fever, muscle aches lasting for 1-2 days (in 1%)
14. **Polio Vaccine (IPV):**
    - Tenderness at the injection site
15. **Rabies Vaccine:**
    - Pain, redness, or tenderness at the injection site (in 30-74%)
    - Malaise, nausea, headache, abdominal pain, dizziness, body aches (in 5-40%)
16. **Shingles (Herpes Zoster; Zostavax) Vaccine:**
    - Redness, swelling, pain, or itching at the injection site (in 33%)
    - Headache (in 10%)
    - Fever over 100.4° F (38.0° C) (in 10%) and fever over 102° F (38.9° C) (in 1-2%)
    - Malaise, nausea, headache, body aches

17. **Smallpox Vaccine:**
    - It is expected and desired that patients develop a red bump (papule) at the vaccination site at 2-5 days; this turns into a pustule and reaches its maximum size at 8-10 days; this scabs over by 14-21 days and leaves a permanent scar.
    - Fever headache, muscle aches.
    - Swelling of nearby lymph nodes.
18. **Tetanus-Diphtheria (Td) Vaccine:**
    - Pain and tenderness at the injection site lasts for 24 to 48 hours (in 50-85%).
    - Mild redness and mild swelling at the injection site (in 20-30%).
    - Fever lasts for 24 to 48 hours (in 5-10%).
    - Malaise, nausea, headache.
19. **Tetanus-Diphtheria-Pertussis (Tdap) Vaccine:**
    - Pain and tenderness at the injection site (in 66%)
    - Mild redness and mild swelling at the injection site (in 20%)
    - Fever over 100.4° F (38.0° C) (in 1%) and fever over 102° F (38.9° C) (in 0.4%)
    - Malaise, nausea, headache, body aches
20. **Yellow Fever Vaccine:**
    - Pain, redness, or tenderness at the injection site.
    - Malaise, nausea, headache, abdominal pain, body aches.
    - These symptoms may occur in 25% of recipients; symptoms typically last 5-10 days.

Rare Adverse Reactions

1. **Anthrax Vaccine:**
    - Anaphylactic reaction (acute severe allergic reaction with wheezing, urticaria, shock). Very rare (1 person in 100,000).
2. **Chickenpox Vaccine:**
    - Anaphylactic reaction (acute severe allergic reaction with wheezing, urticaria, shock). Very rare.
    - Pneumonia. Very rare.
    - Seizure caused by fever (1 case per 1,000 doses of vaccine).
    - Possible association with Guillain-Barré syndrome (1-2 cases per million doses of vaccine).
3. **Hepatitis A (HAV) Vaccine:**
    - Anaphylactic reaction (acute severe allergic reaction with wheezing, urticaria, shock). Very rare.
4. **Hepatitis B (HBV) Vaccine:**
    - Anaphylactic reaction (acute severe allergic reaction with wheezing, urticaria, shock). Estimated at 1 in 300,000 doses of vaccine.
5. **Human Papillomavirus (HPV) Vaccine:**
    - Anaphylactic reaction (acute severe allergic reaction with wheezing, urticaria, shock). Very rare.
6. **H1N1 Influenza Vaccine (Inactivated; Injected):**
    - Anaphylactic reaction (acute severe allergic reaction with wheezing, urticaria, shock). Very rare.
    - In 1976, an earlier version of the swine flu vaccine was associated with cases of Guillain-Barré syndrome (GBS). Flu vaccines since that time have not been clearly linked to GBS.
7. **H1N1 Influenza Intranasal Vaccine:**
    - Anaphylactic reaction (acute severe allergic reaction with wheezing, urticaria, shock). Very rare.
8. **Influenza (TIV; Injected) Vaccine:**
    - Anaphylactic reaction (acute severe allergic reaction with wheezing, urticaria, shock). Very rare.
    - Possible association with Guillain-Barré syndrome (1-2 cases per million doses of vaccine).
9. **Influenza (LAIV; Intranasal) Vaccine:**
    - Anaphylactic reaction (acute severe allergic reaction with wheezing, urticaria, shock). Very rare.
10. **Japanese Encephalitis Vaccine:**
    - Anaphylactic reaction (acute severe allergic reaction with wheezing, urticaria, shock). Rare.
    - Severe allergic reactions with rash, hand, and face swelling; breathing difficulty (about 60 per 10,000).
    - Seizures and other nervous system problems (less than 1 in 50,000).
11. **Measles, Mumps, Rubella (MMR) Vaccine:**
    - Anaphylactic reaction (acute severe allergic reaction with wheezing, urticaria, shock).
    - Encephalitis and encephalopathy.
    - Temporary low platelet count (1 in 30,000 vaccine doses).

12. **Meningococcal Vaccine:**
    - Anaphylactic reaction (acute severe allergic reaction with wheezing, urticaria, shock).
    - Extremely rare (1 person in 1,000,000).
13. **Pneumococcal Vaccine:**
    - Anaphylactic reaction (acute severe allergic reaction with wheezing, urticaria, shock)
14. **Polio Vaccine (IPV):**
    - Severe allergic reaction. Very rare.
15. **Rabies Vaccine:**
    - Hives, joint pain, fever (in 6%).
    - Illness resembling Guillain-Barré syndrome, with complete recovery. Very rare.
16. **Shingles (Herpes Zoster; Zostavax) Vaccine:**
    - No serious reactions have been reported with this vaccine.
    - An anaphylactic reaction (acute severe allergic reaction with wheezing, urticaria, shock) is possible with any new medication.
17. **Smallpox Vaccine:**
    - Inadvertent inoculation is the most common complication. This results when the patient scratches the vaccine pustule and then spreads the vaccinia virus by touching another part of the body. Patients who develop eye pain or redness should see a physician (Reason: possible vaccinia keratitis).
    - Generalized vaccinia is a diffuse vesicular rash (blistering). Usually not serious (self-limited).
    - Hives, erythema multiforme.
    - The OVERALL RATE of these reactions is approximately 1,000 reactions for every 1 million doses of vaccine in patients receiving the vaccine for the first time. The rate is much less for patients being revaccinated.
18. **Tetanus-Diphtheria (Td) Vaccine:**
    - Anaphylactic reaction (acute severe allergic reaction with wheezing, urticaria, shock)
    - Brachial plexus neuropathy (deep ongoing upper arm pain with muscle atrophy and weakness)
    - Guillain-Barré syndrome
    - Sterile abscess
19. **Tetanus-Diphtheria-Pertussis (Tdap) Vaccine:**
    - Anaphylactic reaction (acute severe allergic reaction with wheezing, urticaria, shock)
20. **Yellow Fever Vaccine:**
    - Anaphylactic reaction (acute severe allergic reaction with wheezing, urticaria, shock) (1 in 131,000)
    - Nervous system reactions (approximately 1 in 200,000)

Rare Life-Threatening Reactions

1. **Smallpox Vaccine:**
    - Encephalitis.
    - Eczema vaccinatum, a serious diffuse rash seen in patients with underlying skin disorders (e.g., eczema).
    - Progressive vaccinia (vaccinia necrosum) is a progressive necrosis (skin death) in the area of the vaccination.
    - The OVERALL RATE of life-threatening reactions is approximately 14-52 reactions for every 1 million doses of vaccine in patients receiving the vaccine for the first time. The rate is less for patients being revaccinated. It is estimated that 1 patient in 1 million who receives the vaccine may die as a result; the death rate for revaccination has been estimated as 1 patient in 4 million.

FIRST AID

First Aid Advice for Anaphylaxis—Epinephrine (Pending EMS Arrival):

- If the patient has an epinephrine autoinjector, the patient should use it now.
- Use the autoinjector on the upper outer thigh. You may give it through clothing if necessary.
- Epinephrine is available in autoinjectors under trade names: EpiPen, EpiPen Jr, and Twinject. EpiPen is a single injection. Twinject has a second injection that can be used if there is no improvement after 5 minutes.

First Aid Advice for Anaphylaxis—Benadryl (Pending EMS Arrival):

- Give antihistamine orally NOW if able to swallow.
- Use Benadryl (diphenhydramine; adult dose 50 mg) or any other available antihistamine.

BACKGROUND INFORMATION

General

- Vaccines are generally safe and effective. Minor temporary adverse reactions are common. Serious adverse reactions are rare.
- Vaccinations are given in either the deltoid muscle of the upper arm (usually) or in the anterolateral thigh muscles (rarely). Vaccinations should not be given in the buttocks because studies have shown that such vaccination is not as effective because of the fatty tissue present.

Types of Reactions

- **Local Reaction:** Most local swelling, redness, and pain at the injection site begins within 24 hours of the shot (rarely 24 to 48 hours). It usually lasts 2 or 3 days. Occasionally, localized hives or itching occurs at the injection site; these usually last less than 12 hours. Localized hives do not mean you are allergic to the vaccine.
- **Systemic Reaction:** Fever with most vaccines (e.g., DTaP) begins within 24 hours (rarely 24-48 hours). Headache, myalgias, malaise, and poor appetite can also be seen. Systemic symptoms usually last 1 to 3 days.

Vaccine Information Statements From the CDC:

- Vaccine Information Statements (VISs) are information sheets produced by the Centers for Disease Control and Prevention (CDC) that explain to vaccine recipients the benefits and risks of a vaccine. US federal law requires that a VIS be handed out at the time certain vaccinations are administered. Each VIS is available for viewing and downloading on the Internet at: www.cdc.gov/vaccines/pubs/vis/default.htm.

CDC US National Immunization Hotline

- Trained specialists provide vaccine information; available to patients, nurses, doctors.
- Open 8:00 am-11:00 pm EST, Monday-Friday
- **Toll-free Phone Number:** 800-232-4636 (English and Spanish)

Internet Resources—Recommended Adult Immunization Schedules:

- **United States:** The Advisory Committee on Immunization Practices (ACIP) publishes vaccine recommendations. The most recent adult schedule is available at: www.cdc.gov/vaccines/schedules/hcp/adult.html.
- **Canada:** The National Advisory Committee on Immunization (NACI) publishes vaccine recommendations. These are available at: www.phac-aspc.gc.ca/im/is-cv/index.html. The seventh edition of the *Canadian Immunization Guide* (2006) is available at: www.phac-aspc.gc.ca/publicat/cig-gci/index-eng.php.

US National Vaccine Injury Compensation Program

- In the rare event that a serious reaction has definitely occurred, a federal program has been created to help pay for the injury.
- **Toll-free Phone Number:** 800-338-2382

Combination Vaccines:

- Combination vaccines are popular because they reduce the number of shots a person must receive. Knowing the names and content of combination vaccines allows the triage nurse to address the vaccine reactions of each ingredient.
- **MMR Vaccine:** Measles, mumps, rubella.
- **Comvax:** *Haemophilus influenzae* type b and hepatitis B.
- **Twinrix:** Hepatitis A and B.

INFLUENZA

DEFINITION

- Influenza is a viral respiratory infection that affects the nose, throat, trachea, and bronchi. It is also called the flu.
- Adult thinks he/she has influenza because other family members have it.
- Adult thinks he/she has influenza and it's prevalent in the community.
- Use this guideline only if the patient has symptoms that match Influenza.

Symptoms of Influenza Include:

- There is usually a sudden onset of fever, chills, feeling sick, muscle aches, and headache.
- Respiratory symptoms are similar to a common cold: runny nose, sore throat, and a bad cough.
- The fever is usually higher (102 - 104° F; 38.9 - 40° C) with influenza than with a cold. Headaches and muscle aches are also worse with influenza.

The following groups of individuals are at higher risk for complications from influenza and therefore are considered as HIGH RISK in this protocol:

- Persons 65 years and older
- Children younger than 5 years old
- Children and adolescents (less than 19 years old) who are receiving long-term aspirin therapy (Reason: at risk for Reye syndrome)
- Pregnant women
- Chronic medical conditions, including: cardiovascular (not hypertension), chronic pulmonary conditions (e.g., asthma, emphysema), immunosuppression (e.g., chemotherapy, HIV), renal failure, hematologic (e.g., sickle cell disease), and diabetes mellitus
- Residents of nursing homes and chronic care facilities

TRIAGE ASSESSMENT QUESTIONS

Call EMS 911 Now

- Severe difficulty breathing (e.g., struggling for each breath, speaks in single words)
- Bluish lips or face now
  R/O: hypoxia and need for oxygen
- Shock suspected (e.g., cold/pale/clammy skin, too weak to stand)
  R/O: shock
- Sounds like a life-threatening emergency to the triager

See More Appropriate Protocol

- Severe sore throat pain
  Go to Protocol: Sore Throat on page 241
- Severe cough
  Go to Protocol: Cough on page 66
- Doesn't match the symptoms for Influenza and sounds like a cold
  Go to Protocol: Colds on page 53
- Influenza vaccine reaction is suspected
  Go to Protocol: Immunization Reactions on page 155

Go to ED Now

- Headache and stiff neck (can't touch chin to chest)
  R/O: meningitis
- Chest pain
  Exception: MILD central chest pain, present only when coughing
  R/O: pneumonia, pleurisy

Go to ED Now (or to Office With PCP Approval)

- Difficulty breathing that is not severe and not relieved by cleaning out the nose
  R/O: pneumonia
- Patient sounds very sick or weak to the triager

Go to Office Now

- Fever > 104° F (40.0° C)
  R/O: serious bacterial infection
- Fever > 100.5° F (38.1° C) and over 60 years of age
  R/O: pneumonia
- Fever > 100.5° F (38.1° C) and diabetes mellitus or immunocompromised (e.g., HIV positive, cancer chemotherapy, splenectomy, organ transplant, chronic steroids)
  R/O: pneumonia
- Fever > 100.5° F (38.1° C) and bedridden (e.g., nursing home patient, stroke, chronic illness, recovering from surgery)
  R/O: pneumonia
  Note: may need ambulance transport to ED

Discuss With PCP and Callback by Nurse Within 1 Hour

- HIGH RISK (e.g., age > 64 years, pregnant, HIV+, chronic medical condition) and flu symptoms
  Reason: Treatment with antiviral medication should be considered, especially for symptoms present < 48 hours. PCP may wish to phone in a prescription to the pharmacy. HIGH RISK is defined in Definition area of protocol.

See Today in Office

- Using nasal washes and pain medicine > 24 hours and sinus pain (lower forehead, cheekbone, or eye) persists
  R/O: sinusitis
- Fever present > 3 days (72 hours)
  R/O: bacterial sinusitis, bronchitis, pneumonia
- Fever returns after gone for over 24 hours and symptoms worse (or not improved)
  R/O: bacterial sinusitis, bronchitis, pneumonia
- Earache
  R/O: otitis media

See Today or Tomorrow in Office

- Patient wants to be seen

Discuss With PCP and Callback by Nurse Today

- Patient requests antiviral medicine for influenza and flu symptoms present < 48 hours
  Note: Not a HIGH RISK patient. Patients who are not high risk typically do not require treatment with antiviral medication.

See Within 3 Days in Office

- Nasal discharge present > 10 days
  R/O: bacterial sinusitis, allergic rhinitis
- Cough present > 3 weeks

Home Care

- Probable influenza with no complications and not HIGH RISK (all triage questions negative)
  Reason: Not HIGH RISK. Patients who are not high risk typically do not require treatment with antiviral medication.
- Influenza vaccine, questions about

HOME CARE ADVICE FOR INFLUENZA

General Care Advice

1. **Reassurance:**
   - For most healthy adults, influenza feels like a bad cold. The dangers of influenza for normal, healthy people (under 65 years of age) are overrated.
   - The treatment of influenza depends on your main symptoms. Generally, treatment is the same as for other viral respiratory infections (colds). Bed rest is unnecessary.
2. **Treating the Symptoms of Flu:**
   - **Fever, Muscle Aches, and Headache:** For fever more than 101° F (38.3° C), muscle aches, and headaches, take acetaminophen every 4-6 hours (adults 650 mg) OR ibuprofen every 6-8 hours (adults 400-600 mg).
   - **Sore Throat:** Use throat lozenges, hard candy, or warm chicken broth.
   - **Cough:** Use cough drops.
   - **Hydrate:** Drink extra liquids. If the air in your home is dry, use a humidifier.
3. **No Aspirin:** Do not use aspirin for treatment of fever or pain (Reason: there is an association between influenza and Reye syndrome).
4. **Isolation Is Needed Until After the Fever Is Gone:**
   - The CDC recommends that people with influenza-like illness remain at home until at least 24 hours after they are free of fever (100° F or 37.8°C).
   - Do NOT go to work or school.

- Do NOT go to church, child care centers, shopping, or other public places.
- Do NOT shake hands.
- Avoid close contact with others (hugging, kissing).

5. **Expected Course:** The fever lasts 2-3 days, the runny nose 5-10 days, and the cough 2-3 weeks.
6. **Call Back If:**
   - Fever lasts more than 3 days.
   - Runny nose lasts more than 10 days.
   - Cough lasts more than 3 weeks.
   - You become short of breath or worse.

Treating the Symptoms of Flu—Additional Information

1. **For a Runny Nose With Profuse Discharge: Blow the Nose:**
   - Nasal mucus and discharge helps to wash viruses and bacteria out of the nose and sinuses.
   - Blowing the nose is all that is needed.
   - If the skin around your nostrils gets irritated, apply a tiny amount of petroleum ointment to the nasal openings once or twice a day.
2. **For A Stuffy Nose—Use Nasal Washes:**
   - **Introduction:** Saline (salt water) nasal irrigation is an effective and simple home remedy for treating cold symptoms and other conditions involving the nasal and sinus passages. Nasal irrigation consists of pouring, spraying, or squirting salt water into the nose and then letting it run back out.
   - **How It Helps:** The salt water rinses out excess mucus, washes out any irritants (dust, allergens) that might be present, and moisturizes the nasal cavity.
   - **Methods:** There are several ways to perform nasal irrigation. You can use a saline nasal spray bottle (available over-the-counter), a rubber ear syringe, a medical syringe without the needle, or a Neti Pot.

   Step-by-Step Instructions:
   - **Step 1:** Lean over a sink.
   - **Step 2:** Gently squirt or spray warm salt water into one of your nostrils.
   - **Step 3:** Some of the water may run into the back of your throat. Spit this out. If you swallow the salt water it will not hurt you.
   - **Step 4:** Blow your nose to clean out the water and mucus.
   - **Step 5:** Repeat steps 1-4 for the other nostril. You can do this a couple times a day if it seems to help you.

   How to Make Saline (Salt Water) Nasal Wash:
   - You can make your own saline nasal wash.
   - Add ½ tsp of table salt to 1 cup (8 oz; 240 mL) of warm water.
   - You should use sterile, distilled, or previously boiled water for nasal irrigation.
3. **Coughing Spasms:**
   - Drink warm fluids. Inhale warm mist (Reason: both relax the airway and loosen up the phlegm).
   - Suck on cough drops or hard candy to coat the irritated throat.
4. **For All Fevers:**
   - Drink cold fluids to prevent dehydration.
   - Dress in 1 layer of lightweight clothing and sleep with 1 light blanket.
   - For fevers less than 101° F (38.3° C), fever medicines are usually not necessary.
5. **Pain and Fever Medicines:**
   - For pain or fever relief, take acetaminophen or ibuprofen.
   - Treat fevers above 101° F (38.3° C).
   - The goal of fever therapy is to bring the fever down to a comfortable level. Remember that fever medicine usually lowers fever 2-3° F (1-1.5° C).

   Acetaminophen (e.g., Tylenol):
   - Take 650 mg by mouth every 4-6 hours as needed. Each Regular Strength Tylenol pill has 325 mg of acetaminophen. The most you should take each day is 3,250 mg (10 pills a day).
   - Another choice is to take 1,000 mg every 8 hours. Each Extra Strength Tylenol pill has 500 mg of acetaminophen. The most you should take each day is 3,000 mg (6 pills a day).

Ibuprofen (e.g., Motrin, Advil):

- Take 400 mg by mouth every 6 hours.
- Another choice is to take 600 mg by mouth every 8 hours.

Extra Notes:

- Acetaminophen is thought to be safer than ibuprofen in people over 65 years old.
- Acetaminophen is in many OTC and prescription medicines. It might be in more than one medicine that you are taking. You need to be careful and not take an overdose. An acetaminophen overdose can hurt the liver.
- **Caution:** Do not take acetaminophen if you have liver disease.
- **Caution:** Do not take ibuprofen if you have stomach problems, kidney disease, are pregnant, or have been told by your doctor to avoid this type of anti-inflammatory drug. Do not take ibuprofen for more than 7 days without consulting your doctor.
- Use the lowest amount of medicine that makes your pain or fever better.
- Before taking any medicine, read all the instructions on the package.

Inactivated Influenza Vaccine (TIV)—Flu Shot

1. **General:**
   - Given annually (in September-November) before the onset of influenza season.
   - The vaccine is 70-90% effective in preventing influenza. It is not 100% protective, as the influenza viruses change yearly.
   - The Vaccine Information Statement (VIS) for influenza is available at: www.cdc.gov/vaccines/pubs/vis/downloads/vis-flu.pdf.
2. **Indications for Getting the Influenza Vaccine—Which Adults Should Get a Flu Shot?**
   - All persons 50 years and older.
   - Patient populations at high-risk for complications of influenza: chronic cardiopulmonary conditions (e.g., asthma), immunosuppression (e.g., chemotherapy), renal dysfunction, diabetes, women who will be pregnant during flu season.
   - Patients with chronic medical conditions who reside in nursing home or chronic-care facilities.
   - Healthy persons who could transmit influenza to high-risk patients: health care workers, nursing home employees, and family members.
   - Note that the indications for getting the nasal spray vaccine are slightly different than those for the shot since the nasal spray contains live virus. Refer to the Vaccine Information Statement if additional information is needed.
   - Internet Resource: www.cdc.gov/flu/protect/keyfacts.htm.
3. **Indications—People Who Can Spread Influenza to Those at High Risk:**
   - Health care workers
   - Household contacts and caregivers of children from 0-59 months of age
   - Household contacts and caregivers of persons with medical conditions that put them at higher risk for severe complications from influenza

Live Influenza Vaccine (LAIV)—Nasal Spray

1. **General:**
   - This is a live, attenuated (weakened) virus vaccine to prevent influenza.
   - It is sprayed in the nose.
   - The Vaccine Information Statement (VIS) for the nasal spray flu vaccine is available at: www.cdc.gov/vaccines/pubs/vis/downloads/vis-flulive.pdf.
2. **Indications:** If vaccination is INDICATED, then the intranasal vaccine is an OPTION for vaccination of children and nonpregnant healthy adults from 5 to 49 years of age.

Additional Resources

- **Centers for Disease Control and Prevention:** www.cdc.gov/flu/Influenza; general information and latest recommendations.

BACKGROUND INFORMATION

General

- **Seasonal Epidemic:** Influenza viruses change (or mutate) yearly, which is why some individuals seem to get influenza every year. The influenza virus is spread via airborne droplet, from sneezing and coughing. Influenza epidemics occur commonly between November and March. During these months 5-40% of the population may be affected.
- **Expected Course:** The fever lasts 2-3 days, the runny nose 5-10 days, and the cough 2-3 weeks.
- **Incubation Period:** Spread is rapid because the incubation period is only 24 to 36 hours and the virus is very contagious.
- **Contagiousness:** A person is potentially contagious (virus may be in respiratory secretions) from 1 day prior to and for 7 days after the onset of symptoms (e.g., fever, cough). The CDC recommends that people with influenza-like illness remain at home until at least 24 hours after they are free of fever (100° F [37.8°C]).
- **Complications—Respiratory:** Viral and secondary bacterial pneumonia, COPD, and asthma exacerbations.
- **Complications—Other:** Heart failure, EKG abnormalities, Reye syndrome, poor diabetic control.

Antiviral Medications for Influenza

- **Four Medications Licensed in the United States and Canada:** Amantadine (Symmetrel), rimantadine (Flumadine; not available in Canada), zanamivir (Relenza), and oseltamivir (Tamiflu).
- **Treatment of Influenza:** These medications have been shown to reduce the duration (by 1 day) and severity of flu symptoms. They do not cure the disease nor remove all the symptoms. They must be started within 48 hours of symptom onset.
- **Prevention of Influenza:** These medications can also be taken prophylactically during influenza epidemics to prevent illness in high-risk patients. However, they should not be used as a substitute for vaccination.
- **Internet Resource:** www.cdc.gov/flu/about/qa/antiviral.htm.

Avian Flu

- As of the end of 2012, there have been 0 cases of avian flu in humans in the United States and Canada.
- **Symptoms:** Symptoms of avian flu are similar to influenza: fever, cough, muscle aches, sore throat. Pneumonia and eye infections can sometimes occur.
- **Treatment:** Oseltamivir (Tamiflu) may be helpful in treatment.
- Additional up-to-date information is available on the Internet at: www.cdc.gov/flu/avian.

INSECT BITE

DEFINITION

- Itching, pain, or swelling from an insect bite

Types of Insect Bites

- **Itchy Insect Bites:** Bites of chiggers (harvest mites), fleas, and bedbugs usually cause itchy, red bumps.
- **Painful Insect Bites:** Bites of horseflies, blackflies, deerflies, gnats, harvester ants, blister beetles, and centipedes usually cause a painful, red bump. Although fire ants are members of the *Hymenoptera* or bee family which have stingers on the back of their bodies, most people group them with other ants, which are insects. Within a few hours, fire ant bites can change to blisters or pimples.

TRIAGE ASSESSMENT QUESTIONS

Call EMS 911 Now

- Passed out (i.e., fainted, collapsed and was not responding)
  R/O: anaphylaxis
  Use FIRST AID ADVICE for anaphylaxis.
- Wheezing or difficulty breathing
  R/O: anaphylaxis
  Use FIRST AID ADVICE for anaphylaxis
- Hoarseness, cough, or tightness in the throat or chest
  R/O: anaphylaxis
  Use FIRST AID ADVICE for anaphylaxis
- Swollen tongue or difficulty swallowing
- Life-threatening reaction (anaphylaxis) in the past to same insect bite and < 2 hours since bite
- Sounds like a life-threatening emergency to the triager

See More Appropriate Protocol

- Bee sting(s)
  Go to Protocol: Bee Sting on page 32
- Spider bite(s)
  Go to Protocol: Spider Bite on page 244
- Tick bite(s)
  Go to Protocol: Tick Bite on page 268
- Doesn't sound like an insect bite
  Go to Protocol: Rash or Redness, Localized and Cause Unknown on page 216

Go to ED Now (or to Office With PCP Approval)

- Patient sounds very sick or weak to the triager

Go to Office Now

- SEVERE bite pain and not improved after 2 hours of pain medicine
- Fever and area is red
  R/O: cellulitis, lymphangitis
  Reason: fever and looks infected
- Fever and area is very tender to touch
  R/O: cellulitis, lymphangitis
  Reason: fever and looks infected
- Red streak or red line and length > 2 inches (5 cm)
  R/O: lymphangitis
  Note: lymphangitis looks like a red streak or line originating at the wound and ascending up the arm or leg toward the heart.

See Today in Office

- Red or very tender (to touch) area, and started over 24 hours after the bite
  R/O: cellulitis
- Red or very tender (to touch) area, getting larger over 48 hours after the bite
  R/O: cellulitis

See Today or Tomorrow in Office

- Patient wants to be seen

See Within 3 Days in Office

- SEVERE local itching (i.e., interferes with work, school, activities) and not improved after 24 hours of hydrocortisone cream
- Scab drains pus or increases in size, and not improved after applying antibiotic ointment for 2 days
  R/O: infected sore, impetigo
- Bite starts to look bad (e.g., blister, purplish skin, ulcer)
  R/O: necrotic spider bite (brown recluse, hobo spider) or other cause of skin lesion
- After 14 days the insect bite is not healed
  R/O: low-grade infection, misdiagnosis

Home Care

- ○ Itchy insect bite
- ○ Painful insect bite
- ○ Scab drains pus or increases in size
  R/O: infected sore, impetigo
- ○ West Nile virus, questions about
- ○ Preventing insect bites, questions about

HOME CARE ADVICE

Treatment for Insect Bites

1. **Local Treatment—Itchy Insect Bites (Including All Mosquito Bites)**
   - Apply calamine lotion or a baking soda paste.
   - If the itch is severe, use 1% hydrocortisone cream. Apply 4 times a day until the itch is less severe, then switch to calamine lotion.
   - Try applying firm, sharp, direct, steady pressure to the bite for 10 seconds. A fingernail, pen cap, or other object can be used.
2. **Oral Antihistamine Medication for Severe Itching:** Take an antihistamine by mouth to reduce the itching. Diphenhydramine (Benadryl) is a good choice. The adult dosage of Benadryl is 25-50 mg by mouth and you can take it up to 4 times a day.
   - Do not take antihistamine medications if you have prostate enlargement.
   - Antihistamines may cause sleepiness. Do not drink, drive, or operate dangerous machinery while taking antihistamines.
   - An over-the-counter antihistamine that causes less sleepiness is loratadine (e.g., Alavert or Claritin).
   - Read the package instructions thoroughly on all medications that you take.
3. **Local Treatment—Painful Insect Bites**
   - Rub the bite for 15 to 20 minutes with a cotton ball soaked in a meat tenderizer solution. This will usually relieve the pain (Caution: don't use near the eye).
   - If not available, use a baking soda solution on a cotton ball.
   - If neither is available, apply an ice cube for 20 minutes.
4. **Pain Medicines:**
   - For pain relief, take acetaminophen, ibuprofen, or naproxen.

   Acetaminophen (e.g., Tylenol):
   - Take 650 mg by mouth every 4-6 hours as needed. Each Regular Strength Tylenol pill has 325 mg of acetaminophen. The most you should take each day is 3,250 mg (10 pills a day).
   - Another choice is to take 1,000 mg every 8 hours. Each Extra Strength Tylenol pill has 500 mg of acetaminophen. The most you should take each day is 3,000 mg (6 pills a day).

   Ibuprofen (e.g., Motrin, Advil):
   - Take 400 mg by mouth every 6 hours.
   - Another choice is to take 600 mg by mouth every 8 hours.

   Naproxen (e.g., Aleve):
   - Take 250-500 mg by mouth every 12 hours.

   Extra Notes:
   - Acetaminophen is thought to be safer than ibuprofen or naproxen in people over 65 years old. Acetaminophen is in many OTC and prescription medicines. It might be in more than one medicine that you are taking. You need to be careful and not take an overdose. An acetaminophen overdose can hurt the liver.
   - **Caution:** Do not take acetaminophen if you have liver disease.
   - **Caution:** Do not take ibuprofen if you have stomach problems, kidney disease, are pregnant, or have been told by your doctor to avoid this type of anti-inflammatory drug. Do not take ibuprofen for more than 7 days without consulting your doctor.
   - Use the lowest amount of medicine that makes your pain feel better.
   - Before taking any medicine, read all the instructions on the package
5. **Antibiotic Ointment:** If the insect bite has a scab on it and the scab looks infected, apply an antibiotic ointment 4 times per day.
   - Cover the scab with a Band-Aid to prevent scratching and spread.
   - Repeat washing the sore, the antibiotic ointment, and the Band-Aid 4 times per day until healed.

6. **Expected Course:**
   - Most insect bites are itchy and puffy for several days.
   - Insect bites of the upper face can cause marked swelling around the eye, but this is harmless.
   - Any pinkness or redness usually lasts 3 days.
7. **Call Back If:**
   - Severe pain persists more than 2 hours after pain medicine.
   - Bite looks infected (redness, red streaks, increased tenderness).
   - Redness getting larger and more than 48 hours after the bite.
   - Infected scab doesn't look better after 48 hours of antibiotic ointment.
   - You become worse.

Infected Sore or Scab

1. **Reassurance:**
   - Sometimes a small infected sore can develop at the site of a cut, scratch, insect bite, or sting.
   - The typical appearance is a sore smaller than 1 inch (2.5 cm) in diameter. It is often covered by a soft, honey-yellow or yellow-brown crust or scab. Sometimes the scab may drain a tiny amount of pus or yellow fluid. Usually there is minimal to no pain.
   - Small infected sores usually get better with regular cleansing and use of an antibiotic ointment.
2. **Cleaning:**
   - Wash the area 2-3 times daily with an antibacterial soap and warm water.
   - Gently remove any scab. The bacteria live underneath the scab. You may need to soak the scab off by placing a warm, wet washcloth (or gauze) on the sore for 10 minutes.
3. **Antbiotic Ointment:**
   - Apply an antibiotic ointment 3 times per day.
   - Cover the sore with a Band-Aid to prevent scratching and spread.
   - Use Bacitracin ointment (OTC in United States) or Polysporin ointment (OTC in Canada) or one that you already have.
4. **Avoid Picking:** Avoid scratching and picking. This can worsen and spread a skin infection.
5. **Contagiousness:**
   - Infected sores can be spread by skin-to-skin contact.
   - Wash your hands frequently and avoid touching the sore.
   - **Work and School:** You can attend school or work if it is covered.
   - **Contact Sports:** Generally, you need to receive antibiotic treatment for 3 days before you can return to the sport. There can be no pus or drainage. You should check with your trainer, if there is one for your sports team.
6. **Expected Course:**
   - The sore should stop growing in 1 to 2 days and it should begin improving within 2-3 days.
   - The sore should be completely healed in 7-10 days.
7. **Call Back If:**
   - Fever occurs.
   - Spreading redness or a red streak occurs.
   - Sore increases in size.
   - Sore not improving after 2 days using antibiotic ointment.
   - Sore not completely healed in 7 days (1 week).
   - New sore appears.
   - You become worse.

Preventing Insect Bites

1. **Prevention**
   - Wear long pants and long-sleeved shirts.
   - Avoid being outside when the insect is most active. Many insects that cause itchy bites are most active at sunrise or sunset (e.g., chiggers, no-see-ums, mosquitoes).
   - Insect repellents containing DEET are effective in preventing many itchy insect bites.
2. **DEET—An Insect Repellent**
   - DEET is a very effective insect repellent. It also repels ticks.
   - Higher concentrations of DEET do work better, but there appears to be no benefit in using DEET concentrations above 50%. For children and adolescents, the American Academy of Pediatrics recommends a maximum concentration of 30%. Health Canada recommends using a concentration of 5-30% for adults.
   - Apply to exposed areas of skin. Do not apply to eyes, mouth, or irritated areas of skin. Do not apply to skin that is covered by clothing.

- Remember to wash it off with soap and water when you return indoors.
- DEET can damage clothing made of synthetic fibers, plastics (e.g., eyeglasses), and leather.
- Breastfeeding women may use DEET. No problems have been reported (CDC 2003).
- Read the label carefully.

3. **Picaridin (Also Called KBR 3023):**
   - In 2005 the CDC added picaridin to its list of recommended insect repellents.
   - Evidence indicates that it works just as well as DEET.
   - It has been used in other countries for years, including Europe, Australia, Latin America, and Asia.
   - Read the label carefully.

West Nile Virus Information

1. **Symptoms of WNV:**
   - **No Clinical Symptoms:** 80% of infections.
   - **Mild Febrile Illness:** 20% of infections. Symptoms include fever, headache, body aches, and occasionally a skin rash. These symptoms last 3-6 days and resolve without any treatment (also called WNV fever).
   - **Encephalitis or Viral Meningitis:** 0.7% (1:150) of infections. Symptoms are obvious: high fever, stiff neck, confusion, coma, convulsions, muscle weakness or paralysis. The muscle weakness is often unilateral.
   - **Fatal Outcome:** 10% of those hospitalized.
   - Pediatric cases are generally mild. Most deaths and encephalitis occur in people over age 60.
2. **Diagnosis of WNV:**
   - Mild cases do not need to be diagnosed.
   - Severe cases (with encephalitis and viral meningitis) would all be hospitalized based upon their symptoms, and the disease would be diagnosed by tests on the blood and spinal fluid. These tests are not available for the usual mild infections seen with this virus.
3. **Treatment of WNV:**
   - No special treatment is needed after a mosquito bite.
   - There is no specific treatment or antiviral agent for West Nile virus.
   - Patients who require admission are treated supportively with IV fluids, airway management, and good nursing care.
   - There is no vaccine available to prevent West Nile virus in humans.
4. **WNV—Spread by Mosquito:**
   - The West Nile virus is spread by the bite of a mosquito. The reservoir for the virus is infected birds.
   - Even in an area where West Nile virus has been identified, less than 1% of mosquitoes carry the virus.
   - Transmission is mosquito-to-human.
   - Person-to-person spread does not occur (eg, from kissing, touching, sharing glassware, or sexual intercourse).
   - Mothers with mosquito bites can continue breastfeeding (CDC 2003).
   - **Incubation Period:** 3-14 days after the mosquito bite.

FIRST AID

First Aid Advice for Anaphylaxis—Epinephrine (Pending EMS Arrival):

- If the patient has an epinephrine autoinjector, the patient should use it now.
- Use the autoinjector on the upper outer thigh. You may give it through clothing if necessary.

Epinephrine is available in autoinjectors under trade names: EpiPen, EpiPen Jr, and Twinject. EpiPen is a single injection. Twinject has a second injection that can be used if there is no improvement after 5 minutes.

First Aid Advice for Anaphylaxis—Benadryl (Pending EMS Arrival):

- Give antihistamine orally NOW if able to swallow.
- Use Benadryl (diphenhydramine; adult dose 50 mg) or any other available antihistamine.

First Aid Advice for Anaphylactic Shock (Pending EMS Arrival):

- Lie down with feet elevated.

BACKGROUND INFORMATION

General

- Tetanus vaccination after an insect bite is not necessary.

Anaphylactic Reaction With Insect Bites

- **Definition:** Anaphylaxis is a serious allergic reaction that is rapid in onset and may cause death.
- Anaphylaxis can occur following fire ant stings but rarely with other insects. It mainly occurs with bee, yellow jacket, or wasp stings. Onset usually begins within 20 minutes and almost always by 2 hours. If no symptoms occur by 2 hours, the risk for anaphylaxis is minimal.
- Symptoms include wheezing, hypotension, shock, generalized urticaria (hives), and abdominal cramping.

No-See-Ums

- No-see-ums are tiny bugs that are about 1/10 - 1/15 of an inch (0.16-0.25 cm). They can pass easily through screens. They are attracted to light. They are most active at sunset.
- **Other Names:** They are also called biting midges, punkies, or sand flies.
- **Habitat:** Adults live in wet sand. They are especially common along the seashore and shores of rivers and lakes. They lay their eggs near standing water (margins of ponds, ditches, lakes, muddy edges of a salt marsh).
- **Symptoms:** The initial bite is generally painless. But within 12 hours the bite mark becomes a small red spot that is intensely itchy. Some sensitive people can develop a larger reaction with a swollen itchy spot (hive) 1-2 inches in diameter (2-5 cm). Scratching makes the itching last longer.
- **OTC Treatment for Itching:** Topical hydrocortisone may help; anthistamines reduce the itching.
- **Prevention:** No-see-ums cannot bite through clothing, thus good advice is to wear long pants and long-sleeved shirts. Insect repellents containing DEET also seem to be effective in preventing bites.

Chiggers

- Common chiggers are very tiny bugs that are about 1/150 of an inch (0.017 cm) in size.
- **Other Names:** They are also called harvest mites, red mites, jiggers, or red bugs. They can easily go through screens.
- **Habitat:** Tall grass, berry patches, edge of woods.
- **Symptoms:** The main symptom is intense itching and this peaks on day 2. There are usually tiny red bumps or small hives. Tiny bumps may last for 1-2 weeks.
- **OTC Treatment:** Topical hydrocortisone may help; anthistamines reduce the itching.
- **Prevention:** Avoid areas where chiggers are known to be. Insect repellents containing DEET also seem to be effective in preventing bites.

Bedbugs

- Common bedbugs are small, visible bloodsucking bugs that are about ¼ of an inch (7 mm) in length.
- **Habitat:** During the day bedbugs hide in the corners of mattresses, bed crevices, floors, and walls. At night the bedbugs come out of hiding and feed on their preferred host, humans. The common bedbug is found worldwide.
- **Symptoms:** There is no pain while the bedbug is biting. However, later small red bumps or large itchy wheals (2-20 cm) may develop at the bite site. Occasionally blisters (bulla) can occur at the bite site.
- **OTC Treatment:** Topical hydrocortisone cream and oral anthistamines help reduce the itching.
- Watch for signs of infection.
- **Prevention:** Avoid hotels and hostels where bedbugs have been reported. Check along corners of bedding or mattresses for the presence of these bugs. Wash linens once a week in hot water. DEET and permethrin are effective against bedbugs.

JOCK ITCH

DEFINITION

- A fungus infection that grows on the warm, damp skin of the inner thigh. It is also referred to as tinea cruris.
- Causes an itchy, slowly expanding rash
- Use this guideline only if the patient has symptoms that match Jock Itch.

Symptoms of Jock Itch Include:

- Slowly expanding pink-red rash of inner thigh near genital area; rash is usually symmetrical.
- Itchy and not painful.
- In men does not involve penis or scrotum.
- In women does not involve vulva.

TRIAGE ASSESSMENT QUESTIONS

See More Appropriate Protocol

- Pus or blood from end of penis
  Go to Protocol: Penis and Scrotum Symptoms on page 196
- Pain or burning with passing urine and female
  Go to Protocol: Urination Pain (Female) on page 323
- Pain or burning with passing urine and male
  Go to Protocol: Urination Pain (Male) on page 326
- Rash of penis or scrotum
  Go to Protocol: Penis and Scrotum Symptoms on page 196
- Rash of female genitalia (vulva)
  Go to Protocol: Vulvar Symptoms on page 338
- Pubic lice suspected
  Go to Protocol: Pubic Lice on page 203
- Poison ivy, oak, or sumac suspected as cause
  Go to Protocol: Poison Ivy/Oak/Sumac on page 198

Go to ED Now (or to Office With PCP Approval)

- Patient sounds very sick or weak to the triager
  Reason: not consistent with jock itch, patients feel well

Go to Office Now

- Fever
  R/O: cellulitis

See Today in Office

- Rash is painful to touch
  R/O: cellulitis
- Boil, infected sore, deep ulcer present
  R/O: furuncle, abscess, impetigo, sexually transmitted disease

See Today or Tomorrow in Office

- Female
  Reason: jock itch is less common in women, see physician to confirm
- Diabetes mellitus or immunocompromised (e.g., HIV positive, cancer chemotherapy, transplant patient)
- After week on treatment and rash has not improved
- After 3 weeks on treatment and rash has not completely gone away
- Patient wants to be seen

Home Care

- Mild jock itch in a male

HOME CARE ADVICE FOR JOCK ITCH

1. **Genital Hygiene:**
   - Keep your penis and scrotal area clean. Wash this area once daily with unscented soap and water.
   - After washing, dry the groin area before the feet (Reason: to prevent spread of tinea pedis to groin area).
   - Keep your penis and scrotal area dry.
   - Wear cotton underwear (Reason: breathes and keeps area drier). Avoid nylon or tight-fitting underwear.

2. **Antifungal Cream for Treatment of Jock Itch:** Apply antifungal cream 2 times per day to the area of itching and rash. Apply it to the rash and 1 inch beyond its borders. Continue the cream for at least 7 days after the rash is cleared.
   - Available over-the-counter in United States as clotrimazole (Lotrimin AF) or miconazole (Micatin, Monistat-Derm).
   - Available over-the-counter in Canada as clotrimazole (clotrimazole cream) or miconazole (Micatin Cream, Micozole, Monistat-Derm).
3. **Expected Course:** The rash should clear up completely in 2-3 weeks.
4. **Call Back If:**
   - Rash is not improving after 1 week on treatment.
   - Rash is not completely cleared by 3 weeks.
   - Fever or pain occurs.
   - You become worse.

BACKGROUND INFORMATION

General Information

- Usually caused by the same fungal infection that causes athlete's foot.
- Jock itch, as the name implies, is much more common in men than women.
- Most individuals will be able to treat jock itch effectively using an over-the-counter (OTC) antifungal cream.

KNEE PAIN

DEFINITION

- Pain in the knee
- Not due to a traumatic injury

Pain Severity Is Defined As:

- **Mild (1-3):** Doesn't interfere with normal activities
- **Moderate (4-7):** Interferes with normal activities (e.g., work or school) or awakens from sleep, limping
- **Severe (8-10):** Excruciating pain, unable to do any normal activities, unable to walk

TRIAGE ASSESSMENT QUESTIONS

Call EMS 911 Now

- Sounds like a life-threatening emergency to the triager

See More Appropriate Protocol

- Followed an injury
  Go to Protocol: Trauma, Knee on page 297

Go to ED Now (or to Office With PCP Approval)

- Pain or swelling in one calf
  R/O: DVT
- Patient sounds very sick or weak to the triager

Go to Office Now

- Can't move swollen joint at all
  R/O: un-witnessed trauma, severe joint effusion
- Looks infected (spreading redness, red streak, pus)
  R/O: cellulitis, erysipelas

See Today in Office

- SEVERE pain (e.g., excruciating, unable to walk)
  R/O: forgotten trauma, arthritis
- Very swollen joint
  R/O: forgotten trauma, arthritis
- Blistering rash in area of pain (i.e., dermatomal distribution or "band" or "stripe")
  R/O: herpes zoster
- Looks like a boil, infected sore, or deep ulcer
  R/O: popliteal abscess, MRSA

See Within 3 Days in Office

- MODERATE pain (e.g., symptoms interfere with work or school, limping)
- Swollen knee joint (no fever or redness)
  R/O: degenerative arthritis
- Fluid-filled sack just below kneecap (no fever or redness)
  R/O: prepatellar bursitis
- Knee pain persists > 7 days
- Patient wants to be seen

See Within 2 Weeks in Office

- Knee pain is a chronic symptom (recurrent or ongoing AND lasting > 4 weeks)
  R/O: arthritis, chondromalacia patellae
- Knee stiffness or locking is a chronic symptom (recurrent or ongoing AND lasting > 4 weeks)
  R/O: meniscal cartilage tear, degenerative arthritis
- Knee giving way (or buckling) when walking is a chronic symptom (recurrent or ongoing AND lasting > 4 weeks)
  R/O: occult anterior or posterior cruciate ligament tear, patellar subluxation

Home Care

- Knee pain from overuse or strain (e.g., vigorous activity, running)
  R/O: muscle strain, overuse
- Mild knee pain

HOME CARE ADVICE FOR MILD KNEE PAIN

1. **Knee Pain After Overuse:** Muscle strain and joint irritation are very common following vigorous activity. Such activities include sports like tennis and basketball, jogging, and certain types of work.
   - **Local Cold:** Apply a cold pack or ice bag (wrapped in a moist towel) to the area for 20 minutes. Repeat in 1 hour, then every 4 hours while awake. Continue this for the first 48 hours after an overuse injury (Reason: reduce the swelling and pain).

- **Local Heat:** Beginning 48 hours after an injury, apply a warm washcloth or heating pad for 10 minutes 3 times a day to help increase circulation and improve healing.

2. **Rest Your Knee for the Next Couple Days:** Avoid activities that worsen your pain. Reduce activities that put a lot of strain on the knee joint (e.g., deep knee bends, stair climbing, running).
3. **Pain Medicines:**
   - For pain relief, take acetaminophen, ibuprofen, or naproxen.

   Acetaminophen (e.g., Tylenol):
   - Take 650 mg by mouth every 4-6 hours as needed. Each Regular Strength Tylenol pill has 325 mg of acetaminophen. The most you should take each day is 3,250 mg (10 pills a day).
   - Another choice is to take 1,000 mg every 8 hours. Each Extra Strength Tylenol pill has 500 mg of acetaminophen. The most you should take each day is 3,000 mg (6 pills a day).

   Ibuprofen (e.g., Motrin, Advil):
   - Take 400 mg by mouth every 6 hours.
   - Another choice is to take 600 mg by mouth every 8 hours.

   Naproxen (e.g., Aleve):
   - Take 250-500 mg by mouth every 12 hours.

   Extra Notes:
   - Acetaminophen is thought to be safer than ibuprofen or naproxen in people over 65 years old. Acetaminophen is in many OTC and prescription medicines. It might be in more than one medicine that you are taking. You need to be careful and not take an overdose. An acetaminophen overdose can hurt the liver.
   - **Caution:** Do not take acetaminophen if you have liver disease.
   - **Caution:** Do not take ibuprofen if you have stomach problems, kidney disease, are pregnant, or have been told by your doctor to avoid this type of anti-inflammatory drug. Do not take ibuprofen for more than 7 days without consulting your doctor.
   - Use the lowest amount of medicine that makes your pain feel better.
   - Before taking any medicine, read all the instructions on the package
4. **Expected Course:** If your knee pain does not get better during the next week or if it recurs, then you should make an appointment with your doctor.
5. **Call Back If:**
   - Knee pain persists longer than 7 days.
   - You become worse.

BACKGROUND INFORMATION

Causes of Knee Pain

- Arthritis (e.g., degenerative, gouty, infectious, inflammatory, traumatic)
- **Baker Cyst (Popliteal Cyst):** This is a fluid collection in a cyst that bulges out from the knee joint. Symptoms include painful or painless swelling in the area behind the knee.
- **Bursitis:** Prepatellar bursitis is a fluid-filled sack localized on the inferior aspect of the anterior knee.
- Cellulitis.
- Overuse injury, tendonitis.
- Patellofemoral pain syndrome (chondromalacia patellae).
- Trauma (e.g., contusion, dislocation, fracture, sprain, strain).

Some Signs and Symptoms That Could be Serious

- Severe pain, even slight movement of the knee causes intense pain.
- Knee swelling with fever (possibility of infection of knee joint).
- Unilateral calf pain and/or swelling (possibility of blood clot in leg).

LEG PAIN

DEFINITION

- Pain in the leg(s).
- Not due to a traumatic injury.
- Minor muscle strain and overuse are covered in this guideline.

Pain Severity Is Defined As:

- **Mild (1-3):** Doesn't interfere with normal activities
- **Moderate (4-7):** Interferes with normal activities (e.g., work or school) or awakens from sleep, limping
- **Severe (8-10):** Excruciating pain, unable to do any normal activities, unable to walk

TRIAGE ASSESSMENT QUESTIONS

Call EMS 911 Now

- Looks like a broken bone or dislocated joint (e.g., crooked or deformed)
  R/O: forgotten trauma, pathologic fracture or dislocation
- Sounds like a life-threatening emergency to the triager

See More Appropriate Protocol

- Followed a hip injury
  Go to Protocol: Trauma, Hip on page 295
- Followed a knee injury
  Go to Protocol: Trauma, Knee on page 297
- Followed an ankle or foot injury
  Go to Protocol: Trauma, Ankle and Foot on page 274
- Back pain radiating into leg(s)
  Go to Protocol: Back Pain on page 29
- Knee pain is the main symptom
  Go to Protocol: Knee Pain on page 173
- Leg swelling is the main symptom
  Go to Protocol: Leg Swelling and Edema on page 180

Go to ED Now

- Chest pain
  R/O: DVT, pulmonary embolus
- Difficulty breathing
  R/O: DVT, pulmonary embolus
- Entire foot is cool or blue in comparison to other side
  R/O: iliofemoral arterial occlusion (ischemic foot)
- Unable to walk

Go to ED Now (or to Office With PCP Approval)

- Fever and red area (or area very tender to touch)
  R/O: cellulitis, lymphangitis
- Fever and swollen joint
  R/O: septic arthritis, acute rheumatic fever
- Calf pain in only 1 leg and present > 1 hour
  R/O: deep vein thrombosis (DVT)
- Calf or ankle swelling in only 1 leg
  R/O: deep vein thrombosis
- Calf or ankle swelling in both legs, but one side is definitely more swollen
  R/O: DVT
- History of prior "blood clot" in leg or lungs (i.e., deep vein thrombosis, pulmonary embolism)
  Note: a "blood clot" typically would have required treatment with heparin or coumadin.
  Reason: increased risk of thromboembolism
  R/O: deep vein thrombosis
- History of inherited increased risk of blood clots (e.g., factor 5 Leiden, antithrombin 3, protein C or protein S deficiency, prothrombin mutation)
  Note: Diagnosing such genetic blood disorders would have required prior blood testing.
  Reason: increased risk of thromboembolism
  R/O: pulmonary embolism
- Recent illness requiring prolonged bed rest (immobilization)
  R/O: deep vein thrombosis
- Hip or leg fracture in past 2 months (e.g, or had cast on leg or ankle)
  R/O: deep vein thrombosis
- Cancer treatment in the past 2 months (or has cancer now)
  R/O: deep vein thrombosis
- Recent long-distance travel with prolonged time in car, bus, plane, or train (i.e., within past 2 weeks; 6 or more hours' duration)
  Reason: immobilization during prolonged travel increases risk of deep vein thrombosis
- Patient sounds very sick or weak to the triager

Go to Office Now

- SEVERE pain (e.g., excruciating, unable to do any normal activities)
  Reason: inadequate analgesia
  R/O: sciatica, iliofemoral arterial occlusion
- Red area or streak and large (> 2 in or 5 cm)
  R/O: cellulitis, erysipelas, lymphangitis.
  Note: It may be difficult to determine the rash color in people with darker-colored skin.

See Today in Office

- Painful rash with multiple small blisters grouped together (i.e., dermatomal distribution or "band" or "stripe")
  R/O: herpes zoster
- Looks like a boil, infected sore, deep ulcer, or other infected rash (spreading redness, pus)
  R/O: abscess, venous stasis ulcer, cellulitis
- Localized rash is very painful (no fever)
  R/O: cellulitis, spider bite, bee sting

See Today or Tomorrow in Office

- Numbness in a leg or foot (i.e., loss of sensation)
  R/O: nerve root compression, herniated disk
- Localized pain, redness, or hard lump along vein
  R/O: superficial thrombophlebitis
- Patient wants to be seen

See Within 3 Days in Office

- MODERATE pain (e.g., interferes with normal activities, limping) and present > 3 days
  R/O: sciatica, arthritis
- Swollen joint with no fever or redness
  R/O: degenerative arthritis
- Leg pain which occurs after walking a certain distance and disappears with rest, AND age > 50
  R/O: claudication
- Leg pain in shins (front of lower legs) and it occurs with running or jumping exercise (e.g., jogging, basketball)
  R/O: shin splints, stress fracture

See Within 2 Weeks in Office

- MILD pain persists > 7 days
  R/O: muscle strain, sciatica, arthritis, bursitis
- Leg pain or muscle cramp is a chronic symptom (recurrent or ongoing AND lasting > 4 weeks)
  R/O: night muscle cramps, meralgia paresthetica, varicose veins

Home Care

- Caused by strained muscle
  R/O: muscle strain (pulled muscle)
- Caused by overuse injury from recent vigorous activity (e.g., sports, running, physical work)
  R/O: muscle strain (sore muscles from overuse)
- Caused by transient muscle cramps in the thigh or calf
  R/O: muscle cramps, nocturnal cramps
- Caused by previously diagnosed varicose veins (same pain, worsened by prolonged standing, bulging veins in legs with wormlike appearance)
  R/O: varicose veins
- Leg pain

HOME CARE ADVICE FOR LEG PAIN

Muscle Strain and Overuse

1. **Reassurance—Muscle Strain:**
   - **Definition:** A muscle strain occurs from over-stretching or tearing a muscle. People often call this a "pulled muscle." This muscle injury can occur while exercising, while lifting something, or sometimes during normal activities.
   - **Symptoms:** People often describe a sharp pain or popping when the muscle strain occurs. The muscle pain worsens with movement of the leg (e.g., bending, straightening).
2. **Reassurance—Overuse:**
   - **Definition:** Sore muscles are common following vigorous activity (overuse), especially when your body is not used to this amount of activity (e.g., running, sports, weight lifting, moving furniture).
   - **Symptoms:** People often describe a diffuse soreness and aching in the overused muscles. Often the pain is present in in the same muscles of both legs.
3. **Local Cold for First 48 Hours:**
   - Apply a cold pack or an ice bag (wrapped in a moist towel) to the area for 20 minutes. Repeat in 1 hour, then every 4 hours while awake.
   - Continue this for the first 48 hours after an injury (Reason: to reduce the swelling and pain).

4. **Local Heat**
   - Beginning 48 hours after an injury, apply a warm washcloth or heating pad for 10 minutes 3 times a day.
   - This will help increase circulation and improve healing.
5. **Local Heat (Bathtub Option):** If stiffness persists more than 48 hours, relax in a hot bath for 20 minutes twice a day and gently exercise the involved part under water.
6. **Rest:** Avoid any exercise activity which causes this pain for the next 3 days.
7. **Pain Medicines:**
   - For pain relief, take acetaminophen, ibuprofen, or naproxen.

   Acetaminophen (e.g., Tylenol):
   - Take 650 mg by mouth every 4-6 hours as needed. Each Regular Strength Tylenol pill has 325 mg of acetaminophen. The most you should take each day is 3,250 mg (10 pills a day).
   - Another choice is to take 1,000 mg every 8 hours. Each Extra Strength Tylenol pill has 500 mg of acetaminophen. The most you should take each day is 3,000 mg (6 pills a day).

   Ibuprofen (e.g., Motrin, Advil):
   - Take 400 mg by mouth every 6 hours.
   - Another choice is to take 600 mg by mouth every 8 hours.

   Naproxen (e.g., Aleve):
   - Take 250-500 mg by mouth every 12 hours.

   Extra Notes:
   - Acetaminophen is thought to be safer than ibuprofen or naproxen in people over 65 years old. Acetaminophen is in many OTC and prescription medicines. It might be in more than one medicine that you are taking. You need to be careful and not take an overdose. An acetaminophen overdose can hurt the liver.
   - **Caution:** Do not take acetaminophen if you have liver disease.
   - **Caution:** Do not take ibuprofen if you have stomach problems, kidney disease, are pregnant, or have been told by your doctor to avoid this type of anti-inflammatory drug. Do not take ibuprofen for more than 7 days without consulting your doctor.
   - Use the lowest amount of medicine that makes your pain feel better.
   - Before taking any medicine, read all the instructions on the package.
8. **Expected Course:**
   - **Muscle Strain:** A minor muscle strain usually hurts for 2-3 days. The pain often peaks on day 2. A more severe muscle strain can hurt for 2-4 weeks.
   - **Muscle Overuse:** Sore muscles from overuse usually hurts for 2-4 days. The pain often peaks on day 2.
9. **Call Back If:**
   - Moderate pain (e.g., limping) lasts more than 3 days.
   - Mild pain lasts more than 7 days.
   - You become worse.

Muscle Cramp

1. **Reassurance—Muscle Cramps:**
   - Muscle cramps can occur in the calves and thighs.
   - During attacks, you can break the muscle spasm by stretching the muscle in the direction opposite to how it is being pulled by the cramp or spasm. For example, for a calf cramp, pull the foot and toes backward as far as they will go.
2. **Fluids for Heat Cramps (Occurring During Exercise on a Hot Day):**
   - Drink 1 cup (8 oz; 240 mL) of cold water every 15 minutes for the next 2 hours. Also eat some salty foods (e.g., potato chips or pretzels).
   - OR drink a sports-rehydration drink (e.g., Gatorade or Powerade), which contains sugar and salt.
3. **Prevention:** Future attacks may be prevented by daily stretching exercises of the heel cords. Stand with the knees straight and stretch the ankles by leaning forward against a wall.
4. **Expected Course:**
   - Muscle cramps usually last 5 to 30 minutes. Once the muscle cramp stops, the muscle returns to normal quickly. The pain should go away completely.
   - If you have frequent muscle cramps, then you should call your doctor (call us back) when the office is open. Sometimes the doctor can give medications to reduce the muscle cramps.

5. **Call Back If:**
   - Calf swelling or constant leg pain occur
   - Signs of infection occur (e.g., spreading redness, warmth, fever)
   - You become worse.

Varicose Veins

1. **Reassurance—Varicose Veins:**
   - Appear as bulging winding (wormlike) blue blood vessels in the thigh and lower leg.
   - Patients with varicose veins will sometimes report a mild aching in their legs after a prolonged day of standing or walking. The discomfort should go away with rest and leg elevation.
2. **Varicose Veins—Treatment:**
   - Try to rest and elevate your legs above your heart a couple times each day for 15 minutes.
   - Walking is good for your circulation (Reason: helps pump the blood out of the veins).
   - Avoid prolonged standing in one place.
   - Wear support hose.
   - If you are overweight, talk with your doctor about a weight-loss program.
3. **Call Back If:**
   - Severe pain occurs.
   - Calf swelling or constant calf pain occur.
   - Signs of infection occur (e.g., spreading redness, warmth, fever).
   - You become worse.

Leg Pain—General Care Advice

1. **Pain Medicines:**
   - For pain relief, take acetaminophen, ibuprofen, or naproxen.

   Acetaminophen (e.g., Tylenol):
   - Take 650 mg by mouth every 4-6 hours as needed. Each Regular Strength Tylenol pill has 325 mg of acetaminophen. The most you should take each day is 3,250 mg (10 pills a day).
   - Another choice is to take 1,000 mg every 8 hours. Each Extra Strength Tylenol pill has 500 mg of acetaminophen. The most you should take each day is 3,000 mg (6 pills a day).

   Ibuprofen (e.g., Motrin, Advil):
   - Take 400 mg by mouth every 6 hours.
   - Another choice is to take 600 mg by mouth every 8 hours.

   Naproxen (e.g., Aleve):
   - Take 250-500 mg by mouth every 12 hours.

   Extra Notes:
   - Acetaminophen is thought to be safer than ibuprofen or naproxen in people over 65 years old. Acetaminophen is in many OTC and prescription medicines. It might be in more than one medicine that you are taking. You need to be careful and not take an overdose. An acetaminophen overdose can hurt the liver.
   - **Caution:** Do not take acetaminophen if you have liver disease.
   - **Caution:** Do not take ibuprofen if you have stomach problems, kidney disease, are pregnant, or have been told by your doctor to avoid this type of anti-inflammatory drug. Do not take ibuprofen for more than 7 days without consulting your doctor.
   - Use the lowest amount of medicine that makes your pain feel better.
   - Before taking any medicine, read all the instructions on the package.
2. **Call Back If:**
   - Moderate pain (e.g. limping) lasts more than 3 days.
   - Mild pain lasts more than 7 days.
   - Signs of infection occur (e.g., spreading redness, warmth, fever).
   - You become worse.

BACKGROUND INFORMATION

Causes

- **Deep Vein Thrombosis (DVT):** This is a serious and unfortunately common problem. The deep veins of the leg become obstructed with blood clots. Symptoms include calf pain and swelling, localized redness, and warmth. Risk factors for developing a DVT include: prolonged immobilization (e.g., recent surgery, prolonged travel), local injury (e.g., femur fracture), and an increased tendency to clot (e.g., pregnancy, cancer patients).
- **Muscle Cramps:** Brief pains (1 to 15 minutes) may be due to muscle spasms. Foot or calf muscles are especially prone to cramps that awaken from sleep. The pain should resolve completely after an episode of muscle spasm.
- **Muscle Strain (Pulled Muscle):** A muscle strain occurs from over-stretching or tearing a muscle. This muscle injury can occur while exercising, while lifting something, and sometimes during normal activities. This is also referred to as a "pulled muscle."
- **Muscle Strain (Sore Muscles From Overuse):** Continuous acute pains (2 to 7 days) are often due to over-strenuous activities or forgotten muscle injuries from recent exercise or work-related activities.
- **Sciatica:** Sciatic pain is a common cause of leg pain in adults. Sciatic pain is pain that radiates from the back down into the leg, sometimes as far as the foot. It is cause by pressure on the spinal nerve roots from a herniated disk or from spinal arthritis.
- **Shin Splints:** This is an overuse injury typically from a jumping or running sport activity like jogging, aerobics, basketball, or gymnastics. Symptoms include pain in the shin area, especially during the sports activity.
- **Varicose Veins:** Appear as bulging, winding (wormlike) blue blood vessels in the thigh and lower leg. Patients with varicose veins will sometimes report a mild aching in their legs after a prolonged day of standing or walking. The discomfort usually subsides with rest and leg elevation. Sometimes a varicose vein can become thrombosed and inflamed (hard and red). This may cause localized pain but generally is not serious. Varicose veins occur more commonly in women.
- **Viral Illness:** Mild to moderate bilateral diffuse muscle aches can occur with many viral illnesses.
- **Other Causes:** Unwitnessed fracture, arthritis, arterial occlusion, skin infection (cellulitis, erysipelas), bursitis, and meralgia paresthetica.

Caution: Deep Vein Thrombosis (DVT)

- Consider the possibility of DVT in anyone with unexplained leg swelling and pain, especially if symptoms are predominantly unilateral.
- **Risk Factors:** Include venous stasis (e.g., casting, long-distance travel, prolonged bed rest), leg/venous injury (e.g., fracture, prior DVT, leg surgery), and hypercoagulable states (e.g., pregnancy, cancer).

LEG SWELLING AND EDEMA

DEFINITION

- Swelling of the leg(s) or generalized edema of body
- Pedal edema (bilateral swelling of feet and ankles)
- Not due to a traumatic injury.

TRIAGE ASSESSMENT QUESTIONS

Call EMS 911 Now

- Sounds like a life-threatening emergency to the triager

See More Appropriate Protocol

- Chest pain
  Go to Protocol: Chest Pain on page 48
- Small area of swelling and followed an insect bite to the area
  Go to Protocol: Insect Bite on page 166
- Knee injury
  Go to Protocol: Trauma, Knee on page 297
- Ankle or foot injury
  Go to Protocol: Trauma, Ankle and Foot on page 274

Go to ED Now

- Difficulty breathing at rest
  R/O: CHF, PE
- Entire foot is cool or blue in comparison to other side
  R/O: arterial occlusion

Go to ED Now (or to Office With PCP Approval)

- SEVERE swelling (e.g., swelling extends above knee, entire leg is swollen, weeping fluid)
  Reason: severe edema (3-4+), evaluation needed
- Pain or swelling in one calf
  R/O: DVT
- Bilateral calf swelling, but one side more swollen
  R/O: DVT
  Exception: long-standing difference between legs
- Cast on leg or ankle and has increasing pain
  R/O: cast swelling (may need it bivalved) or DVT
- Can't walk or can barely stand (new onset)
- Patient sounds very sick or weak to the triager

Go to Office Now

- Swelling of face, arm, or hands
  Exception: slight puffiness of fingers during hot weather
  R/O: renal disease, low protein state
- Looks infected (e.g., spreading redness, red streak, pus)
  R/O: cellulitis, erysipelas
- Looks like a boil, infected sore, or deep ulcer
  R/O: abscess, MRSA
- Pregnant > 20 weeks and sudden weight gain (i.e., > 2 lb, 1 kg in 1 week)
  R/O: preeclampsia

See Today in Office

- MODERATE swelling of both ankles (e.g., swelling extends up to the knees) AND new onset or worsening
  Reason: edema 2+, diagnostic evaluation or change in management may be needed
- Difficulty breathing with exertion AND worsening or new onset
  R/O: CHF
- Patient wants to be seen

See Within 3 Days in Office

- MILD swelling of both ankles (i.e., pedal edema) AND new onset or worsening

See Within 2 Weeks in Office

- MILD swelling of both ankles (i.e., pedal edema) and worsened by hot weather
  R/O: heat edema
- Mild swelling of both ankles and varicose veins
- Mild swelling of both ankles and chronic (unchanged)
  R/O: venous insufficiency

HOME CARE ADVICE FOR LEG SWELLING AND EDEMA (Pending Office Visit)

1. **Heat Edema:** Many individuals experience heat edema during the first few days of hot weather or after traveling to a warmer climate. There may be mild swelling of the feet and ankles and some puffiness of the fingers. Typically, your body adjusts to the higher temperatures (acclimatizes) in a couple of days and the swelling resolves.
2. **Varicose Veins:** Appear as bulging, winding (wormlike) blue blood vessels in the thigh and lower leg. Patients with varicose veins often report a mild swelling in their legs after a prolonged day of standing or walking. The swelling usually subsides with rest and leg elevation.
3. **Varicose Veins—Treatment:**
   - Try to rest and elevate your legs above your heart a couple times each day for 15 minutes.
   - Walking is good for your circulation (Reason: helps pump the blood out of the veins).
   - Avoid prolonged standing in one place.
   - Support hose may be helpful. Put them on first thing in the morning when the swelling is least.
4. **Expected Course:** If your leg swelling does not get better during the next week or if it recurs, make an appointment with your doctor.
5. **Call Back If:**
   - Swelling becomes worse.
   - Swelling becomes red or painful to the touch.
   - Calf pain occurs and becomes constant.
   - You become worse.

BACKGROUND INFORMATION

Causes of Bilateral Swelling of the Leg:

- Congestive heart failure (right-sided)
- Heat edema
- Idiopathic edema
- Liver failure and other low protein conditions
- Lymphedema
- Pregnancy
- Renal failure
- Venodilating drug—e.g., nifedipine
- Venous insufficiency or venous stasis

Causes of Unilateral Swelling of the Leg:

- **Bypass Surgery:** After saphenous vein harvesting from leg for coronary artery bypas surgery (CABG)
- **Cellulitis:** Localized swelling, redness, and tenderness
- **Deep Vein Thrombosis (DVT):** Calf swelling and tenderness
- **Insect Bites:** Localized swelling, often itchy
- **Leg Paralysis (e.g., From Stroke):** Chronic swelling of extremity from disuse
- **Lymphedema:** Lymphatic obstruction from malignancy, radiation therapy, or surgery

Definition—Pitting Edema:

- Press firmly with your thumb and hold for 5 seconds. If a visible indentation persists after the thumb is removed, then pitting edema exists.
- Edema usually shows up first in the lower (dependent) extremities, where it is initially seen in the feet or ankles.

Caution—Deep Vein Thrombosis (DVT):

- Consider the possibility of DVT in anyone with unexplained leg swelling and pain, especially if symptoms are predominantly unilateral.
- Risk factors include immobility (e.g., casting, long-distance travel, prolonged bed rest), leg/venous injury (e.g., fracture, prior DVT, leg surgery), and hypercoagulable states (e.g., pregnancy, cancer).

LYMPH NODES, SWOLLEN

DEFINITION

- Increased size of a lymph node in the neck, occipital area, armpit, or groin.
- Normal nodes are usually < 1 cm (½ inch) across (size of pea or baked bean).

Estimating Size:

- **Pea or Pencil Eraser:** ¼ inch or 6 mm
- **Marble:** 0.5 inch or 12 mm
- **Dime:** 0.75 inch or 18 mm
- **Quarter:** 1 inch or 2.4 cm
- **Ping-pong Ball:** 1.6 inches or 4.0 cm
- **Golf Ball:** 1.7 inches or 4.3 cm
- **Tennis Ball:** 2.6 inches or 6.7 cm

TRIAGE ASSESSMENT QUESTIONS

Call EMS 911 Now

- Sounds like a life-threatening emergency to the triager

See More Appropriate Protocol

- Sore throat is the main symptom and has swollen node in the neck that is < 1 inch (2.5 cm) in size
  Go to Protocol: Sore Throat on page 241

Go to ED Now (or to Office With PCP Approval)

- Node is in the neck and causes difficulty breathing
  R/O: impingement on airway
- Patient sounds very sick or weak to the triager

Go to Office Now

- Node is in the neck and can't swallow fluids
  R/O: retropharyngeal abscess
- Fever > 103° F (39.4° C)
  R/O: bacterial infection
- Lump or swelling in groin and pulsating (like heartbeat)
  R/O: femoral artery aneurysm
- Single large node and size > 1 inch (2.5 cm)
  R/O: bacterial adenitis
- Overlying skin is red
  R/O: bacterial adenitis

See Today in Office

- Rapid increase in size of node over several hours
  R/O: bacterial adenitis
- Tender node in the groin and has a sore, scratch, cut, or painful red area on that leg
  R/O: bacterial adenitis
- Tender node in the armpit and has a sore, scratch, cut, or painful red area on that arm
  R/O: bacterial adenitis
- Tender node in the neck and also has a sore throat with minimal/no runny nose or cough
  R/O: strep pharyngitis, mono (infectious mononucleosis)
- Fever present > 3 days (72 hours)
  R/O: bacterial adenitis, mono

See Today or Tomorrow in Office

- Large nodes at multiple locations
  R/O: malignancy, sarcoidosis, systemic illness
- Very tender to the touch but no fever
  R/O: low-grade bacterial adenitis
- Patient wants to be seen

See Within 2 Weeks in Office

- Large node present > 2 weeks
  R/O: malignancy, sarcoidosis
- Normal-sized node (i.e. < 1 cm, <½ in) present > 2 weeks, but patient is worried about cancer
  R/O: malignancy

Home Care

- Mildly swollen lymph node present < 2 weeks, and has cold symptoms (e.g., runny nose, cough, sore throat)
- Normal-sized lymph node (i.e., < 1 cm, < ½ inch)

HOME CARE ADVICE FOR LYMPH NODES, SWOLLEN

1. **Swollen Lymph Nodes From a Viral Infection:**
    - Viral throat infections and colds can cause lymph nodes in the neck to double in size. Slight enlargement and mild tenderness means the lymph node is fighting the infection and doing a good job.
    - **Treatment:** Usually no treatment is necessary.
    - **Expected Course:** After the infection is gone, the nodes slowly return to normal size over 1 to 2 weeks. However, they will not ever completely disappear.
    - **Contagiousness:** Swollen lymph nodes are not contagious.
2. **Normal Lymph Nodes:**
    - A pea-sized lymph node (smaller than ½ inch or 1 cm) is usually a normal lymph node.
    - **Expected Course:** Small normal-sized lymph nodes should not get any larger over time. Lymph nodes can temporarily swell and become tender when you have an infection. But after the infection is gone, the lymph node should shrink back to normal size.
3. **Pain and Fever Medicines:**
    - For pain or fever relief, take acetaminophen or ibuprofen.
    - Treat fevers above 101° F (38.3° C).
    - The goal of fever therapy is to bring the fever down to a comfortable level. Remember that fever medicine usually lowers fever 2-3° F (1-1.5° C).

    Acetaminophen (e.g., Tylenol):
    - Take 650 mg by mouth every 4-6 hours as needed. Each Regular Strength Tylenol pill has 325 mg of acetaminophen. The most you should take each day is 3,250 mg (10 pills a day).
    - Another choice is to take 1,000 mg every 8 hours. Each Extra Strength Tylenol pill has 500 mg of acetaminophen. The most you should take each day is 3,000 mg (6 pills a day).

    Ibuprofen (e.g., Motrin, Advil):
    - Take 400 mg by mouth every 6 hours.
    - Another choice is to take 600 mg by mouth every 8 hours.

    Extra Notes:
    - Acetaminophen is thought to be safer than ibuprofen in people over 65 years old. Acetaminophen is in many OTC and prescription medicines. It might be in more than one medicine that you are taking. You need to be careful and not take an overdose. An acetaminophen overdose can hurt the liver.
    - **Caution:** Do not take acetaminophen if you have liver disease.
    - **Caution:** Do not take ibuprofen if you have stomach problems, kidney disease, are pregnant, or have been told by your doctor to avoid this type of anti-inflammatory drug. Do not take ibuprofen for more than 7 days without consulting your doctor.
    - Use the lowest amount of medicine that makes your pain or fever better.
    - Before taking any medicine, read all the instructions on the package.
4. **Call Back If:**
    - Node enlarges to more than 1 inch (2.5 cm) in size.
    - Overlying skin becomes red.
    - Fever more than 103° F (39.4° C) occurs.
    - You become worse or are worried about a lymph node.

BACKGROUND INFORMATION

General

- Lymph nodes are round bean-shaped structures that assist the lymphatic system in fighting infection.
- Normally lymph nodes are less than 1 cm (½ inch) in size. Lymph nodes enlarge and become tender when an infection is present.
- Children and adolescents generally have larger lymph nodes than adults.

Location of Lymph Nodes

- Occipital (posterior lower scalp)
- Cervical (neck)
- Supraclavicular (just above collar bone)
- Axillary (armpit)
- Epitrochlear (just above elbow)
- Inguinal (groin crease at top of thigh)

Causes of Lymph Node Swelling

- **Infection:** Viral, bacterial, or fungal infections can cause lymph nodes to become swollen and tender. Infection is the most common cause of lymph node swelling. The cervical (neck) nodes are most commonly involved because of respiratory and throat infections. Enlarged nodes in the armpit or groin are often reacting to a skin infection in the involved extremity. Lymph nodes in the groin can become swollen when there is a leg infection or an STD.
- **Malignancy:** Malignancy is a less common cause of lymph node enlargement. However, any persistently enlarged nontender lymph node could possibly be a sign of malignancy (cancer, lymphoma, leukemia).
- Medications
- **Other:** e.g., collagen vascular disease, sarcoidosis, HIV.

Caution—Hernia:

- Groin hernias usually bulge out with straining (lifting, coughing, bowel movement) and subside with rest (laying down quietly). Painful swelling in this area requires immediate evaluation because of the possibility that the hernia is incarcerated (trapped) and strangulated (ischemic).

MENSTRUAL PERIOD, MISSED OR LATE

DEFINITION

- **Late Menstrual Period:** 5 or more days overdue compared to usual menstrual cycle
- **Missed Menstrual Period:** No menstrual flow for > 6 weeks

TRIAGE ASSESSMENT QUESTIONS

Call EMS 911 Now

- Sounds like a life-threatening emergency to the triager

See More Appropriate Protocol

- Abdominal pain is present
  Go to Protocol: Abdominal Pain (Female) on page 1
- STD exposure and prevention, questions about
  Go to Protocol: STD Exposure and Prevention on page 249

Go to ED Now (or to Office With PCP Approval)

- Patient sounds very sick or weak to the triager

See Today in Office

- Patient wants to be seen

See Within 3 Days in Office

- Pregnant and ANY of the following:
  - Has an IUD
  - Prior history of ectopic pregnancy
  - Previous tubal surgery (e.g., tubal ligation)
  - History of infertility
  - *Reason: higher risk for ectopic pregnancy*
  - Wants a pregnancy test done in the office

See Within 2 Weeks in Office

- Pregnant
- Recent weight loss (e.g., more than 10 pounds or 20 kg)
  R/O: excessive dieting, eating disorder, medical disorder
- Age > 40 years
  R/O: menopause
- Has missed 2 or more periods in a row
  Reason: needs evaluation
- Missed period has occurred 2 or more times in the last year and the cause is not known
  Reason: needs diagnosis determined, possible further workup

Home Care

- Pregnancy suspected or possible
  Reason: needs a home pregnancy test
- Recent stress (e.g., new school/job/home/marriage, relationship problems)
  Reason: possible stress-related secondary amenorrhea
- Menstrual period, missed or late (all triage questions negative)

HOME CARE ADVICE FOR MISSED OR LATE MENSTRUAL PERIOD

1. **Pregnancy Test, When in Doubt:**
   - If there is any possibility of pregnancy, obtain and use a urine pregnancy test from the local drugstore.
   - Follow the instructions included in the package.
2. **Stress:** Stress can interrupt normal menstrual periods. Try to reduce your stress by talking about it with a friend or family member. Try to avoid or decrease stressors. If this is not effective, seek help from a counselor or talk with your doctor.
3. **Call Back If:**
   - Pregnancy test is positive.
   - You have difficulties with the home pregnancy test.
   - New symptoms suggest pregnancy (e.g., morning sickness, breast tenderness/swelling).
   - You need help coping with stress.
   - You become worse.

BACKGROUND INFORMATION

General Information

- The first day of menstrual bleeding is considered the first day of a new menstrual cycle.
- Menstrual bleeding typically lasts 3-7 days.
- Ovulation generally occurs around day 14 of the cycle.
- The length of the menstrual cycle varies from woman to woman. The range is from 24 to 35 days. The average is 28 days.

Causes

- Pregnancy is the most important cause. This needs to be considered and ruled out in every woman who has a missed or late period.
- Recent pregnancy.
- Stress.
- Dieting, exercise, and weight loss.
- Menopause.
- Polycystic ovarian disease.
- Birth control pills.
- DepoProvera injection.
- Pituitary and other endocrine disorders.

Home Urine Pregnancy Tests

- Home urine pregnancy tests are inexpensive, accurate, and easy to use. Most drugstores sell these tests over-the-counter.
- Urine pregnancy tests can often diagnose pregnancy during the week after the first missed period (2 weeks after ovulation).
- Use of a first-morning urine specimen is recommended because the urine HCG concentration is highest in the morning.
- When a home pregnancy test is negative but there is still a high suspicion of pregnancy, the woman should either repeat the test in 3-5 days or go to her doctor's office for testing.
- The urine pregnancy test can sometimes be falsely negative if the urine specimen is grossly bloody. A small amount of blood (e.g., blood-tinged urine) should not interfere with the accuracy of the test.
- More information is available at: www.womenshealth.gov/publications/our-publications/fact-sheet/pregnancy-tests.cfm.

NECK PAIN OR STIFFNESS

DEFINITION

- Complains of neck pain in the back, side, or front of the neck.
- Not due to a known traumatic injury.
- Minor muscle strain and overuse are covered in this guideline.

Pain Severity Is Defined As:

- **Mild (1-3):** Doesn't interfere with normal activities
- **Moderate (4-7):** Interferes with normal activities or awakens from sleep
- **Severe (8-10):** Excruciating pain, unable to do any normal activities

TRIAGE ASSESSMENT QUESTIONS

Call EMS 911 Now

- Shock suspected (e.g., cold/pale/clammy skin, too weak to stand)
  R/O: shock
  FIRST AID: Lie down with the feet elevated.
- Similar pain previously and it was from "heart attack"
  R/O: myocardial infarction
- Similar pain previously from "angina" and not relieved by nitroglycerin
  R/O: cardiac ischemia, myocardial infarction
- Difficult to awaken or acting confused (e.g., disoriented, slurred speech)
  R/O: meningitis, encephalitis
- Sounds like a life-threatening emergency to the triager

See More Appropriate Protocol

- Chest pain
  Go to Protocol: Chest Pain on page 48
- Lymph node in the neck is swollen or painful to the touch
  Go to Protocol: Lymph Nodes, Swollen on page 182
- Sore throat is the main symptom
  Go to Protocol: Sore Throat on page 241

Go to ED Now (or to Office With PCP Approval)

- Difficulty breathing or unusual sweating (e.g., sweating without exertion)
  R/O: cardiac ischemia
- Chest pain lasting longer than 5 minutes
  Reason: chest pain is a high-risk complaint; referral for evaluation
- Stiff neck (can't touch chin to chest) and has headache
  R/O: meningitis or SAH
- Stiff neck (can't touch chin to chest) and fever
  R/O: meningitis
- Weakness of an arm or hand
  R/O: nerve root compression
- Problems with bowel or bladder control
  R/O: cord compression
- Patient sounds very sick or weak to the triager

Go to Office Now

- SEVERE pain (e.g., excruciating, unable to do any normal activities)
- Head is twisting to one side (or ask, "Is it turning against your will?")
  R/O: acute dystonic reaction.
  Note: occurs as a side effect when taking medications like Compazine (prochlorperazine), Reglan (metoclopramide), Haldol (haloperidol), et.al.
- Fever > 103° F (39.4° C)
- Fever > 100.5° F (38.1° C) and IVDA (intravenous drug abuse)
  R/O: bacterial illness, epidural abscess
- Fever > 100.5° F (38.1° C) and has diabetes mellitus or a weakened immune system (e.g., HIV positive, cancer chemotherapy, organ transplant, splenectomy, chronic steroids)

See Today in Office

- Numbness in an arm or hand (i.e., loss of sensation)
  R/O: nerve root compression
- Rash in same area as pain (may be described as "small blisters")
  R/O: herpes zoster
- High-risk adult (e.g., history of cancer, HIV, or IV drug abuse)
  R/O: malignancy, metastasis, epidural abscess
- Patient wants to be seen

See Today or Tomorrow in Office

- Tenderness in front of neck over windpipe
  R/O: thyroiditis

See Within 3 Days in Office

- MODERATE neck pain (e.g., interferes with normal activities like work or school)
- Pain shoots (radiates) into arm or hand
  R/O: cervical radiculopathy, herniated cervical disk
- Neck pain persists > 2 weeks

See Within 2 Weeks in Office

- Neck pain is a chronic symptom (recurrent or ongoing AND lasting > 4 weeks)
- Age > 50 and no prior history of similar neck pain
  Reason: higher risk of pathology

Home Care

- ○ Neck pain or stiffness
- ○ Neck pain from twisting, bending, or lifting injury

HOME CARE ADVICE FOR MILD NECK PAIN

1. **Reassurance:** Prolonged turning of the head or working in an awkward position can cause muscle pain in the back of the neck. With treatment, the pain usually resolves in 1 to 2 weeks.
2. **Local Cold or Heat:** During the first 2 days after a mild injury, apply a cold pack or an ice bag (wrapped in a towel) for 20 minutes 4 times a day. After 2 days, apply a heating pad or hot water bottle to the most painful area for 20 minutes whenever the pain flares up. Wrap hot water bottles or heating pads in a towel to avoid burns.
3. **Sleep:**
   - Sleep on your back or side, not on your abdomen.
   - Sleep with a neck collar—use a foam neck collar (from a pharmacy) OR a small towel wrapped around the neck (Reason: keep the head from moving too much during sleep).
4. **Stretching Exercises:**
   - After 48 hours of protecting the neck, begin gentle stretching exercises.
   - Improve the tone of the neck muscles with 2 or 3 minutes of gentle stretching exercises per day such as touching the chin to each shoulder, touching the ear to each shoulder, and moving the head forward and backward.
   - Don't apply any resistance during these stretching exercises.
5. **Pain Medicines:**
   - For pain relief, take acetaminophen, ibuprofen, or naproxen.

   Acetaminophen (e.g., Tylenol):
   - Take 650 mg by mouth every 4-6 hours as needed. Each Regular Strength Tylenol pill has 325 mg of acetaminophen. The most you should take each day is 3,250 mg (10 pills a day).
   - Another choice is to take 1,000 mg every 8 hours. Each Extra Strength Tylenol pill has 500 mg of acetaminophen. The most you should take each day is 3,000 mg (6 pills a day).

   Ibuprofen (e.g., Motrin, Advil):
   - Take 400 mg by mouth every 6 hours.
   - Another choice is to take 600 mg by mouth every 8 hours.

   Naproxen (e.g., Aleve):
   - Take 250-500 mg by mouth every 12 hours.

   Extra Notes:
   - Acetaminophen is thought to be safer than ibuprofen or naproxen in people over 65 years old. Acetaminophen is in many OTC and prescription medicines. It might be in more than one medicine that you are taking. You need to be careful and not take an overdose. An acetaminophen overdose can hurt the liver.
   - **Caution:** Do not take acetaminophen if you have liver disease.
   - **Caution:** Do not take ibuprofen if you have stomach problems, kidney disease, are pregnant, or have been told by your doctor to avoid this type of anti-inflammatory drug. Do not take ibuprofen for more than 7 days without consulting your doctor.
   - Use the lowest amount of medicine that makes your pain feel better.
   - Before taking any medicine, read all the instructions on the package

6. **Good Body Mechanics:**
   - **Lifting:** Stand close to the object to be lifted. Keep your back straight and lift by bending your legs. Ask for help if needed.
   - **Sleeping:** Sleep on a firm mattress.
   - **Sitting:** Avoid sitting for long periods of time without a break. Avoid slouching. Place a pillow or towel behind your lower back for support.
   - **Computer Screen:** Place at eye level.
   - **Posture:** Maintain good posture.
7. **Avoid:** Avoid triggers that overstress the neck such as working with the neck turned or bent backward, carrying heavy objects on the head, carrying heavy objects with one arm (instead of both arms), standing on the head, contact sports, or even friendly wrestling.
8. **Call Back If:**
   - Numbness or weakness occurs.
   - Bowel or bladder problems occur.
   - Pain persists for more than 2 weeks.
   - You become worse.

BACKGROUND INFORMATION

Causes

- **Muscle Strain:** Acute neck pain is often from strained neck muscles caused by sleeping in an awkward position, cradling a telephone between neck and shoulder for extended conversation, painting a ceiling, reading in bed, reaching for something that was difficult to get, sitting in the front of a movie theater, looking at something that requires extreme bending or turning of neck, prolonged typing, etc.
- **Muscle Tension/Spasm:** Muscle tension neck pain is one of the most common causes of acute neck pain. It is seen in every age group and is related to stressful situations in the workplace and at home. The pain may radiate into the upper back and into the scalp. Frequently, patients with this type of tension neck pain will report that the discomfort is worse toward the end of the day. Therapy for this type of pain should be directed at stress reduction, good posture, and gentle neck exercises.
- **Pharyngitis:** Pain in the front or side of the neck is usually due to a sore throat (pharyngitis) or from swollen lymph nodes.
- Degenerative arthritis.
- Inflammatory arthritis (e.g., rheumatoid arthritis).
- Muscle aches (myalgia) from viral syndrome, URI.
- Poor posture.
- Anxiety, stress, depression.

Serious Causes

- Acute coronary syndrome
- Meningitis
- Subarachnoid hemorrhage
- Epidural abscess
- Epidural hematoma
- Thyroiditis
- Cancer

Stiff Neck

- Callers are frequently concerned about a stiff neck and the possibility of meningitis.
- The stiff neck that accompanies meningitis is the result of inflammation of the spinal cord membranes. Patients with meningitis are typically unable to touch the chin to their chest because of pain.
- Patients with muscle strain or myalgia may also describe some neck stiffness. Such patients are usually able to touch their chin to their chest but have difficulty putting the chin to each shoulder (can't rotate the neck). In addition, the neck muscles are often painful to the touch.

Caution—Cardiac Ischemia

- The most life-threatening cause of acute neck pain is cardiac ischemia.
- Rarely, patients may present with anterior neck pain as the sole symptom of a myocardial infarction. Usually there will be other associated symptoms of cardiac ischemia: chest pain, shortness of breath, nausea, and/or diaphoresis.
- Cardiac ischemia should be suspected in any patients with risk factors for cardiac disease. These include: hypertension, smoking, diabetes, hyperlipidemia, a strong family history of heart disease, and age > 50.

NEUROLOGIC DEFICIT

DEFINITION

- Weakness or paralysis of the face, arm, or leg
- Numbness of the face, arm, or leg
- Loss of speech, garbled or confused speech
- Not due to a known traumatic injury

TRIAGE ASSESSMENT QUESTIONS

Call EMS 911 Now

- Difficult to awaken or acting confused (e.g., disoriented, slurred speech)
  R/O: stroke, subarachnoid hemorrhage (SAH)
- New neurologic deficit that is present NOW, sudden onset of ANY of the following:
  - Weakness of the face, arm, or leg on one side of the body
  - Numbness of the face, arm, or leg on one side of the body
  - Loss of speech or garbled speech
    R/O: stroke
    Exception: Bell palsy suspected (i.e., weakness only one side of the face, developing over hours to days, no other symptoms)
- Sounds like a life-threatening emergency to the triager

See More Appropriate Protocol

- Confusion, disorientation, or hallucinations is the main symptom
  Go to Protocol: Confusion (Delirium) on page 60
- Dizziness is main symptom
  Go to Protocol: Dizziness on page 92
- Followed a head injury within last 3 days
  Go to Protocol: Trauma, Head on page 290

Go to ED Now (or to Office With PCP Approval)

- Headache (with neurologic deficit)
  R/O: stroke, SAH
- Can't use hand normally (e.g., hold a glass of water)
  Reason: significant deficit requiring urgent evaluation
- Can't walk or can barely walk
  Reason: significant weakness or ataxia
- Back pain with numbness (loss of sensation) in groin or rectal area
  R/O: cauda equina syndrome
- Unable to urinate (or only a few drops) and bladder feels very full
  R/O: urinary retention, cauda equina syndrome
- Loss of control of bowel or bladder (i.e., incontinence) of new onset
  R/O: spinal cord lesion
- Patient sounds very sick or weak to the triager

Go to Office Now

- Neurologic deficit that was transient (now gone), ANY of the following:
  - Weakness of the face, arm, or leg on one side of the body
  - Numbness of the face, arm, or leg on one side of the body
  - Loss of speech or garbled speech
  - Note: transient tingling from foot or hand "falling asleep" from prolonged sitting or laying on arm may best be triaged to home care disposition. Use nursing judgment.
- Neurologic deficit of gradual onset, ANY of the following:
  - Weakness of the face, arm, or leg on one side of the body
  - Numbness of the face, arm, or leg on one side of the body
  - Loss of speech or garbled speech
    R/O: brain tumor, spinal cord lesion, TIA
- Bell palsy suspected (i.e., weakness only one side of the face, developing over hours to days, no other symptoms)
  Reason: clinical evaluation; treatment with oral corticosteroids may be indicated
- Tingling (e.g., pins and needles) of the face, arm, or leg on one side of the body, that is present now
  Exceptions: chronic/recurrent symptom lasting > 4 weeks or tingling from known cause (e.g., bumped elbow, carpal tunnel syndrome, pinched nerve, frostbite)

See Today in Office

- Neck pain (with neurologic deficit)
  R/O: herniated disk
- Back pain (with neurologic deficit)
  R/O: herniated disk
- Patient wants to be seen

See Within 3 Days in Office

- Loss of speech or garbled speech is a chronic symptom (recurrent or ongoing problem lasting > 4 weeks)
- Weakness of arm or leg is a chronic symptom (recurrent or ongoing problem lasting > 4 weeks)
- Numbness or tingling in one or both hands is a chronic symptom (recurrent or ongoing problem lasting > 4 weeks)
  R/O: peripheral neuropathy, carpal tunnel syndrome
- Numbness or tingling in one or both feet is a chronic symptom (recurrent or ongoing problem lasting > 4 weeks)
  R/O: peripheral neuropathy

Home Care

- ○ Transient tingling in hand (e.g., pins and needles) after prolonged laying on arm
- ○ Transient tingling in foot (e.g., pins and needles) after prolonged sitting with legs crossed
- ○ Transient numbness (or tingling or burning) in hand and fingers after bumped elbow
  R/O: "bruised funny bone"

HOME CARE ADVICE FOR NEUROLOGIC DEFICIT

1. **Transient Tingling in Hand (e.g., Pins and Needles) After Prolonged Laying on Arm:**
   - **Description:** Many people note that if they lay down for a prolonged period on an arm, the hand becomes numb. People describe this as "their hand falling asleep." Direct pressure on one of the nerves in the arm is what causes this.
   - **Expected Course:** Tingling should go away after several minutes of stretching and gentle movement of the arm.
2. **Transient Tingling in Foot (e.g., Pins and Needles) After Prolonged Sitting With Legs Crossed:**
   - **Description:** Many people note that if they sit for a prolonged period with legs crossed, their foot becomes numb. People describe this as "their foot falling asleep." Direct pressure on nerves in the leg from sitting in an unusual position is what causes this.
   - **Expected Course:** Tingling should go away after several minutes of stretching and gentle movement of the leg.
3. **Bruised "Funny Bone":**
   - **Description:** A direct blow to the inner side of the posterior elbow can cause numbness, tingling, and burning in the hand. The involved fingers are usually the middle, ring, and little fingers. Your funny bone is actually a nerve (ulnar) which wraps around the posterior part of your elbow.
   - **Expected Course:** Symptoms from bruising your funny bone usually last only a few minutes. If the symptoms last longer than 30 minutes or if this problem seems to happen to you frequently, then you should see the doctor for evaluation.
4. **Call Back If:**
   - Symptoms do not go away within 30 minutes.
   - You become worse.

BACKGROUND INFORMATION

Causes

- **Bell Palsy:** Unilateral face weakness due to a facial nerve palsy. The main symptom is a crooked smile.
- Brain tumor.
- Guillain-Barré syndrome.
- Head trauma with intracranial bleeding (e.g, epidural or subdural hematoma).
- Hemiplegic or hemisensory migraine.
- Meningitis, encephalitis.
- Multiple sclerosis.
- Neuropathy.
- Spinal cord lesion (e.g., tumor, disc protrusion, epidural abscess).
- Stroke ("brain attack," cerebrovascular accident, CVA)
- Subarachnoid hemorrhage.
- TIA (transient ischemic attack).
- **Todd Paralysis:** Temporary unilateral weakness after a seizure.
- Transverse myelitis.

Stroke (Brain Attack)

- "Brain attack" is a new layperson term being used to describe a stroke. This term originated from the need to emphasize to patients the urgency of a stroke and the need for immediate evaluation.
- **Signs:** Signs of a brain attack include sudden onset of weakness or numbness of one side of the body, sudden loss of vision, sudden loss of speech, or sudden dizziness and unsteadiness. With thrombotic or embolic strokes there is usually minimal or no headache.
- **Cause:** A brain attack occurs when one of the blood vessels to the brain becomes blocked. This keeps blood from flowing to that part of the brain. Permanent damage can result.
- **Treatment—Thrombolytic (e.g., TPA, Alteplase):** There are thrombolytic medications ("clotbusters") that can be used to treat some patients with a brain attack. However, the thrombolytic must be given within 3-4.5 hours of symptom onset. Because of this narrow window only about 2-3% of all stroke patients qualify to receive this medication.

Transient Ischemic Attack (TIA)

- **Definition:** Some patients have a warning attack in which there are symptoms of a stroke but the symptoms go away after a few minutes or hours.
- **Signs:** Signs of a TIA are the same as for a stroke. They include sudden onset of weakness or numbness of one side of the body, sudden loss of vision, sudden loss of speech, or sudden dizziness and unsteadiness.
- **Cause:** A TIA occurs when one of the blood vessels to the brain becomes temporarily blocked. This keeps blood from flowing to that part of the brain.
- **Triage:** These patients require urgent evaluation as they remain at risk for having a permanent stroke.

NOSEBLEED

DEFINITION

- Bleeding from 1 or both nostrils
- Not due to a traumatic injury
- Includes follow-up calls about nasal packing placed by health care providers to control bleeding

TRIAGE ASSESSMENT QUESTIONS

Call EMS 911 Now

- Fainted (passed out), or too weak to stand following large blood loss
  R/O: impending shock
  FIRST AID: Lie down with feet elevated.
- Sounds like a life-threatening emergency to the triager

See More Appropriate Protocol

- Nosebleed followed nose injury
  Go to Protocol: Trauma, Nose on page 304

Go to ED Now (or to Office With PCP Approval)

- Bleeding present > 30 minutes and using correct method of direct pressure
  R/O: posterior nosebleed, coagulopathy
- Bleeding now and second call after being instructed in correct technique of direct pressure
  R/O: posterior nosebleed, coagulopathy
- Light-headedness or dizziness
  R/O: excessive blood loss
- Pale skin (pallor) of new onset or worsening
  R/O: excessive blood loss
- Has nasal packing (inserted by health care provider to control bleeding) and now has new rash
  R/O: toxic shock syndrome
- Has nasal packing and now has bleeding around the packing
  Exception: few drops or ooze
  Reason: may need to be repacked or have nasal cautery
- Patient sounds very sick or weak to the triager

Go to Office Now

- Large amount of blood has been lost (e.g., 1 cup)
  R/O: anemia

See Today in Office

- Bleeding recurs 3 or more times in 24 hours despite direct pressure
- Taking Coumadin (warfarin), Pradaxa (dabigatran), or known bleeding disorder (e.g., thrombocytopenia)
  Reason: higher risk of serious bleeding; may need for testing of INR, ProTime, or platelet count
- Has skin bruises or bleeding gums that are not caused by an injury
  R/O: bleeding disorder
- Has nasal packing and now has fever > 100.5° F (38.1° C)
  R/O: sinusitis
- Patient wants to be seen

See Within 3 Days in Office

- Has nasal packing (inserted by health care provider to control bleeding)
  Reason: nasal packing needs removal 2-3 days after placement

See Within 2 Weeks in Office

- Hard-to-stop nosebleeds are a chronic symptom (recurrent or ongoing AND lasting > 4 weeks)
  R/O: bleeding disorder
- Easy bleeding present in other family members

Home Care

- Mild to moderate nosebleed and bleeding has stopped now
- Bleeding present < 30 minutes and using correct method of direct pressure
- Nosebleed and needs instruction in correct technique of applying direct pressure

HOME CARE ADVICE FOR MILD NOSEBLEED

1. **Reassurance:**
   - Nosebleeds are common.
   - It sounds like a routine nosebleed that we can treat at home.
   - You should be able to stop the bleeding if you use the correct technique.
   - Remember to sit up and lean forward to keep the blood from running down the back of your throat.
2. **Treating a Nosebleed—Pinch the Nostrils:**
   - First blow the nose to clear out any large clots.
   - Sit up and lean forward (Reason: blood makes people choke if they lean backwards).
   - Gently squeeze the soft parts of the lower nose (nostrils) together. Use your thumb and your index finger in a pinching manner. Do this for 15 minutes. Use a clock or watch to measure the time. Your goal is to apply continuous pressure to the bleeding point.
3. **Treating a Nosebleed—Inserting a Gauze With Decongestant Nose Drops:**
   - If applying pressure fails, insert a gauze wet with decongestant nose drops (or petroleum jelly) (Reason: the gauze helps to apply pressure and the nose drops shrink the blood vessels).
   - Then repeat the process of gently squeezing the lower nose for 10 minutes.
   - **Example Decongestant Medication:** Afrin (oxymetazoline) nasal spray is available over-the-counter and is a nasal decongestant.
4. **Caution—Nasal Decongestants:**
   - Do not use this medication if you have high blood pressure, heart disease, or prostate enlargement. Do not take these medications if you are pregnant. Do not take these medications if you have used an MAO inhibitor such as isocarboxazid (Marplan), phenelzine (Nardil), rasagiline (Azilect), selegiline (Eldepryl, Emsam), or tranylcypromine (Parnate) in the past 2 weeks. Life-threatening side effects can occur.
   - Do not use these medications for more than 3 days (Reason: rebound nasal congestion).
   - Read the package instructions thoroughly on all medications that you use.
5. **Prevention:**
   - Dry air in your house or workplace can increase the chance of nosebleeds occurring. If the air is dry, use a humidifier in your bedroom to keep the nose from drying out. You can also apply petroleum jelly to the center wall (septum) inside the nose twice daily to reduce cracking and to promote healing.
   - Bleeding can start again if you rub your nose or blow the nose too hard. Avoid touching your nose and nose picking. Avoid blowing the nose.
   - Do not take aspirin or other anti-inflammatory medications (e.g., ibuprofen, Advil, Motrin, Aleve), unless you have been instructed to by your physician.
6. **Expected Course:**
   - Over 99% of nosebleeds will stop following 15 minutes of direct pressure if you press on the right spot.
   - After swallowing blood from a nosebleed, you may feel nauseated because the blood can irritate your stomach. You may also later pass a dark stool that contains the blood.
7. **Call Back If:**
   - Nosebleed lasts longer than 30 minutes with using direct pressure.
   - Light-headedness or weakness occurs.
   - Nosebleeds become worse.
   - You become worse.

FIRST AID

First Aid Advice for Nosebleed:

- First blow the nose to clear out any large blood clots.
- Placing your thumb and index finger over each side of the soft lower portion of the nose, firmly pinch the nostrils together. Pinch the nostrils together for 10-15 minutes.
- Lean slightly forward; this keeps the blood from trickling down the back of your throat.

BACKGROUND INFORMATION

General Information

- Most nosebleeds (90%) originate from the front part of the nose (anterior nasal septum). Thus, most nosebleeds will stop when pressure is correctly applied over the bleeding area. The correct method is to squeeze the soft parts of the nose using thumb and index finger, thus applying pressure inside of the nose. Hold for 10-15 minutes.
- Leading causative factors for nosebleeds include upper respiratory infections (colds) and nose picking. There is a higher incidence of nosebleeds in the 60- to 80-year-old age group. Individuals in this age group often have a couple of causative factors for bleeding. A typical elderly adult with a nosebleed might be 72, have high blood pressure, and be exposed to dry winter air.

Risk Factors

- **Environmental:** Environmental factors include temperature and dryness of the air.
- **Local:** Local factors include URI, nasal drug inhalation, nasal tumors, septal deviation, too vigrous nose blowing, and nose picking.
- **Systemic:** Systemic factors include hypertension, arteriosclerosis, and coagulopathies.
- **Medications:** Certain medications can increase bleeding: aspirin, NSAIDs (e.g., ibuprofen, naproxen), heparin, Coumadin, Plavix (clopidogrel).

PENIS AND SCROTUM SYMPTOMS

DEFINITION

- Penis symptoms include rash, pain, discharge, itching, and swelling.
- Scrotum symptoms include rash and itching.
- Not due to a traumatic injury.

TRIAGE ASSESSMENT QUESTIONS

Call EMS 911 Now

- Sounds like a life-threatening emergency to the triager

See More Appropriate Protocol

- Pain or burning with passing urine is main symptom
  Go to Protocol: Urination Pain (Male) on page 326
- Pubic lice suspected
  Go to Protocol: Pubic Lice on page 203
- STD exposure and prevention, question about
  Go to Protocol: STD Exposure and Prevention on page 249

Go to ED Now (or to Office With PCP Approval)

- Large amount of blood from end of penis
  R/O: urinary retention, UTI
- Foreskin pulled back and stuck (not circumcised)
  R/O: paraphimosis
- Fever > 100.5° F (38.1° C)
  R/O: UTI, epididymitis
- Unable to urinate (or only a few drops) and bladder feels very full
  R/O: acute urinary retention
- Painful erection present > 2 hours
  R/O: priapism
- Patient sounds very sick or weak to the triager

Go to Office Now

- Severe pain or burning with passing urine
  R/O: UTI, severe urethritis
- Entire penis is swollen (i.e., edema)
  R/O: CHF, anasarca
- Looks infected (e.g., draining sore, spreading redness)
  R/O: cellulitis

See Today in Office

- Pain or burning with passing urine
  R/O: UTI, urethritis
- Blood in urine (red, pink, or tea-colored)
  R/O: tumor, kidney stone
- Pus (white, yellow) or bloody discharge from end of penis
  R/O: GC or chlamydia urethritis, UTI
- Swollen foreskin (not circumcised)
  R/O: balanoposthitis
- Tiny water blisters rash, 3 or more
  R/O: herpes simplex, pustules
- Antibiotic treatment > 3 days for STD (e.g., penile discharge from gonorrhea, chlamydia) and painful urination not improved
  R/O: resistant organism
- Patient wants to be seen

See Today or Tomorrow in Office

- SEVERE itching (i.e., interferes with work or school)
  R/O: poison ivy, pubic lice
- Painless rash (e.g., redness, tiny bumps, sore) present > 24 hours
  R/O: contact dermatitis, skin cancer, genital warts
- Patient is worried about a sexually transmitted disease (STD)
  Reason: relieve fear and prevent spread of STD
- ALL other penis/scrotum symptoms
  Exception: painless rash < 24 hours' duration
  R/O: skin cancer, pubic lice

Home Care

- Painless rash (e.g., mild redness, tiny bumps, small sore) present < 24 hours
  R/O: contact dermatitis, abrasion

HOME CARE ADVICE FOR PENIS SYMPTOMS

1. **Causes of Mild Rash:**
   - **Irritation From a Chemical Product:** Perfumed soaps, latex condoms.
   - Irritation from a plant (e.g., poison ivy, evergreen), chemicals (e.g., insecticides), fiberglass, detergents.
   - Early finding of sexually transmitted disease (STD).
   - Small friction burns can occur from intercourse (if inadequate lubrication).
2. **Cleaning:** Wash the area once thoroughly with unscented soap and water to remove any irritants.
3. **Genital Hygiene:**
   - Keep your penis and scrotal area clean. Wash once daily with unscented soap and water.
   - Keep your penis and scrotal area dry. Wear cotton underwear.
4. **Call Back If:**
   - Rash spreads or becomes worse.
   - Rash lasts more than 1 day.
   - Fever occurs.
   - You become worse.

BACKGROUND INFORMATION

Causes

- Bladder infection (cystitis).
- Contact dermatitis (e.g., latex condoms, lubricants, spermicides, perfumed soaps).
- Irritation (small friction burns) after sexual intercourse or masturbation (inadequate lubrication).
- Poison ivy, oak, or sumac rash.
- Priapism.
- Skin cancer. STDs (e.g., herpes simplex, syphilis, chancroid, LGV, pubic lice, genital warts).
- Trauma.
- Any preexisting skin disorders/rashes can also occur on the penis and scrotum (e.g., psoriasis, eczema, drug rashes).

Priapism

- **Definition:** Priapism is defined as an erection that lasts longer than 4 hours.
- **Symptoms:** Prolonged, unwanted, usually painful erection.
- **Causes:** Sickle cell anemia, certain medications.
- **Treatment:** Erections lasting longer than 4 hours may require specialized treatment in an emergency department.

Erectile Dysfunction

- **Definition:** Erectile dysfunction is defined as an inability to achieve or maintain an erection. Approximately 40% of men between the ages of 40 and 70 have problems with erectile dysfunction.
- **Causes:** In most cases there is a medical (organic, nonpsychiatric) cause. The main cause is atherosclerotic disease and thus risk factors are similar to those for heart disease (hypertension, obesity, smoking, diabetes). Other medical causes include neurologic (spinal cord injury, cerebral disease), hormonal (e.g., hypothyroidism), and pharmacologic (especially antihypertensive medications).

PDE5 Inhibitor Drugs for Erectile Dysfunction

- There are 3 oral drugs that are now available by prescription for treatment of erectile dysfunction: Viagra (sildenafil), Levitra (vardenafil), and Cialis (tadalafil).
- These 3 medicationas are in a class called phosphodiesterase (PDE5) inhibitors.
- **Side Effects:** Priapism (very rare), vision loss in one eye (very rare), vision changes (e.g., changes in color), headache, indigestion, flushing.
- **Warnings:** Using PDE5 drugs and nitrates at the same time can cause a sudden and possibly serious drop in blood pressure. Men who use PDE5 drugs should not take any medicines called "nitrates" or "nitroglycerin." For similar reasons, recreational drugs called "poppers," like amyl nitrate and butyl nitrate, must be avoided.

POISON IVY/OAK/SUMAC

DEFINITION

- A very itchy, blistering rash caused by contact with the poison ivy plant, or by contact with poison oak or poison sumac.
- Use this guideline only if the patient has symptoms that match Poison Ivy.

Symptoms of Poison Ivy (and Poison Oak and Poison Sumac) Include:

- The rash is extremely itchy.
- Localized redness, swelling, and weeping blisters.
- Rash is located on exposed body surfaces (eg, the hands) or areas touched by the hands (e.g., the face or genitals).

TRIAGE ASSESSMENT QUESTIONS

See More Appropriate Protocol

- Doesn't match the symptoms of poison ivy, oak, or sumac
  Go to Protocol: Rash or Redness, Localized and Cause Unknown on page 216

Go to ED Now

- Difficulty breathing or severe coughing following exposure to burning weeds

Go to ED Now (or to Office With PCP Approval)

- Patient sounds very sick or weak to the triager

Go to Office Now

- Fever and bright red area or streak (from open poison ivy sores)
  R/O: cellulitis, lymphangitis
- Increasing redness around poison ivy and larger than 2 inches (5 cm)
  R/O: cellulitis

See Today in Office

- SEVERE itching interferes with normal activities (e.g., work or school) or prevents sleep
  Reason: probably needs prednisone
- Rash involves more than ¼ of the body
  Reason: probably needs prednisone
- Face, eyes, lips, or genitals are involved
  Reason: may need oral prednisone if more than a small area of rash
- Big blisters or oozing sores
- Severe poison ivy reaction in the past
- Taking oral steroids more than 24 hours and rash becoming worse
  R/O: wrong diagnosis
- Patient wants to be seen

See Today or Tomorrow in Office

- Poison ivy rash lasts > 3 weeks
  R/O: wrong diagnosis

Home Care

- Poison Ivy, oak, or sumac with no complications

HOME CARE ADVICE FOR MILD RASH FROM POISON IVY, OAK, OR SUMAC

1. **Hydrocortisone Cream for Itching:**
   - Apply 1% hydrocortisone cream 4 times a day to reduce itching. Use it for 5 days.
   - Keep the cream in the refrigerator (Reason: it feels better if applied cold).
   - Available over-the-counter in United States as 0.5% and 1% cream.
   - Available over-the-counter in Canada as 0.5% cream.
2. **Local Cold:** Soak the involved area in cool water for 20 minutes or massage it with an ice cube as often as necessary to reduce itching and oozing.
3. **Oral Antihistamine Medication for Itching:** Take an antihistamine by mouth to reduce the itching. Diphenhydramine (Benadryl) is available over-the-counter. Adult dose is 25-50 mg. Take it up to 4 times a day.
   - Do not take antihistamine medications if you have prostate enlargement.
   - Antihistamines may cause sleepiness. Do not drink, drive, or operate dangerous machinery while taking antihistamines.
   - An over-the-counter antihistamine that causes less sleepiness is loratadine (e.g., Alavert or Claritin).

- Read the package instructions thoroughly on all medications that you take.

4. **Avoid Scratching:** Cut your fingernails short and try not to scratch so as to prevent a secondary infection from bacteria.
5. **New Blisters Appear:** If new blisters occur several days after the first ones, you probably have had ongoing contact with the irritating plant oil. To prevent recurrences: bathe all dogs and wash all clothes and shoes that were with you on the day of exposure.
6. **Contagiousness:** Poison ivy or oak is not contagious to others.
7. **Expected Course:** Usually lasts 2 weeks. Treatment reduces the severity of the symptoms, not how long they last.
8. **Call Back If:**
   - Rash lasts longer than 3 weeks.
   - It looks infected.
   - You become worse.

BACKGROUND INFORMATION

General

- Poison Ivy, poison sumac, and poison oak are 3 plants that can cause an itchy red rash in sensitive individuals. The oil contained in the plant leaves irritates the skin. The redness and blistering from the rash are often arranged in streaks or lines, because the leaves brush across the body in a line as an individual walks past.
- **Onset:** Following a first-time exposure, the onset time for the rash is 1 to 2 weeks. For recurrences, the onset is 8 to 48 hours after the individual was in a forest or field.

Preventing the Rash

- **Avoid Exposure:** Avoid exposure to these plants, especially if you have had a bad reaction in the past.
- **Wash Skin:** If you are exposed, remove the irritating plant oil from your skin as soon as possible. Wash the exposed part of your body with soap and water within 30 minutes. Wash your clothes in warm soapy water.
- **IvyBlock:** An over-the-counter cream that you put on your skin before walking in the woods. It coats the skin and acts as a barrier to the irritating oil of the poison ivy/oak/sumac plants and prevents the rash from occurring. More information is available at www.ivyblock.com.

Rule of Nines for Estimating Body Surface Area (BSA):

- Each part of the body contributes a predictable portion of the total BSA:
  - **Head and Neck:** 9%
  - **Each Arm:** 9%
  - **Anterior Chest and Abdomen:** 18%
  - **Entire Back:** 18%
  - **Each Leg:** 18%
  - **Genital Region:** 1%

Wild Parsnip Photodermatitis

- **Definition:** The juice (sap) from broken stems and leaves of the wild parsnip can cause a photosensitivity rash in everyone. It is a 2-step reaction. First, the juice comes into contact with skin. Second, that area of skin is exposed to daylight (sun or cloudy day).
- **Symptoms:** Approximately 24-48 hours after wild parsnip juice and light exposure, a painful localized rash with blisters appears on the area of the skin that was exposed to the juice. Of note, while the rash of poison ivy is much more itchy, the rash from wild parsnip is more painful and burning.
- **Expected Course:** Rash usually fades after a couple days.
- **Treatment:** None known.
- **Complications:** Can leave a scar at the site.
- **Prevention:** Learn what the plant looks like. Avoid contact. Wash exposed surfaces afterward. Avoid any sun exposure for 2 days after skin contact or where sun-protecting clothing.
- **Internet Resources:** A nicely written article on this is available at: dnr.wi.gov/wnrmag/html/stories/2000/jun00/parsnip.htm. Photographs of wild parsnip are present on the Wisconsin Botanical Information System at www.botany.wisc.edu/wisflora/scripts/detail.asp?SpCode=PASSAT.

POISONING

DEFINITION

- Swallows a drug, chemical, plant, or other possibly poisonous substance.
- Occasionally a poisonous gas is absorbed across the lungs or irritates the lungs (e.g., ammonia, chlorine).
- Rarely a poisonous chemical is absorbed across the skin (e.g., organophospates found in some insecticides).

Excluded:

- Chemical in eye. Use Eye, Chemical In protocol on page 108.

TRIAGE ASSESSMENT QUESTIONS

Call EMS 911 Now

- Severe difficulty breathing (e.g., struggling for each breath, speaks in single words)
- Bluish lips or face now
  R/O: hypoxia and need for oxygen
- Seizure
- Difficult to awaken or acting confused (e.g., disoriented, slurred speech)
  R/O: overdose, shock
- Shock suspected (e.g., cold/pale/clammy skin, too weak to stand)
  R/O: shock
  FIRST AID: Lie down with the feet elevated.
- Intentional overdose and suicidal thoughts or ideas
  Reason: suicidal ideation/gesture/attempt
- Suicide attempt, known or suspected
  Reason: suicidal ideation/gesture/attempt
- Sounds like a life-threatening emergency to the triager

See More Appropriate Protocol

- Poisonous substance or chemical in eye
  Go to Protocol: Eye, Chemical In on page 108

Go to ED Now

- HARMFUL SUBSTANCE or ACID or ALKALI ingestion (e.g., toilet cleaners, drain cleaners, lye, Clinitest tablets, ammonia, bleaches) AND any symptoms (e.g., mouth pain, sore throat, breathing difficulty)
- PETROLEUM PRODUCT ingestion (e.g., kerosene, gasoline, benzene, furniture polish, lighter fluid) AND any symptoms (e.g., breathing difficulty, coughing, vomiting)

Call Poison Center Now

- HARMFUL SUBSTANCE or ACID or ALKALI ingestion (e.g., toilet cleaners, drain cleaners, lye, Clinitest tablets, ammonia, bleaches) AND NO symptoms
- PETROLEUM PRODUCT ingestion (e.g., kerosene, gasoline, benzene, furniture polish, lighter fluid) AND NO symptoms
- Carbon monoxide exposure suspected
- Mercury spill (e.g., broken glass thermometer, broken spiral CFL lightbulb)
- Patient or caller provides unclear information about type or amount of substance
- ALL OTHER HARMFUL SUBSTANCES (e.g., nearly all drugs, plants, and chemicals)
  Exception: harmless substances or harmless overdose such as double dose of OTC drug or antibiotic

See Today in Office

- Patient wants to be seen

Home Care

- ○ HARMLESS SUBSTANCE (nontoxic) ingestion (all triage questions negative)
- ○ HARMLESS OVERDOSE (nontoxic) of OTC drug or antibiotic (all triage questions negative)
- ○ Poison-proofing your home, questions about

HOME CARE ADVICE FOR HARMLESS SUBSTANCE OR OVERDOSE

General Information

1. **Accidental Ingestion of a Harmless Substance**
   - You were lucky this time. What have you learned? What are you going to change?
   - It is time to poison-proof your home.
2. **Accidental Harmless Overdose of OTC Drug or Antibiotic:** You did receive too much medication, but there shouldn't be any side effects. Think about ways that you can avoid this in the future. For example:
   - Use a form or a notepad to write down the names of your medications, the amounts, and times you are supposed to take them.
   - Obtain a pill dispenser (can obtain a plastic dispenser with compartments from pharmacy)
   - Discard unused and outdated pill bottles.
3. **Avoid Vomiting:** Do not induce vomiting. Ipecac is unnecessary.
4. **Call Back If:**
   - You have any more questions
   - You become worse.

Questions About Mercury Spills (e.g., Broken Glass Thermometer or Broken Spiral CFL Lightbulb)

1. **Mercury Spills—What Not to Do:**
   - DO NOT use a vacuum cleaner to clean up mercury. The vacuum cleaner will spread the mercury into the air.
   - DO NOT sweep up mercury with a broom. It will break the mercury into tiny drops and spread them apart.
   - DO NOT pour mercury down the drain. It is poisonous to the environment.
2. **Internet Resource About Mercury Spills:**
   - The US EPA has a Web site on handling mercury spills: www.epa.gov/mercury/spills/index.htm. Information is provided on broken thermometers and broken compact fluourescent lightbulbs (CFLs).
   - Snopes.com has a brief information page on broken CFLs at: www.snopes.com/medical/toxins/cfl.asp.

Additional Poisoning Resources

1. **Poison-Proofing Your Home**
   - The American Association of Poison Control Centers has prepared a guide to preventing poisonings at home.
   - It is available online at www.1-800-222-1222.info/poisonPrevention/documents/homediag.pdf.
2. **Medication Safety**
   - A guide to medication safety from the Agency for Healthcare Research and Quality (AHRQ) is available online at: www.ahrq.gov/consumer/safemeds/yourmeds.htm.

FIRST AID

First Aid Advice for Carbon Monoxide Exposure:

Immediately move to fresh air.

- Go outdoors (best).
- Or move to an open door/window (in extreme weather conditions).

First Aid Advice for Swallowed Acids or Alkalies:

- Remove any solid poisons out of the mouth (spit them out or rescuer can sweep them out with a finger).
- Drink ½ cup (120 mL) of water (or milk) to rinse out the esophagus.
- Avoid vomiting (Reason: if these agents are vomited, additional damage can occur to the esophagus).

First Aid Advice for Swallowed Petroleum Product:

- Do not eat or drink anything.
- Avoid vomiting (Reason: If these hydrocarbon agents are vomited, additional damage can occur to the lungs from aspiration).

First Aid Advice for Swallowed Other Poisonous Substances:

- Remove any solid poisons out of the mouth (spit them out or rescuer can sweep them out with a finger).
- Avoid vomiting (Do not use syrup of ipecac).

US Poison Center Number: 1-800-222-1222

- This is the telephone number for every poison center in the United States.
- It connects you automatically with the local poison center.

BACKGROUND INFORMATION

Poisoning and Overdose—Telephone Triage Assessment and Disposition:

Poisoning and overdose can be **accidental** or **intentional.** Accidental poisoning is more common in children. Children explore their world with enthusiastic curiosity. There is a natural tendency to put things in their mouth. In contrast, intentional poisoning or overdose is more common in adults. Sometimes adults take an overdose of a medicine on purpose to relieve pain or other symptoms. Sometimes adults take medicines or other substances to get high or feel better. Regardless, the triager should always be suspicious of the possibility of suicidality in adults with an intentional poisoning or overdose.

Any patient who has attempted suicide or is threatening self-harm now needs to be seen immediately for evaluation.

Based on the substance ingested, the triager should place the patient in one of the following categories:

- **Harmful Substances (e.g., Acid, Alkali, Petroleum Products)**
- **Potentially Harmful Substances or Unknown**
- **Harmless Substances**
- **Harmless Overdose**

Harmful Substances—Acids, Alkalis, and Petroleum Products:

Each of the substances in this category is extremely harmful. All individuals who have swallowed one of these substances and has any symptoms should be sent to the ED for evaluation and treatment.

Even individuals without symptoms will probably require ED evaluation. If the individual has no symptoms, is not suicidal, and the exposure sounds less concerning, a referral to a poison center may be appropriate.

- **Strong Acids and Alkalis:** Examples are toilet bowl cleaners, drain cleaners, lye, automatic dishwasher detergent, and Clinitest tablets.
- **Other Alkalis:** Examples are ammonia, bleaches, and chemical hair removers (e.g., Nair).
- **Petroleum Products:** Examples are kerosene, gasoline, benzene, furniture polish, and lighter fluid.

Potentially Harmful Substances or Unknown

This category includes nearly all prescription medicines, chemicals, and plants. Referral or call transfer to a poison center is recommended.

- **Prescription Medicines:** The following prescription drugs are especially dangerous if a person takes too much: barbiturates, clonidine, digoxin (Lanoxin), high blood pressure medicines, narcotics, tricyclic antidepressants, and warfarin (Coumadin).
- **Over-the-counter (OTC) Medicines:** Two dangerous OTC medicines are iron and aspirin. Acetaminophen (eg, Tylenol) can also be dangerous if taken as an overdose.
- **Chemicals**
- **Plants**

Harmless Substances (Nonpoisonous)

The following substances are completely harmless if tasted or swallowed. A disposition of home care is appropriate and the caller should be reassured. When in doubt, the triager should refer the caller to a poison center.

- **Cosmetics:** Lipstick, rouge, mascara. Deodorants and hair sprays are usually harmless, unless they contain alcohol. Perfumes always contain alcohol and can be harmful.
- **Glue:** White, arts and crafts.
- **Miscellaneous:** Candles, cooking lard or grease, dirt, glow products (glow sticks), mercury in glass thermometers (safe if swallowed but dangerous if inhaled), silica granules (in desiccant packets).
- **Mouth Products:** Breath mints, chewing gum, toothpaste.
- **Paints:** Watercolor paints and water-based paints.
- **Pet Products:** Dog or cat food, cat litter (earth or clay), stool.
- **Skin Care Products:** Corn starch baby powder (talcum powder can be harmful), hand lotions (creams or ointments), petroleum jelly, shaving cream, suntan lotion. Creams and ointments containing the following OTC medicines are safe: antibiotic, steroid, antifungal, anti-yeast and diaper rash creams and ointments.
- **Soaps:** Hand soaps (liquid or bar), shampoo.
- **Writing Products:** Chalk, crayons, pen and marker ink, lead pencils (which are actually graphite).

The US National Capital Poison Center (www.poison.org) maintains a list of nonpoisonous plants at www.poison.org/prevent/plants.asp.

Harmless Overdose (Nonpoisonous)

- **OTC Medications:** Taking twice the recommended dose of an OTC medicine (e.g., cough or cold medicines, pain or fever medicines, vitamin pills) on a one-time basis is harmless.
- **Antibiotic:** Taking an extra dose of a prescription antibiotic is harmless.

When in doubt, the triager should refer the caller to a poison center.

PUBIC LICE

DEFINITION

- A genital area infection with tiny gray bugs called lice.
- Use this guideline only if the patient has symptoms that match Pubic Lice.

Symptoms of Pubic Lice Include:

- Itching of the pubic area is the main symptom.
- Gray bugs (lice) are 1/16-inch (1-2 mm) long, move quickly, and are difficult to see.
- Nits (white or tan eggs) cemented to hair shafts near the skin (usually within ½ inch or 12 mm). Unlike dandruff or sand, nits can't be shaken off the hair shafts.

TRIAGE ASSESSMFOR PUBIC LICE

See More Appropriate Protocol

● Doesn't match the symptoms for lice, and insect bite suspected
Go to Protocol: Insect Bite on page 166

● Doesn't match the symptoms for lice
Go to Protocol: Rash or Redness, Localized and Cause Unknown on page 216

See Today in Office

● Looks infected (e.g., pus, soft scabs, open sores)
R/O: superinfection with staph or strep

● New or unusual vaginal discharge (e.g., odorous, yellow, green, or foamy-white)
Reason: patient also may have vaginitis from another sexually transmitted disease (STD)

● White or yellow discharge from penis
Reason: sounds like patient also may have urethritis (another STD)

See Today or Tomorrow in Office

● Diagnosis of lice is uncertain

● Pubic lice or nits recurs within 1 month
Reason: resistant pubic lice or reinfection

● More than 3 hours since completing treatment and moving lice are seen in the pubic hair
Reason: probably resistant lice

● Patient wants to be seen

See Within 3 Days in Office

● All other patients with pubic lice
Reason: to make certain that the patient has no other STD

HOME CARE ADVICE FOR PUBIC LICE (Pending Office Visit)

1. **Nix:** Buy Nix anti-lice creme rinse (permethrin).
   - Pour about 2 ounces (60 mL) of the creme onto previously washed and towel-dried pubic hair. Add a little warm water to work up a lather. Be sure to work the creme into all the hair down to the roots.
   - Leave the Nix on for a full 20 minutes or it won't kill all the lice (10 minutes is not enough).
   - Rinse the hair thoroughly and dry it with a towel. Repeat the Nix treatment in 1 week to kill any nits that were missed.
2. **Dead Nits:** Wait 3 or more hours after Nix treatment is completed before removing the dead nits (Reason: let Nix permeate the nits). The nits can be loosened using a mixture of half vinegar and half warm water. After wetting the hair with this solution, cover the hair with a towel for 30 minutes. Then remove the dead nits by back-combing with a special nit comb or pull them out individually.
3. **Pregnancy and Breastfeeding:** According to the Centers for Disease Control and Prevention, women who are pregnant or who are breastfeeding can be treated with products containing permethrin (e.g., Nix).
4. **Contagiousness:** Pubic lice are very contagious. Pubic lice are transmitted by skin-to-skin contact during sexual intercourse (they cannot jump). You should have no sexual intercourse until 2 weeks after successful treatment.
5. **Sexual Contacts:** Any sexual partners that you have had during the last month will also need treatment even if they don't see any obvious lice.

6. **Expected Course:** With 2 treatments, all lice and nits should be killed. A recurrence usually means that there has been another contact with an infected person; the shampoo wasn't left on for 20 minutes; or the treatment wasn't repeated in 7 days. There are no lasting problems from having lice and they do not carry other diseases. Even after successful treatment, itching of the pubic area may persist for 1-2 weeks.
7. **Other Shampoos:** If any of the pyrethrin anti-lice shampoos (A200 Clear, R&C, Pronto, or RID) are used, they must be applied to dry hair. Reapplication in 7 days to prevent reinfection is also required. Do not use these products if you are pregnant or breastfeeding.
8. **Pregnancy Test, When in Doubt:**
   - If there is any possibility of pregnancy, obtain and use a urine pregnancy test from the local drugstore.
   - Follow the instructions included in the package.
9. **STD National Hotline:**
   - The American Social Health Association national STD hotline provides information on sexually transmitted diseases (STDs) such as chlamydia, gonorrhea, HPV/genital warts, herpes, and HIV/AIDS. Specialists can provide general information, referrals to local clinics, and written materials about STDs and disease prevention.
   - Toll-free number (English): (800) 227-8922.
   - Toll-free number (Spanish): (800) 344-7432.
   - Their Web site is at: www.ashastd.org.
10. **Call Back If:**
    - Pregnancy test is positive or if you have difficulties with the home pregnancy test.
    - You become worse.

BACKGROUND INFORMATION

General

- Slight redness may be present in the pubic area from scratching.
- Adult lice survive 3 weeks in the pubic area but only 24 hours once off the human body.
- The nits (eggs) are easier to see than the lice because they are white and very numerous.
- Nits hatch into lice in about 1 week. Off the body, they can survive up to 2 weeks.
- Nits that are > 1 cm from the skin are empty egg cases and very white in color.

Cause

- Pubic lice are tiny wingless insects which live only on human beings.
- The primary mode of transmission is via the skin-to-skin contact that occurs during sexual intercourse. Lice are very contagious. There is a 95% chance of transmission during a single episode of sexual intercourse.
- Rarely they may be transmitted via objects (i.e., fomites) such as infected bed linens or toilet seats.
- Pubic lice are annoying but cause no serious health problems.
- They are also referred to as "crabs."
- Up to 30% of individuals with pubic lice have another sexually transmitted disease.

OTC Treatment of Public Lice

There are 2 medications that can be purchased OTC which are effective in treating pubic lice. The package instructions should be followed closely. They are:

- 1% permethrin (i.e., Nix)
- Pyrethrin with piperonyl butoxide (e.g., RID, A200 Clear, R&C, Pronto)

Prescription Medications for Treatment of Pubic Lice

- 5% permethrin (i.e., Elimite)
- Lindane (i.e., Kwell, Kwellada, Hexit)
- Malathion (i.e., Ovide)

Pubic Lice in Pregnancy

- Women who are pregnant or breastfeeding can be treated with permethrin (Nix) (CDC).
- Permethrin is considered a category B drug in pregnancy.

Internet Resources on Sexually Transmitted Disease (STD, STI)

- **Australia:** Information on sexually transmitted infection is provided by the Australian government at: www.sti.health.gov.au/internet/sti/publishing.nsf.
- **Canada—Public Health Agency of Canada:** Sexually transmitted infections (STI), sexual health facts, and information for the public is available at: www.phac-aspc.gc.ca/std-mts/faq_e.html.
- **United States:** American Social Health Association answers to questions about teen sexual health and sexually transmitted diseases are available at: www.iwannaknow.org.
- **United States:** Centers for Disease Control and Prevention sexually transmitted diseases treatment guidelines available at: www.cdc.gov/std/treatment/2010 or www.cdc.gov/mmwr/preview/mmwrhtml/rr5912a1.htm.

PUNCTURE WOUND

DEFINITION

- Skin is punctured by a narrow, pointed object.

TRIAGE ASSESSMENT QUESTIONS

Call EMS 911 Now

- Shock suspected (e.g., cold/pale/clammy skin, too weak to stand)
  R/O: shock
  FIRST AID: Lie down with the feet elevated.
- Puncture on the head, neck, chest, back, or abdomen that sounds life-threatening to triager
  FIRST AID: Apply direct pressure with a clean cloth.
- Sounds like a life-threatening emergency to the triager

See More Appropriate Protocol

- Caused by an animal bite
  Go to Protocol: Animal Bite on page 13
- Skin is cut or scraped, not punctured
  Go to Protocol: Trauma, Skin on page 310
- Puncture wound of eye or eyelid
  Go to Protocol: Trauma, Eye on page 280
- Foreign body is still in the skin (e.g., splinter, sliver, fishhook)
  Go to Protocol: Skin, Foreign Body on page 236

Go to ED Now

- Puncture on the head, neck, chest, abdomen, or overlying a joint and it could be deep
  R/O: internal injury or penetration of joint
- Needlestick from used or discarded injection needle
  Exception: clean, unused needle
- High-pressure injection injury (e.g., from grease gun or paint gun, usually work-related)
  Reason: deep tissue damage exceeds superficial injury

Go to ED Now (or to Office With PCP Approval)

- Tip of the object is broken off and missing
  R/O: foreign body that needs removal
- Sensation of something still in the wound
  R/O: retained foreign body (FB)
- Foot puncture that hurts too much to walk on (i.e., unable to bear weight, severe limp)
  R/O: retained foreign body, deep tissue injury
- Sharp object was very dirty (e.g., barnyard)
  Reason: need for wound irrigation or debridement
- Dirt (debris) can be seen in the wound, not removed with 15-minute scrubbing
  Reason: additional scrubbing in ED or office may be needed
- Occurs on bare foot and setting was dirty
  Reason: need for wound irrigation or debridement
- No previous tetanus shots
  Reason: May need TIG
- Sounds like a serious injury to the triager

Go to Office Now

- Severe pain
  R/O: deep puncture or FB
- Looks infected (e.g., red area, red streak, pus)
  R/O: cellulitis, lymphangitis
- Finger puncture and entire finger swollen
  R/O: tenosynovitis, felon

See Today in Office

- Pain or swelling present > 5 days
- No tetanus booster in > 5 years
- Patient wants to be seen

See Today or Tomorrow in Office

- After 14 days and wound isn't healed
  R/O: low-grade infection
- Puncture wound on foot and patient has diabetes mellitus
  Reason: increased risk of foot infection
- Puncture through shoe (e.g., tennis shoe) and into bottom of foot
  Reason: wound check

Home Care

- Minor puncture wound

HOME CARE ADVICE FOR MINOR PUNCTURE WOUND

1. **Cleaning:**
   - Wash the wound with soap and warm water for 15 minutes.
   - If there is any dirt or debris, scrub the wound back and forth with a washcloth to remove it.
2. **Trimming:** Cut off any flaps of loose skin that seal the wound and interfere with drainage or removing debris. Use fine scissors after cleaning them with rubbing alcohol.
3. **Antibiotic Ointment:** Apply an antibiotic ointment and a Band-Aid to reduce the risk of infection. Wash the area and reapply an antibiotic ointment every 12 hours for 2 days.
4. **Pain Medicines:**
   - For pain relief, take acetaminophen, ibuprofen, or naproxen.

   Acetaminophen (e.g., Tylenol):
   - Take 650 mg by mouth every 4-6 hours as needed. Each Regular Strength Tylenol pill has 325 mg of acetaminophen. The most you should take each day is 3,250 mg (10 pills a day).
   - Another choice is to take 1,000 mg every 8 hours. Each Extra Strength Tylenol pill has 500 mg of acetaminophen. The most you should take each day is 3,000 mg (6 pills a day).

   Ibuprofen (e.g., Motrin, Advil):
   - Take 400 mg by mouth every 6 hours.
   - Another choice is to take 600 mg by mouth every 8 hours.

   Naproxen (e.g., Aleve):
   - Take 250-500 mg by mouth every 12 hours.

   Extra Notes:
   - Acetaminophen is thought to be safer than ibuprofen or naproxen in people over 65 years old. Acetaminophen is in many OTC and prescription medicines. It might be in more than one medicine that you are taking. You need to be careful and not take an overdose. An acetaminophen overdose can hurt the liver.
   - **Caution:** Do not take acetaminophen if you have liver disease.
   - **Caution:** Do not take ibuprofen if you have stomach problems, kidney disease, are pregnant, or have been told by your doctor to avoid this type of anti-inflammatory drug. Do not take ibuprofen for more than 7 days without consulting your doctor.
   - Use the lowest amount of medicine that makes your pain feel better.
   - Before taking any medicine, read all the instructions on the package.
5. **Expected Course:** Puncture wounds seal over in 1 to 2 hours. Pain should resolve within 2 days.
6. **Call Back If:**
   - Dirt in the wound persists after 15 minutes of scrubbing.
   - It begins to look infected (redness, red streaks, tenderness, pus, fever).
   - Pain becomes severe.
   - You become worse.

FIRST AID

First Aid Advice for Bleeding:
Apply direct pressure to the entire wound with a clean cloth.

First Aid Advice for Shock:
Lie down with feet elevated.

BACKGROUND INFORMATION

General Information

- **Needlesticks:** Any needlestick from a used or discarded needle should be reported immediately to the doctor. In some cases, medicines should be started to prevent transmission of the HIV (AIDS) virus.

Foot Punctures Through Athletic Shoes:

- Puncture wounds into the bottom of the foot have a risk of infection of approximately 4%. This increases to 25% in patients with puncture wounds through athletic (tennis) shoes into the bottom of the foot near the toes. Pain persisting greater than 4-5 days after the injury is suggestive of infection.
- **Pencil Lead Punctures:** Pencil lead is actually graphite (harmless), not poisonous lead. Even colored leads are nontoxic. However, they will cause a tattoo and should be scrubbed out.

Common Causes

- **Animal Bite:** See Animal Bite protocol on page 13.
- Fishhook.
- Marine creatures.
- Nail.
- Needlestick.
- Pen.
- Pencil.
- Pin.
- Sewing needle.
- **Splinter:** See Skin, Foreign Body protocol on page 236.
- Toothpick.

Tetanus Booster

- **Clean Puncture Wound: Every 10 Years:** Patients with clean puncture wounds and who have previously had 3 or more tetanus shots (full series), need a booster every 10 years. CLEAN punctures mean that both the skin and object were clean. Examples of clean punctures include a puncture wound from an unused injection needle, a sewing needle, a thumb tack, or a safety pin.
- Obtain tetanus booster within 72 hours.
- **Dirty Puncture Wound: Every 5 Years:** Patients with dirty wounds need a booster every 5 years. Puncture wounds should be considered DIRTY if either the object or the skin was dirty. Examples of dirty puncture wounds include pencils (saliva), any sharp object on the floor, and if the punctured skin was contaminated with soil, saliva, or feces. Obtain tetanus booster within 24 hours.

RASH, WIDESPREAD AND CAUSE UNKNOWN

DEFINITION

- Rash over most of the body (widespread or generalized).
- Occasionally just on hands, feet, and buttocks—but symmetrical.
- Cause of rash is unknown.
- Red or pink rash (erythema).
- Smooth (macular) or slightly bumpy (papular).
- Small spots, large spots, or solid red.

TRIAGE ASSESSMENT QUESTIONS

Call EMS 911 Now

- Sudden onset of rash (within last 2 hours) and difficulty with breathing or swallowing
  R/O: anaphylaxis, angioedema
- Difficult to awaken or acting confused (e.g., disoriented, slurred speech)
  R/O: toxic shock syndrome or septic shock, meningitis
- Fever and purple or blood-colored spots or dots
  R/O: meningococcemia, Rocky Mountain spotted fever
  Note: it may be difficult to determine the rash color in people with darker-colored skin.
- Too weak or sick to stand
  R/O: meningococcemia
- Life-threatening reaction (anaphylaxis) in the past to similar substance (e.g., food, insect bite/sting, chemical, etc.) and < 2 hours since exposure
- Sounds like a life-threatening emergency to the triager

See More Appropriate Protocol

- Insect bites suspected
  Go to Protocol: Insect Bite on page 166
- Sunburn suspected
  Go to Protocol: Sunburn on page 262
- Hives suspected
  Go to Protocol: Hives on page 152
- Drug rash suspected and started taking new medicine within last 2 weeks
  Exception: antihistamine, eyedrops, ear drops, decongestant, or other OTC cough/cold medicines
  Go to Protocol: Rash, Widespread on Drugs (Drug Reaction) on page 212

Go to ED Now (or to Office With PCP Approval)

- Bright red, sunburn-like rash and current tampon use
  R/O: toxic shock syndrome, staph or strep exotoxin rash
- Bright red, sunburn-like rash and current tampon use or nasal packing
  R/O: toxic shock syndrome, staph or strep exotoxin rash
  Note: It may be difficult to determine the rash color in people with darker-colored skin.
- Bright red, sunburn-like rash and wound infection or recent surgery
  R/O: toxic shock syndrome, staph or strep exotoxin rash
- Bright red skin that peels off in sheets
  R/O: TENS, scalded skin syndrome
- Stiff neck (can't touch chin to chest)
  R/O: meningitis
- Patient sounds very sick or weak to the triager

Go to Office Now

- Fever
  R/O: bacterial or rickettsial illness
- Face becomes swollen
  Reason: may need steroids
- Headache
  R/O: Rocky Mountain spotted fever
- Purple or blood-colored spots or dots (no fever)
  R/O: purpura or petechiae, vasculitis.
  Note: in comparison to other red rashes, petechiae and purpura do not temporarily blanch (fade) when pressure is applied to a spot. It may be difficult to determine the rash color in people with darker-colored skin.
- Joint pain or swelling
  R/O: gonococcemia
- Sores in mouth
  R/O: Stevens-Johnson syndrome, chickenpox
- Rash looks like large or small blisters (i.e., fluid-filled bubbles or sacs on the skin)
  R/O: Stevens-Johnson syndrome, erythema multiforme, TENS, disseminated herpes zoster

Callback by PCP or Subspecialist Within 1 Hour

- Pregnant
- Rash began within 4 hours of a new prescription medication
  R/O: allergic reaction

See Today in Office

- Severe itching
- Sore throat
  R/O: scarlet fever
- Ring-like appearance of rash (or ask, "Does it look like a 'target' or 'bull's-eye'?")
  R/O: target lesions of erythema multiforme
- Patient wants to be seen

See Today or Tomorrow in Office

- Mild widespread rash
  R/O: allergy, viral exanthem

HOME CARE ADVICE FOR WIDESPREAD RASHES (Pending Office Visit)

1. **Reassurance:** There are many causes of widespread rashes and most of the time they are not serious. Common causes include viral illness (e.g., cold viruses) and allergic reactions (to a food, medicine, or environmental exposure).
2. **For Non-Itchy Rashes:** No treatment is necessary, except for heat rashes, which respond to cool baths.
3. **For Itchy Rashes:**
   - Wash the skin once with gentle non-perfumed soap to remove any irritants. Rince the soap off thoroughly.
   - You may also take an oatmeal (Aveeno) bath or take an anithistamine medication by mouth to help reduce the itching.
4. **Oatmeal Aveeno Bath for Itching:** Sprinkle contents of one Aveeno packet under running faucet with comfortably warm water. Bathe for 15-20 minutes, 1-2 times daily. Pat dry with a towel. Do not rub the rash.
5. **Oral Antihistamine Medication for Itching:**
   - Take an antihistamine like diphenhydramine (Benadryl) for widespread rashes that itch. The adult dosage of Benadryl is 25-50 mg by mouth 4 times daily.
   - An over-the-counter antihistamine that causes less sleepiness is loratadine (e.g., Alavert or Claritin).
   - **Caution:** This type of medication may cause sleepiness. Do not drink alcohol, drive, or operate dangerous machinery while taking antihistamines. Do not take these medications if you have prostate enlargement.
   - Read the package instructions thoroughly on all medications that you take.
6. **Contagiousness:** Avoid contact with pregnant women until a diagnosis is made. Most viral rashes are contagious (especially if a fever is present). You can return to work or school after the rash is gone or when your doctor says it is safe to return with the rash.
7. **Expected Course:** Most viral rashes disappear within 48 hours.
8. **Call Back If:**
   - You become worse.

FIRST AID

First Aid Advice for Anaphylaxis—Epinephrine (Pending EMS Arrival):

- If the patient has an epinephrine autoinjector, the patient should use it now.
- Use the autoinjector on the upper outer thigh. You may give it through clothing if necessary. Epinephrine is available in autoinjectors under trade names: EpiPen, EpiPen Jr, and Twinject. EpiPen is a single injection. Twinject has a second injection that can be used if there is no improvement after 5 minutes.

First Aid Advice for Anaphylaxis—Benadryl (Pending EMS Arrival):

- Give antihistamine orally NOW if able to swallow.
- Use Benadryl (diphenhydramine; adult dose 50 mg) or any other available antihistamine.

BACKGROUND INFORMATION

General Information

- Three widespread rashes that individuals may be able to recognize are: hives, insect bites, and sunburn. If present, use that protocol. If not, use this protocol.
- An adult with FEVER and RASH should seek medical attention immediately. There are a number of serious infections that can present in this manner. Examples of serious infections iclude meningococcemia, gonococcemia, endocarditis, and Rocky Mountain spotted fever.
- It is difficult to assess rash color in people with darker-colored skin. When this situation occurs, simply ask the caller to describe what they see.

Fever and Rash

- **Toxic Shock Syndrome:** The rash is a widespread erythroderma (painless "sunburn") that usually fades in 72 hours. It is followed by skin desquamation (peeling), especially of the palms and soles. Other signs and symptoms of the syndrome include fever, muscle aches, vomiting or diarrhea, multiorgan dysfunction (liver, kidney), confusion, shock, and death. Those at risk include menstruating women using tampons, postsurgical patients, and patients with nasal packings.
- **Rocky Mountain Spotted Fever:** This is a tick-borne disease most commonly seen along the south Atlantic seaboard and in the south-central states. The rash usually starts as red spots on the hands and wrists and then becomes petechial (does not blanch with pressure). The rash occurs 2-14 days after a tick bite. Associated symptoms include headache and muscle aches.
- **Meningococcemia:** Is a rapidly fatal infectious disease that presents with fever, rash, headache, and stiff neck.
- **Gonococcemia:** The skin rash may first appear on the hands and feet as red pales (small raised spots) that then become pus-filled. Associated symptoms include fever and joint pain.
- **Endocarditis:** Is a bacterial infection of the heart. Risk factors for developing endocarditis include IV drug abuse, valvular heart disease, artificial heart valves, and indwelling IV catheters.

RASH, WIDESPREAD ON DRUGS (DRUG REACTION)

DEFINITION

- A widespread rash begins within 2 weeks of starting a new medication.
- The rash is most commonly red or pink spots that are smooth (macular) or slightly bumpy (papular).
- Other drug rashes that can occur include blisters (vesicles), skin redness (erythroderma), erythema nodosum, hives (urticaria), and pustules.
- May or may not be itchy

Included:

- Drug rashes from prescription medications
- Drug rashes from nonsteroidal anti-inflammatory drugs (NSAIDs)
- Niacin flushing

Excluded:

- Do not use this protocol if the rash is thought to be caused by taking over-the-counter (OTC) medications like antihistamines, decongestants, cough/cold medicines, eyedrops, or nose drops.
- Instead use the Rash, Widespread and Cause Unknown protocol on page 209.

TRIAGE ASSESSMENT QUESTIONS

Call EMS 911 Now

- Difficulty breathing or wheezing
  R/O: anaphylaxis, angioedema
- Hoarseness or cough that started soon after first dose of drug
  R/O: anaphylaxis, angioedema
- Swollen tongue that started soon after first dose of drug
- Fever and purple or blood-colored spots or dots
  R/O: meningococcemia, Rocky Mountain spotted fever
  Note: it may be difficult to determine the rash color in people with darker-colored skin.
- Too weak or sick to stand
  R/O: toxic shock syndrome or septic shock, meningitis
- Sounds like a life-threatening emergency to the triager

See More Appropriate Protocol

- Rash is only on 1 part of the body (localized)
  Go to Protocol: Rash or Redness, Localized and Cause Unknown on page 216
- New medicine is antihistamine, ear drops, eyedrops, decongestant, or other OTC cough/cold medicine
  Go to Protocol: Rash, Widespread and Cause Unknown on page 209
  Reason: these medicines rarely cause rashes

Go to ED Now

- Swollen tongue

Go to ED Now (or to Office With PCP Approval)

- Widespread hives and onset < 2 hours of exposure to first dose of drug
  R/O: allergic reaction
  Note: No history of life-threatening reaction and no anaphylactic symptoms
- Patient sounds very sick or weak to the triager

Go to Office Now

- Fever
  R/O: infectious cause
- Face becomes swollen
  Reason: may need steroids
- Purple or blood-colored spots or dots (no fever)
  R/O: purpura or petechiae, vasculitis
  Note: in comparison to other red rashes, petechiae and purpura do not temporarily blanch (fade) when pressure is applied to a spot. It may be difficult to determine the rash color in people with darker-colored skin.
- Joint pain or swelling
  R/O: gonococcemia
- Sores in mouth
  R/O: Stevens-Johnson syndrome
- Rash looks like large or small blisters (i.e., fluid filled bubbles or sacs on the skin)
  R/O: Stevens-Johnson syndrome, TENS, disseminated herpes zoster, chickenpox

Callback by PCP or Subspecialist Within 1 Hour

- Pregnant
- Rash beginning within 4 hours of a new prescription medication
  R/O: allergic drug reaction

See Today in Office

- Hives
  R/O: allergic drug reaction
- All other patients with widespread rash taking a new medication
  R/O: allergic drug reaction
- Patient wants to be seen

Discuss With PCP and Callback by Nurse Today

- NIacin flush suspected

HOME CARE ADVICE FOR WIDESPREAD RASH ON DRUGS (DRUG REACTION) (Pending Office Visit)

1. **Reassurance:** There are many causes of widespread rashes and most of the time they are not serious. Common causes include viral illness (e.g., cold viruses) and allergic reactions (to a food, medicine, or environmental exposure).
2. **Stopping the Medication:**
   - If medication is an antibiotic—stop the medication (Reason: possible allergy).
   - If rash is hives or is very itchy—stop the medication (Reason: possible allergy).
   - If the medication is an OTC drug—stop the medication (Reason: medicine is not essential).
   - Other rashes and prescription medications—continue the medication (Reason: lower likelihood of allergic drug reaction).
3. **For Non-Itchy Rashes:** No treatment is necessary.
4. **For Itchy Rashes:** Wash the skin once with soap to remove any irritants. Use Benadryl or take an Aveeno bath to reduce the itching.
5. **Oral Antihistamine Medication for Itching:**
   - Take an antihistamine like diphenhydramine (Benadryl) for widespread rashes that itch. The adult dosage of Benadryl is 25-50 mg by mouth 4 times daily.
   - An over-the-counter antihistamine that causes less sleepiness is loratadine (e.g., Alavert or Claritin).
   - **Caution:** This type of medication may cause sleepiness. Do not drink alcohol, drive, or operate dangerous machinery while taking antihistamines. Do not take these medications if you have prostate enlargement.
   - Read the package instructions thoroughly on all medications that you take.
6. **Oatmeal Aveeno Bath for Itching:** Sprinkle contents of one Aveeno packet under running faucet with comfortably warm water. Bathe for 15-20 minutes, 1-2 times daily. Pat dry with a towel. Do not rub the rash.
7. **Contagiousness:** Avoid contact with pregnant women until a diagnosis is made. Most viral rashes are contagious (especially if a fever is present). Allergic drug rashes are not contagious.
8. **Call Back If:**
   - You become worse.

FIRST AID

First Aid Advice for Anaphylaxis—Epinephrine (Pending EMS Arrival):

- If the patient has an epinephrine autoinjector, the patient should use it now.
- Use the autoinjector on the upper outer thigh. You may give it through clothing if necessary. Epinephrine is available in autoinjectors under trade names: EpiPen, EpiPen Jr, and Twinject. EpiPen is a single injection. Twinject has a second injection that can be used if there is no improvement after 5 minutes.

First Aid Advice for Anaphylaxis—Benadryl (Pending EMS Arrival):

- Give antihistamine orally NOW if able to swallow.
- Use Benadryl (diphenhydramine; adult dose 50 mg) or any other available antihistamine.

BACKGROUND INFORMATION

Cutaneous Drug Reactions (Drug Rashes)

- Rashes are one of the most common adverse reactions to drugs.
- **Incidence:** Adults are more likely than children to have an allergic reaction to a medication. Of course, adults are more frequently taking multiple medications.
- **Onset:** Most drug rashes begin within 2 weeks of starting a medicine. In fact, if any new skin condition occurs within 2 weeks of starting a new medication, the medication should be considered as a possible cause. Occasionally, drug rashes begin after the drug is stopped. For example, a rash might appear 10 days after starting a 7-day course of antibiotic treatment.
- **Symptoms:** The rash is most commonly red or pink spots that are smooth (macular) or slightly bumpy (papular). Other drug rashes that can occur include blisters (vesicles), skin redness (erythroderma), erythema nodosum, hives (urticaria), and pustules. Most drug rashes have associated itching. Localized rashes are less likely to be caused by drugs.
- **Diagnosis:** Determining the cause of a rash is often very difficult. Rashes from drug reactions often look similar to rashes from other causes (e.g., viral rashes). Usually the health care provider takes into consideration how likely a specific drug is to cause a rash and the rash appearance.
- **Treatment:** The patient should stop taking the drug that caused the rash. The patient can take oral antihistamine medications (e.g., diphenhydramine/Benadryl) if there is severe itching. Health care providers may prescribe oral prednisone for severe drug rashes.
- **Expected Course:** A drug rash will almost always improve simply by stopping the drug that caused it. However, depending on the type of rash it might take from a couple days (e.g., urticarial rash from ibuprofen) to 2-3 weeks (e.g., maculopapular rash from ampicillin) to get better.

Risk Factors for Developing a Drug Rash

- Older age; possibly from cumulative exposure
- Personal history of any prior drug allergy
- Family history of any drug allergy
- **Certain Concurrent Illnesses:** Cytomegalovirus or Epstein-Barr virus (mononucleosis) infections, AIDS, liver or renal disease

Drugs Most Likely to Cause Rashes

- **Angiotensin-Converting Enzyme (ACE) Inhibitors:** Examples include: enalapril (Vasotec, Renitec), lisinopril (Prinivil, Zestril), and benazepril (Lotensin)
- Allopurinol
- **Antibiotics:** Examples include penicillins (e.g., amoxicillin, ampicillin) and sulfa antibiotics (e.g., trimethoprim-sulfamethoxazole/Bactrim).
- **Anticonvulsants:** Examples include phenytoin (Dilantin)
- Antilipids
- Aspirin
- **Diuretics:** Examples include hydrochlorothiazide (HCTZ) and furosemide (e.g., Lasix).
- Nonsteroidal anti-inflammatory drugs (NSAIDs): Examples include ibuprofen (e.g., Motrin, Advil), naproxen (e.g., Aleve, Naprosyn), and ketorolac (Toradol).
- Oral contraceptives

Drugs Least Likely to Cause Rashes

- Over-the-counter (OTC; non-prescription) medicines rarely cause a rash. Here is a list of drugs least likely to be the cause of a rash.
  - Aminophylline
  - Antacids (e.g., Mylanta)
  - Acetaminophen (e.g., Tylenol)
  - Ear drops, prescription and OTC
  - Eye drops, prescription and OTC
  - Meperidine
  - Nitroglycerin
  - Prednisone, prednisolone
  - Propranolol
  - Spironolactone

Types of Cutaneous Drug Reactions (Drug Rashes)

Maculopapular eruptions are the most common cutaneous drug reactions. The rash has widespread pink and red macules (smooth-flat spots) and papules (bumpy-raised spots).

- Acneiform (pustular) eruptions
- Alopecia
- Erythema multiform-like eruptions
- Erythema nodosum
- Erythroderma
- Fixed drug eruption
- Hypertrichosis
- Maculopapular (exanthematous) eruptions
- Photosensitivity
- Phototoxic
- Pityriasis rosea-like eruptions
- Serum sickness
- Skin pigmentation
- Stevens-Johnson syndrome
- Toxic epidermal necrolysis
- Vasculitis
- Vesicles and blisters

Definition of Hives

- Itchy swollen patches that appear suddenly
- Patches change shape and location frequently; any one patch generally only lasts for a few hours, then fades away.
- Sizes of patches vary from ½ inch to several inches across.

Niacin Flush

- Niacin (nicotinic acid) is used in the treatment of hyperlipidemia. Perhaps as many as 80% of people who take niacin experience skin flushing. It is a well-known side effect.
- **Symptoms:** Flushing (deep red coloration) of the face and upper body occur approximately 20-60 minutes after taking niacin. Occasionally the skin flush spreads to the arms. Most people also report an accompanying sensation of warmth and itching. Usually the flushing lasts less than 1 hour.
- **Treatment:** Taking an adult aspirin or other nonsteroidal anti-inflammatory medication (e.g., ibuprofen) may help; however, the flushing goes away by itself within 1 hour.
- **Prevention:** Taking an adult aspirin or other nonsteroidal anti-inflammatory medication (if there are no contraindications) 30 minutes before the niacin reduces the degree of flushing. Extended-release niacin causes less flushing than regular niacin. Individuals taking niacin should avoid alcohol, spicy foods, hot beverages, and hot baths/showers right after taking niacin as these factors can increase the likelihood of flushing occurring.
- **Expected Course:** People who continue to take niacin for several weeks report that the flushing seems to happen less.

Anaphylaxis—Anaphylactic Reactions

- **Definition:** Anaphylaxis is a serious allergic reaction that is rapid in onset and may cause death.
- **Onset:** Generally, the shorter the interval between the allergen exposure (e.g., food, drug, or sting) and the onset of the first systemic symptoms, the more serious the reaction will be. Anaphylaxis usually starts within 20 minutes and always by 2 hours. If no symptoms occur by 2 hours, the risk for anaphylaxis has passed.
- **Symptoms—Systemic:** By definition, an anaphylactic reaction must include respiratory (e.g., wheezing or stridor), cardiovascular (e.g., fainting), or CNS (e.g., confusion) symptoms.
- **Symptoms—Cutaneous:** Hives or another itchy rash is often present (over 80%). The appearance of cutaneous symptoms (hives or facial swelling) may be a precursor to anaphylaxis.
- **Causes:** Foods (especially peanuts, tree nuts, fish, and shellfish), drugs (especially antibiotics and NSAIDs), and stings are the most common causes of anaphylaxis.

Caution—Fever:

- An adult with FEVER and RASH should seek medical attention immediately. A number of serious infections present in this manner.

RASH OR REDNESS, LOCALIZED AND CAUSE UNKNOWN

DEFINITION

- Rash or redness on one part of the body (localized or clustered).
- Cause of rash is unknown.

Includes:

- Localized areas of redness or skin irritation.
- Rash may be smooth (macular) or slightly bumpy (papular).
- Rash may look like small spots, large spots, or solid red.

TRIAGE ASSESSMENT QUESTIONS

Call EMS 911 Now

- Sounds like a life-threatening emergency to the triager

See More Appropriate Protocol

- Possible contact with poison ivy or oak
  Go to Protocol: Poison Ivy/Oak/Sumac on page 198
- Insect bite(s) suspected
  Go to Protocol: Insect Bite on page 166
- Athlete's foot suspected (i.e., itchy rash between the toes)
  Go to Protocol: Athlete's Foot on page 27
- Jock itch suspected (i.e., itchy rash on inner thighs near genital area)
  Go to Protocol: Jock Itch on page 171
- Wound infection suspected (i.e., pain, spreading redness, or pus; in a cut, puncture, scrape, or sutured wound)
  Go to Protocol: Wound Infection on page 344
- Rash of external female genital area (vulva)
  Go to Protocol: Vulvar Symptoms on page 338
- Rash of penis or scrotum
  Go to Protocol: Penis and Scrotum Symptoms on page 196
- Small spot, skin growth, or mole
  Go to Protocol: Skin Lesion (Moles or Growths) on page 239

Go to ED Now (or to Office With PCP Approval)

- Fever and localized purple or blood-colored spots or dots that are not from injury or friction
  R/O: early meningococcemia
  Note: it may be difficult to determine the rash color in people with darker-colored skin.
- Fever and localized rash is very painful
  R/O: cellulitis
- Patient sounds very sick or weak to the triager

Go to Office Now

- Looks like a boil, infected sore, deep ulcer, or other infected rash (spreading redness, red streak, pus)
  R/O: cellulitis, erysipelas, abscess

See Today in Office

- Painful rash and has multiple small blisters grouped together in one area of body (i.e., dermatomal distribution or "band" or "stripe")
  R/O: herpes zoster
- Localized rash is very painful (no fever)
  R/O: spider bite, bee sting
- Localized purple or blood-colored spots or dots that are not from injury or friction (no fever)
  R/O: bleeding disorder, petechiae, vasculitis.
  Note: it may be difficult to determine the rash color in people with darker-colored skin.
- Lyme disease suspected (e.g., bull's-eye rash or tick bite/exposure)
  R/O: erythema chronicum migrans
- Patient wants to be seen

See Today or Tomorrow in Office

- Tender bumps in armpits
  R/O: hidradenitis suppurativa
- Pimples (localized) and no improvement after using care advice
- Severe localized itching persists after 2 days of steroid cream and antihistamines
  R/O: poison ivy, contact dermatitis

Callback by PCP Today

- Applying cream or ointment and it causes severe itch, burning, or pain
  R/O: severe contact dermatitis

See Within 3 Days in Office

- Localized rash present > 7 days
  R/O: contact dermatitis, eczema, ringworm

See Within 2 Weeks in Office

- Red, moist, irritated area between skinfolds (or under larger breasts)
  R/O: intertrigo
  Note: see Background Information.

Home Care

- ○ Mild localized rash
- ○ Pimples (localized)

HOME CARE ADVICE

General Care Advice for Mild Localized Rash

1. **Avoid the Cause:** Try to find the cause. Consider irritants like a plant (e.g., poison ivy or evergreens), chemicals (e.g., solvents or insecticides), fiberglass, a new cosmetic, or new jewelry (called contact dermatitis). A pet may be carrying the irritating substance (e.g., with poison ivy or poison oak).
2. **Avoid Soap:** Wash the area once thoroughly with soap to remove any remaining irritants. Thereafter avoid soaps to this area. Cleanse the area when needed with warm water.
3. **Local Cold:** Apply or soak in cold water for 20 minutes every 3 to 4 hours to reduce itching or pain.
4. **Hydrocortisone Cream for Itching:** If the itch is more than mild, apply 1% hydrocortisone cream 4 times a day to reduce itching. Use it for 5 days.
   - Keep the cream in the refrigerator (Reason: it feels better if applied cold).
   - Available over-the-counter in United States as 0.5% and 1% cream.
   - Available over-the-counter in Canada as 0.5% cream.
   - **Caution:** Do not use hydrocortisone cream on suspected athlete's foot, jock itch, ringworm, or impetigo.
5. **Avoid Scratching:** Try not to scratch. Cut your fingernails short.
6. **Contagiousness:** Adults with localized rashes do not need to miss any work or school.
7. **Expected Course:** Most of these rashes pass in 2 to 3 days.
8. **Call Back If:**
   - Rash spreads or becomes worse.
   - Rash lasts longer than 1 week.
   - You become worse.

General Care Advice for Pimples

1. **Reassurance:** A pimple is a tiny, superficial infection without any redness. Pimples can occur with acne or friction.
2. **Cleaning:** Wash the infected area with an antibacterial soap and warm water 3 times a day.
3. **Antibiotic Ointment:** Apply antibiotic ointment (OTC) to the infected area 3 times per day.
4. **Call Back If:**
   - Redness occurs.
   - Fever occurs.
   - More pimples occur.
   - You become worse.

BACKGROUND INFORMATION

General Information

- Three localized rashes that individuals may be able to recognize are: athlete's foot, insect bites, and poison ivy. If present, use that protocol. If not, use this protocol.
- The main cause of a new localized rash is often skin contact with some irritant.
- The main cause of a persistent localized rash is often contact dermatitis, which is an allergic reaction to skin contact with some substance.
- Cellulitis is the medical term for an infection of the skin. There is spreading redness. The skin is also painful, tender to touch, and warm. There may or may not be any drainage or discharge. Antibiotic treatment is required.

Contact Dermatitis

Contact dermatitis is a common cause of persistent localized rashes. Contact dermatitis usually presents as localized raised red spots or a red area. Occasionally it progresses to localized blisters (e.g., poison ivy). The contact dermatitis rash is itchy.

Contact dermatitis is an allergic skin reaction that occurs after repeated contacts with the allergic substance. Once sensitized to a substance, however, reactions occur 12 to 24 hours after exposure. The location of the rash may suggest the cause.

- **Poison Ivy or Oak:** Exposed areas (e.g., hands, forearms)
- **Nickel (Metal):** Neck from necklaces, earlobe from earrings, belly button from metal snaps inside pants, wrist from wrist watch
- **Tanning Agents in Leather:** Tops of the feet from shoes or hands after wearing leather gloves
- **Preservatives in Creams, Lotions, Sunscreens, Shampoos:** Site of application
- **Neomycin in Antibiotic Ointment:** Site of application

Contact Dermatitis From Nickel

- **Definition:** Over 10% of adults have an allergy to nickel-containing metals. Nickel is often present in less-expensive jewelry. Even gold posts should be avoided immediately after a piercing because even higher-quality gold can contain trace amounts of nickel.
- **Symptoms:** People with nickel allergy can get an itchy rash where the metal touches their skin: finger (rings), earlobes (earrings), neck (neck chains), mid-abdomen (metal fasteners on jeans or belt buckle), wrist (bracelets and wrist watches).
- **Diagnosis:** See doctor if diagnosis is uncertain.
- **Treatment:** Avoid further contact with nickel. Apply a small amount of hydrocortisone cream 3 times a day for 7 days to the red-itchy area.
- **Expected Course:** Once the person stops wearing the nickel-containing jewelry, the redness and itching should go away in 7-14 days.
- **Prevention:** Avoid nickel-containing jewelry. Piercing jewelry should be made of hypoallergenic metal. Examples of metals that cause the least amount of allergy are stainless steel, titanium, platinum, palladium, and niobium. Titanium has the least risk of allergic reaction.

Intertrigo

- **Symptoms:** Erythematous and macerated (moist) areas between skin folds. Sometimes the patient may experience mild burning discomfort or itching.
- **Location:** The most common area is under the breasts. However, in obese individuals it can happen in multiple other areas of the body wherever skin folds over and creates a moist pocket. In obese individuals another common area is where the abdomen overlaps onto the upper thigh.
- **Risk Factors:** Obesity, heat, humidity, sweating, occlusive clothing, and diabetes.
- **Complications:** May become infected with yeast; a secondary baterial infection of the skin can sometimes occur.
- **Treatment:** Reducing the moisture in the area is the most important thing to do. Strategies for accomplishing this include wearing loose clothing, drying area with warm hair dryer or fan, keeping skin folds open to the air with a towel, and losing weight. Sometimes antifungal cream is helpful.

RECTAL BLEEDING

DEFINITION

- Blood-colored material mixed in with the stool or passed separately
- Bloody or maroon-colored stools
- Tarry-black stools (melena)
- Includes calls about: blood just on toilet paper, few drops into toilet water, or streaks on surface of normal formed BM

TRIAGE ASSESSMENT QUESTIONS

Call EMS 911 Now

- Passed out (i.e., fainted, collapsed and was not responding)
  R/O: shock
  FIRST AID: Lie down with the feet elevated.
- Shock suspected (e.g., cold/pale/clammy skin, too weak to stand)
  R/O: shock
  FIRST AID: Lie down with the feet elevated.
- Vomiting red blood or black (coffee ground) material
- Sounds like a life-threatening emergency to the triager

See More Appropriate Protocol

- Diarrhea is main symptom
  Go to Protocol: Diarrhea on page 89
- Rectal symptoms
  Go to Protocol: Rectal Symptoms on page 222

Go to ED Now (or to Office With PCP Approval)

- Severe dizziness (e.g., unable to stand, requires support to walk, feels like passing out now)
  R/O: significant blood loss, anemia
- Pale skin (pallor) of new onset or worsening
  R/O: anemia from GI bleeding
- Bloody, black, or tarry bowel movements
  R/O: ischemic colitis, obstruction
- Severe abdominal pain
- Constant abdominal pain lasting > 2 hours
  R/O: ischemic colitis, acute abdomen
- Rectal foreign body (inserted or swallowed)
- Patient sounds very sick or weak to the triager

Go to Office Now

- High-risk adult (e.g., prior surgery on aorta, abdominal aortic aneurysm)
  R/O: aortoenteric fistula
- Taking Coumadin (warfarin), Pradaxa (dabigatran), or known bleeding disorder (e.g., thrombocytopenia)
  Reason: higher risk of serious bleeding; may need for testing of INR, ProTime, or platelet count
- Colonoscopy in past 72 hours
  R/O: post-polypectomy bleeding

See Today in Office

- Blood passed alone without any stool
  R/O: rectal polyp, diverticulosis
- History of radiation therapy to lower abdomen or pelvis
  R/O: radiation proctitis
- History of cancer of rectum or intestines (colon)
  R/O: possibility of recurrence
- All other patients with rectal bleeding
  Exception: blood just on toilet paper, few drops, streaks on surface of normal formed BM
- Patient wants to be seen

See Within 2 Weeks in Office

- Normal formed BM with a few streaks or drops of blood on surface of BM
  R/O: hemorrhoids, anal fissure
- Rectal bleeding is minimal (e.g., blood just on toilet paper, a few drops in toilet bowl)
  R/O: hemorrhoids, anal fissure

HOME CARE ADVICE FOR RECTAL BLEEDING (Pending Office Visit)

1. **Warm Sitz Baths Twice a Day:**
   - Sit in a warm saline bath for 20 minutes 2 times daily to cleanse the rectal area and to promote healing.
   - You can add 2 ounces (57 grams) of table salt or baking soda to each tub of water.
2. **General Instructions for Treating and Preventing Constipation:**
   - Eat a high-fiber diet.
   - Drink adequate liquids.
   - Exercise regularly (even a daily 15-minute walk!).
   - Get into a rhythm—try to have a BM at the same time each day.
   - Don't ignore your body's signals to have a BM.
   - Avoid enemas and stimulant laxatives.
3. **High-Fiber Diet:** A high-fiber diet will help improve your intestinal function and soften your BMs. The fiber works by holding more water in your stools:
   - Try to eat fresh fruit and vegetables at each meal (peas, prunes, citrus, apples, beans, corn).
   - Eat more grain foods (bran flakes, bran muffins, graham crackers, oatmeal, brown rice, and whole wheat bread).
4. **Stool Softener for Hard Bowel Movements:**
   - Stool softeners help reduce rectal pain during bowel movements.
   - Colace (docusate sodium) is available OTC. Adult dosage 100 mg PO qd.
   - Discuss with PCP before using in pregnancy.
   - Read the package instructions and warnings.
5. **Treatment of Rectal Itching and Irritation:**
   - The main treatment for rectal itching is keeping the rectal area clean and dry, and avoiding excessive rubbing or scratching. Loose cotton underwear helps keep the area dry.
   - **Cleansing After a Bowel Movement:** Cleanse the anus with warm water after each bowel movement. Use wet cotton or tissue. Pat the area dry using unscented toilet paper. Avoid rubbing area with toilet paper.
   - **Topical Hydrocortisone Cream Twice a Day:** Apply 1% hydrocortisone ointment (OTC) bid to reduce irritation (e.g., Anusol-HC, Preparation H Hydrocortisone).
   - **Prevention:** Avoid scented toilet products. Keep rectal area clean and dry.
6. **Call Back If:**
   - Bleeding increases in amount.
   - Bleeding occurs 3 or more times after treatment begins.
   - You become worse.

FIRST AID

First Aid Advice for Shock:
Lie down with the feet elevated.

BACKGROUND INFORMATION

Causes:

- **Anal Fissure:** A small crack or tear in the skin of the anus. It may result from passing hard BMs or from having frequent diarrheal BMs. Symptoms include pain during and immediately after having a BM, mild rectal bleeding, and rectal itching.
- **Colon and Rectal Causes:** Examples include cancer, polyps, angiodysplasia, inflammatory bowel disease, diverticulosis, ischemic colitis, and infection.
- **Hemorrhoids (aka "Piles"):** Are enlarged veins that may be just inside (internal) or outside (external) the rectal opening (anus). Risk factors for developing hemorrhoids include chronic constipation and pregnancy. Individuals with hemorrhoids complain of a small amount (drops, 1-2 tsp) of bright red rectal bleeding with bowel movements (BMs) and may also note localized pain or irritation.
- **Rectal Foreign Body:** May cause tearing of the rectal mucosa.
- **Upper Gastrointestinal Causes:** Examples include peptic ulcer disease and esophageal varices.

Stool Appearance:

- **Bright Red Blood Just on Toilet Paper:** The least serious patient complaint. It almost always signifies that the bleeding is coming from the anus. The 2 most common causes of this type of bleeding are hemorrhoids and anal fissures.
- **Bright Red Blood on the Surface of a Formed BM:** This generally signifies bleeding from the anus or just inside the rectum. This can be caused by hemorrhoids or anal fissures, but may also be caused by more serious entities like cancer and polyps.
- **Blood Mixed in With a BM:** This generally signifies some type of disease process in the colon or rectal area. Examples of diseases that can cause this include colon cancer, colon polyps, diverticulosis, and ulcerative colitis.
- **Blood Mixed With Diarrheal Stool:** Various intestinal infections and ischemic colitis can present like this.
- **Tarry-black BM:** This almost always represents upper gastrointestinal bleeding from the stomach or esophagus. Stomach acid breaks down the blood and turns it black.

Red or Black Stools That Aren't Blood:

- **Red:** Red Jell-O, red Kool-Aid, red cereals, tomato juice or soup, cranberries, red licorice, red medicines.
- **Black:** Bismuth (e.g., Pepto-Bismol), iron, licorice, Oreo cookies, cigarette ashes, charcoal, grape juice. Bile can look black to the uninitiated. Having the caller smear a piece of stool on white paper and looking at it under a bright light often confirms that the color is actually dark green.

RECTAL SYMPTOMS

DEFINITION

- Rash, pain, itching, swelling, and other symptoms of the rectal area (anus)

TRIAGE ASSESSMENT QUESTIONS

Call EMS 911 Now

- Sounds like a life-threatening emergency to the triager

See More Appropriate Protocol

- Diarrhea is main concern
  Go to Protocol: Diarrhea on page 89
- Constipation is main concern (e.g., pain or discomfort caused by passage of hard BMs)
  Go to Protocol: Constipation on page 63
- Blood in or on bowel movement is main concern
  Go to Protocol: Rectal Bleeding on page 219

Go to ED Now (or to Office With PCP Approval)

- Sexual assault
  R/O: sexual assault, rectal injury from foreign body
- Injury to rectum
  R/O: sexual assault, rectal injury from foreign body
- Patient sounds very sick or weak to the triager

Go to Office Now

- Severe rectal pain
  R/O: abscess, herpes
- Rectal pain or redness and fever > 100.5° F (38.1° C)
  R/O: cellulitis, abscess
- Acute onset rectal pain and constipation (straining with rectal pressure or fullness), which is not relieved by sitz bath or suppository
  R/O: fecal impaction

See Today in Office

- Moderate-severe rectal pain (i.e., interferes with school, work, or sleep)
  R/O: thrombosed hemorrhoid, abscess, STD
- Moderate-severe rectal itching (i.e., interferes with school, work, or sleep)
  R/O: contact dermatitis, poison ivy, pinworms
- Last bowel movement (BM) > 4 days ago
  R/O: fecal impaction
- Rectal area looks infected (e.g., draining sore, spreading redness)
  R/O: abscess, cellulitis, STD
- Rash of rectal area (e.g., open sore, painful tiny water blisters, unexplained bumps)
  R/O: STD
- Caller is worried about a sexually transmitted disease (STD)
  Reason: prevent spread of STD or relieve fear

See Today or Tomorrow in Office

- Home treatment > 3 days for rectal pain and not improved
  R/O: thrombosed hemorrhoid, anal fissure, abscess
- Home treatment for > 3 days for rectal itching and not improved
  R/O: pruritis ani, contact dermatitis, cancer, STD
- Patient wants to be seen

See Within 2 Weeks in Office

- Recurrent episodes of unexplained rectal pain, but NO rectal symptoms now
  R/O: proctalgia fugax
- Painless lump in rectal area
  R/O: hemorrhoid, condyloma, anal cancer

Home Care

- Acute onset rectal pain and constipation (i.e., straining with rectal pressure or fullness) that is untreated
  R/O: fecal impaction
- Mild rectal pain
  R/O: hemorrhoids, fissure
- Mild rectal itching
  R/O: contact dermatitis

HOME CARE ADVICE FOR RECTAL SYMPTOMS

1. **Treatment of Acute Rectal Pain Due to Fecal Impaction:**
   - **Sitz Bath:** Take a 20-minute bath in warm water. Add 2 oz (57 grams) of baking soda to the bath water. This is also called a sitz bath and it often helps relax the anal sphincter and release the bowel movement (BM).
   - **Suppository:** If the sitz bath does not work, try 1 or 2 glycerin rectal suppositories, which you can get over-the-counter (OTC) at your local pharmacy.
   - **Enema:** An enema should be used rarely and only after other measures have not worked. How to give an enema: [1] Patient should lie on his/her side with knees pulled up. [2] The tip of the enema tube should be lubricated with Vaseline and inserted 1 to 2 inches (3-5 cm) into the rectum. [3] The enema fluid should be delivered gradually. The patient should try to hold the enema fluid inside for a few minutes.
   - **Expected Course:** Acute rectal pain should be completely relieved by these instructions. If the discomfort does not go away, you will need to be seen.
2. **Treatment of Mild Rectal Pain:**
   - Rectal pain and irritation can often be caused by either hemorrhoids or a tiny tear in the rectal opening (anal fissure). Small drops of blood can sometimes be seen on the toilet paper or stool in people with hemorrhoids or rectal irritation from hard bowel movements.
   - **Warm Sitz Bath Twice a Day:** Sit in a warm saline bath for 20 minutes bid to cleanse the area and to promote healing. Add 2 ounces (57 grams) of table salt or baking soda to each tub of water. Afterwards, gently pat area dry with unscented toilet paper.
   - **Topical Hydrocortisone Twice a Day:** After taking a sitz bath and drying your rectal area, apply 1% hydrocortisone ointment (OTC) bid to reduce irritation. Hydrocortisone is found in various OTC hemorrhoid medications (e.g., Anusol-HC, Preparation H Hydrocortisone, Analpram-HC Cream).
3. **Treatment of Mild Rectal Itching:**
   - The main treatment for rectal itching is keeping the rectal area clean and dry, and avoiding excessive rubbing or scratching. Loose cotton underwear helps keep the area dry.
   - **Cleansing After a Bowel Movement:** Cleanse the anus with warm water after each bowel movement. Use wet cotton or tissue. Pat the area dry using unscented toilet paper. Avoid rubbing area with toilet paper.
   - **Topical Hydrocortisone Twice a Day:** Apply 1% hydrocortisone ointment (OTC) bid to reduce irritation (e.g., Anusol-HC, Preparation H Hydrocortisone).
   - **Prevention:** Avoid scented toilet products. Keep rectal area clean and dry.
4. **Call Back If:**
   - Severe rectal pain or itching.
   - Acute rectal pain due to fecal impaction is not completely relieved after treatment.
   - Rectal pain or itching persists more than 3 days.
   - Rectal bleeding (i.e., more than just a few drops on toilet paper from wiping).
   - You become worse.

BACKGROUND INFORMATION

General:

- The anus and skin around it is very sensitive because of a rich nerve supply. Pain or itching at this site can be intense.
- The passage of large, hard stools or diarrhea stools causes most of the normal symptoms. Dried stool left on the skin can be very irritating.

Common Causes of Rectal Pain:

- Anal fissure
- Fecal impaction
- Hemorrhoids—thrombosed
- Perirectal abscess and fistula
- Proctalgia fugax (severely painful muscle spasm of rectal area)
- Sexually transmitted disease (e.g., herpes simplex)

Common Causes of Rectal Itching (Pruritis Ani):

- Contact dermatitis (e.g., scented toilet products)
- Foods (e.g., citrus fruit, coffee, spices, tomatoes)
- Hemorrhoids
- Pinworms
- Poison ivy
- Pruritis ani (primary, no other cause found)
- Skin disorders (e.g., psoriasis, seborrhea, skin cancer)

Hemorrhoids (Piles):

- **Definition:** Abnormally enlarged veins in the rectal (anal) canal.
- **Internal Hemorrhoids:** Are located just inside the rectum. Symptoms include pain, bleeding, and itching. Sometimes internal hemorrhoids can protrude (prolapse) out of the rectal opening; patients may then describe a fullness in this area after a bowel movement.
- **External Hemorrhoids:** Are located just outside the rectal opening. Symptoms include pain, bleeding, and itching. External hemorrhoids can be thrombosed (clotted, hard, painful tense blue lump) or not thrombosed (soft flesh-colored lump).
- **Causes:** Constipation, obesity, pregnancy, sitting for long periods, diarrhea, straining to lift heavy objects.
- **Treatment:** Includes sitz bath, hemorrhoid cream, stool softeners. Thrombosed hemorrhoids may need to be surgically excised.
- **Prevention:** Good bowel habits including: adequate liquid intake (8 glasses of water daily), regular exercise, high-fiber diet, having bowel movement at same time each day.

Pruritis Ani:

- **Definition:** A general term meaning anal itching. It is a common and bothersome symptom.
- **Causes:** In most cases itching is caused by irritation of the sensitive anal nerve endings from residual stool or scented toilet products. Hemorrhoids can also cause itching. Occasionally, certain foods can cause itching. Rarely, persistent itching can be caused by skin disorders or rectal cancer.
- **Treatment:** The main treatment for rectal itching is to keep the rectal area clean, dry, and to avoid excessive rubbing or scratching. Loose cotton underwear helps keep the area dry. OTC hydrocortisone cream can also reduce itching.
- **Prevention:** Avoid scented toilet products. Keep rectal area clean and dry.

SEIZURE

DEFINITION

- A seizure (convulsion) occurs.

Symptoms of a Seizure Include:

- During a generalized seizure, the victim loses consciousness, becomes stiff, and has jerking of the arms and legs.
- During a partial (focal) seizure, jerking of an arm or leg on one side occurs.
- Most seizures last < 5 minutes.

TRIAGE ASSESSMENT QUESTIONS

Call EMS 911 Now

- First seizure ever
  R/O: stroke, brain tumor
- Epileptic seizure (in adult with known epilepsy) and continues > 5 minutes
  Reason: increased risk of status epilepticus
- Two or more seizures and stays confused between seizures
  R/O: status epilepticus
- Bluish lips or face now
  FIRST AID: Begin mouth-to-mouth breathing if breathing stops.
  Note: most adults breathe adequately during a seizure; a red-purple coloration of face is common.
- Head injury caused the seizure
  R/O: concussion, cerebral contusion, subdural/ epidural, or intracerebral hemorrhage
- Pregnant or postpartum (<1 month)
  Reason: higher-risk situation (mother and fetus). Consider eclampsia if third trimester.
- Known poisoning or overdose
- Seizure in a swimming pool
  R/O: aspiration
  FIRST AID: Remove victim from swimming pool.
- Known diabetic
  R/O: hypoglycemia
- Unresponsive (can't be awakened) after the seizure stops and persists > 5 minutes
  R/O: stroke, head trauma, overdose
- Acting confused (e.g., disoriented, slurred speech) after the seizure stops and persists > 30 minutes
  R/O: stroke, head trauma, overdose
- Sounds like a life-threatening emergency to the triager

Go to ED Now

- Second seizure occurs on the same day
  R/O: low anticonvulsant drug level
- Fever > 99.5° F (37.5° C)
  R/O: meningitis
- Severe headache
  R/O: meningitis, intracerebral hemorrhage
  Note: most seizure victims will have a headache after a seizure.
- High-risk adult (e.g., alcohol or drug abuse)
  R/O: alcohol withdrawal seizure

Go to ED Now (or to Office With PCP Approval)

- Wants to sleep after the seizure and persists much longer than usual
  Reason: prolonged postictal sleepiness
- Patient sounds very sick or weak to the triager

See Today in Office

- Not on or ran out of seizure medicines (anticonvulsants)
  Reason: needs to be on anticonvulsant medications

See Today or Tomorrow in Office

- Stopped taking seizure medicines (anticonvulsants)
  Reason: patient education
  Note: needs to resume anticonvulsant medications
- Epileptic seizures occur frequently (several per week)
  R/O: low anticonvulsant drug level
- Patient wants to be seen

Home Care

- Seizure lasting < 5 minutes with a history of prior seizure(s), and taking anticonvulsants
  Reason: brief seizure in patient on anticonvulsants

HOME CARE ADVICE FOR SEIZURE

1. **Reassurance:** This seizure did not last very long and there is a history of prior seizures. There is no need to go to the emergency room for every seizure.
2. **Anticonvulsant Medication:** If the seizure victim missed a dose of seizure medicine in the last 2 days, he/she should take that missed dose now.
3. **Anticonvulsant Medication Levels:**
   If patient takes phenytoin (Dilantin), carbamazepine (Tegretol), valproic acid (Depakene, Depakote), or phenobarbital, THEN:
   - You should have the blood levels of your seizure medication(s) checked periodically.
   - If it has been more than 1 month, then we should arrange to get your medication levels checked this week.
4. **Headache:**
   - Most people after a seizure will have a headache.
   - If the seizure has stopped and the person is now awake and alert, it is OK to treat the headache with acetaminophen (Tylenol; 650-1,000 mg by mouth).
5. **Postictal Period:**
   - Most seizure victims will be confused and groggy for a period of time after the seizure stops.
   - Immediately after the seizure, the seizure victim will be very sleepy and may have noisy breathing.
   - Gradually, the seizure victim will become more and more alert.
   - Usually, the seizure victim is fully alert within 1-2 hours.
6. **Sleep:**
   - Let the seizure victim sleep if he/she wishes (Reason: the brain is temporarily exhausted, and sleep is restorative).
   - Check the individual frequently for any breathing problems.
7. **Expected Course:** After a brief seizure, most people feel normal within 1 to 2 hours.
8. **Call Back If:**
   - Another seizure occurs.
   - Fever or severe headache.
   - Stays confused (e.g., disoriented or slurred speech) more than 30 minutes.
   - Wants to sleep more than 2 hours (or longer than usual).
   - Patient becomes worse or you have more questions.

FIRST AID

First Aid Advice for Seizure—Do Protect the Victim:

- Lay the seizing person on the ground, preferably on his/her side.
- Place a pillow or soft item under the head.
- Remove glasses.
- Move lamps, chairs, etc. away from person to prevent injury.
- Stay with victim until help arrives.

First Aid Advice for Seizure—Do Not:

- **Do Not:** Put your finger or any object into the victim's mouth. This is unnecessary and can cut the mouth, injure a tooth, cause vomiting, or result in a serious bite of your finger.
- **Do Not:** Try to restrain or hold the patient down.
- **Do Not:** Try to resuscitate the victim just because breathing stops momentarily for 5 to 10 seconds. Breathing never looks normal during the seizure, but it's adequate if the color is not bluish.

BACKGROUND INFORMATION

Types of Seizures

- **Generalized:** A generalized seizure involves the whole brain. The victim loses consciousness, becomes stiff, and has bilateral jerking of the arms and legs.
- **Partial:** A partial (focal) seizure involves only part of the brain. Jerking of an arm or leg on one side of the body occurs, with no loss of consciousness.
- **Complex:** A complex seizure is characterized by a period of abnormal behavior with associated confusion. There are no jerking movements.
- **Febrile:** Seen in children, not in adults.

- **Status Epilepticus:** The victim has a prolonged seizure (>30 minutes) or does not awaken between 2 separate seizures.

Causes

- Alcohol withdrawal.
- Brain tumor.
- **Eclampsia:** Women in their third trimester of pregnancy can develop hypertension (preeclampsia) and rarely seizures (eclampsia).
- **Epilepsy:** Most seizures occur in adults already known to have epilepsy (recurrent seizure disorder).
- Head injury.
- Heatstroke.
- **Hypoxia:** Cerebral hypoxia can cause seizures.
- **Infection:** Examples include meningitis, encephalitis.
- **Low Drug Levels:** The most common cause of a seizure in an epileptic is noncompliance with anticonvulsant medications.
- **Metabolic:** Examples include hypoglycemia and hyponatremia.
- **Stroke:** This can be either cerebral infarction or hemorrhage.

Epilepsy

- **Definition:** Epilepsy is a recurrent seizure disorder. Many individuals with epilepsy wear medical identification (e.g., MedicAlert bracelet). If there is no medical ID and no other information available to confirm epilepsy, then the triager should assume that a seizure is a first seizure.
- **Triage Disposition:** A person with epilepsy does not need to come into the ED if the following conditions are met: seizure less than 5 minutes AND returns to consciousness AND is not pregnant or diabetic AND there is no injury.
- **Treatment:** Anticonvulsant medications can reduce the frequency of seizures.

Postictal Symptoms

After experiencing a brief generalized (grand mal) seizure lasting less than 5 minutes, many adults with epilepsy will have postictal symptoms for up to 2 hours afterward. During the initial several minutes of this postictal period the patient will be in a postictal coma; the patient is unresponsive to painful stimuli and has loud snoring respirations. For up to 15-30 minutes after a seizure the patient may have postictal confusion; the patient should demonstrate gradually improving alertness and orientation. For up to 2 hours after a seizure the patient may have postictal sleepiness; with verbal stimuli, the patient can be awakened and is not confused but may return to sleep when left alone. A headache is a common complaint. A patient whose postictal symptoms last longer than these time periods may have a complication (e.g., head trauma, drug overdose, stroke, status epilepticus, etc.). Because of potential complications, the following cutoffs are used in this guideline for seeing postictal adults following a brief generalized seizure:

- Postictal coma > 5 minutes
- Postictal confusion > 30 minutes
- Postictal sleepiness > 2 hours, or longer than usual

SEXUAL ASSAULT OR RAPE

DEFINITION

- Sexual intercourse by force

TRIAGE ASSESSMENT QUESTIONS

Call EMS 911 Now

- Someone is threatening violence now
  Reason: need police involvement
- Major blood loss and has fainted or too weak to stand
  R/O: impending shock
- Major bleeding (e.g., actively dripping or spurting) and can't be stopped
  FIRST AID: Apply direct pressure to the entire wound with a clean cloth.
- Sounds like a life-threatening emergency to the triager

Go to ED Now

- Injuries needing medical treatment
- Sexual assault within last 5 days
  Reason: evidence collection (semen, DNA)
- Attempted sexual assault within last 5 days
  Reason: evidence collection (semen, DNA)
- Suspected victim of rape drug (e.g., GHB, ketamine, Rohypnol) and within last 5 days
  Reason: urine drug testing

See Today in Office

- Sexual assault > 5 days ago and has symptoms or minor injuries
- Patient wants to be seen

Call Local Agency Today

- Sexual assault > 5 days ago and no symptoms nor injuries
  Reason: referral to rape crisis center for counseling and support

HOME CARE ADVICE (Pending Further Evaluation)

General Information

1. **Helpful Telephone Numbers:**
   - **Police Department:** XXX-XXX-XXXX
   - **Rape Crisis Center:** XXX-XXX-XXXX
   - **Rape, Abuse & Incest National Network (RAINN) hotline:** 1-800-656-HOPE (4673)
2. **Call Back If:**
   - You have any other question or if I can help you in any way.
   - You become worse.

Instructions for Patients Being Sent in to ED for Sexual Assault Exam

1. **Preserve the Evidence:**
   - Don't bathe.
   - Following vaginal intercourse, don't douche or change your tampon.
   - Following oral intercourse, don't eat, drink, or brush the teeth.
   - Bring any articles of clothing that may contain blood or semen.
2. **Bring Clothes:**
   - If the victim has not changed clothes since the assault, then bring a change of clothes to put on at the hospital.
3. **Support:**
   - I'm glad you called.
   - Encourage the victim to seek medical evaluation and help.
   - Encourage the victim to bring a family member or friend for support.

Emergency Contraceptive Pills (ECP)

1. **ECP:**
   - Emergency contraceptive pills are very effective in preventing pregnancy after unprotected sexual intercourse. Emergency contraceptive pills can reduce the pregnancy rate by 75-88%.
   - They are also sometimes called "morning-after pills," but you do not have to take them just in the morning.

- The sooner the pills are started, the better they work. The pills must be started within 120 hours (5 days) and ideally within 72 hours (3 days) of the unprotected sexual intercourse.
- Emergency contraceptive pills do not prevent sexually transmitted diseases.

2. **ECP—Effectiveness (Statistics for Women in Second or Third Week of Cycle):**
   - **No Treatment:** 8 out of 100 women will get pregnant.
   - **Treatment 72-120 Hours After Intercourse:** 3-4 out of 100 women will get pregnant.
   - **Treatment Within 72 Hours After Intercourse:** 1-2 out of 100 women will get pregnant.
3. **ECP—Side Effects:**
   - **Nausea:** 30-60 %
   - **Vomiting:** 5-20 %
   - **Abdominal Pain:** 10-20%
   - **Fatigue and Headache:** 10-20%
   - **Change in Menstrual Bleeding Onset or Amount:** 50%
4. **ECP—Contraindications:**
   - Pregnancy known or suspected
   - Abnormal vaginal bleeding and cause is unknown
5. **ECP—No Increased Risk of Birth Defects:**
   - Emergency contraceptive pills do not cause any birth defects.
6. **ECP—Dosage for Plan B (Levonorgestrel):**
   - **Availability:** You can get Plan B without a prescription at most pharmacies. Contact your local pharmacy to determine if they have and provide this pill.
   - **Dosage:** Take 1 pill now and 1 pill in 12 hours.
   - **Cost:** The typical cost of ECP is $20-30.

Additional Internet Resources

1. Rape, Abuse & Incest National Network (RAINN) has a hotline that victims of sexual assault can call: 1-800-656-HOPE (4673) (www.rainn.org).
2. RAINN has a search engine for locating a local counseling center for a victim of sexual assault: www.rainn.org.
3. National Protocol for Sexual Assault Medical Forensic Examinations of Adults/Adolescents. US Department of Justice. Available at: www.safeta.org/protocol/protocolHome.cfm.
4. National Sexual Violence Resource Center (877-739-3895 or 717-909-0710) (www.nsvrc.org).

BACKGROUND INFORMATION

General

- The victim is usually female (96%).
- Between 60%-80% of the time the victim knows the assailant.
- Approximately 40% of the time the assault occurs in the victim's or assailant's home.
- **Physical Examination:** General body trauma is more commonly found than genital trauma. General body injuries are usually minor and include contusions, abrasions, and lacerations.
- **Evidence Collection:** Many jurisdictions currently use 72 hours after the assault as the standard cutoff time for collecting evidence. Evidence collection beyond that point is still possible, especially with recent advances in DNA testing. Because of this, some jurisdictions have extended the standard cutoff time (e.g., up to 5 days).
- **Pregnancy Risk After Sexual Assault:** The risk of pregnancy after sexual assault is between 2-5%. Emergency (morning-after) contraceptive pills can prevent pregnancy. The sooner the pills are started, the better they work. The pills must be started within 120 hours (5 days) and ideally within 72 hours (3 days) of the unprotected sexual intercourse.

Emergency Contraceptive Pills—Availability

- Emergency contraceptive pills are 95% effective at preventing unintended pregnancy if taken within 24 hours of unprotected intercourse and 85% effective if taken within 72 hours. The sooner the emergency contraception pills are taken, the more effective they are.
- **Availability in the United States:** On August 24, 2006, Plan B (levonorgestrel) was approved by the FDA for nonprescription sale in pharmacies to women and men 18 and older in the United States.
- **Availability in Canada:** On April 19, 2005, the Canadian Ministry of Health approved the sale of Plan B (levonorgestrel) without prescription in pharmacies in Canada.

Emergency Contraceptive Pills—Important Internet Resources

- **The Emergency Contraception Website:** http://ec.princeton.edu. This is a very useful website with answers to many FAQs. This Web site also lists physicians and clinics in the United States and Canada that provide emergency contraceptive pills.
- **Canadian Paediatric Society Adolescent Health Committee Position Statement:** www.cps.ca/english/statements/AM/ah10-02.htm

Rape Drugs

- **Definition:** There are several drugs that are referred to as "rape drugs" because they are used by rapists to make a victim confused or unconscious. The drugs are typically put into the victim's drink without the victim's knowledge or consent. The drugs can be tasteless, colorless, and odorless; the victim does not know that she (or he) is being drugged.
- **Alternate Term:** Drug-facilitated sexual assault.
- **Symptoms:** Victims report waking up feeling drugged or more hung over than expected. Victims sometimes report amnesia: they may remember taking a drink but then can't remember what happened after that. Sometimes victims report that they feel like someone had sex with them but they cannot remember anything more.
- **Examples of Rape Drugs:** GHB, ketamine, Rohypnol (flunitrazepam).
- **Urine Testing for Rape Drugs:** Date rape drugs can be detected in the urine. However, the body metabolizes these drugs very quickly and the drug may be difficult to detect in as little as 12 hours.
- **Alcohol and Alcohol-Facilitated Sexual Assault:** Approximately 30-75% of victims of sexual assault have been drinking alcohol. Thus, there is a correlation between alcohol intoxication and the risk of sexual assault.

SINUS PAIN AND CONGESTION

DEFINITION

- Sensation of fullness, pressure, and pain on the face overlying a sinus cavity (e.g., above the eyebrow, behind the eye, around the eye, or over the cheekbone).
- Pain or pressure may be bilateral but more often is unilateral (on one side of the face).
- Associated symptoms are a blocked nose, nasal discharge, and/or postnasal drip.

Pain Severity Is Defined As:

- **Mild (1-3):** Doesn't interfere with normal activities
- **Moderate (4-7):** Interferes with normal activities (e.g., work or school) or awakens from sleep
- **Severe (8-10):** Excruciating pain, unable to do any normal activities

TRIAGE ASSESSMENT QUESTIONS

Call EMS 911 Now

● Sounds like a life-threatening emergency to the triager

Go to ED Now

● Difficulty breathing, and not from stuffy nose (e.g., not relieved by cleaning out the nose)
R/O: pneumonia

Go to ED Now (or to Office With PCP Approval)

● Severe headache and has fever
R/O: bacterial frontal sinusitis, cavernous sinus thrombosis, meningitis

● Patient sounds very sick or weak to the triager

Go to Office Now

● Severe sinus pain
R/O: bacterial sinusitis

● Severe headache
R/O: cavernous sinus thrombosis, meningitis

● Redness or swelling on the cheek, forehead, or around the eye
R/O: sinusitis with overlying cellulitis, osteomyelitis, preseptal cellulitis

● Fever > 103° F (39.4° C)
R/O: sinusitis, pneumonia

● Fever > 100.5° F (38.1° C) and over 60 years of age
R/O: pneumonia, sinusitis.

● Fever > 100.5° F (38.1° C) and has diabetes mellitus or a weakened immune system (e.g., HIV positive, cancer chemotherapy, organ transplant, splenectomy, chronic steroids)
R/O: pneumonia, sinusitis

● Fever > 100.5° F (38.1° C) and bedridden (e.g., nursing home patient, stroke, chronic illness, recovering from surgery)
R/O: pneumonia, sinusitis
Note: may need ambulance transport to ED

See Today in Office

● Fever present > 3 days (72 hours)
R/O: bacterial sinusitis

● Fever returns after gone for over 24 hours and symptoms worse or not improved
R/O: bacterial sinusitis, bronchitis, pneumonia

● Sinus pain (not just congestion) and fever
R/O: bacterial sinusitis

● Earache
R/O: ear infection

See Today or Tomorrow in Office

● Sinus congestion (pressure, fullness) present > 10 days
R/O: bacterial sinusitis, allergic rhinitis

● Nasal discharge present > 10 days
R/O: bacterial sinusitis, allergic rhinitis

● Using nasal washes and pain medicine > 24 hours and sinus pain (lower forehead, cheekbone, or eye) persists
R/O: bacterial sinusitis, allergic rhinitis

● Lots of coughing
R/O: cough triggered by sinusitis

● Patient wants to be seen

Home Care

○ Sinus congestion as part of a cold, present < 10 days

HOME CARE ADVICE FOR MILD SINUS PAIN AND CONGESTION

General Care Advice for Mild Sinus Pain and Congestion

1. **Reassurance:**
   - Sinus congestion is a normal part of a cold.
   - Usually home treatment with nasal washes can prevent an actual bacterial sinus infection.
   - Antibiotics are not helpful for the sinus congestion that occurs with colds.
2. **For a Runny Nose With Profuse Discharge: Blow the Nose:**
   - Nasal mucus and discharge helps to wash viruses and bacteria out of the nose and sinuses.
   - Blowing the nose is all that is needed.
   - If the skin around your nostrils gets irritated, apply a tiny amount of petroleum ointment to the nasal openings once or twice a day.
3. **For a Stuffy Nose—Use Nasal Washes:**
   - **Introduction:** Saline (salt water) nasal irrigation is an effective and simple home remedy for treating cold symptoms and other conditions involving the nasal and sinus passages. Nasal irrigation consists of pouring, spraying, or squirting salt water into the nose and then letting it run back out.
   - **How It Helps:** The salt water rinses out excess mucus, washes out any irritants (dust, allergens) that might be present, and moisturizes the nasal cavity.
   - **Methods:** There are several ways to perform nasal irrigation. You can use a saline nasal spray bottle (available over-the-counter), a rubber ear syringe, a medical syringe without the needle, or a Neti Pot.

   Step-by-Step Instructions:
   - **Step 1:** Lean over a sink.
   - **Step 2:** Gently squirt or spray warm salt water into one of your nostrils.
   - **Step 3:** Some of the water may run into the back of your throat. Spit this out. If you swallow the salt water it will not hurt you.
   - **Step 4:** Blow your nose to clean out the water and mucus.
   - **Step 5:** Repeat steps 1-4 for the other nostril. You can do this a couple times a day if it seems to help you.

   How to Make Saline (Salt Water) Nasal Wash:
   - You can make your own saline nasal wash.
   - Add ½ tsp of table salt to 1 cup (8 oz; 240 mL) of warm water.
   - You should use sterile, distilled, or previously boiled water for nasal irrigation.
4. **Hydration:** Drink plenty of liquids (6-8 glasses of water daily). If the air in your home is dry, use a cool mist humidifier
5. **Cold Medicines:** Most "cold" medicines are not helpful. They can't remove dried mucus from the nose. Antihistamines are only helpful if you also have nasal allergies. Antibiotics are not helpful unless you develop an ear or sinus infection.
6. **Nasal Decongestants for a Very Stuffy Nose:**
   - If you have a very stuffy nose, nasal decongestant medicines can shrink the swollen nasal mucosa and allow for easier breathing. If you have a very runny nose, these medicines can reduce the amount of drainage. They may be taken as pills by mouth or as a nasal spray.
   - Most people do NOT need to use these medicines. If your nose feels blocked, you should try using nasal washes first.
   - Pseudoephedrine (Sudafed) is available OTC in pill form. Typical adult dosage is two 30-mg tablets every 6 hours. Read package instructions.
   - Phenylephrine (Sudafed PE) is available OTC in pill form. Typical adult dosage is two 30-mg tablets every 6 hours. Read package instructions.
   - Oxymetazoline nasal drops (Afrin) are available OTC. Clean out the nose before using. Spray each nostril once, wait 1 minute for absorption, and then spray a second time. Read package instructions.
   - Phenylephrine nasal drops (Neo-Synephrine) are available OTC. Clean out the nose before using. Spray each nostril once, wait 1 minute for absorption, and then spray a second time. Read package instructions.

7. **Pain and Fever Medicines:**
   - For pain or fever relief, take acetaminophen or ibuprofen.
   - Treat fevers above 101° F (38.3° C).
   - The goal of fever therapy is to bring the fever down to a comfortable level. Remember that fever medicine usually lowers fever 2-3° F (1-1.5° C).

   Acetaminophen (e.g., Tylenol):
   - Take 650 mg by mouth every 4-6 hours as needed. Each Regular Strength Tylenol pill has 325 mg of acetaminophen. The most you should take each day is 3,250 mg (10 pills a day).
   - Another choice is to take 1,000 mg every 8 hours. Each Extra Strength Tylenol pill has 500 mg of acetaminophen. The most you should take each day is 3,000 mg (6 pills a day).

   Ibuprofen (e.g., Motrin, Advil):
   - Take 400 mg by mouth every 6 hours.
   - Another choice is to take 600 mg by mouth every 8 hours.

   Extra Notes:
   - Acetaminophen is thought to be safer than ibuprofen in people over 65 years old. Acetaminophen is in many OTC and prescription medicines. It might be in more than one medicine that you are taking. You need to be careful and not take an overdose. An acetaminophen overdose can hurt the liver.
   - **Caution:** Do not take acetaminophen if you have liver disease.
   - **Caution:** Do not take ibuprofen if you have stomach problems, kidney disease, are pregnant, or have been told by your doctor to avoid this type of anti-inflammatory drug. Do not take ibuprofen for more than 7 days without consulting your doctor.
   - Use the lowest amount of medicine that makes your pain or fever better.
   - Before taking any medicine, read all the instructions on the package.

8. **Expected Course:**
   - Sinus congestion from viral upper respiratory infections (colds) usually lasts 5-10 days.
   - Occasionally a cold can worsen and turn into bacterial sinusitis. Clues to this are sinus symptoms lasting longer than 10 days, fever lasting longer than 3 days, and worsening pain. Bacterial sinusitis may need antibiotic treatment.
9. **Call Back If:**
   - Severe pain persists longer than 2 hours after pain medicine.
   - Sinus pain persists longer than 1 day after starting treatment using nasal washes.
   - Sinus congestion (fullness) persists longer than 10 days.
   - Fever lasts longer than 3 days.
   - You become worse.

Neti Pot for Sinus Symptoms

1. **Neti Pot**
   - The Neti Pot is a small ceramic or plastic pot with a narrow spout. It looks like a small teapot. Two manufacturers of the Neti Pot are the Himalayan Institute in Pennsylvania and SinuCleanse in Wisconsin.
   - **How It Helps:** The Neti Pot performs nasal washing (also called nasal irrigation or "jala neti"). The salt water rinses out excess mucus, washes out any irritants (dust, allergens) that might be present, and moisturizes the nasal cavity.
   - **Indications:** The Neti Pot is widely used as a home remedy to relieve conditions such as colds, sinus infections, and hay fever (nasal allergies).
   - **Adverse Reactions:** None. Though, not everyone likes the sensation of pouring water into their nose.

2. **Neti Pot Step-by-Step Instructions:**
   - **Step 1:** Follow the directions on the salt package to make warm salt walter.
   - **Step 2:** Lean forward and turn your head to one side over the sink. Keep your forehead slightly higher than your chin.
   - **Step 3:** Gently insert the spout of the Neti Pot into the higher nostril. Put it far enough so that it forms a comfortable seal.
   - **Step 4:** Raise the Neti Pot gradually so the salt water flows in through your higher nostril and out of the lower nostril. Breathe through your mouth.
   - **Step 5:** When the Neti Pot is empty, blow your nose to clean out the water and mucus.
   - **Step 6:** Some of the water may run into the back of your throat. Spit this out. If you swallow the salt water it will not hurt you.
   - **Step 7:** Refill the Neti Pot and repeat on the other side. Again, exhale vigorously to clear the nasal passages.

   How to Make Saline (Salt Water) Nasal Wash:
   - You can make your own saline nasal wash.
   - Add ½ tsp of table salt to 1 cup (8 oz; 240 mL) of warm water.
   - You should use sterile, distilled, or previously boiled water for nasal irrigation.

BACKGROUND INFORMATION

Causes of Sinus Pain and Congestion

- Sinus opening(s) becomes blocked by an infection or nasal allergy.
- **Viral Sinusitis:** Sinusitis can occur as part of a viral upper respiratory infection (e.g., rhinosinusitis or the "common cold"). The viral infection and inflammation of the lining of the nose can also affect the lining of all the paranasal sinuses.
- **Bacterial Sinusitis:** Approximately 1-2% of viral sinusitis cases progress to become bacterial sinusitis; one or more of the sinuses affected with viral sinusitis becomes secondarily infected with bacteria. Distinguishing symptoms are symptoms lasting longer than 10 days, increasing sinus pain, and the return of fever.
- **Allergic Sinusitis:** When an allergen (e.g., pollen) activates the lining of the nose (allergic rhinitis), sinus congestion may occur due to swelling of the sinus passage openings (ostia). Symptoms suggesting an allergic etiology include sneezing, itchy nose, clear nasal discharge, and itchy watery eyes.
- **Rhinitis Medicamentosa:** Prolonged continuous use (> 5 days) of decongestant nose drops can lead to "rebound' congestion where the nose becomes even more stuffy.

Treatment of Sinusitis

- **Viral Sinusitis:** Saline nasal washes. Antibiotics are not helpful.
- **Bacterial Sinusitis:** Saline nasal washes. Oral antibiotics may be needed.
- **Allergic Sinusitis (Hay Fever):** Oral antihistamines can relieve mild to moderate symptoms. Examples include diphenhydramine (Benadryl), loratadine (Claritin, Alavert), fexofenadine (Allegra), and cetirizine (Zyrtec). Nasal corticosteroid sprays are probably the most effective treatment for allergic rhinitis. Saline nasal washes are also helpful.

Site of Pain and Sinus Involved

- Ethmoid sinusitis causes pain between or behind the eyes.
- Maxillary sinusitis causes pain in the area of the zygomatic arch, cheek, or upper teeth.
- Frontal sinusitis causes pain above the eyebrow or frontal headaches.

Color of Nasal Discharge With Colds

- The nasal discharge normally changes color during different stages of a cold.
- It starts as a clear discharge and later becomes cloudy.
- Sometimes it becomes yellow or green colored for a few days, and this is still normal.
- Intermittent yellow or green discharge is more common with sleep, antihistamines, or low humidity (Reason: all of these events reduce the production of normal nasal secretions).
- Yellow or green nasal secretions suggest the presence of a bacterial sinusitis ONLY if they occur in combination with [1] sinus pain OR [2] drainage persists > 10 days without improvement.
- Nasal secretions only need treatment with nasal washes when they block the nose and interfere with breathing through the nose. During a cold, if nasal

breathing is noisy but the caller can't see blockage in the nose, it usually means the dried mucus is farther back. Nasal washes can remove it.

Nasal Washes (Nasal Irrigation) for Sinus Symptoms

- **Introduction:** Saline (salt water) nasal irrigation is an effective and simple home remedy for treating cold symptoms and other conditions involving the nasal and sinus passages. Nasal irrigation consists of pouring, spraying, or squirting salt water into the nose and then letting it run back out.
- **How It Helps:** The salt water rinses out excess mucus, washes out any irritants (dust, allergens) that might be present, and moisturizes the nasal cavity.
- **Indications:** Nasal irrigation appears to be an effective treatment for chronic sinusitis. It may also help reduce sinus symptoms from acute viral upper respiratory infection (colds), irritant rhinitis (e.g., dust from the workplace), and allergic rhinitis (hay fever). Some doctors recommend it for rhinitis of pregnancy.
- **Adverse Reactions:** Nasal irrigation is safe and there are no serious adverse effects. However, not everyone likes the sensation of having water in their nose.
- **Methods:** There are several ways to perform nasal irrigation. None has been proven to be better than any other. Methods include use of a nasal spray bottle (available OTC), a rubber ear syringe, a Waterpik set on low, a 5- to 20-cc medical syringe without the needle, or a Neti Pot.
- **How to Make Salt Water for Nasal Irrigation:** Add ½ teaspoon of table salt to 1 cup (8 oz; 240 mL) of warm water.

Neti Pot for Sinus Symptoms

- The Neti Pot is a small ceramic or plastic pot with a narrow spout. It looks like a small teapot. Two manufacturers of the Neti Pot are the Himalayan Institute in Pennsylvania and SinuCleanse in Wisconsin.
- **How It Helps:** The Neti Pot performs nasal washing (also called nasal irrigation or "jala neti"). The salt water rinses out excess mucus, washes out any irritants (dust, allergens) that might be present, and moisturizes the nasal cavity.
- **Indications:** The Neti Pot is widely used as a home remedy to relieve conditions such as colds, sinus infections, and hay fever (nasal allergies).
- **Adverse Reactions:** None. Nasal irrigation with a Neti Pot is safe and there are no serious adverse effects. However, not everyone likes the sensation of having salt water poured into their nose.

Neti Pot and Primary Amebic Meningoencephalitis (PAM)

- Primary amebic meningoencephalitis (PAM) is caused by *Naegleria fowleri,* the so-called "brain-eating ameba." This is an extremely rare infection. There were 32 cases in the United States between 2001 and 2010.
- The majority of the cases of PAM have occurred in the southern United States and were linked to swimming or bathing in freshwater lakes, rivers, and ponds containing this ameba. The ameba can also be found in hot springs, geothermal water sources, and poorly maintained swimming pools.
- In 2011 there were 2 cases of PAM in Louisiana that occurred after nasal irrigation with a Neti Pot. These 2 cases suggest—but are not definite proof—that the nasal irrigation fluid that the individuals used was somehow contaminated with the *Naegleria fowleri* ameba.
- The Centers for Disease Control and Prevention (CDC) recommends that individuals should use distilled, sterile, or previously boiled water for nasal irrigation. It's also important to rinse the irrigation device after each use and leave open to air-dry.

Nasal Decongestants

Use only if the sinus is still blocked after nasal washes.

- **Caution:** These medications should not be taken by individuals with high blood pressure, heart disease, or prostate enlargement. These medications should not be used for more than 3 days (Reason: rebound nasal congestion).
- **Caution:** The individual may currently be taking a decongestant medication and not know it or not have told the triager.
- Commonly used decongestants include Allegra-D, Benadryl Allergy and Congestion, Claritin-D, Dimetapp, Duratuss, Entex, ephedrine, pseuo-ephedrine, Rondec, Semprex-D, Sudafed, Triaminic, and many others.

SKIN, FOREIGN BODY

DEFINITION

- Patient reports a foreign body (e.g., splinter, fishhook, sliver of glass) embedded in the skin.

Symptoms of a Foreign Body in the Skin Include:

- **Pain:** Most tiny slivers (e.g., cactus spine, stinging nettles, fiberglass spicules) are in the superficial skin and do not cause much pain. Deeper or perpendicular foreign bodies are usually painful to pressure.
- **Foreign Body Sensation:** Often adult patients may report the sensation of something being in the skin ("I feel something there").

TRIAGE ASSESSMENT QUESTIONS

Call EMS 911 Now

● Sounds like a life-threatening emergency to the triager

See More Appropriate Protocol

● Puncture wound (and no current foreign body)
Go to Protocol: Puncture Wound on page 206

Go to ED Now (or to Office With PCP Approval)

● Severe pain
Reason: home attempts to remove may push it in deeper

● Deeply embedded FB (e.g., needle or toothpick in foot)
Reason: home attempts to remove may push it in deeper

● FB has a barb (e.g., fishhook)
Reason: need special technique to remove

● FB is a BB
Reason: needs incision to remove

● Dirt (debris) can be seen in the wound, not removed with 15-minute scrubbing
Reason: additional scrubbing in the ED or office may be needed

● Sounds like a serious injury to the triager

Go to Office Now

● FB is clear (glass or plastic)
Reason: difficult to see for removal

● Caller cannot remove FB

● Caller reluctant to take out FB

● Wound looks infected (e.g., spreading redness, red streak, pus)
R/O: cellulitis, lymphangitis

See Today in Office

● Deep puncture wound and no tetanus booster in > 5 years

● Patient wants to be seen

See Today or Tomorrow in Office

● Minor sliver, splinter, or thorn (removable) and patient has diabetes mellitus
Reason: diabetic neuropathy and decreased resistance to infection
Note: more urgent evaluation is needed if the foreign body is not removable.

Home Care

○ Minor sliver, splinter, or thorn that needs removal
Reason: patient should be able to remove this FB at home

○ Tiny plant stickers (e.g., cactus spines, stinging nettles) or fiberglass spicules that need removal
Reason: patient should be able to remove this FB at home

○ Tiny superficial pain-free slivers
Reason: do not need removal

HOME CARE ADVICE FOR MINOR SKIN FOREIGN BODIES

Removing Slivers, Splinters, and Thorns

1. **Needle and Tweezers:**
   - You can remove slivers, splinters, or thorns with a needle and tweezers.
   - Check the tweezers beforehand to be certain the ends (pickups) meet exactly (if they do not, bend them).
   - Sterilize the tools with rubbing alcohol or a flame.

- Clean the skin surrounding the sliver briefly with rubbing alcohol before trying to remove it. Be careful not to push the splinter in deeper. If you don't have rubbing alcohol, use soap and water, but don't soak the area if FB is wood (Reason: can cause swelling of the splinter).

2. **Step-by-Step Instuctions:**
   - **Step 1:** Use the needle to completely expose the end of the sliver. Use good lighting. A magnifying glass may help.
   - **Step 2:** Then grasp the end firmly with the tweezers and pull it out at the same angle that it went in. Getting a good grip the first time is especially important with slivers that go in perpendicular to the skin or those trapped under the fingernail.
3. **Additional Instructions:**
   - For slivers under a fingernail, sometimes a wedge of the nail must be cut away with fine scissors to expose the end of the sliver.
   - Superficial horizontal slivers (where you can see all of it) usually can be removed by pulling on the end. If the end breaks off, open the skin with a sterile needle along the length of the sliver and flick it out.
4. **Antibiotic Ointment:** Apply an antibiotic ointment (OTC) to the area once after removal to reduce the risk of infection.
5. **Tetanus Booster:**
   - If your last tetanus shot was given over 10 years ago, you need a booster.
   - You should try to get this booster shot within the next couple days.
6. **Call Back If:**
   - Can't get it all out.
   - Removed it, but pain becomes worse.
   - Starts to look infected.
   - You become worse.

Removing Tiny Plant Stickers (e.g., Cactus Spines, Stinging Nettles) or Fiberglass Spicules

1. **Tiny Plant Stickers:** Plant stickers (e.g., stinging nettles), cactus spines, or fiberglass spicules are difficult to remove. Usually they break when pressure is applied with tweezers.
2. **Tape:** First try to remove the small spines or spicules by touching the area lightly with packaging tape or another very sticky tape.
3. **Wax Hair Remover (If Tape Does Not Work):**
   - Warm up the wax in your microwave for 10 seconds and apply a layer over the spicules (or fiberglass). Cover it with the cloth strip that came in the hair remover package. Let it air-dry for 5 minutes or accelerate the process with a hair dryer. Then peel it off with the spicules. Most will be removed. The others will usually work themselves out with normal shedding of the skin.
   - You can also try all-purpose white glue, but it's far less effective.
4. **Tetanus Booster:**
   - If your last tetanus shot was given over 10 years ago, you need a booster.
   - You should try to get this booster shot within the next couple days.
5. **Call Back If:**
   - Can't get it all out and it's painful.
   - Starts to look infected.
   - You become worse.

Tiny Superficial Pain-Free Slivers

1. **Tiny, Pain-Free Slivers:** If superficial slivers are numerous, tiny, and pain-free, they can be left in. Eventually they will work their way out with normal shedding of the skin or the body will reject them by forming a tiny little pimple.
2. **Tetanus Booster:**
   - If your last tetanus shot was given over 10 years ago, you need a booster.
   - You should try to get this booster shot within the next couple days.
3. **Call Back If:**
   - Starts to look infected.
   - You become worse.

BACKGROUND INFORMATION

Types of Foreign Bodies

- Fiberglass spicules
- **Fishhooks:** May have a barbed point that make removal difficult
- Glass
- **Metallic Foreign Bodies:** Bullets, BBs, nails, sewing needles, pins, tacs
- Pencil lead-graphite
- Plastic
- **Wood-Organic:** Splinters, cactus spines, thorns, toothpicks
- Other

Pencil Punctures

- There's no danger of lead poisoning. Pencil leads are made of graphite and clay, not lead.
- Sometimes the graphite dust can leave a tiny black stain (tattoo) in the puncture wound.

Diagnosis—Foreign Bodies With X-ray Films

- **Metal:** X-ray films are helpful in localization of metallic foreign bodies. Even tiny pieces of metal will usually show up on x-rays.
- **Glass:** Glass is radiopaque (meaning visible on x-ray) and so x-ray films can be helpful. However, tiny pieces of glass (< 2 mm) cannot usually be seen on x-ray.
- **Wood-Organic:** Organic materials like wood are radiolucent and usually do not show up on x-ray.

Treatment—Need for Removal

- Most small superficially located skin foreign bodies can be removed at home. Examples include splinters, cactus spines, fiberglass spicules, and pieces of glass.
- A general principle is that if an FB needs to be removed in a medical setting, it's better for the patient to get seen sooner, before the FB becomes hidden by swelling or pushed in more deeply by the patient.
- **BBs:** BBs from an air gun usually lodge superficially and generally need to be removed by making a tiny incision (with local anesthesia).
- **Bullets:** Of course anyone with an acute bullet wound needs to be evaluated on an emergency basis! Interestingly though, most bullets and bullet fragments are not removed unless they are interfering with bodily function or causing ongoing pain.
- **Glass and Metal FBs:** Glass and metal are inert, which means that they do not react with human tissue and generally do not become infected. If the FB is causing pain it will need to be removed. Sometimes a tiny (< 2 mm) painless glass or metal FB is not removed by the treating physician because removal would cause more problems than leaving the FB where it is.
- **Wood-Organic:** Organic FBs like wood splinters or thorns can cause infection if they are not removed.

SKIN LESION (MOLES OR GROWTHS)

DEFINITION

- Small bump, lump, spot, growth, or pigmented area of skin
- Moles, skin tags, warts included
- Questions about skin cancer included

TRIAGE ASSESSMENT QUESTIONS

Go to ED Now (or to Office With PCP Approval)

- Patient sounds very sick or weak to the triager

Go to Office Now

- Fever and bump is tender to touch
  R/O: abscess

See Today in Office

- Looks infected (e.g., spreading redness, pus, red streak)
  R/O: cellulitis, lymphangitis
- Looks like a boil, infected sore, or deep ulcer
  R/O: abscess, boil/furuncle, impetigo, ulcer

See Today or Tomorrow in Office

- Caller cannot describe it clearly

See Within 3 Days in Office

- Patient wants to be seen

See Within 2 Weeks in Office

- Skin growth or mole and 2 sides do not look the same (it is asymmetric)
  R/O: skin cancer
- Skin growth or mole and border is irregular or blurry
  R/O: skin cancer
- Skin growth or mole and changes color or it has more than one color
  R/O: skin cancer
- Skin growth or mole and it is larger than a pencil eraser or increasing in size
  R/O: skin cancer
- Skin growth or mole and bleeds
  R/O: skin cancer
- Sticks up out of the skin (elevated), and feels rough to the touch
  R/O: skin cancer, wart, skin tag, seborrheic keratosis
- Flat waxy-yellow patch near eyelids
  R/O: xanthelasma
- Scar that is growing larger
  R/O: keloid
- Caller is uncertain what it is
  Reason: obtain diagnosis

Home Care

- Freckles
- Small growth or mole that is unchanged in size or appearance

HOME CARE ADVICE FOR SKIN LESION (MOLES OR GROWTHS)

1. **Freckles:**
   - Tend to be inherited and are more common in individuals with fair skin.
   - Increase with sun exposure.
2. **Monthly Skin Self-Examination:**
   - Some doctors recommend that you perform a skin self-examination once a month.
   - Stand in front of a mirror. Examine every inch of your skin for new moles or changes in old ones.
3. **Skin Health:**
   - Avoid sun exposure. Use sunscreen or wear protective clothing: long-sleeve shirts.
   - Stay in the shade during the middle of the day. Wear a wide-brimmed hat to keep the sun off your face and neck.
   - Do not go to tanning salons. Tanning booths also cause skin damage.
4. **Call Back If:**
   - Fever or pain occurs.
   - Any change in the mole or growth.
   - You become worse.

BACKGROUND INFORMATION

Causes

- Abscess, boils (furuncles or carbuncles)
- Birthmarks
- Freckles
- Keloid
- Lipoma
- Moles
- Sebaceous cysts
- Seborrheic keratosis
- **Skin Cancer:** Malignant melanoma, basal cell, squamous cell
- Skin tags
- Warts
- Xanthelasma

Is It a Mole or Could It Be Melanoma? The Following Are Signs of Possible Malignant Melanoma (Skin Cancer):

- **A—Symmetry:** The shape of the mole is not round and 2 sides of a mole do not look the same.
- **B—Border:** The borders of the mole are irregular, blurry, or look like they are "leaking" pigment into the adjacent skin.
- **C—Color:** A mole which changes color or contains more than one color.
- **D—Diameter:** Size larger than a pencil eraser (> 6 mm or > 0.25 inches).
- **E—Elevation:** Moles that are rough and are raised above the skin surface.

Other Possible Signs of Skin Cancer:

- A new skin growth or mole
- A skin growth or mole that bleeds or feels irritated
- An enlarging skin lesion in sun-damaged areas of skin—possible basal cell cancer or squamous cell cancer

SORE THROAT

DEFINITION

- Pain, discomfort, or raw feeling of the throat, especially when swallowing

Pain Severity Is Defined As:

- **Mild (1-3):** Doesn't interfere with eating or normal activities
- **Moderate (4-7):** Interferes with eating some solids and normal activities
- **Severe (8-10):** Excruciating pain, interferes with most normal activities
- **Severe Dysphagia:** Can't swallow liquids, drooling

TRIAGE ASSESSMENT QUESTIONS

Call EMS 911 Now

- ● Severe difficulty breathing (e.g., struggling for each breath, speaks in single words)
  R/O: airway obstruction
- ● Sounds like a life-threatening emergency to the triager

See More Appropriate Protocol

- ● Productive cough is main symptom
  Go to Protocol: Cough on page 66
- ● Runny nose is main symptom
  Go to Protocol: Colds on page 53

Go to ED Now (or to Office With PCP Approval)

- ● Drooling or spitting out saliva (because can't swallow)
  R/O: epiglottitis
- ● Unable to open mouth completely
  R/O: peritonsillar abscess
- ● Drinking very little and has signs of dehydration (e.g., no urine > 12 hours, very dry mouth, very light-headed)
- ● Patient sounds very sick or weak to the triager

Go to Office Now

- ● Difficulty breathing (per caller) but not severe
  R/O: swollen tonsils that are touching
- ● Fever > 104° F (40.0° C)
- ● Refuses to drink anything for > 12 hours
  R/O: tonsillitis, abscess

See Today in Office

- SEVERE sore throat pain
  R/O: strep pharyngitis
- Pus on tonsils (back of throat) and swollen neck lymph nodes ("glands")
  R/O: strep pharyngitis
- Earache also present
  R/O: peritonsillar abscess, tonsillitis
- Widespread rash (especially chest and abdomen)
  R/O: scarlet fever
- Diabetes mellitus or immunocompromised (e.g., HIV positive, cancer chemotherapy, splenectomy, organ transplant)
  R/O: candidal pharyngitis
- History of rheumatic fever
- Patient wants to be seen

See Today or Tomorrow in Office

- Fever present > 3 days (72 hours)

Strep Test Only Visit Today or Tomorrow

- Patient requesting a strep throat test
  R/O: strep pharyngitis
- Strep exposure within last 10 days
- Sore throat is the main symptom and persists > 48 hours
- Sore throat with cough/cold symptoms present > 5 days

Home Care

- ○ Sore throat
  Reason: probably viral pharyngitis

HOME CARE ADVICE FOR MILD SORE THROAT

1. **For Relief of Sore Throat Pain:**
   - Sip warm chicken broth or apple juice.
   - Suck on hard candy or a throat lozenge (over-the-counter).
   - Gargle warm salt water 3 times daily (1 teaspoon of salt in 8 oz or 240 mL of warm water).
   - Avoid cigarette smoke.

2. **Pain Medicines:**
   - For pain relief, take acetaminophen, ibuprofen, or naproxen.

   Acetaminophen (e.g., Tylenol):
   - Take 650 mg by mouth every 4-6 hours as needed. Each Regular Strength Tylenol pill has 325 mg of acetaminophen. The most you should take each day is 3,250 mg (10 pills a day).
   - Another choice is to take 1,000 mg every 8 hours. Each Extra Strength Tylenol pill has 500 mg of acetaminophen. The most you should take each day is 3,000 mg (6 pills a day).

   Ibuprofen (e.g., Motrin, Advil):
   - Take 400 mg by mouth every 6 hours.
   - Another choice is to take 600 mg by mouth every 8 hours.

   Naproxen (e .g., Aleve):
   - Take 250-500 mg by mouth every 12 hours.

   Extra Notes:
   - Acetaminophen is thought to be safer than ibuprofen or naproxen in people over 65 years old. Acetaminophen is in many OTC and prescription medicines. It might be in more than one medicine that you are taking. You need to be careful and not take an overdose. An acetaminophen overdose can hurt the liver.
   - **Caution:** Do not take acetaminophen if you have liver disease.
   - **Caution:** Do not take ibuprofen if you have stomach problems, kidney disease, are pregnant, or have been told by your doctor to avoid this type of anti-inflammatory drug. Do not take ibuprofen for more than 7 days without consulting your doctor.
   - Use the lowest amount of medicine that makes your pain feel better.
   - Before taking any medicine, read all the instructions on the package
3. **Fever Medicines:**
   - For fevers above 101° F (38.3° C) take acetaminophen or ibuprofen.
   - The goal of fever therapy is to bring the fever down to a comfortable level. Remember that fever medicine usually lowers fever 2 degrees F (1 - 1½ degrees C).

   Acetaminophen (e.g., Tylenol):
   - Take 650 mg by mouth every 4-6 hours. Each Regular Strength Tylenol pill has 325 mg of acetaminophen.
   - Another choice is to take 1,000 mg every 8 hours. Each Extra Strength Tylenol pill has 500 mg of acetaminophen.
   - The most you should take each day is 3,000 mg.

   Ibuprofen (e.g., Motrin, Advil):
   - Take 400 mg by mouth every 6 hours.
   - Another choice is to take 600 mg by mouth every 8 hours.
   - Use the lowest amount that makes your pain feel better.

   Extra Notes:
   - Acetaminophen is thought to be safer than ibuprofen in people over 65 years old. Acetaminophen is in many OTC and prescription medicines. It might be in more than one medicine that you are taking. You need to be careful and not take an overdose. An acetaminophen overdose can hurt the liver.
   - **Caution:** Do not take acetaminophen if you have liver disease.
   - **Caution:** Do not take ibuprofen if you have stomach problems, kidney disease, are pregnant, or have been told by your doctor to avoid this type of anti-inflammatory drug. Do not take ibuprofen for more than 7 days without consulting your doctor.
   - Before taking any medicine, read all the instructions on the package.
4. **Soft Diet:** Cold drinks and milk shakes are especially good (Reason: swollen tonsils can make some foods hard to swallow).
5. **Liquids:** Adequate liquid intake is important to prevent dehydration. Drink 6-8 glasses of water per day.
6. **Contagiousness:** You can return to work or school after the fever is gone and you feel well enough to participate in normal activities. If your doctor determines that you have strep throat, then you will need to take an antibiotic for 24 hours before you can return.
7. **Expected Course:** Sore throats with viral illnesses usually last 3 or 4 days.

8. Call Back If:
- Sore throat is the main symptom and it lasts longer than 24 hours.
- Sore throat is mild but lasts longer than 4 days.
- Fever lasts longer than 3 days.
- You become worse.

BACKGROUND INFORMATION

General Information
- Sore throat is one of the most common reasons patients go to the doctor's office.
- The medical term for a throat infection is pharyngitis or tonsillopharyngitis.

Causes of Sore Throat
- **Colds:** Most sore throats are from a cold or other viral infection. The presence of a cough, hoarseness, or nasal symptoms points to a cold or viral infection as the cause of the sore throat.
- **Strep Throat:** In adults, approximately 10-20% of sore throats are caused by the *Streptococcus* (strep) bacteria. Streptococcal pharyngitis is the only commonly occurring bacteria for which antibiotic therapy is definitely indicated.
- **Mono:** Infectious mononucleosis is primarily seen in young adults, causing 5-10% of the sore throats in that population. It should be suspected in young adults with fever, sore throat, swollen lymph nodes, and a negative strep throat culture. A blood test called a monospot can help make the diagnosis. There is no antibiotic treatment.
- **Other Common Causes:** Include dry air, smoking, postnasal drip, and yelling. Sexually transmitted diseases (e.g., gonorrhea) can also cause pharyngitis.

Empiric Therapy for Presumed Strep Pharyngitis
- Some physicians are willing to initiate antibiotic therapy for presumed strep pharyngitis over the telephone. Remember, most sore throats are not caused by strep.
- **Should Be Present:** [1] Pus on tonsils (back of throat) AND [2] fever > 101° F (38.3° C) AND [3] swollen neck lymph nodes ("glands").
- **Should Be Absent (or Minimal):** Cough, runny nose, hoarseness.
- **Typical Antibiotic Prescription:** Penicillin (PCN VK 500 mg PO BID for 10 days). If allergic to penicillin, erythromycin (e.g., erythromycin base 500 mg PO QID for 10 days) can be used. The dosage of erythromycin depends on the type prescribed.

What Patients Really Want: Pain Relief
A study was performed with 298 patients (adolescents and adults) who saw their PCP for chief complaint of "sore throat." They were asked to rank the importance of 13 reasons for visiting their PCP. Here are the pertinent results:
- #1 reason was to establish the cause of the sore throat (Note: pharyngitis as part of a cold can usually be determined by telephone).
- #2 was pain relief (Note: can absolutely be provided by telephone).
- #3 was information on the expected course of the illness (Note: can usually be provided by telephone).
- **Surprise:** Hopes for an antibiotic was #11.
- **Summary:** If we meet the caller's request for pain relief, we may be able to prevent unnecessary ED and office visits.
- Reference: *Ann Fam Med.* 2006;4(6):494–499.

SPIDER BITE

DEFINITION

- Bite from a spider seen on the skin
- Onset of spider bite symptoms (redness, pain, swelling) and a spider is seen in close proximity

TRIAGE ASSESSMENT QUESTIONS

Call EMS 911 Now

- Difficulty breathing or swallowing
  R/O: anaphylactic shock
- Difficult to awaken or acting confused (e.g., disoriented, slurred speech)
  R/O: anaphylactic shock
- Pale cold skin and very weak (e.g., can't stand)
  R/O: shock
- Sounds like a life-threatening emergency to the triager

See More Appropriate Protocol

- Not a spider bite
  Go to Protocol: Insect Bite on page 166

Go to ED Now

- Black widow (or brown widow) spider bite and local skin changes
- Abdominal pain, chest tightness, or other muscle cramps
  R/O: black or brown widow spider
- Urine is brown, black, or red in color
  R/O: brown recluse spider bite with hemolysis
- Vomiting
  R/O: systemic venom reaction

Go to ED Now (or to Office With PCP Approval)

- Patient sounds very sick or weak to the triager

Go to Office Now

- SEVERE bite pain and not improved after 2 hours of pain medicine
- Rash elsewhere on body that developed after spider bite
  R/O: hives, systemic venom reaction
- Fever and area is red
  R/O: cellulitis, lymphangitis
  Reason: fever and looks infected
- Fever and area is very tender to touch
  R/O: cellulitis, CA-MRSA, abscess
  Reason: fever and looks infected
- Red streak or red line and length > 2 inches (5 cm)
  R/O: lymphangitis
  Note: lymphangitis looks like a red streak or line originating at the wound and ascending up the arm or leg toward the heart.

See Today in Office

- Red or very tender (to touch) area, and started over 24 hours after the bite
  R/O: cellulitis
- Red or very tender (to touch) area, getting larger over 48 hours after the bite
  R/O: cellulitis
- Eye irritation after handling or touching a tarantula
  R/O: foreign body (hairs) keratoconjunctivitis or ophthalmia nodosa
- Patient wants to be seen

See Today or Tomorrow in Office

- Diabetic with spider bite wound on foot
  Reason: diabetic neuropathy and decreased resistance to infection

See Within 3 Days in Office

- Scab drains pus or increases in size, and not improved after applying antibiotic ointment for 2 days
  R/O: infected sore, impetigo
- Bite starts to look bad (e.g., blister, purplish skin, ulcer)
  R/O: necrotic spider bite (brown recluse, hobo spider) or other cause of skin lesion

Home Care

- Nonserious spider bite
- Scab drains pus or increases in size
  R/O: infected sore, impetigo
- Prevention of spider bites, questions about

HOME CARE ADVICE

Nonserious Spider Bite

1. **Cleaning:** Wash the bite thoroughly with antibacterial soap and warm water.
2. **Pain Medicines:**
   - For pain relief, take acetaminophen, ibuprofen, or naproxen.

   Acetaminophen (e.g., Tylenol):
   - Take 650 mg by mouth every 4-6 hours as needed. Each Regular Strength Tylenol pill has 325 mg of acetaminophen. The most you should take each day is 3,250 mg (10 pills a day).
   - Another choice is to take 1,000 mg every 8 hours. Each Extra Strength Tylenol pill has 500 mg of acetaminophen. The most you should take each day is 3,000 mg (6 pills a day).

   Ibuprofen (e.g., Motrin, Advil):
   - Take 400 mg by mouth every 6 hours.
   - Another choice is to take 600 mg by mouth every 8 hours.

   Naproxen (e.g., Aleve):
   - Take 250-500 mg by mouth every 12 hours.

   Extra Notes:
   - Acetaminophen is thought to be safer than ibuprofen or naproxen in people over 65 years old. Acetaminophen is in many OTC and prescription medicines. It might be in more than one medicine that you are taking. You need to be careful and not take an overdose. An acetaminophen overdose can hurt the liver.
   - **Caution:** Do not take acetaminophen if you have liver disease.
   - **Caution:** Do not take ibuprofen if you have stomach problems, kidney disease, are pregnant, or have been told by your doctor to avoid this type of anti-inflammatory drug. Do not take ibuprofen for more than 7 days without consulting your doctor.
   - Use the lowest amount of medicine that makes your pain feel better.
   - Before taking any medicine, read all the instructions on the package
3. **Expected Course:** Some swelling and pain for 1 to 2 days. It shouldn't be any worse than a bee sting.
4. **Call Back If:**
   - Severe bite pain persists longer than 2 hours after pain medicine.
   - Abdominal pains or muscle spasms occur.
   - Local pain lasts more than 2 days (48 hours).
   - Bite begins to look infected.
   - You become worse.

Infected Sore or Scab

1. **Reassurance:**
   - Sometimes a small infected sore can develop at the site of a cut, scratch, insect bite, or sting.
   - The typical appearance is a sore smaller than 1 inch (2.5 cm) in diameter. It is often covered by a soft, honey-yellow or yellow-brown crust or scab. Sometimes the scab may drain a tiny amount of pus or yellow fluid. Usually there is minimal to no pain.
   - Small infected sores usually get better with regular cleansing and use of an antibiotic ointment.
2. **Cleaning:**
   - Wash the area 2-3 times daily with an antibacterial soap and warm water.
   - Gently remove any scab. The bacteria live underneath the scab. You may need to soak the scab off by placing a warm, wet washcloth (or gauze) on the sore for 10 minutes.
3. **Antbiotic Ointment:**
   - Apply an antibiotic ointment 3 times per day.
   - Cover the sore with a Band-Aid to prevent scratching and spread.
   - Use bacitracin ointment (OTC in United States) or Polysporin ointment (OTC in Canada) or one that you already have.
4. **Avoid Picking:** Avoid scratching and picking. This can worsen and spread a skin infection.
5. **Contagiousness:**
   - Infected sores can be spread by skin-to-skin contact.
   - Wash your hands frequently and avoid touching the sore.
   - **Work and School:** You can attend school or work if it is covered.

- **Contact Sports:** Generally, you need to receive antibiotic treatment for 3 days before you can return to the sport. There can be no pus or drainage. You should check with your trainer, if there is one for your sports team.

6. **Expected Course:**
   - The sore should stop growing in 1 to 2 days and it should begin improving within 2-3 days.
   - The sore should be completely healed in 7-10 days.
7. **Call Back If:**
   - Fever occurs.
   - Spreading redness or a red streak occurs.
   - Sore increases in size.
   - Sore not improving after 2 days using antibiotic ointment.
   - Sore not completely healed in 7 days (1 week).
   - New sore appears.
   - You become worse.

Preventing Spider Bites

1. **Prevention—Outdoors:**
   - Be especially careful around wood piles and when clearing brush.
   - Wear long pants with the pants tucked into your socks.
   - Wear long-sleeved shirts and use gloves.
   - DEET is a very effective insect repellent. It also repels spiders.
2. **Prevention—Indoors:**
   - Remove spiderwebs.
   - Make certain that doorways and windows are effectively sealed and insulated.
3. **Using DEET-Containing Insect Repellents When Outdoors:**
   - DEET is a very effective insect repellent. It also repels spiders.
   - Higher concentrations of DEET do work better—but there appears to be no benefit in using DEET concentrations above 50%. For children and adolescents, the American Academy of Pediatrics recommends a maximum concentration of 30%. Health Canada recommends using a concentration of 5-30% for adults.
   - Apply to exposed areas of skin. Do not apply to eyes, mouth, or irritated areas of skin. Do not apply to skin that is covered by clothing.
   - Remember to wash it off with soap and water when you return indoors.
   - DEET can damage clothing made of synthetic fibers, plastics (e.g., eyeglasses), and leather.
   - Breastfeeding women may use DEET. No problems have been reported (CDC 2003).

FIRST AID

First Aid Advice for Shock:

Lie down with feet elevated.

First Aid Advice for Spider Bite (Localized Symptoms Only):

- Wash bite wound with soap and water.
- Apply a cold pack to the area of the bite for 10-20 minutes.

First Aid Advice for Black Widow Spider Bite:

- Wash bite wound with soap and water.
- Apply a cold pack to the area of the bite for 10-20 minutes.
- If possible, capture the spider and place it in a jar (for spider identification).

First Aid Advice for Brown Recluse Spider Bite:

- Wash bite wound with soap and water.
- Apply a cold pack to the area of the bite for 10-20 minutes.
- If possible, capture the spider and place it in a jar (for spider identification).

BACKGROUND INFORMATION

General

- There are approximately 20,000+ species of spiders in the world.
- In the United States and Canada, there are 2 species which cause bites in humans of medical importance: the black widow *(Latrodectus)* and the brown recluse *(Loxosceles)*.
- Patients sometimes incorrectly believe that they sustained a spider bite, when instead a minor break in the skin instead simply became infected with *Staphylococcus aureus*. An infection with CA-MRSA must be considered as a possible cause of any infected-appearing "spider bite."

Types of Spider Bites

1. **Black Widow Spider Bite**
   - **Description:** A shiny, jet-black spider with long legs (total size 1 inch). A red (or orange) hourglass-shaped marking may be on its underside (not present in all *Latrodectus* species).
   - **Habitat:** Found throughout North America, except Alaska and the far north.
   - **Symptoms—Bite Wound:** The black widow spider produces one of nature's most potent neurotoxic venoms. The bite causes immediate moderate to severe pain; there is usually minimal to no local reaction.
   - **Symptoms—Systemic:** Severe muscle cramps are present by 1 to 6 hours and last 24 to 48 hours. Other possible symptoms include abdominal pain, vomiting, restlessness, hypertension, and weakness.
   - **Treatment—Local Wound Care:** Wash bite with soap and water. Apply an ice pack.
   - **Treatment—Medications:** Tetanus prophylaxis should be provided. Parenteral analgesics may be needed for pain and benzodiazepines for muscle spasms. There is a *Latrodectus* antivenin that is indicated for severe symptoms, seizures, or uncontrolled hypertension.
   - **Expected Course:** All symptoms usually resolve over 2-3 days. Death may occur rarely; a bite is more serious in a small child; multiple spider bites are also more serious.
   - **Special Note:** Many bite wounds are "dry bites" (no venom injected into skin) because the fangs are small.
2. **Brown Widow Spider Bite**
   - The brown widow spider is related to the black widow and is also a member of *Latrodectus (Latrodectus geometricus).*
   - **Habitat:** First appeared in North America in 1980. Has been reported in the southern United States (Florida, Georgia, Louisiana, Texas, California).
   - **Symptoms:** Brown widow spider bites are thought to be less serious than those from black widows.
   - **Treatment:** Same as for black widow spiders.
3. **Brown Recluse Spider Bite**
   - Also known as the "violin" or "fiddleback" spider.
   - **Description:** A brown spider with long legs (total size ½ inch). Dark violin-shaped marking on top of its head (not present in all *Loxosceles* species).
   - **Habitat:** Found in the southern, southwestern, and midwestern United States.
   - **Symptoms—Bite Wound:** The spider produces a venom which causes cell destruction and blood cell breakdown. The bite is initially painless or there is mild stinging discomfort. Localized aching, itching, and blister formation develops in 4 to 8 hours. The center becomes bluish and depressed (craterlike) over 2 to 3 days. A deep necrotic ulcer may develop.
   - **Symptoms—Systemic:** Systemic symptoms include fever, vomiting, and myalgias (but no life-threatening symptoms).
   - **Red, White, and Blue Sign:** These bites have some distinguishing features. They are very painful. The puncture mark left by the spider's fangs is off-center. The bite progresses to 3 concentric red, white, and blue zones. The outer zone is red (erythema). The middle zone is white (ischemia). The inner zone is blue, suggesting impending necrosis. By contrast, the necrotic lesion of cutaneous anthrax is painless and does not have the red, white, and blue sign. (Source: Dr Edwin Masters, Cape Girardeau, Missouri.)
   - **Treatment—Local Wound Care:** Cleansing of wound with soap and water, cold pack.
   - **Treatment—Medications:** Tetanus prophylaxis should be provided.
   - **Expected Course:** Most necrotic ulcers heal over 1 to 8 weeks. Permanent scarring occurs in 10-15%. Skin damage sometimes requires skin grafting.

4. **Tarantulas**
   - **Habitat:** Tarantulas are found in the southern United States (e.g., desert southwest).
   - **Symptoms—Bite Wound:** Mild stinging with minimal local inflammation. No skin necrosis occurs.
   - **Symptoms—Eye:** Some genera of tarantula have urticating hairs that can come off. Like a little piece of fiberglass, they can penetrate human skin and cause itching and redness. If they lodge in the cornea they can cause foreign body keratoconjunctivitis or ophthalmia nodosa.
   - **Symptoms—Systemic:** None.
   - **Treatment—Local Wound Care:** Cleansing of bite wound with soap and water, cold pack, oral analgesics. Obtaining a tetanus booster is appropriate if it has been longer than 10 years.
   - **Treatment—Eye Irritation:** Individuals with eye irritation or redness after handling a tarantula should be referred to an ophthalmologist for a slit-lamp examination of the eye,
   - **Expected Course:** Bite wounds heal completely. Eye problems generally resolve under the close follow-up care of an ophthalmologist.
5. **Minor (Non-Dangerous) Spider Bites:**
   - More than 50 spiders in the United States and Canada have venom and can cause minor, localized, nonserious reactions. Many single, unseen, and unexplained painful bites that occur during the night can be due to spiders.
   - **Symptoms—Bite Wound:** The bites are painful and mildly swollen for 1 or 2 days (much like a bee sting).
   - **Symptoms—Systemic:** None.
   - **Treatment—Local Wound Care:** Cleansing of bite wound with soap and water, cold pack, oral analgesics. Obtaining a tetanus booster is appropriate if it has been longer than 10 years.
   - **Expected Course:** Bite wounds heal completely.

Brown Recluse Spider Vs Anthrax

- **Brown Recluse Spider and the Red, White, and Blue Sign:** Brown recluse bites have some distinguishing features. Initially there may be mild stinging pain or no discomfort. The puncture mark left by the spider's fangs is off-center. The bite progresses to 3 concentric red, white, and blue zones. The outer zone is red (erythema). The middle zone is white (ischemia). The inner zone is blue, suggesting impending necrosis.
- **Anthrax:** By contrast, the necrotic lesion of cutaneous anthrax is painless and does not have the red, white, and blue sign.
- **Source:** Dr Edwin Masters, Cape Girardeau, Missouri.

Community Acquired Methicillin-Resistant Staphylococcus aureus *(CA-MRSA)*

- *Staphylococcus aureus* is a bacteria that can cause a variety of skin infections including pimples, boils, abscesses, cellulitis, wound infections, and impetigo. It can also cause more serious infections like staphylococcal pneumonia, sepsis, and toxic shock syndrome.
- In the 1960s strains of *S aureus* that were resistant to penicillin-type antibiotics started appearing in hospitals and health care settings. These were referred to as methicillin-resistant *S aureus* (MRSA) infections.
- More recently, strains of penicillin-resistant *S aureus* have increasingly become the cause of skin infections in healthy individuals in the community. These are now being referred to as community acquired methicillin-resistant *S aureus* (CA-MRSA) infections. There have been outbreaks in athletes (e.g., wrestling teams) and in prison populations.
- CA-MRSA requires treatment with specific types of antibiotics.
- More information about CA-MRSA is available at www.cdc.gov/mrsa/index.html.

STD EXPOSURE AND PREVENTION

DEFINITION

- Seeking information about how to prevent sexually transmitted diseases (STD)

TRIAGE ASSESSMENT QUESTIONS

See More Appropriate Protocol

- Rash or sores on penis or scrotum
  Go to Protocol: Penis and Scrotum Symptoms on page 196
- Rash or sores on female genital area (vulvar area)
  Go to Protocol: Vulvar Symptoms on page 338

Go to ED Now

- Forced to have sex (sexual assault or rape) in the past 3 days

Go to ED Now (or to Office With PCP Approval)

- Sexual intercourse (in the past 72 hours) with someone who was diagnosed with HIV
- Female and ANY of the following:
  - Fever and burning (pain) with urination
  - Constant lower abdominal pain lasting more than 2 hours
  - Unable to urinate for more than 4 hours, and bladder feels very full
- Male and ANY of the following:
  - Fever and burning (pain) with urination
  - Fever and testicle pain or swelling
  - Unable to urinate for more than 4 hours, and bladder feels very full

See Today in Office

- Forced to have sex (sexual assault or rape) > 3 days ago
- Female and ANY of the following:
  - Burning (pain) with urination
  - Unexplained lower abdominal pain
  - Abnormal color of vaginal discharge (i.e., yellow, green, gray)
  - Bad-smelling vaginal discharge
- Male with ANY of the following:
  - Burning (pain) with urination
  - Pus (white, yellow) or bloody discharge from end of penis
  - Testicle pain or swelling
- Rectal discharge or unusual rectal pain or itching
- Patient wants to be seen

See Within 3 Days in Office

- Patient is worried about a sexually transmitted disease (STD)
  Reason: relieve fear and prevent spread of STD
- Sexual intercourse (oral, vaginal, or anal) with someone who was diagnosed with a sexually transmitted disease (STD)
  Reason: will need to be tested and treated

Home Care

- Questions about preventing STDs

HOME CARE ADVICE ABOUT STD PREVENTION

1. **General Condom Information:**
   - LATEX CONDOMS ARE THE ONLY EFFECTIVE WAY TO PREVENT STDs DURING SEXUAL INTERCOURSE.
   - You can also use condoms during oral sex.
2. **Obtaining a Condom:**
   - Buy latex rubber condoms. Persons who are allergic to latex can use a polyurethane (plastic) condom. Never use condoms made from animal skins; they can leak.
   - You can get condoms at public health clinics (often free), drugstores, supermarkets, and via the Internet. You do not need a prescription.
3. **Storing Condoms:**
   - Store condoms at room temperature. Avoid extreme heat, extreme cold, or sunlight.
   - You might want to keep a condom in your wallet or purse; this way it is ready and available.

4. Putting on a Condom—Instructions:
- Hold the condom at the tip to squeeze out the air.
- Roll the condom all the way down the erect penis (do not try to put a condom on a soft penis).
- If you use a lubricant during sex, make sure it is water-based (e.g., K-Y Liquid, Astroglide). Do not use petroleum jelly (Vaseline), vegetable oil (Crisco), or baby oil; these can cause a condom to break.

5. Taking Off a Condom—Instructions:
- After sex, hold onto the condom while the penis is being pulled out.
- The penis should be pulled out while still erect, so that sperm (semen) doesn't leak out of the condom.

6. Female Condoms
- There are female condoms (e.g., Reality) that you can also buy without a prescription.
- A female condom is a polyurethane (plastic) sheath that is placed inside the vagina.

7. STD National Hotline
- The American Social Health Association National STD Hotline provides information on sexually transmitted diseases (STDs), such as chlamydia, gonorrhea, HPV/genital warts, herpes, and HIV/AIDS. Specialists can provide general information, referrals to local clinics, and written materials about STDs and disease prevention.
- Toll-free number (English): (800) 227-8922
- Toll-free number (Spanish): (800) 344-7432
- The Web site is: www.ashastd.org.

8. Pregnancy Test, When in Doubt:
- If there is any possibility of pregnancy, obtain and use a urine pregnancy test from the local drugstore.
- Follow the instructions included in the package.

9. Call Back If:
- Pregnancy test is positive or if you have difficulties with the home pregnancy test.
- You become worse.

BACKGROUND INFORMATION

General Information
- A sexually transmitted disease is an infection that is transmitted through sexual intercourse (vaginal, anal, oral). It is also sometimes referred to as a sexually transmitted infection (STI).
- Examples of STDs include chlamydia, gonorrhea, genital herpes, HIV, pubic lice, and trichomonas.
- Some STDs can be cured with antibiotics (e.g., gonorrhea, chlamydia).
- Some STDs cannot cured, but the symptoms can be reduced (e.g., herpes, HIV) by taking prescription medications.

Transmission
- Most STDs are transmitted by exchange of body fluids (e.g., semen, vaginal secretions, or blood) during oral, anal, or vaginal sex.
- Also can occur following direct contact with any sores/lesions during sex.
- A latex condom acts as barrier and is effective at preventing STDs.

Abstinence and Other "Safe" Sexual Activities
There are only two 100% effective means of avoiding STDs:
- Abstaining from sexual intercourse and from oral sex.
- A truly monogamous (one sexual partner only) and long-standing relationship between 2 uninfected partners.
- Sexual behaviors that are considered safe (and do not usually transmit STDs) include holding hands, hugging, touching, and kissing (as long as there are no sores on the lips or in the mouth).
- Touching semen during mutual masturbation generally is safe.

Behaviors That Do Not Prevent STDs

- Douching the vagina or showering after sex does not prevent STDs.
- Withdrawal (when a man pulls his penis out before he ejaculates) is not a way to prevent STDs or pregnancy.
- Having an STD once does not prevent one from getting it again.
- Using the birth control pill, birth control patch, or DepoProvera shots do not prevent STDs. A condom should be used to protect against STDs.

Internet Resources on Sexually Transmitted Diseases (STD, STI)

- **Australia:** Information on sexually transmitted infection is provided by the Australian government at: www.sti.health.gov.au/internet/sti/publishing.nsf.
- **Canada—Public Health Agency of Canada:** Sexually transmitted infections (STI), sexual health facts, and information for the public at: www.phac-aspc.gc.ca/std-mts/faq_e.html.
- **United States:** American Social Health Association answers to questions about teen sexual health and sexually transmitted diseases are available at: www.iwannaknow.org
- **United States:** Centers for Disease Control and Prevention sexually transmitted diseases treatment guidelines available at: www.cdc.gov/std/treatment/2010 or www.cdc.gov/mmwr/preview/mmwrhtml/rr5912a1.htm.

STREP THROAT TEST (FOLLOW-UP CALL)

DEFINITION

- Strep throat culture or rapid strep test done and results called to triage nurse by the lab, PCP, or adult caller.
- Patient has been previously triaged by triage nurse or examined by PCP.
- In most cases, the triage nurse needs to call the patient.

TRIAGE ASSESSMENT QUESTIONS

See More Appropriate Protocol

- Sore throat symptoms are much worse
  Go to Protocol: Sore Throat on page 241

Go to ED Now (or to Office With PCP Approval)

- Patient sounds very sick or weak to the triager

See Today or Tomorrow in Office

- Patient wants to be seen

Discuss With PCP and Callback by Nurse Today

- Positive throat culture or rapid stress test (according to lab, PCP, caller, etc.) AND NO standing order to call in prescription for antibiotic
  Reason: antibiotic prescription needed

Home Care

- Positive throat culture or rapid strep test (according to lab, PCP, caller, etc.) AND standing order
  Reason: antibiotic prescription needed
- Rapid strep test negative and symptoms not worse
- Strep throat culture negative and symptoms not worse

HOME CARE ADVICE

Positive Rapid Strep Test or Strep Throat Culture

1. **Strep Throat Culture Positive:** Your throat culture was positive: You have strep throat. Strep throat is treated with antibiotics.
2. **Rapid Strep Test Positive:** Your rapid strep test was positive: You have strep throat. Strep throat is treated with antibiotics.
3. **Antibiotic Presciption for Strep Throat:**
   - Penicillin (PCN VK 500 mg PO BID for 10 days).
   - **Penicillin Allergy:** If allergic to penicillin, erythromycin (erythromycin base 500 mg PO QID for 10 days). Erythromycin can cause nausea and vomiting in some people. Another alternative for penicillin allergic patients is Zithromax (a 5-day Z-Pak).
4. **Contagiousness:** After taking antibiotics for 24 hours, the disease is no longer considered contagious and you can return to work or school.
5. **Expected Course:** Antibiotic treatment should make you feel much better within 48 hours.
6. **Call Back If:**
   - Fever lasts more than 2 days on antibiotics.
   - Symptoms last more than 3 days on antibiotics.
   - You become worse.

Negative Rapid Strep Test or Strep Throat Culture

1. **Strep Throat Culture Negative:** Your throat culture was negative, so you don't have strep. Most sore throats are caused by a virus and are just part of a cold.
2. **Rapid Strep Test Negative:** Your rapid strep test was negative. Most sore throats are caused by a virus and are just part of a cold.
3. **No Antibiotics:** Antibiotics are not helpful for viral sore throats.
4. **Expected Course:** Sore throats with viral illnesses usually last 3 or 4 days.
5. **Contagiousness:** You can return to work or school after the fever is gone and you feel well enough to participate in normal activities.
6. **Call Back If:**
   - Fever lasts more than 3 days.
   - You become worse.

General Care Advice for Sore Throat

1. **For Relief of Sore Throat Pain:**
   - Sip warm chicken broth or apple juice.
   - Suck on hard candy or a throat lozenge (over-the-counter).
   - Gargle warm salt water 3 times daily (1 teaspoon of salt in 8 oz or 240 mL of warm water).
   - Avoid cigarette smoke.
2. **Pain Medicines:**
   - For pain relief, take acetaminophen, ibuprofen, or naproxen.

   Acetaminophen (e.g., Tylenol):
   - Take 650 mg by mouth every 4-6 hours as needed. Each Regular Strength Tylenol pill has 325 mg of acetaminophen. The most you should take each day is 3,250 mg (10 pills a day).
   - Another choice is to take 1,000 mg every 8 hours. Each Extra Strength Tylenol pill has 500 mg of acetaminophen. The most you should take each day is 3,000 mg (6 pills a day).

   Ibuprofen (e.g., Motrin, Advil):
   - Take 400 mg by mouth every 6 hours.
   - Another choice is to take 600 mg by mouth every 8 hours.

   Naproxen (e.g., Aleve):
   - Take 250-500 mg by mouth every 12 hours.

   Extra Notes:
   - Acetaminophen is thought to be safer than ibuprofen or naproxen in people over 65 years old. Acetaminophen is in many OTC and prescription medicines. It might be in more than one medicine that you are taking. You need to be careful and not take an overdose. An acetaminophen overdose can hurt the liver.
   - **Caution:** Do not take acetaminophen if you have liver disease.
   - **Caution:** Do not take ibuprofen if you have stomach problems, kidney disease, are pregnant, or have been told by your doctor to avoid this type of anti-inflammatory drug. Do not take ibuprofen for more than 7 days without consulting your doctor.
   - Use the lowest amount of medicine that makes your pain feel better.
   - Before taking any medicine, read all the instructions on the package
3. **Fever Medicines:**
   - For fevers above 101° F (38.3° C) take acetaminophen or ibuprofen.
   - The goal of fever therapy is to bring the fever down to a comfortable level. Remember that fever medicine usually lowers fever 2 degrees F (1 - 1½ degrees C).

   Acetaminophen (e.g., Tylenol):
   - Take 650 mg by mouth every 4-6 hours. Each Regular Strength Tylenol pill has 325 mg of acetaminophen.
   - Another choice is to take 1,000 mg every 8 hours. Each Extra Strength Tylenol pill has 500 mg of acetaminophen.
   - The most you should take each day is 3,000 mg.

   Ibuprofen (e.g., Motrin, Advil):
   - Take 400 mg by mouth every 6 hours.
   - Another choice is to take 600 mg by mouth every 8 hours.
   - Use the lowest amount that makes your pain feel better.

   Extra Notes:
   - Acetaminophen is thought to be safer than ibuprofen in people over 65 years old. Acetaminophen is in many OTC and prescription medicines. It might be in more than one medicine that you are taking. You need to be careful and not take an overdose. An acetaminophen overdose can hurt the liver.
   - **Caution:** Do not take acetaminophen if you have liver disease.
   - **Caution:** Do not take ibuprofen if you have stomach problems, kidney disease, are pregnant, or have been told by your doctor to avoid this type of anti-inflammatory drug. Do not take ibuprofen for more than 7 days without consulting your doctor.
   - Before taking any medicine, read all the instructions on the package.
4. **Soft Diet:** Cold drinks and milk shakes are especially good (Reason: swollen tonsils can make some foods hard to swallow).

5. **Liquids:** Adequate liquid intake is important to prevent dehydration. Drink 6-8 glasses of water per day.
6. **Call Back If:**
   - Fever lasts more than 3 days.
   - You become worse.

BACKGROUND INFORMATION

General

- Sore throat is one of the most common reasons why patients go to the doctor's office.
- The medical term for a throat infection is pharyngitis or tonsillopharyngitis.

Causes of a Sore Throat

- **Colds:** Most sore throats are from a cold or other viral infection.
- **Strep:** In adults, approximately 10-20% of sore throats are caused by the strep bacteria. Streptococcal pharyngitis is the only commonly occurring bacteria for which antibiotic therapy is definitely indicated.
- **Mono:** Infectious mononucleosis is primarily seen in young adults, causing 5-10% of the sore throats in this population. It should be suspected in young adults with fever, sore throat, cervical adenopathy, and a negative strep throat culture. A blood test called a monospot can help make the diagnosis. There is no antibiotic treatment.
- **Other:** Other common causes include dry air, smoking, postnasal drip, allergies, singing, and yelling. Sexually transmitted diseases (e.g., gonorrhea) can also cause pharyngitis.

Streptococcal Pharyngitis (Strep Throat)

- **Cause:** Strep throat is a type of bacterial pharyngitis caused by group A beta-hemolytic *Streptococcus*.
- **Symptoms:** The main symptom is sore throat and pain with swallowing. Other symptoms can include fever, headache, swollen lymph nodes, nausea, and malaise.
- **Physical Examination:** Examination of the throat typically shows redness and exudate (pus) on the tonsils.
- **Diagnosis:** Strep throat culture and/or rapid strep test. In adults the diagnosis is often made by health care providers clinically, without testing.
- **Treatment:** Since this is caused by a bacteria, antibiotic treatment is needed. Penicillin, amoxicillin, and erythromycin are the first-line antibiotics used for treatment of this infection.
- **Complications:** Complications are rare; they include: peritonsillar abscess, acute rheumatic fever, and post-streptococcal glomerulonephritis.

Strep Throat—Return to Work or School:

- Adults can return to work or school after taking antibiotics for 24 hours and the fever is gone.

Strep Throat—Risk of Secondary Cases in the Family

- A recent research study from Australia followed 202 families who had a child with acute strep pharyngitis. A secondary case of strep pharyngitis occurred in 43% of these families.
- **Significance:** Strep pharyngitis is readily transmitted to siblings and even parents.
- **Reference:** Danchin 2007.

SUBSTANCE ABUSE AND DEPENDENCE

DEFINITION

- Caller has questions or concerns about substance abuse (drug abuse).
- Substance abuse is using (huffing, ingesting, injecting, smoking, snorting) any drug or alcohol with the intention of experiencing euphoria or other mind-altering sensations.

TRIAGE ASSESSMENT QUESTIONS

Call EMS 911 Now

- Coma (e.g., not moving, not talking, not responding to stimuli)
  R/O: overdose, occult head trauma
- Difficult to awaken or acting confused (e.g., disoriented, slurred speech)
  R/O: overdose, occult head trauma
- Seeing, hearing, or feeling things that are not there (i.e., visual, auditory, or tactile hallucinations)
  R/O: hallucinations
- Slow, shallow, and weak breathing
  R/O: impending respiratory arrest
- Seizure
  R/O: overdose, hypoxia
- Violent behavior or threatening to kill someone
  R/O: homicidal ideation
- Sounds like a life-threatening emergency to the triager

See More Appropriate Protocol

- Suicide thoughts, threats, and attempts: questions or concerns about
  Go to Protocol: Suicide Concerns on page 259
- Other significant medical symptom is present: see that protocol (e.g., chest pain, headache, vomiting)
  Go to Relevant Protocol
- Alcohol use, abuse, or dependence: question or problem related to
  Go to Protocol: Alcohol Use and Abuse and Dependence on page 9

Go to ED Now

- Bizarre, paranoid, or confused behavior
  R/O: drug-induced psychosis, current drug intoxication
- Feeling very shaky (i.e., visible tremors of hands)
  R/O: withdrawal
- Pregnant and symptoms of narcotic withdrawal (e.g., vomiting, severe muscle cramps)
  Reason: effect of withdrawal on fetus

Go to ED Now (or to Office With PCP Approval)

- Fever > 100.5° F (38.1° C) and IVDA (intravenous drug abuse)
  R/O: bacterial endocarditis from IVDA
- Patient sounds very anxious or agitated
  R/O: anxiety, drug intoxication, withdrawal symptoms
- Patient sounds very sick or weak to the triager

See Today in Office

- White of the eyes have turned yellow (i.e., jaundice)
  R/O: hepatitis, cirrhosis of the liver
- Fever > 101.5° F (38.6° C)
  R/O: bacterial illness

See Today or Tomorrow in Office

- Patient wants to be seen

Callback by PCP Today

- Pregnant and admits to substance abuse problem
  Reason: risk to fetus

Call Local Agency Today

- Alcohol or drug abuse, known or suspected
  Reason: needs evaluation and counseling
- Inhalant abuse (e.g., huffing), known or suspected
  Note: examples include adhesives (glue, rubber cement), aerosols (spray paint, hair spray), solvents (nail polish remover), and cleaning agents (spot remover). See Background Information.
- Requesting admission for susbtance (drug) abuse
- Requesting to talk with a counselor (mental health worker, psychiatrist, etc.)
- Drug use interferes with work or school

Home Care

- ○ Substance abuse, questions about
- ○ Urine drug tests, questions about

HOME CARE ADVICE

General Information

1. **Local Substance Abuse Treatment Program:**
   - If available, local alcohol treatment program: xxx-xxx-xxxx.
   - If available, local psychiatric crisis service at _______ hospital: xxx-xxx-xxxx.
2. **Urine Drug Testing:**
   - Urine drug tests may be helpful in 3 situations:
     1) Where a drug's identity is needed to treat an acutely intoxicated adult (i.e., with symptoms);
     2) As part of an ongoing drug rehabilitation program;
     3) As a required drug screening evaluation for work.
   - **Positive Tests:** False-positive tests are possible. A physician should be involved in the interpretation of positive drug screen results.
   - **Negative Tests:** Negative tests do not mean there is not a drug problem; simply that no drugs are detected at the time of the test, or that someone has tampered with the urine sample.
3. **Urine Drug Testing—Time Detectable:**
   - **Alcohol:** 1 day
   - **Amphetamine:** 8-24 hours
   - **Barbiturates:** 2-10 days
   - **Benzodiazepines:** 2-7 days
   - **Cocaine:** 1-4 days
   - **Codeine:** 1-2 days
   - **Gamma Hydroxybutyrate (GHB; Rohypnol):** 1-3 days; special test required
   - **Heroin:** 1-4 days
   - **Inhalants:** Not detected
   - **LSD:** 8 hours
   - **Marijuana:** Single use 1-7 days; chronic use 1-4 weeks
   - **MDMA (Ecstasy):** Not detected
   - **Methamphetamine:** 1-2 days
   - **Morphine:** 1-3 days
   - **Phencyclidine (PCP):** 1-7 days
4. **Call Back If:**
   - You have more questions about substance abuse.
   - You become worse.

Additional Resources

1. **Canada—Internet Resources**
   - **Canadian Network of Substance Abuse and Allied Professionals:** This Web site lists treatment agencies for each of the provinces in Canada. Available at: www.cnsaap.ca/Eng/CanadianLandscape/Pages/default.aspx.
   - **New Brunswick:** Department of Health and Wellness Addiction Services (www.gnb.ca/0378/addiction-e.asp). Services offered by region.
   - **Newfoundland and Labrador:** Newfoundland and Labrador Addictions Services (www.health.gov.nl.ca/health/addictions/services.html). Services offered by region.
   - **Northwest Territories:** Nats`ejée K`éh Treatment Centre (www.natsejeekeh.org). The phone number is 867-874-6699.
   - **Ontario—Drug and Alcohol Registry of Treatment (DART):** This is an online database of treatment programs offered in Ontario. It is searchable by name, municipality, Local Health Integration Network (LHIN), provincial service category, and/or specific population group. Available at: www.drugandalcoholhelpline.ca. The phone number for the helpline is 800-565-8603.
2. **Narcotics Anonymous:**
   - Narcotics Anonymous is "a nonprofit fellowship or society of men and women for whom drugs had become a major problem. We...meet regularly to help each other stay clean....We are not interested in what or how much you used... but only in what you want to do about your problem and how we can help."
   - Membership is open to any drug addict, regardless of the particular drug or combination of drugs used.
   - Chapters of Narcotics Anonymous are present in every state in the United States and in many countries of the world. Each has a local contact phone number.
   - More information is available at: www.na.org.

3. **United States—National Institute on Drug Abuse (NIDA):**
   - There is extensive information on drug abuse provided on the NIDA Web site (www.drugabuse.gov).
   - There is a useful and well-organized chart of commonly abused drugs available at: www.drugabuse.gov/drugs-abuse/commonly-abused-drugs/commonly-abused-drugs-chart.
4. **United States—Substance Abuse and Mental Health Services Administration (SAMHSA):**
   - This governmental agency works to improve the quality and availability of substance abuse prevention, alcohol and drug addiction treatment, and mental health services.
   - More information available at: www.samhsa.gov.
5. **United States—SAMHSA Treatment Referral Line:**
   - SAMHSA Treatment Referral Routing Service (samhsa.gov/treatment) is a "confidential, free, 24-hour-a-day, 365-day-a-year, information service, in English and Spanish, for individuals and family members facing substance abuse and mental health issues. This service provides referrals to local treatment facilities, support groups, and community-based organizations. Callers can also order free publications and other information in print on substance abuse and mental health issues."
   - The phone number is 800-662-HELP (4357).
6. **United States—SAMHSA Substance Abuse Treatment Facility Locator:**
   - SAMHSA has a Web tool for finding local drug abuse treatment programs.
   - This locator is available at: http://findtreatment.samhsa.gov.

BACKGROUND INFORMATION

General Information

- Chemical dependency/addiction is a disease and can be treated. Medical detox followed by 12-step/educational services can be successful in helping a patient to recover.
- Addiction can occur to legal/prescription drugs.

Priorities in Substance Abuse Triage

- The triager should first evaluate the drug abuse patient for medical life threats, suicidal ideation, physical injuries, and any active medical complaints. If this evaluation is negative, then the triager should refer the patient for substance abuse counseling.
- On average, addicts have been wanting to seek help for 7 or more years. It is important to acknowledge this and provide support while helping them with the next step. The next step is often referring the caller to a local substance abuse program, the CSAT hotline, or a local chapter of Narcotics Anonymous.
- Families and friends often call with questions and concerns. Generally, treatment will not be effective unless the addict themself wants help. Encourage the family to seek supportive services for themselves.
- Names and content of street drugs are ever-changing. Do not focus on the name of the drug. Instead, engage the caller to determine symptoms and the impact of the drug on day-to-day living.

Common Illegal Drugs of Abuse, Their Street Names, and Route of Use:

- **Cocaine** (coke, crack, rock): Inject/smoke/snort.
- **Heroin** (smack, horse, junk): Inject/smoke/snort.
- **LSD** (acid, microdot, blotter): Ingest.
- **Marijuana** (grass, pot, reefer, weed, blunts): Smoke/ingest.
- **Methamphetamine** (crank, crystal, ice, glass, meth): Inject/smoke/ingest/snort.
- **PCP/phencyclidine** (angel dust, embalming fluid, rocket fuel): Inject/ingest/smoke.
- For a comprehensive listing of over 2000 street drug names, see www.whitehouse.gov/ondcp.

Types of Drugs

- **Anabolic Steroids:** Used to enhance athletic performance, strength, or physical appearance. May cause mania, delusions, hallucinations, or over-aggressiveness ("steroid rage").
- **Designer Drugs:** Designer drugs are synthetic chemical modifications of commonly abused drugs. The most well-known one is Ecstasy (MDMA), a designer amphetamine. It is a stimulant

and a hallucinogen. Users describe initial anxiety and nausea, followed by relaxation, euphoria, and feelings of enhanced emotional insight. Very popular in the dance-club setting. Can lead to death associated with hyperthermia.

- **Dextromethorphan:** Can cause a LSD-like picture (visual hallucinations, confusion, excitation). It can also cause coma and death. Dextromethorphan (DM) is present in OTC cough medicines.
- **Dissociatives (Ketamine, Phencyclidine/PCP):** Cause perceptual alterations and hallucinations.
- **Hallucinogens/Psychedelics (LSD, Mescaline):** Cause visual hallucinations, perceptual alterations, and a dreamlike state.
- **Inhalants (Toluene/Glue, Gasoline, Butane, Trichloroethane/Typewriter Correction Fluid):** Can cause giddiness or euphoria. Can also rarely cause sudden death from cardiac arrhythmias.
- **Marijuana:** Marijuana is the most commonly used illegal drug. Over 40% of high school seniors have tried marijuana. It's the only illegal drug with virtually no lethal potential except from secondary accidents. Hence, patients with mild symptoms (mellow euphoria) don't need to be seen on an emergency basis. Marijuana sold on the streets today is much stronger than it was in the 1960s/1970s. Marijuana causes euphoria and in higher concentrations can be associated with paranoia, delusions, and hallucinations.
- **Narcotics/Opiates (Heroin, Morphine, Codeine, Pentazocine, Methadone):** Cause sedation and euphoria. Overdose can cause profound respiratory depression, coma, and death. Withdrawal from opiates is not life-threatening. However, the withdrawal symptoms are extremely uncomfortable (i.e., yawning, nausea, vomiting, diarrhea, muscle cramps).
- **Sedative-Hypnotics/Depressants (Barbiturates, Benzodiazepines, Tranquilizers):** Cause sedation, drowsiness and euphoria. Can cause coma and death.
- **Stimulants (Cocaine, Crack Cocaine, Amphetamine, Methamphetamine):** Causes hyperalertness, stimulation, restlessness, and euphoria. Can cause stroke, coma, arrhythmias, and death.

Inhalant Abuse

- Inhaling (huffing) chemical vapors is the most common form of substance abuse from age 12-15 (Reason: solvents are cheap and readily available).
- **Types of Inhalants:** Toluene from glue, butane from lighters, gasoline, paints, paint thinners, hair spray, air fresheners, and hundreds more. The latest dangerous fad is "dusting": inhaling the Freon propellants in computer keyboard cleaners.
- **Symptoms:** Inhaling these substances from a rag soaked with them (often in a plastic bag) can give a 3-minute "high" (dizziness, giddiness, even euphoria). Acute neurologic symptoms are common: altered mental status, slurred speech, ataxia.
- **Complications:** Chronic inhalant use can permanently damage the white matter of the brain (memory, etc.) On rare occasions, inhalants have caused sudden death from cardiac arrhythmias, sometimes even the first time they are used.
- Clues that should alert family, friends, and parents to inhalant abuse include:
  - Breath or clothing that smells like chemicals; paint or glue on face, fingers, or clothing; rashes around the mouth.

Psychiatric Symptoms From Substance Abuse

- Drug withdrawal and drug intoxication can mimic medical and psychiatric disorders.
- **Anxiety:** Sometimes anxiety symptoms may represent withdrawal symptoms from depressant medications such as opiates (e.g., heroin) or sedative-hypnotics (e.g., alcohol, benzodiazepines). Anxiety attacks can occur during intoxication with stimulants (e.g., cocaine) and hallucinogens (e.g., LSD).
- **Depression:** Many individuals with drug abuse have symptoms of depression. Cocaine addicts experience a profound period of depression ("crash") after a cocaine binge.
- **Polydrug Abuse:** Many individuals abuse more than one drug at a time. For example, as many as 75% of individuals with cocaine abuse will also have alcohol dependence.
- **Suicidal Ideation:** It is appropriate to directly ask a patient about intent to harm himself or end his own life. Such questions will not provoke a suicide attempt and may instead give the patient a chance to unburden himself.

SUICIDE CONCERNS

DEFINITION

- Patient or caller has questions or concerns about suicide thoughts, threats, or attempts.

TRIAGE ASSESSMENT QUESTIONS

Call EMS 911 Now

- Patient has attempted suicide
  R/O: physical injury or overdosage
  Note: if patient is alone, another triage nurse should call EMS 911.
- Patient is threatening suicide
  Reason: suicidal ideation
  Note: if patient is alone, another triage nurse should call EMS 911
- Sounds like a life-threatening emergency to the triager

See More Appropriate Protocol

- Depression is the main concern and is not threatening suicide
  Go to Protocol: Depression on page 74

Call Local Agency Now

- Recurrent thoughts of death (e.g., "life is not worth living") and is not threatening suicide
  R/O: major depression
- Has lethal plan (e.g., overdose, gunshot) and access (e.g., hoarding pills, firearm in house), but is not threatening suicide
- Patient sounds very upset or severely depressed (e.g., multiple symptoms of depression)

See Today in Office

- Patient wants to be seen

Call Local Agency Today

- Patient is evasive or refuses to answer questions regarding intent to harm themselves
- Requesting to talk with a counselor (mental health worker, psychiatrist, etc.)

HOME CARE ADVICE (Pending Further Evaluation)

General Information

1. **Reassurance:**
   - It sounds like you are feeling helpless. I am glad you had the courage to call.
   - Let me help you with the next step.
   - Encourage the caller to talk about his/her problems and feelings. Offer hope.
2. **Suicidal Ideation Or Suicide Attempt:**
   All patients with a suicide attempt or threat should be seen immediately for an evaluation even if they have no medical symptoms.
   - **Patient Is Alone:** Triager should stay on the phone with the patient until EMS or the police arrive and take over. Have a coworker call EMS 911. Trace the call if needed.
   - **Patient Is Not Alone:** If caller is with a friend or family member, ask this person to call EMS 911 now. Ask this person to make sure patient doesn't have access to medications or firearms; request that he/she not leave the patient alone.
3. **Local Agency or Suicide Hotline Phone Numbers:**
   - If available, local suicide hotline or crisis phone number: xxx-xxx-xxxx.
   - If available, local psychiatric crisis service at ________ hospital: xxx-xxx-xxxx.
   - US National Suicide Hotline Toll-free Crisis Phone: 888-SUICIDE (784-2433).
4. **Call Back If:**
   - You feel like harming yourself or feel more depressed.
   - Situation becomes worse.

Additional Resources

1. **United States—Crisis and Suicide Hotline:**
   - Kristin Brooks Hope Center: National Hopeline Network
   - www.hopeline.com
   - National crisis hotline in the United States for suicide intervention: 800-442-HOPE (4673) and 800-SUICIDE (784-2433).

2. **United States—Vet2Vet Veterans Crisis Hotline**
   - www.veteranscall.us
   - 877-VET2VET (838-2838)
   - "This a toll-free line targeted to the population of returning armed forces men and women and veterans from previous conflicts and wars."
3. **United States—Substance Abuse and Mental Health Services Administration (SAMHSA) Treatment Referral Line:**
   - SAMHSA Treatment Referral Routing Service (http://samhsa.gov/treatment) is a "confidential, free, 24-hour-a-day, 365-day-a-year, information service, in English and Spanish, for individuals and family members facing substance abuse and mental health issues. This service provides referrals to local treatment facilities, support groups, and community-based organizations. Callers can also order free publications and other information in print on substance abuse and mental health issues."
   - The phone number is 800-662-HELP (4357).
4. **United States—NAMI Information HelpLine:**
   - National Alliance on Mental Illness
   - "NAMI is dedicated to the eradication of mental illnesses and to the improvement of the quality of life of all whose lives are affected by these diseases....The National Alliance for the Mentally Ill (NAMI) is a network of local support groups for the mentally ill and their families..."
   - The NAMI Helpline is an information and referral source for locating community mental health programs. National toll-free phone number: 800-950-NAMI (6264). Monday through Friday, 10:00 am- 6:00 pm, Eastern time.
   - www.nami.org.
5. **United States—Mood Disorders Organizations:**
   - Anxiety and Depression Association of America (ADAA).
   - There is a "Find a Therapist" link on the home page.
   - www.adaa.org.
   - Telephone: 240-485-1001.
6. **Canada—Internet Resources**
   - **Canadian Network of Substance Abuse and Allied Professionals:** This Web site lists treatment agencies for each of the provinces in Canada. Available at: www.cnsaap.ca/Eng/CanadianLandscape/Pages/default.aspx.
   - **New Brunswick:** Department of Health and Wellness Addiction Services (www.gnb.ca/0378/addiction-e.asp). Services offered by region.
   - **Newfoundland and Labrador:** Newfoundland and Labrador Addictions Services (www.health.gov.nl.ca/health/addictions/services.html). Services offered by region.
   - **Northwest Territories:** Nats`ejée K`éh Treatment Centre (www.natsejeekeh.org). The phone number is 867-874-6699.
   - **Ontario: Drug and Alcohol Registry of Treatment (DART):** This is an online database of treatment programs offered in Ontario. It is searchable by name, municipality, Local Health Integration Network (LHIN), provincial service category, and/or specific population group. Available at: www.drugandalcoholhelpline.ca. The phone number for the helpline is 800-565-8603.
7. **Canada—Mood Disorder Organizations**
   - **Ontario:** Mood Disorders Association of Ontario (MDAO)—888-486-8236
   - www.mooddisorders.ca

BACKGROUND INFORMATION

General

- **Alternatives:** Suicidal patients often feel they have no alternatives. It is important for the triager to offer hope and to show such patient how they can get help.
- **Intent:** It is appropriate to directly ask patients about their intent to harm themselves or end their own life. Such questions will not provoke a suicide attempt and may instead give patients a chance to unburden themselves. Any patient who is threatening self-harm now needs to be seen immediately for evaluation.

- **Plan:** This refers to the extent to which the patient has prepared for a suicide attempt. Does the patient have a specific method in mind (e.g., gun, knife, overdose)? Does the patient have access to the verbalized method (e.g., hoarded pills, firearm in house)? Access to lethal methods increases the risk of suicide attempt and death. Generally, a patient with a specific plan is considered at higher suicide risk than a patient who is threatening suicide but has no plan.

Risks for Suicide Attempt

- Prior treatment for or diagnosis of mental health or chemical dependence problem
- **Addiction:** Alcohol, drug, gambling
- Serious or chronic medical illness
- **Lack of Social Support:** Living alone, divorced, widowed
- **Recent Losses:** Recent bereavement, separation, divorce, unemployment
- Prior suicide attempt
- Family history of completed suicide
- **Age:** Greater than 60 or less than 25 years old

Risks for Suicide Completion (Death)

- Older
- Male
- Living alone
- Physical illness
- Access to lethal methods, such as a gun

Dos for the Triager

- Do ask about suicidal thoughts; be direct in questioning.
- Do assess for access to lethal methods (pills, gun).
- Do listen and show interest.
- Do utilize friends and family.
- Do show support for courage to call.
- Do offer hope.
- Do show you care.

Don'ts for the Triager

- Don't try to cheer the patient up (e.g., jokes).
- Don't be judgmental.

SUNBURN

DEFINITION

- Red, painful skin following sun exposure.
- The pain and swelling starts at 4 hours, peaks at 24 hours, and improves after 48 hours.
- Sunburn to the cornea (ultraviolet keratitis) is included in this guideline.

Sunburn Pain Severity Is Defined As:

- **Mild (1-3):** Doesn't interfere with normal activities
- **Moderate (4-7):** Interferes with normal activities or awakens from sleep
- **Severe (8-10):** Excruciating pain, unable to do any normal activities

TRIAGE ASSESSMENT QUESTIONS

Call EMS 911 Now

- Difficult to awaken or acting confused (e.g., disoriented, slurred speech)
  R/O: heatstroke, shock
- Passed out (i.e., fainted, collapsed and was not responding)
  R/O: heat exhaustion or dehydration
- Sounds like a life-threatening emergency to the triager

See More Appropriate Protocol

- Sunburn-like rash BUT minimal or no sun exposure
  Go to Protocol: Rash, Widespread and Cause Unknown on page 209
- Heatstroke, sunstroke, or heat exhaustion suspected
  Go to Protocol: Heat Exposure (Heat Exhaustion and Heatstroke) on page 146

Go to ED Now (or to Office With PCP Approval)

- Too weak to stand
  R/O: heat exhaustion
- Fever > 103° F (39.4° C)
  R/O: impending heatstroke
- Blisters (second-degree burn) covering > 10% BSA
- Patient sounds very sick or weak to the triager

See Today in Office

- SEVERE sunburn pain
  Reason: may need narcotic analgesic
- Severe eye pain or blurred vision that follows sun exposure (welding or other significant light exposure)
  R/O: ultraviolet photokeratitis needing patching
  Note: photokeratitis can occur after exposure to the sun, tanning lamps, and broken mercury vapor lamps.
- Looks infected (e.g., fever, pus, red streaks, spreading redness)
  Reason: may need antibiotics

See Today or Tomorrow in Office

- Patient wants to be seen

Discuss With PCP and Callback by Nurse Today

- Sunburn following brief sun exposure and taking photosensitizing drug (e.g., tetracycline, doxycycline, elidel, protopic, griseofulvin, sulfa drugs)

See Within 3 Days in Office

- Blisters on the face
  Reason: cosmetic concerns
- Blisters (second-degree burn) covering > 2% BSA (i.e., more than 2 palms)
- Blister larger than 1 inch (2.5 cm)

Home Care

- Mild sunburn
- Mild eye symptoms that follows sun exposure (or other significant light exposure)
  Reason: probably mild ultraviolet photokeratitis
  Note: photokeratitis can occur after exposure to the sun, tanning lamps, and broken mercury vapor lamps.
- Sunscreen and protection from the sun, questions about

HOME CARE ADVICE

Mild Sunburn

1. **Ibuprofen for Pain:** For pain relief, begin taking ibuprofen (e.g., Advil, Motrin) as soon as possible. Adult dosage is 400 mg every 6 hours. If anti-inflammatory agents such as ibuprofen are begun within 6 hours of sun exposure and continued for 2 days, they can greatly reduce your discomfort. If you can't take ibuprofen, use acetaminophen (e.g., Tylenol) instead.
   - Do not take ibuprofen if you have stomach problems, kidney disease, are pregnant, or have been told by your doctor to avoid this type of anti-inflammatory drug. Do not take ibuprofen for more than 7 days without consulting your doctor.
   - Do not take acetaminophen if you have liver disease.
   - Read the package instructions thoroughly on all medications that you take.
2. **Hydrocortisone Cream:** Apply 1% hydrocortisone cream as soon as possible and then 3 times a day for 2 days. If begun early, it may reduce swelling and pain. If you don't have any hydrocortisone cream, use a moisturizing cream until you can get some.
   - Keep the cream in the refrigerator (Reason: it feels better if applied cold).
   - Available over-the-counter in United States as 0.5% and 1% cream.
   - Available over-the-counter in Canada as 0.5% cream.
3. **Cool Baths:** Apply cool compresses to the burned area several times a day to reduce pain and burning. For larger sunburns, give cool baths for 10 minutes (Caution: avoid any chill). Add 2 oz (60 g) baking soda per tub. Avoid soap on the sunburn.
4. **Extra Fluids:** Drink extra water on the first day to replace the fluids lost into the sunburn and to prevent dehydration and dizziness.
5. **Broken Blisters:**
   - For broken blisters, trim off the dead skin with fine scissors (Reason: these hidden pockets can become a breeding ground for infection).
   - Apply antibiotic ointment (e.g., bacitracin) to the raw skin under broken blisters. Reapply twice daily for 3 days.
   - **Caution:** Leave intact blisters alone (Reason: the intact blister protects the skin and allows it to heal).
6. **Expected Course:** Pain usually stops after 2 or 3 days. Skin flaking and peeling usually occur 5-7 days after the sunburn.
7. **Call Back If:**
   - Pain becomes severe and not improved after taking pain medication.
   - Pain does not improve after 3 days.
   - Sunburn looks infected.
   - You become worse.

Mild Photokeratitis

1. **Photokeratitis (Sunburn of Cornea):**
   - **Definition:** Photokeratitis can be thought of as a sunburn of the cornea. Exposure to intense light can cause corneal irritation (keratitis), especially if a person uses inadequate eye protection.
   - **Causes:** This is most commonly seen in individuals with inadequate eye protection while outside on a bright sunny day (e.g., water sports, snow skiing). It can also occur in individuals who do not use eye protection while using a tanning booth. This can also occur in welders.
2. **Eye Treatment:**
   - Apply cool wet compresses to the eyes.
   - Try to rest with your eyes closed.
   - Do not wear contacts until your eyes are completely better.
   - Avoid rubbing your eyes.
3. **Expected Course:**
   - Symptoms should disappear completely over the next 24 hours. There should be no permanent damage to the cornea.
   - You can prevent future eye symptoms from sun exposure by wearing sunglasses.
4. **Call Back If:**
   - Severe pain occurs.
   - Pain persists more than 24 hours.
   - Pus or yellow/green discharge occurs.
   - Blurred vision occurs.
   - You become worse.

How to Prevent Sunburn

1. **Prevention—Reduce Sun Exposure:**
   - Try to avoid all sun exposure between 10:00 am and 3:00 pm.
   - You can get a sunburn while swimming. Water only blocks the ultraviolet radiation a little.
2. **Prevention—Clothing:**
   - Wear a wide-brimmed hat; it protects your face and neck from the sun.
   - Wear shirts with long sleeves when outdoors and pants that go down to at least your knees.
3. **Prevention—Use Sunscreen:**
   - Apply sunscreen to areas that can't be protected by clothing. Generally, an adult needs about 1 oz (30 g) of sunscreen lotion to cover the entire body.
   - You should reapply the sunscreen every 2-4 hours. You should also reapply after swimming, exercising, or sweating.
   - A sunscreen with a rating of SPF 15 to 30 should be used. Sunscreens with ratings higher than 30 provide minimal additional protection.
   - Sunscreens help prevent sunburn but do not completely prevent skin damage. Thus, sun exposure can still increase your risk of skin aging and skin cancer.
4. **Vitamins C and E:** Vitamins C and E have anti-oxidant properties, which means they help prevent sun damage to cells in your skin. Taking vitamins C and E by mouth may partially reduce the sunburn reaction.
   - **Adult Dosage of Vitamin C (Ascorbic Acid):** 2 grams by mouth once a day.
   - **Adult Dosage of Vitamin E (D-Alpha-Tocopherol):** 1,000 IU by mouth once a day.
   - **Caution:** Prevention is the key. Remember to reduce sun exposure and use sunscreens.
   - Read the package instructions thoroughly on all medications that you take.

Questions About Sunglasses

1. **The Sun and Your Eyes:**
   - The cornea can also get sunburned. This can cause eye pain, watery eyes, difficulty looking at lights, and blurred vision.
   - Long-term sun exposure can also cause eye cataracts.
2. **Sunglasses:**
   - You can protect your eyes from the sun by wearing sunglasses.
   - When you buy sunglasses, look for glasses that block 99-100% of the full ultraviolet (UV) spectrum.

FIRST AID

First Aid Advice for Heatstroke or Sunstroke:

- Call EMS 911 immediately.
- Move to a cool, shady area. If possible, move into an air-conditioned place.
- Remove excess clothing or equipment (e.g., sports gear, protective work uniforms).
- Sponge the entire body surface with cool water (as cool as tolerated without shivering). If available, place ice packs on the neck, armpits, and groin. Fan the patient to increase evaporation.
- Keep the feet elevated to counteract shock.
- If the patient is awake, give as much cold water or sports drink (e.g., Gatorade, Powerade) as he or she can tolerate.
- Fever medicines are of no value for heatstroke.

First Aid for Heat Exhaustion:

- Put the patient in a cool place. Lie down with the feet elevated.
- Undress patient (except for underwear) so the body surface can give off heat.
- Sponge the entire body surface continuously with cool water (as cool as tolerated without shivering). Fan the patient to increase evaporation.
- After 2 or 3 glasses of water, drive the patient in to be seen. During the drive, provide unlimited amounts of water.

BACKGROUND INFORMATION

General Information

- Sunburn may cause a first-degree (redness and pain) or a second-degree (blistering) burn to the sun-exposed areas of the body.
- The triager should document the percentage of body surface area (BSA) involvement of blistering.
- Long-term sun exposure increases the risk for skin cancer and causes aging of the skin. Long-term sun exposure can also cause eye cataracts.
- Vitamins C and E are antioxidants. Taking vitamins C and E by mouth may partially reduce the sunburn reaction (Eberlein-Konig). More research is needed to prove whether there is any true benefit.

Degrees of Sunburn

- **First Degree:** Most sunburn is a first-degree burn which turns the skin pink or red. The pain and swelling starts at 4 hours, peaks at 24 hours, and improves after 48 hours.
- **Second Degree:** Prolonged sun exposure can cause blistering and a second-degree burn.
- **Third Degree:** Sunburn never causes a third-degree burn or scarring.

Causes of Sunburn

- **Broken Mercury-Vapor Lamps (Overhead Lighting):** Damaged mercury-vapor (metal halide) lamps are known to cause outbreaks of UV-radiation "sunburns" and photokeratitis (corneal irritation).
- Tanning lamps.
- The sun.

Photokeratitis (Sunburn of Cornea)

- **Definition:** Photokeratitis can be thought of as a sunburn of the cornea. Exposure to intense light can cause corneal irritation (keratitis), especially if a person uses inadequate eye protection.
- **Pain:** Usually bilateral eye pain; tearing; light bothers eyes.
- **Vision Loss:** Usually minimal vision change (haziness) to none. More severe photokeratitis can cause blurred vision; all patients with blurred vision require medical evaluation; in skiers this is referred to as snow blindness.
- **Causes:** This is most commonly seen in individuals with inadequate eye protection while outside on a bright sunny day (e.g., water sports, snow skiing). It can also occur in individuals who do not use eye protection while using a tanning booth. This can also occur in welders.

Rule of Nines for Estimating Burn Size

- Each part of the body contributes a predictable portion of the total body surface area (BSA).
- **Head and Neck:** 9%
- **Each Arm:** 9%
- **Anterior Chest and Abdomen:** 18%
- **Entire Back:** 18%
- **Each Leg:** 18%
- **Genital Region:** 1%

Rule of Palms for Estimating Burn Size:

- A person's palm (not including the fingers) represents 1% of the total body surface area (BSA).
- For example, if a person had blistering of the left shoulder the size of 2 palms, the total area of blistering would be 2% of the BSA.

Caution—Toxic Shock Syndrome:

- The rash is a widespread erythroderma (painless "sunburn") that usually fades in 72 hours. It is followed by skin desquamation (peeling), especially of the palms and soles.
- Other signs and symptoms of the syndrome include fever, muscle aches, vomiting or diarrhea, multiorgan dysfunction (liver, kidney), confusion, shock, and death.
- Those at risk include menstruating women using tampons, postsurgical patients, and patients with nasal packings.
- Patients suspected of having this condition should be seen immediately.

SUTURE OR STAPLE QUESTIONS

DEFINITION

- Questions about sutured or stapled wounds

TRIAGE ASSESSMENT QUESTIONS

Call EMS 911 Now

- Major abdominal surgical wound and visible internal organs
- Sounds like a life-threatening emergency to the triager

See More Appropriate Protocol

- Wound looks infected
  Go to Protocol: Wound Infection on page 344
- New cut and caller wonders if it needs stitches
  Go to Protocol: Trauma, Skin on page 310

Go to ED Now (or to Office With PCP Approval)

- Bleeding won't stop after 10 minutes of direct pressure (using correct technique)
- Patient sounds very sick or weak to the triager

Go to Office Now

- Major surgical wound that is starting to open up
  R/O: dehiscence (Site: if possible, refer to surgeon who performed surgery)
- Wound gaping open and < 48 hours since sutures placed
  Reason: may re-suture

See Today in Office

- Wound gaping open and length of opening > ½ inch (6 mm)
- Wound gaping open and on face
  R/O: cosmetic concerns
- Suture removal is overdue
- Suture came out early and > 48 hours since sutures placed, and caller wants wound checked

See Today or Tomorrow in Office

- Patient wants to be seen

See Within 3 Days in Office

- Numbness extends beyond the wound edges and lasts > 8 hours

Home Care

- Suture came out early and > 48 hours since sutures placed
- Care of sutured wound, questions about
- Suture removal date, questions about

HOME CARE ADVICE

General Care Advice for the Sutured or Stapled Wound

1. **Suture Care for a Normal Sutured Wound:**
   - Can get wound wet (e.g., bathing or swimming) after 24 hours.
   - Apply antibiotic ointment 3 times a day (Reason: to prevent infection and a thick scab).
   - Cleanse with warm water once daily or if it becomes soiled.
   - Change wound dressing when wet or soiled.
   - Dressing no longer needed when edge of wound closed (usually 48 hours).
   - **Exception:** Dressing needed to prevent sutures from catching on clothing.
2. **Removal Date:** Guidelines for when particular sutures (stitches) or staples should be removed:
   - **Face:** 4-5 days
   - **Neck:** 7 days
   - **Scalp:** 7-10 days
   - **Chest or Abdomen:** 7-10 days
   - **Arms and Back of Hands:** 7-10 days
   - **Legs and Top of Feet:** 10 days
   - **Back:** 10 days
   - **Palms and Soles:** 12-14 days
   - **Overlying a Joint:** 12-14 days
3. **Removal Delays:** Don't miss your appointment for removing stitches. Stitches removed late can leave unnecessary skin marks and occasionally cause scarring. Delays also makes suture removal more difficult.
4. **Suture Out Early:** If the sutures come out early, reinforce the wound with tape or butterfly Band-Aids until the office visit.

5. **Wound Protection:** After removal of sutures:
   - Protect the wound from injury during the following month.
   - Avoid sports that could reinjure the wound. If a sport is essential, apply tape before playing.
   - Allow the scab to fall off on its own. Do not try to remove it.
6. **Pain Medicines:**
   - For pain relief, take acetaminophen, ibuprofen, or naproxen.

   Acetaminophen (e.g., Tylenol):
   - Take 650 mg by mouth every 4-6 hours as needed. Each Regular Strength Tylenol pill has 325 mg of acetaminophen. The most you should take each day is 3,250 mg (10 pills a day).
   - Another choice is to take 1,000 mg every 8 hours. Each Extra Strength Tylenol pill has 500 mg of acetaminophen. The most you should take each day is 3,000 mg (6 pills a day).

   Ibuprofen (e.g., Motrin, Advil):
   - Take 400 mg by mouth every 6 hours.
   - Another choice is to take 600 mg by mouth every 8 hours.

   Naproxen (e.g., Aleve):
   - Take 250-500 mg by mouth every 12 hours.

   Extra Notes:
   - Acetaminophen is thought to be safer than ibuprofen or naproxen in people over 65 years old. Acetaminophen is in many OTC and prescription medicines. It might be in more than one medicine that you are taking. You need to be careful and not take an overdose. An acetaminophen overdose can hurt the liver.
   - Caution: Do not take acetaminophen if you have liver disease.
   - Caution: Do not take ibuprofen if you have stomach problems, kidney disease, are pregnant, or have been told by your doctor to avoid this type of anti-inflammatory drug. Do not take ibuprofen for more than 7 days without consulting your doctor.
   - Use the lowest amount of medicine that makes your pain feel better.
   - Before taking any medicine, read all the instructions on the package
7. **Call Back If:**
   - Looks infected.
   - Fever.
   - Sutures come out early.
   - You become worse.

Preventing Scars—Questions About

1. **Scarring:**
   - Scarring is unfortunately a natural part of the healing process after a cut or wound from surgery or trauma.
   - The more serious the injury and the larger the wound/cut, the greater the likelihood of scarring.
   - Almost all cuts that require closure with sutures, staples, or skin glue will heal with some scarring.
   - Some people are more prone to scarring than others.
2. **Preventing Scarring:**
   - Be certain to get the sutures removed during the time frame that your doctor recommended (Reason: if you leave them in too long they can leave "railroad tracks").
   - Avoid getting a sunburn in this area for 2 months.
   - Avoid reinjuring this area.
   - Some people apply vitamin E lotion (or cream) to a healing wound to prevent scarring.
   - Research has not shown that this helps.

FIRST AID

First Aid Advice for Bleeding:

Apply direct pressure to the entire wound with a clean cloth.

First Aid Advice for Surgical Wound That Is Opening Up:

Cover wound with a clean gauze or dressing.

BACKGROUND INFORMATION

Sutures or Staples That Fall Out

Sutures that pull out early are one of patients' main reasons for calling. The following rules generally apply:

- **Face:** If the wound is on the face and it has reopened, the patient should be seen regardless of how long it's been since the sutures were placed.
- **Body:** If the wound is elsewhere on the body, the patient should be seen if the wound is gaping and the sutures were placed less than 48 hours ago. After 48 hours, re-suturing is rarely done (except on the face). After 48 hours, have the caller reinforce the wound with tape.

Suture Removal Date

Guidelines for when particular sutures (or staples) should be removed:

- **Face:** 4-5 days
- **Neck:** 7 days
- **Scalp:** 7-10 days
- **Chest, Abdomen, and Back:** 7-10 days
- **Arms and Back of Hands:** 7 days
- **Legs and Top of Feet:** 10 days
- **Fingers and Toes:** 10-14 days
- **Palms and Soles:** 12-14 days
- **Overlying a Joint:** 12-14 days
- **Note:** If patient recalls that the doctor told them a different time frame, have patient call PCP or surgeon during normal office hours to confirm.

Numbness of Skin Near a Laceration

- **Local Anesthesia—Duration of Action:** Duration of numbness from local anesthesia depends on what type of local anesthesia was used. Numbness can last from 1 to 8 hours.
- **Numbness From the Laceration Itself:** Some people report a small area of numbness right along the edges of the sutured wound. This can last 1 to 3 weeks.
- **Nerve Injury:**. Sometimes a cut can be deep enough that it cuts an important nerve. This should be suspected if the the area of numbness extends beyond just the edges of the wound and lasts more than 8 hours. An example of this would be a digital nerve injury of the finger; the patient might report persisting numbness of one side of the finger. A patient with a suspected nerve injury should be referred to their doctor within 3 days.

TICK BITE

DEFINITION

- A tick (small brown bug) is attached to the skin.
- A tick recently was removed from the skin.

TRIAGE ASSESSMENT QUESTIONS

See More Appropriate Protocol

- Not a tick bite
  Go to Protocol: Insect Bite on page 166

Go to ED Now (or to Office With PCP Approval)

- Patient sounds very sick or weak to the triager

Go to Office Now

- Fever or severe headache occurs, 2 to 14 days following the bite
  R/O: Rocky Mountain spotted fever
- Widespread rash occurs, 2 to 14 days following the bite
- Can't remove live tick (after using home care advice)
  Reason: needs removal to prevent disease
- Can't remove tick's head that was broken off in the skin (after using home care advice)
  Reason: tick's mouthparts need removal to prevent localized infection or granuloma
  Note: If the removed tick is moving, it was completely removed.
- Fever and area is red
  R/O: cellulitis, lymphangitis
  Reason: fever and looks infected
- Fever and area is very tender to touch
  R/O: cellulitis, lymphangitis
  Note: skin infection is rare after a tick bite.
- Red streak or red line and length > 2 inches (5 cm)
  R/O: lymphangitis
  Note: lymphangitis looks like a red streak or line originating at the wound and ascending up the arm or leg toward the heart. Rare after a tick bite.

See Today in Office

- Red ring or bull's-eye rash occurs around a deer tick bite
  R/O: Lyme disease
- Probable deer tick that was attached > 24 hours (or tick appears swollen, not flat)
  Reason: consider antibiotic prophylaxis, especially if Lyme disease prevalent in the area
- Patient wants to be seen

Home Care

- Tick bite with no complications
- Prevention of tick bites and insect repellents (e.g., DEET), questions about
  R/O: cellulitis, lymphangitis
  Reason: fever and looks infected
  Note: skin infection is rare after a tick bite.

HOME CARE ADVICE

Home Care Advice for Tick Bite

1. **Wood Tick Removal:**
   - Use a pair of tweezers and grasp the wood tick close to the skin (on its head). Pull the wood tick straight upward without twisting or crushing it. Maintain a steady pressure until it releases its grip.
   - If tweezers aren't available, use fingers, a loop of thread around the jaws, or a needle between the jaws for traction.
   - **Note:** Covering the tick with petroleum jelly, nail polish, or rubbing alcohol doesn't work. Neither does touching the tick with a hot or cold object.
2. **Tiny Deer Tick Removal:**
   - Deer ticks are very small and need to be scraped off with a credit card edge or the edge of a knife blade.
   - Place tick in a sealed container (e.g., glass jar, Ziploc plastic bag), in case your doctor wants to see it.
3. **Tick's Head Removal:**
   - If the wood tick's head breaks off in the skin, it must be removed. Clean the skin. Then use a sterile needle to uncover the head and lift it out or scrape it off.
   - If a very small piece of the head remains, the skin will eventually slough it off.

4. **Antibiotic Ointment:** Wash the wound and your hands with soap and water after removal to prevent catching any tick disease. Apply an over-the-counter antibiotic ointment (e.g., bacitracin) to the bite once.
5. **Expected Course:** Tick bites normally do not itch or hurt. That is why they often go unnoticed.
6. **Call Back If:**
    - You can't remove the tick or the tick's head.
    - Fever or rash occur in the next 2 weeks.
    - Bite begins to look infected.
    - You become worse.

How to Prevent a Tick Bite

1. **Prevention—General:**
    - Prevention is important if you are hiking in tick-infested areas.
    - Wear long pants and a long shirt. Tuck your shirt into your pants. Tuck the cuffs of your pants into your socks or boots. Light-colored clothing is better because the ticks can be seen more easily.
    - Inspect your entire body and your clothing every couple hours. Favorite places are in the hair, so be certain to check your scalp, neck, armpits, and groin.
    - A shower at the end of a hike will help rinse off any tick that is not firmly attached.
2. **Prevention With Insect Repellent—DEET:**
    - DEET is a very effective tick repellent. It also repels mosquitoes and other bugs.
    - Apply to exposed areas of skin. Do not apply to eyes, mouth, or irritated areas of skin. Remember to wash it off with soap and water when you return indoors.
    - Pregnant and breastfeeding women may use DEET. No problems have been reported (Centers for Disease Control and Prevention).
    - Be certain to read the package instructions on any product that you use.
3. **Prevention With Insect Repellent For Your Clothing—Permethrin:**
    - Permethrin-containing products (e.g., Duranon, Permanone, and Congo Creek Tick Spray) are highly effective mosquito repellents. They also repel ticks.
    - An advantage over using DEET is that they are applied to and left on clothing instead of skin. Apply it to clothes before putting them on. You can also put it on other outdoor items (shoes, mosquito screen, sleeping bags).
    - Do not apply permethrin to skin (Reason: it is rapidly degraded on contact with skin).
    - Be certain to read the package instructions on any product that you use.

BACKGROUND INFORMATION

General

- The bite is painless and doesn't itch, so ticks may go unnoticed for a few days. Ticks eventually fall off on their own after sucking blood for 3 to 6 days.
- Ticks can transmit many diseases, including Lyme disease, Rocky Mountain spotted fever (RMSF), Colorado tick fever, and relapsing fever.
- After feeding on blood, ticks become quite swollen and easier to see.

Types of Ticks

- The DEER TICK (black-legged tick) is between the size of a poppy seed (pinhead) and an apple seed, and is the tick that usually transmits Lyme disease. A southern form of Lyme disease can be caused by contact with the lone star tick (this is a large tick).
- The LONE STAR TICK is the size of a watermelon seed. The lone star tick is the same size and the most common vector for erlichiosis (HME; human monocytic ehrlichiosis). It also occasionally transmits Lyme disease.
- The WOOD TICK (dog tick) is the size of a watermelon seed and can sometimes transmit Rocky Mountain spotted fever and Colorado tick fever.

Lyme Disease

- Lyme disease has become the most common tick-borne illness in the United States. The risk of Lyme disease following a recognized deer tick bite is approximately 1%.
- **Endemic Areas:** Lyme disease is common (i.e., endemic) in only certain areas of the United States. Over 90% of Lyme disease occurs in the following 11 states: Connecticut, Rhode Island, New York, Pennsylvania , Delaware , New Jersey, Maryland, Massachusetts, Maine, Wisconsin, and Minnesota.
- **Erythema Migrans Rash:** The majority of cases of Lyme disease start with erythema migrans (bull's-eye rash) at the site of the tick bite. The rash can occur days to weeks (typically 7-10 days) after a tick bite. Treatment with antibiotics is indicated if this rash appears. Mild flu-like symptoms may accompany the erythema migrans rash, including: fever, chills, headaches, muscle aches, and fatigue.
- **Vaccine:** There is no Lyme disease vaccine currently available. The vaccine manufacturer discontinued production in 2002 because of insufficent consumer demand.

Antibiotic Prophylaxis After Deer Tick Bite

- Research has demonstrated that the risk of Lyme disease is zero for attachments of less than 24-48 hours or if the tick appears flat (not swollen or engorged from feeding).
- Deer ticks go through 3 states in their life cycle: larval, nymphal, and adult. During the nymphal and adult states they may attach to humans, feed, and potentially transmit Lyme disease. Transmission occurs more often in the nymphal stage, presumably because the nymphal tick is smaller, more easily missed, and thus remains attached for a longer period of time.
- A recent article showed that a single 200-mg dose of doxycycline was effective at preventing Lyme disease if given within 72 hours of a deer tick bite (Nadelman et al, 2001).
- Thus, prophylactic antibiotic may sometimes be indicated in the following circumstances: [1] deer tick AND [2] has been attached for more than 24 hours or appears swollen (engorged from feeding) AND [3] Lyme disease is relatively common in the region.

How to Remove a Wood Tick

- **Best Method—Tweezers:** Use a tweezers and grasp the wood tick close to the skin (on its head). Pull the wood tick straight upward without twisting or crushing it. Maintain a steady pressure until it releases its grip. If tweezers aren't available, use fingers, a loop of thread around the jaws, or a needle between the jaws for traction. Research (Needham 1985) has demonstrated that this is the best method for tick removal.
- **Methods That Do Not Work:** Covering a tick with petroleum jelly, 70% rubbing alcohol, or fingernail polish does not work. Touching a tick with a red-hot match does not work. Source: Needham 1985.

How to Remove a Tiny Deer Tick

- Deer ticks are very small and need to be scraped off with a credit card edge or the edge of a knife blade.

How to Remove Seed Ticks (Turkey Ticks, Turkey Mites)

- "Seed ticks," "turkey ticks," and "turkey mites" are all layperson terms for the larval stage of the lone star tick. A female tick can lay several thousand eggs at a time. These eggs hatch at about the same time. If a potential host (animal, human) brushes past, hundreds of these tiny larvae can attach nearly simultaneously.
- It is believed that seed ticks do not spread any disease. This makes sense because they are at the larval stage and have not yet eaten a blood meal from an animal.
- **Symptoms:** A person will note tens or hundreds of tiny poppy seed-sized moving black dots on his or her skin.
- **How to Remove Seed Ticks:** Various removal strategies have been described. Probably the best way to remove seed ticks that are newly attached is to take a shower and use soap and a washcloth.
- Packaging tape or any adhesive tape will also work. You should be able to see the seed ticks on the tape after you pull the tape off the skin. Using tweezers is unnecessary and tedious.

TOOTHACHE

DEFINITION

- Pain or discomfort in a tooth
- Not due to a traumatic injury

Pain Severity Is Defined As:

- **Mild (1-3):** Doesn't interfere with chewing
- **Moderate (4-7):** Interferes with chewing, interferes with normal activities, awakens from sleep
- **Severe (8-10):** Unable to eat, unable to do any normal activities, excruciating pain

TRIAGE ASSESSMENT QUESTIONS

Call EMS 911 Now

- Pale cold skin and very weak (can't stand)
  R/O: shock
- Similar pain previously and it was from "heart attack"
  R/O: cardiac ischemia, myocardial infarction
- Similar pain previously and it was from "angina" and not relieved by nitroglycerin
  R/O: cardiac ischemia, myocardial infarction
- Sounds like a life-threatening emergency to the triager

See More Appropriate Protocol

- Chest pain
  Go to Protocol: Chest Pain on page 48
- Toothache followed tooth injury
  Go to Protocol: Trauma, Tooth on page 317

Go to ED Now (or to Office With PCP Approval)

- Patient sounds very sick or weak to the triager

Go to Office Now

- Face is swollen
  R/O: dental abscess with secondary facial cellulitis
- Fever
  R/O: dental abscess

Call Dentist Now

- SEVERE toothache pain

Call Dentist Today

- Toothache present > 24 hours
  R/O: tooth decay, enamel fracture
- Brown cavity visible in the painful tooth
  R/O: tooth decay
- Red or yellow lump present at the gumline of the painful tooth
  R/O: periapical gum abscess
- Lost crown
  Reason: replace crown. See FIRST AID.
- Lost filling
  Reason: replace filling. See FIRST AID.
- Broken braces wire or end of braces wire is jabbing into gum, cheek, or tongue
  Reason: fix orthodontia wire. See FIRST AID.
- Patient wants to be seen

Home Care

- Minor toothache present < 24 hours

HOME CARE ADVICE FOR MILD TOOTHACHE

1. **Reassurance:** Most toothaches are temporary and due to a sensitive tooth. If the pain becomes worse or does not resolve in 24 hours, it could be due to a small cavity.
2. **Floss:** Floss on either side of the painful tooth to remove any wedged food.
3. **Pain Medicines:**
   - For pain relief, take acetaminophen, ibuprofen, or naproxen.

   Acetaminophen (e.g., Tylenol):
   - Take 650 mg by mouth every 4-6 hours as needed. Each Regular Strength Tylenol pill has 325 mg of acetaminophen. The most you should take each day is 3,250 mg (10 pills a day).
   - Another choice is to take 1,000 mg every 8 hours. Each Extra Strength Tylenol pill has 500 mg of acetaminophen. The most you should take each day is 3,000 mg (6 pills a day).

   Ibuprofen (e.g., Motrin, Advil):
   - Take 400 mg by mouth every 6 hours.
   - Another choice is to take 600 mg by mouth every 8 hours.

   Naproxen (e.g., Aleve):
   - Take 250-500 mg by mouth every 12 hours.

Extra Notes:

- Acetaminophen is thought to be safer than ibuprofen or naproxen in people over 65 years old. Acetaminophen is in many OTC and prescription medicines. It might be in more than one medicine that you are taking. You need to be careful and not take an overdose. An acetaminophen overdose can hurt the liver.
- **Caution:** Do not take acetaminophen if you have liver disease.
- **Caution:** Do not take ibuprofen if you have stomach problems, kidney disease, are pregnant, or have been told by your doctor to avoid this type of anti-inflammatory drug. Do not take ibuprofen for more than 7 days without consulting your doctor.
- Use the lowest amount of medicine that makes your pain feel better.
- Before taking any medicine, read all the instructions on the package

4. **Local Cold:** Apply an ice pack to the painful jaw for 20 minutes.
5. **Expected Course:** Most minor causes of toothache resolve in less than a day.
6. **Call Your Dentist If:**
   - Toothache persists longer than 24 hours.
   - The toothache becomes worse.

FIRST AID

First Aid Advice for Lost Crown

- Obtain some over-the-counter dental cement from your local pharmacy.
- Coat the inside of the crown with the dental cement.
- Place the crown back over the tooth.

Notes:

- You can use dental adhesive if you cannot obtain dental cement.
- Remember to see your dentist as soon as possible.

First Aid Advice for Lost Filling

- Push a piece of sugarless chewing gum into the cavity hole.

Notes:

- You can use over-the-counter dental cement instead of chewing gum.
- Remember to see your dentist as soon as possible.

First Aid Advice for Pain From Braces Wire Poking Cheek, Gum, or Tongue

- Cover the end of the wire with orthodontic wax or a cotton ball.

BACKGROUND INFORMATION

The main cause of toothache is tooth decay (cavities). Complications of tooth decay can also cause pain. For example, a periapical abscess (pus pocket) can develop around the base of tooth with a cavity.

Dental Causes of Toothache

- **Dental Caries (Tooth Decay):** Pulpitis, periapical abscess
- Food stuck between teeth
- Losts crown
- Lost filling
- **Periodontal Disease (Gum Disease):** Gingivitis, periodontal abscess, pericoronitis
- Tooth fracture (broken or cracked tooth)

Other Causes of Toothache

- Canker sore (aphthous ulcer)
- Cardiac ischemia
- Ludwig angina
- Sinusitis
- TMJ syndrome
- Trigeminal neuralgia

Complications of Tooth Decay

- Cellulitis of the cheek.
- Periapical dental abscess.
- **Ludwig Angina:** This serious infection is a rapidly progressive cellulitis of the floor of the mouth that usually is a complication of a dental abscess or tooth extraction. The presenting symptoms are fever, a swollen/tender tongue, and difficulty swallowing.
- Submandibular lymphadenitis.

Caution—Cardiac Ischemia

- Rarely patients may present with toothache or jaw pain as the sole symptom of a myocardial infarction. Usually there will be other associated symptoms of cardiac ischemia: chest pain, shortness of breath, nausea, and/or diaphoresis.
- Cardiac ischemia should be suspected in any patients with risk factors for cardiac disease. These include: hypertension, smoking, diabetes, hyperlipidemia, a strong family history of heart disease, and age > 50.

TRAUMA, ANKLE AND FOOT

DEFINITION

- Injuries to a bone, muscle, joint, or ligament of the ankle and foot.
- Associated skin and soft tissue injuries are also included.

TRIAGE ASSESSMENT QUESTIONS

Call EMS 911 Now

- Major bleeding (actively dripping or spurting) that can't be stopped
  FIRST AID: Apply direct pressure to the entire wound with a clean cloth.
- Amputation or bone sticking through the skin
  FIRST AID: Apply direct pressure to the entire wound with a clean cloth.
- Injury looks like a dislocated joint (crooked or deformed)
  R/O: dislocation, fracture
- Sounds like a life-threatening emergency to the triager

See More Appropriate Protocol

- Wound looks infected
  Go to Protocol: Wound Infection on page 344
- Caused by an animal bite
  Go to Protocol: Animal Bite on page 13
- Puncture wound of foot
  Go to Protocol: Puncture Wound on page 206
- Toe injury is main concern
  Go to Protocol: Trauma, Toe on page 314

Go to ED Now

- Bullet, stabbed by knife, or other serious penetrating wound
  FIRST AID: If penetrating object still in place, don't remove it.

Go to ED Now (or to Office With PCP Approval)

- Can't stand (bear weight) or walk (e.g., 4 steps)
  R/O: fracture, severe sprain
- Skin is split open or gaping (or length > ½ inch or 12 mm)
  R/O: need for sutures
- Bleeding won't stop after 10 minutes of direct pressure (using correct technique)
- Dirt in the wound and not removed after 15 minutes of scrubbing
  Reason: needs irrigation or debridement
- Numbness (new loss of sensation) of toe(s)
- Looks infected (e.g., spreading redness, pus, red streak)
  R/O: cellulitis, lymphangitis
- Sounds like a serious injury to the triager

See Today in Office

- Severe pain (e.g., excruciating)
  R/O: fracture, severe sprain
- Limping
- A "snap" or "pop" was heard at the time of injury
  R/O: ligament tear
- Suspicious history for the injury
  R/O: domestic violence or elder abuse
- Large swelling or bruise (> 2 inches or 5 cm)
- Patient wants to be seen

See Today or Tomorrow in Office

- Diabetes
  Reason: diabetic neuropathy reduces pain of fracture and wound infection
- High-risk adult (e.g., age > 60, osteoporosis, chronic steroid use)
  Reason: greater risk of fracture in patients with osteoporosis
- Wound and no tetanus booster in > 5 years (Or greater than 10 years for clean cuts)

See Within 3 Days in Office

- Injury and pain has not improved after 3 days
- Injury is still painful or swollen after 2 weeks

Home Care

- Minor ankle or foot injury
  R/O: bruise, strain, or sprain

HOME CARE ADVICE FOR MINOR BRUISE, SPRAIN, OR STRAIN

1. **Treatment of Minor Bruise (e.g., Direct Blow to Ankle or Foot):**
   - Apply a cold pack or an ice bag (wrapped in a moist towel) for 20 minutes each hour for 4 consecutive hours (20 minutes of cooling followed by 40 minutes of rest for 4 hours in a row). 48 hours after the injury, use local heat for 10 minutes 3 times each day to help reabsorb the blood.
   - Rest the injured part as much as possible for 48 hours.
2. **Treatment of Minor Sprains and Strains of Foot and Ankle:**
   - **First Aid:** Wrap with a snug elastic bandage. Apply an ice pack (crushed ice in a plastic bag covered with a moist towel) to reduce bleeding, swelling, and pain.
   - Treat with RICE (rest, ice, compression, and elevation) for the first 24 to 48 hours.
   - REST the injured leg for 24 hours. You may return to normal activity after 24 hours of rest if the activity does not cause pain.
   - Continue to apply crushed ICE packs for 10-20 minutes every hour for the first 4 hours. Then apply ice for 10-20 minutes 4 times a day for the first 2 days.
   - Apply COMPRESSION by wrapping the injured part with a snug, elastic bandage for 48 hours. If you experience numbness, tingling, or increased pain in the injured part, the bandage may be too tight. Loosen the bandage wrap.
   - Keep injured ankle or foot ELEVATED and at rest for 24 hours. Keep your foot up on a pillow and stay off your feet as much as possible.
3. **Pain Medicines:**
   - For pain relief, take acetaminophen, ibuprofen, or naproxen.

   Acetaminophen (e.g., Tylenol):
   - Take 650 mg by mouth every 4-6 hours as needed. Each Regular Strength Tylenol pill has 325 mg of acetaminophen. The most you should take each day is 3,250 mg (10 pills a day).
   - Another choice is to take 1,000 mg every 8 hours. Each Extra Strength Tylenol pill has 500 mg of acetaminophen. The most you should take each day is 3,000 mg (6 pills a day).

   Ibuprofen (e.g., Motrin, Advil):
   - Take 400 mg by mouth every 6 hours.
   - Another choice is to take 600 mg by mouth every 8 hours.

   Naproxen (e.g., Aleve):
   - Take 250-500 mg by mouth every 12 hours.

   Extra Notes:
   - Acetaminophen is thought to be safer than ibuprofen or naproxen in people over 65 years old. Acetaminophen is in many OTC and prescription medicines. It might be in more than one medicine that you are taking. You need to be careful and not take an overdose. An acetaminophen overdose can hurt the liver.
   - **Caution:** Do not take acetaminophen if you have liver disease.
   - **Caution:** Do not take ibuprofen if you have stomach problems, kidney disease, are pregnant, or have been told by your doctor to avoid this type of anti-inflammatory drug. Do not take ibuprofen for more than 7 days without consulting your doctor.
   - Use the lowest amount of medicine that makes your pain feel better.
   - Before taking any medicine, read all the instructions on the package
4. **Expected Course:** Pain and swelling usually begin to improve 2 or 3 days after an injury. Swelling is usually gone in 7 days. Pain may take 2 weeks to completely resolve.
5. **Call Back If:**
   - Pain becomes severe.
   - Pain does not improve after 3 days.
   - Pain or swelling lasts more than 2 weeks.
   - You become worse.

FIRST AID

First Aid Advice for Bleeding:

Apply direct pressure to the entire wound with a clean cloth.

First Aid Advice for Penetrating Object:

If penetrating object still in place, don't remove it.

First Aid Advice for Shock:

Lie down with feet elevated.

First Aid Advice for a Sprain or Twisting Injury of Ankle or Foot:

- Apply a cold pack or an ice bag (wrapped in a moist towel) to the area for 20 minutes.
- Wrap area with an elastic bandage.

First Aid Advice for Suspected Fracture or Dislocation of Ankle or Foot:

- Do not remove the shoe.
- Immobilize the ankle and foot by wrapping them with a soft splint (e.g., a pillow, a rolled-up blanket, a towel).
- Use tape to keep this splint in place.

Transport of an Amputated Body Part:

- Briefly rinse amputated part with water (to remove any dirt).
- Place amputated part in plastic bag (to protect and keep clean).
- Place plastic bag containing part in a container of ice (to keep cool and preserve tissue).

BACKGROUND INFORMATION

Types of Foot and Ankle Injuries

- **Achilles Tendon Rupture:** There is pain in the Achilles tendon (area above heel and behind ankle). There is weakness or inability to extend the foot (e.g., can't stand on tiptoes).
- **Contusion:** A direct blow or crushing injury results in bruising of the skin, muscle, and underlying bone.
- Cuts, abrasions.
- Dislocations (bone out of joint).
- Fractures (broken bones).
- **Sprains:** Stretches and tears of ligaments.
- **Strains:** Stretches and tears of muscles (e.g., pulled muscle).

TRAUMA, ELBOW

DEFINITION

- Injuries to a bone, muscle, joint, or ligament of the elbow.
- Associated skin and soft tissue injuries are also included.

TRIAGE ASSESSMENT QUESTIONS

Call EMS 911 Now

- Major bleeding (actively dripping or spurting) that can't be stopped
  FIRST AID: Apply direct pressure to the entire wound with a clean cloth.
- Amputation or bone sticking through the skin
- Serious injury with multiple fractures
- Bullet, stabbed by knife, or other serious penetrating wound
  FIRST AID: If penetrating object still in place, don't remove it.
- Sounds like a life-threatening emergency to the triager

See More Appropriate Protocol

- Wound looks infected
  Go to Protocol: Wound Infection on page 344
- Shoulder injury
  Go to Protocol: Trauma, Shoulder on page 307
- Hand or wrist injury
  Go to Protocol: Trauma, Hand and Wrist on page 287

Go to ED Now

- Injury looks like a broken bone or dislocated joint (crooked or deformed)

Go to ED Now (or to Office With PCP Approval)

- Can't bend injured elbow at all
  R/O: fracture
- Skin is split open or gaping (or length > ½ inch or 12 mm)
  R/O: need for sutures
- Bleeding won't stop after 10 minutes of direct pressure (using correct technique)
- Dirt in the wound and not removed after 15 minutes of scrubbing
  Reason: needs irrigation or debridement
- Numbness (loss of sensation) of finger(s), present now
  R/O: nerve injury
- Sounds like a serious injury to the triager

See Today in Office

- Severe pain (e.g., excruciating)
- Can't move injured elbow normally (i.e., bend or straighten completely)
  R/O: minor fracture
- Large swelling or bruise (> 2 inches or 5 cm)
- Suspicious history for the injury
  R/O: domestic violence or elder abuse
- Patient wants to be seen

See Today or Tomorrow in Office

- High-risk adult (e.g., age > 60, osteoporosis, chronic steroid use)
  Reason: greater risk of fracture in patients with osteoporosis
- Wound and no tetanus booster in > 5 years (or greater than 10 years for clean cuts)

See Within 3 Days in Office

- Pain has not improved after 3 days
- Injury is still painful or swollen after 2 weeks

Home Care

- Minor elbow injury
  R/O: bruise, strain, or sprain

HOME CARE ADVICE FOR TRAUMA, ELBOW

1. **Treatment of a Bruise (e.g., Direct Blow to Elbow):**
   - Apply a cold pack or an ice bag (wrapped in a moist towel) to the area for 20 minutes each hour for 4 consecutive hours (20 minutes of cooling followed by 40 minutes of rest for 4 hours in a row).
   - Rest the injured part as much as possible for 48 hours.
   - 48 hours after the injury, use local heat for 10 minutes 3 times each day to help reabsorb the blood.
2. **Treatment of Sprains and Strains:**
   - **First Aid:** Wrap with a snug elastic bandage. Apply an ice pack (crushed ice in a plastic bag covered with a moist towel) to reduce bleeding, swelling, and pain.
   - Treat with RICE (rest, ice, compression, and elevation) for the first 24 to 48 hours.
   - REST the injured part for 24 hours. You may return to normal activity after 24 hours of rest if the activity does not cause pain.
   - Continue to apply crushed ICE packs for 10-20 minutes every hour for the first 4 hours. Then apply ice for 10-20 minutes 4 times a day for the first 2 days.
   - Apply COMPRESSION by wrapping the injured part with a snug, elastic bandage for 48 hours. If you experience numbness, tingling, or increased pain in the injured part, the bandage may be too tight. Loosen the bandage wrap.
   - Keep injured arm ELEVATED and at rest for 24 hours. Put your arm on a pillow positioned
   - above heart level.
3. **Pain Medicines:**
   - For pain relief, take acetaminophen, ibuprofen, or naproxen.

   Acetaminophen (e.g., Tylenol):
   - Take 650 mg by mouth every 4-6 hours as needed. Each Regular Strength Tylenol pill has 325 mg of acetaminophen. The most you should take each day is 3,250 mg (10 pills a day).
   - Another choice is to take 1,000 mg every 8 hours. Each Extra Strength Tylenol pill has 500 mg of acetaminophen. The most you should take each day is 3,000 mg (6 pills a day).

   Ibuprofen (e.g., Motrin, Advil):
   - Take 400 mg by mouth every 6 hours.
   - Another choice is to take 600 mg by mouth every 8 hours.

   Naproxen (e.g., Aleve):
   - Take 250-500 mg by mouth every 12 hours.

   Extra Notes:
   - Acetaminophen is thought to be safer than ibuprofen or naproxen in people over 65 years old. Acetaminophen is in many OTC and prescription medicines. It might be in more than one medicine that you are taking. You need to be careful and not take an overdose. An acetaminophen overdose can hurt the liver.
   - **Caution:** Do not take acetaminophen if you have liver disease.
   - **Caution:** Do not take ibuprofen if you have stomach problems, kidney disease, are pregnant, or have been told by your doctor to avoid this type of anti-inflammatory drug. Do not take ibuprofen for more than 7 days without consulting your doctor.
   - Use the lowest amount of medicine that makes your pain feel better.
   - Before taking any medicine, read all the instructions on the package
4. **Expected Course:** Pain and swelling usually begin to improve 2 or 3 days after an injury. Swelling is usually gone in 7 days. Pain may take 2 weeks to completely resolve.
5. **Call Back If:**
   - Pain becomes severe.
   - Pain does not improve after 3 days.
   - Pain or swelling lasts more than 2 weeks.
   - You become worse.

FIRST AID

First Aid Advice for Bleeding:

Apply direct pressure to the entire wound with a clean cloth.

First Aid Advice for Penetrating Object:

If penetrating object still in place, don't remove it (Reason: removal could increase bleeding).

First Aid Advice for Shock:

Lie down with feet elevated.

First Aid Advice for Suspected Fracture or Dislocation of the Elbow:

- Use a sling to support the arm. Make the sling with a triangular piece of cloth.
- Or, at the very least, the patient can support the injured arm with the other hand or a pillow.

BACKGROUND INFORMATION

Types of Elbow Injuries:

- Bone bruise from a direct blow (e.g., elbow)
- Dislocations (bone out of joint)
- Fractures (broken bones)
- Muscle overuse injuries from sports or exercise (e.g., tennis elbow)
- Muscle bruise from a direct blow
- **Sprains:** Stretches and tears of ligaments
- **Strains:** Stretches and tears of muscles (e.g., pulled muscle)
- Traumatic olecranon bursitis

Bruised "Funny Bone"

- A direct blow to the near side of the posterior elbow can cause numbess, tingling, and burning in the hand. The involved fingers are usually the middle, ring, and pinky (little).
- The "funny bone" is actually a nerve (ulnar) which wraps around the posterior part of your elbow.
- Symptoms from bruising your funny bone usually last only a few minutes. If the symptoms last longer than 30 minutes or if this problem seems to happen too frequently, then the patient will need to see the doctor for evaluation.

What to Suture

- Any cut that is split open or gaping probably needs sutures. Cuts longer than ½ inch (1 cm) usually need sutures. Any open wound that may need sutures should be evaluated by a physician regardless of the time that has passed since the initial injury.

Tetanus Booster

- **Clean Cuts and Scrapes: Every 10 Years:** Patients with clean MINOR wounds AND who have previously had 3 or more tetanus shots (full series), need a booster every 10 years. Examples of minor wounds include a superficial abrasion or a shallow cut from a clean knife blade. Obtain booster within 72 hours.
- **Dirty Wounds: Every 5 Years:** Patients with dirty wounds need a booster every 5 years. Examples of dirty wounds include those contaminated with soil, feces, saliva, and more serious wounds from deep punctures, crushing, and burns. Obtain booster within 72 hours.

TRAUMA, EYE

DEFINITION

- Injuries to the eye, eyelid, and area around the eye

TRIAGE ASSESSMENT QUESTIONS

Call EMS 911 Now

- Knocked unconscious > 1 minute
  R/O: concussion
- Sounds like a life-threatening emergency to the triager

See More Appropriate Protocol

- Wound looks infected
  Go to Protocol: Wound Infection on page 344
- Foreign body in the eye
  Go to Protocol: Eye, Foreign Body on page 111
- Head injury is the primary problem
  Go to Protocol: Trauma, Head on page 290

Go to ED Now

- Vision is blurred or lost in either eye
  R/O: acute hyphema
- Double vision or unable to look upward
  R/O: blowout fracture
- Bloody or cloudy fluid behind the cornea (clear part)
  R/O: acute hyphema

Go to ED Now (or to Office With PCP Approval)

- Object hit the eye at high speed (e.g., from a lawn mower)
  R/O: penetrating injury or foreign body
- Sharp object hit the eye (e.g., metallic chip)
- Any cut on the eyelid or eyeball
  R/O: eyeball perforation
- Skin is split open or gaping (length > ¼ inch or 6 mm)
  R/O: need for sutures
- Bleeding won't stop after 10 minutes of direct pressure (using correct technique)
- Two black eyes (both sides)
  R/O: "raccoon eyes" from basilar skull fracture
- Sounds like a serious injury to the triager

Go to Office Now

- Severe pain
  R/O: penetrating injury or foreign body
- Constant tearing or blinking
- Patient keeps the eye covered or refuses to open it
  R/O: corneal abrasion

See Today in Office

- Suspicious history for the injury
  R/O: domestic violence or elder abuse
- Large swelling or bruise (wider than 2 inches, 5 cm) at the site of the injury
- Eyelids swollen shut
- Scratch on white of the eye (sclera)
- Patient wants to be seen

See Today or Tomorrow in Office

- Wound and no tetanus booster in > 5 years (or greater than 10 years for clean cuts)

See Within 3 Days in Office

- Pain has not improved after 3 days
  R/O: small fracture
- Pain or swelling persisting > 7 days

Home Care

- Minor eye injury
  R/O: superficial cut or abrasion, bruise
- Minor flame-shaped bruise on sclera (white part of eyeball)
  R/O: small subconjunctival hemorrhage

HOME CARE ADVICE FOR MINOR INJURIES OF THE EYE

1. **Treatment of Superficial Cuts and Scrapes (Abrasions) to Eyelid or Area Around Eye:**
   - Apply direct pressure with a sterile gauze or clean cloth for 10 minutes to stop any bleeding.
   - Wash the wound with soap and water for 5 minutes (protect the eye with a clean cloth).
   - Apply an antibiotic ointment. Cover large scrapes with a Band-Aid or dressing. Change daily.

2. **Treatment of Swelling or Bruise With Intact Skin:**
   - Apply an ice pack to the area for 20 minutes each hour for 4 consecutive hours.
   - 48 hours after the injury, use local heat for 10 minutes 3 times each day to help reabsorb the blood.
3. **Treatment of Subconjunctival Hemorrhage** (flame-shaped bruise of the white area of eyeball): No specific treatment is required. It usually goes away in 2-3 weeks.
4. **Pain Medicines:**
   - For pain relief, take acetaminophen, ibuprofen, or naproxen.

   Acetaminophen (e.g., Tylenol):
   - Take 650 mg by mouth every 4-6 hours as needed. Each Regular Strength Tylenol pill has 325 mg of acetaminophen. The most you should take each day is 3,250 mg (10 pills a day).
   - Another choice is to take 1,000 mg every 8 hours. Each Extra Strength Tylenol pill has 500 mg of acetaminophen. The most you should take each day is 3,000 mg (6 pills a day).

   Ibuprofen (e.g., Motrin, Advil):
   - Take 400 mg by mouth every 6 hours.
   - Another choice is to take 600 mg by mouth every 8 hours.

   Naproxen (e.g., Aleve):
   - Take 250-500 mg by mouth every 12 hours.

   Extra Notes:
   - Acetaminophen is thought to be safer than ibuprofen or naproxen in people over 65 years old. Acetaminophen is in many OTC and prescription medicines. It might be in more than one medicine that you are taking. You need to be careful and not take an overdose. An acetaminophen overdose can hurt the liver.
   - **Caution:** Do not take acetaminophen if you have liver disease.
   - **Caution:** Do not take ibuprofen if you have stomach problems, kidney disease, are pregnant, or have been told by your doctor to avoid this type of anti-inflammatory drug. Do not take ibuprofen for more than 7 days without consulting your doctor.
   - Use the lowest amount of medicine that makes your pain feel better.
   - Before taking any medicine, read all the instructions on the package
5. **Call Back If:**
   - Pain becomes severe.
   - Pain does not improve after 3 days.
   - Changes in vision.
   - You become worse.

FIRST AID

First Aid Advice for Bleeding:
- Apply direct pressure to the entire wound with a clean cloth.
- Try to avoid pressure on the eyeball.

First Aid Advice for Penetrating Object:
If penetrating object still in place, don't remove it (Reason: removal could cause bleeding or more damage).

First Aid Advice for Shock:
Lie down with feet elevated.

BACKGROUND INFORMATION

Vision and Trauma to the Eye
- The main concern in all eye injuries is whether the vision is damaged.
- It is important to test vision in both eyes. If there has been no damage to the vision, then most likely there is no serious injury to the eyeball. Test vision at home by covering each eye in turn and looking at a near object and then a distant object. Is the vision blurred in comparison to normal?

Common Injuries to the Eye and Orbital Area
- **Black Eye:** Bruising and purple discoloration of the eyelids and upper cheek is referred to as a black eye. Usually it is the result of a direct blow to this area (e.g., a punch). It gets worse for the first couple days. It usually goes away in 2-3 weeks.
- **Corneal Abrasion (Scratch):** A corneal abrasion is one of the most common eye injuries. The typical mechanism is an accidental scratch from a fingernail, piece of paper, or the branch of a tree. It can be quite painful. Generally, a minor corneal abrasion will heal in 1-2 days; it is treated with antibiotic eyedrops and (sometimes) patching.

- **Eye Laceration, Puncture Wound:** Penetrating eye injuries are always very serious. They may be caused by a sharp object (laceration) or from a small object traveling at high speed (puncture wound with intraocular foreign body).
- **Eyelid Laceration, Puncture Wound:** Always consider the possibility that the wound went through the eyelid into the eye.
- **Hyphema:** Blood is visible inside the front portion of eye (anterior chamber) just behind the cornea. This finding is serious and can occur with either blunt or penetrating eye trauma.
- **Orbital Fracture (Blowout Fracture):** The bony walls of the socket in which the eye sits are somewhat thin and can be fractured with blunt trauma. The appearance is similar to a black eye. The pain and swelling are usually worse, and sometimes the patient may complain of double vision.
- **Subconjunctival Hemorrhage:** This is the medical term for a flame-shaped bruise of the white area of the eyeball, which sometimes occurs after a direct blow to the eye. It looks as though a red patch was "painted" on to the eye. It usually goes away in 2-3 weeks.

Unilateral Dilated Pupil (Anisocoria)

- Anisocoria is the medical term for unequal pupil sizes.
- **Normal Variant:** Most commonly unequal pupils are a normal variant. Approximately 10% of the population has anisocoria. This is almost always the reason in alert individuals without other serious neurologic symptoms. One simple way to check to see if someone always has anisocoria is to look at a driver's license photo or other photo that shows the pupils.
- **Local Eye Trauma (Traumatic Mydriasis):** Blunt trauma to one eye can cause unilateral dilation of the pupil (traumatic mydriasis). Associated symptoms will include eye pain, eye redness, blurred vision, and photophobia.
- **As a Sign of Brain Stem Herniation:** A unilaterally dilated pupil in the setting of head trauma always raises the concern about brain hemorrhage (intracranial hematoma, swelling, and herniation). A dilated pupil from brain herniation is always accompanied by altered mental status, severe headache, and other neurologic symptoms. Thus, if a patient is comatose AND has a unilateral widely dilated pupil, brain stem herniation should be suspected.

What to Suture

- Any cut that is split open or gaping probably needs sutures. Cuts on the face longer than ¼ inch (6 mm) usually need sutures. Any open wound that may need sutures should be evaluated by a physician regardless of the time that has passed since the initial injury.

Caution: Associated Head and Neck Trauma

- Head trauma should be considered in all patients with a facial injury. Signs of significant head injury include loss of consciousness, amnesia, unsteady walking, confusion, and slurred speech.
- Neck trauma should also be considered in all patients with a facial injury. Concerning findings include: numbness, weakness, and neck pain.
- After using the Trauma, Eye protocol, if the triager or caller has remaining concerns about head or neck trauma, then the patient also should be triaged using the Trauma, Head protocol on page 290.

TRAUMA, FINGER

DEFINITION

- Injuries to finger(s).
- Finger injuries include cuts, abrasions, jammed finger, smashed finger, fingernail injury, subungual hematoma, dislocations, and fractures.

TRIAGE ASSESSMENT QUESTIONS

Call EMS 911 Now

- Major bleeding (actively dripping or spurting) that can't be stopped
  FIRST AID: Apply direct pressure to the entire wound with a clean cloth.
- Sounds like a life-threatening emergency to the triager

See More Appropriate Protocol

- Wound looks infected
  Go to Protocol: Wound Infection on page 344
- Caused by animal bite
  Go to Protocol: Animal Bite on page 13

Go to ED Now

- Amputation
  FIRST AID: Apply direct pressure to the entire wound with a clean cloth.
- High-pressure injection injury (e.g., from paint gun, usually work-related)
  Reason: deep tissue damage may exceed superficial injury

Go to ED Now (or to Office With PCP Approval)

- Looks like a broken bone (e.g., crooked or deformed)
- Looks like a dislocated joint (e.g., crooked or deformed)
- Skin is split open or gaping (or length > ½ inch or 12 mm)
  R/O: need for sutures
- Cut or scrape is very deep (e.g., can see bone or tendons)
  R/O: tendon injury
- Bleeding won't stop after 10 minutes of direct pressure (using correct technique)
  R/O: need for sutures
- Dirt in the wound and not removed after 15 minutes of scrubbing
  Reason: needs irrigation or debridement
- Cut with numbness (loss of sensation) of finger
  R/O: digital nerve laceration
- Fingernail is partially torn from a crush injury
  Exception: torn nail from catching it on something
- Sounds like a serious injury to the triager

Go to Office Now

- Looks infected (e.g., spreading redness, pus, red streak)
  R/O: cellulitis, lymphangitis
- Fingernail is completely torn off
- Base of fingernail has popped out from under skin fold (cuticle)
  Reason: needs to be reinserted under the skin

See Today in Office

- Severe pain
  R/O: fracture
- Moderate-severe pain and blood present under the nail (usually > 50% of nail bed)
  R/O: severe subungual hematoma needing drainage
- Finger joint can't be opened (straightened) or closed (bent) completely
  R/O: fracture, tendon injury
- Suspicious history for the injury
  R/O: domestic violence or elder abuse
- Patient wants to be seen

See Today or Tomorrow in Office

- Injury interferes with work or school
- Wound and no tetanus booster in > 5 years (or greater than 10 years for clean cuts)

See Within 3 Days in Office

- Pain has not improved after 3 days
- Injury is still painful or swollen after 2 weeks

Home Care

- Minor finger injury
  R/O: minor bruise or sprain, scrapes, small subungual hematoma

HOME CARE ADVICE FOR MILD INJURIES OF FINGER

1. **Treatment of Cuts, Scratches, and Scrapes (Abrasions):**
   - Apply direct pressure for 10 minutes to stop any bleeding.
   - Wash the wound with soap and water for 5 minutes.
   - Scrub out any dirt gently with a washcloth.
   - Cut off any pieces of dead loose skin using fine scissors (clean scissors with rubbing alcohol before and after use).
   - Apply an antibiotic ointment, covered by a Band-Aid or dressing. Change daily.
2. **Treatment of Bruised Finger:** Soak the finger in cold water for 20 minutes.
3. **Treatment of Jammed Finger:**
   - **Caution:** Be certain range of motion is normal (can bend and straighten each finger).
   - Soak the finger in cold water for 20 minutes.
   - If the pain is more than mild, protect it by buddy-taping it to the next finger.
4. **Treatment of Smashed or Crushed Fingertip:**
   - Apply an ice bag to the area for 20 minutes.
   - Wash the finger with soap and water for 5 minutes.
   - Trim any small pieces of torn dead skin with a scissors cleaned with rubbing alcohol.
   - Cover any cuts with an antibiotic ointment and Band-Aid. Change daily.
5. **Treatment of Subungual Hematoma (Blood Under the Nail):** Apply an ice bag to the area for 20 minutes.
6. **Torn Nail (From Catching It on Something):**
   - For a cracked nail without rough edges, leave it alone.
   - For a large flap of nail that is almost torn through, use a sterile scissors to cut it off along the line of the tear (Reason: pieces of nail will catch on objects and tear further).
   - Apply an antibiotic ointment and cover with a Band-Aid. Change daily.
   - After about 7 days, the nail bed should be covered by new skin and no longer hurt. It takes about 6-12 weeks for a fingernail to grow back completely.
7. **Pain Medicines:**
   - For pain relief, take acetaminophen, ibuprofen, or naproxen.

   Acetaminophen (e.g., Tylenol):
   - Take 650 mg by mouth every 4-6 hours as needed. Each Regular Strength Tylenol pill has 325 mg of acetaminophen. The most you should take each day is 3,250 mg (10 pills a day).
   - Another choice is to take 1,000 mg every 8 hours. Each Extra Strength Tylenol pill has 500 mg of acetaminophen. The most you should take each day is 3,000 mg (6 pills a day).

   Ibuprofen (e.g., Motrin, Advil):
   - Take 400 mg by mouth every 6 hours.
   - Another choice is to take 600 mg by mouth every 8 hours.

   Naproxen (e.g., Aleve):
   - Take 250-500 mg by mouth every 12 hours.

   Extra Notes:
   - Acetaminophen is thought to be safer than ibuprofen or naproxen in people over 65 years old. Acetaminophen is in many OTC and prescription medicines. It might be in more than one medicine that you are taking. You need to be careful and not take an overdose. An acetaminophen overdose can hurt the liver.
   - **Caution:** Do not take acetaminophen if you have liver disease.
   - **Caution:** Do not take ibuprofen if you have stomach problems, kidney disease, are pregnant, or have been told by your doctor to avoid this type of anti-inflammatory drug. Do not take ibuprofen for more than 7 days without consulting your doctor.
   - Use the lowest amount of medicine that makes your pain feel better.
   - Before taking any medicine, read all the instructions on the package
8. **Call Back If:**
   - Cut or scrape looks infected (redness, red streak, or pus).
   - Pain becomes severe.
   - Pain does not improve after 3 days.
   - Pain or swelling lasts more than 2 weeks.
   - You become worse.

FIRST AID

First Aid Advice for Bleeding:

Apply direct pressure to the entire wound with a clean cloth.

First Aid Advice for Penetrating Object:

If penetrating object still in place, don't remove it (Reason: removal could increase bleeding).

First Aid Advice for Shock:

Lie down with feet elevated.

First Aid Advice for a Sprain of the Finger:

- Remove any rings or jewelry from the injured finger.
- Tape the injured finger to the finger next to it (this is called a buddy splint).
- Apply a cold pack or an ice bag (wrapped in a moist towel) to the area for 20 minutes.

First Aid Advice for Suspected Fracture or Dislocation of the Finger:

- Remove any rings or jewelry from the injured finger.
- Tape the injured finger to the finger next to it (this is called a buddy splint).
- Apply a cold pack or an ice bag (wrapped in a moist towel) to the area for 20 minutes.

First Aid Advice for Transport of an Amputated Finger:

- Briefly rinse amputated part with water (to remove any dirt).
- Place amputated part in plastic bag (to protect and keep clean).
- Place plastic bag containing part in a cup of ice water (to keep cool and preserve tissue).

BACKGROUND INFORMATION

Type of Finger Injuries

1. **Cuts, Abrasions (Skinned Knuckles), and Bruises:** The most common injuries.
2. **Jammed Finger:**
   - **Description:** The end of a straightened finger or thumb receives a blow (usually from a ball). The energy is absorbed by the ligaments (sprain) and the finger joints. For jammed fingers, always check carefully that the injured person can fully straighten (extend) the end of the finger. If the person cannot straighten the finger, the diagnosis may be a mallet finger; see below.
3. **Mallet Finger:**
   - **Description:** The injured person will report that he or she is not able to straighten the end of the finger (DIP joint) completely.
   - **Mechanism:** The most common mechanism is being jammed by a ball (e.g., playing softball without a glove).
   - **Pathology:** This occurs because of either a tear of the extensor tendon at the DIP joint or an avulsion fracture where the extensor tendon attaches to the distal phalanx.
4. **Crushed or Smashed Fingertip (e.g., Slammed Door, Machine Accident):**
   - **Minor Injuries:** The most common injuries are bruising, a blood blister, or a small cut.
   - **Moderate Injuries:** Lacerations of skin or nail bed that require suturing. Fractures of the fingertip (distal phalanx) can occur and are painful but usually not serious. There is a slight risk for osteomyelitis if there is an open wound overlying the fractured bone.
   - **Major Injuries:** Severe crush injuries, amputation, or near-amputation.
5. **Fingernail Injury:**
   - Most fingernail injuries are not in and of themselves serious.
   - **Nail Bed Laceration:** With significant crush injuries (e.g., slammed door, machine accident) a minor injury of the nail may be covering up a major laceration of the nail bed. If the nail bed is lacerated, suturing may be required to prevent a future deformed fingernail. Sometimes the surgeon or ER doctor will use the old nail during the repair; this is the reason the patient should bring the nail.
6. **Finger Amputation:** Patients with this type of injury need to go to the emergency department. In some cases reimplantation is possible. In most cases, a repair-revision of the remaining portion of the finger is the best surgical treatment.

7. **Subungual Hematoma (Bruised Fingernail)**
   - **Definition:** Bleeding under the nail.
   - **Mechanism:** Usually caused by a crush injury from a door or a heavy object falling on the finger while it is on a firm surface.
   - **Treatment of a Small Subungal Hematorma:** Small subungual hematomas have blood under less than 50% of the nail. Pain is mild to moderate. Treatment consists of pain medications, application of cold packs, and time. After a couple days the pain will feel better. The bruising disappears over 2-4 weeks.
   - **Treatment of a Large Subungal Hematorma:** Large subungual hematomas have blood under more than 50% of the nail. Pain can be moderate to severe and throbbing. The doctor may need to drill (or burn) a tiny hole in the nail to reduce the pressure and to relieve pain. Additional treatment consists of pain medications and application of cold packs. Many of these patients will lose the nail sometime in the next couple weeks.
8. **Fractures or Dislocations**
   - **Fractures:** Fractures of the finger can occur and are painful but usually not serious. If there is no deformity, most can be treated with a simple finger splint. There is a slight risk for osteomyelitis if there is an open wound overlying the fractured bone.
   - **Dislocation:** The injured person will report pain and visible deformity of one of the finger joints. Treatment consists of reducing the dislocation and splinting.

What to Suture

- Any cut that is split open or gaping probably needs sutures. Cuts longer than ½ inch (1 cm) usually need sutures. Any open wound that may need sutures should be evaluated by a physician regardless of the time that has passed since the initial injury.

Tetanus Booster

- **Clean Cuts and Scrapes: Every 10 Years:** Patients with clean MINOR wounds AND who have previously had 3 or more tetanus shots (full series), need a booster every 10 years. Examples of minor wounds include a superficial abrasion, a shallow cut from a clean knife blade, or a small glass cut sustained while washing dishes. Obtain booster within 72 hours.
- **Dirty Wounds: Every 5 Years:** Patients with dirty wounds need a booster every 5 years. Examples of dirty wounds include those contaminated with soil, feces, saliva, and more serious wounds from deep punctures, crushing, and burns. Obtain booster within 72 hours.

TRAUMA, HAND AND WRIST

DEFINITION

- Injuries to a bone, muscle, joint, or ligament in the hand.
- Associated skin and soft tissue injuries are also included.

TRIAGE ASSESSMENT QUESTIONS

Call EMS 911 Now

- Major bleeding (actively dripping or spurting) that can't be stopped
  FIRST AID: Apply direct pressure to the entire wound with a clean cloth.
- Amputation or bone sticking through the skin
  FIRST AID: Apply direct pressure to the entire wound with a clean cloth.
- Sounds like a life-threatening emergency to the triager

See More Appropriate Protocol

- Finger injury is main concern
  Go to Protocol: Trauma, Finger on page 283
- Caused by an animal bite
  Go to Protocol: Animal Bite on page 13
- Wound looks infected
  Go to Protocol: Wound Infection on page 344

Go to ED Now

- Bullet, stabbed by knife, or other serious penetrating wound
  FIRST AID: If penetrating object still in place, don't remove it.
- High-pressure injection injury (e.g., from paint gun, usually work-related)
  Reason: deep tissue damage may exceed superficial injury

Go to ED Now (or to Office With PCP Approval)

- Injury looks like a broken bone or dislocated joint (crooked or deformed)
  R/O: fracture, dislocation
- Skin is split open or gaping (or length > ½ inch or 12 mm)
  R/O: need for sutures
- Bleeding won't stop after 10 minutes of direct pressure (using correct technique)
- Dirt in the wound and not removed after 15 minutes of scrubbing
  Reason: needs irrigation or debridement
- Numbness (loss of sensation) of finger(s)
  R/O: nerve injury
- Sounds like a serious injury to the triager

Go to Office Now

- Looks infected (e.g., spreading redness, pus, red streak)
  R/O: cellulitis, lymphangitis

See Today in Office

- Severe pain
  R/O: fracture, severe sprain
- Large swelling or bruise (> 2 inches or 5 cm)
- Suspicious history for the injury
  R/O: domestic violence or elder abuse
- Patient wants to be seen

See Today or Tomorrow in Office

- Injury interferes with work or school
- High-risk adult (e.g., age > 60, osteoporosis, chronic steroid use)
  Reason: greater risk of fracture in patients with osteoporosis
- Wound and no tetanus booster in > 5 years (or greater than 10 years for clean cuts)

See Within 3 Days in Office

- Injury and pain has not improved after 3 days
- Injury is still painful or swollen after 2 weeks

Home Care

- ○ Minor wrist or hand injury
  R/O: bruise, strain, or sprain

HOME CARE ADVICE FOR MINOR INJURIES OF HAND AND WRIST

1. **Treatment of Bruise (e.g., Direct Blow to Hand or Wrist):**
   - Apply a cold pack or an ice pack (wrapped in a moist towel) to the area for 20 minutes each hour for 4 consecutive hours (20 minutes of cooling followed by 40 minutes of rest for 4 hours in a row).
   - 48 hours after the injury, use local heat for 10 minutes 3 times each day to help reabsorb the blood.
   - Rest the injured part as much as possible for 48 hours.
2. **Treatment of Sprains and Strains:**
   - **First Aid:** Wrap with a snug elastic bandage. Apply an ice pack (crushed ice in a plastic bag covered with a moist towel) to reduce bleeding, swelling, and pain.
   - Treat with RICE (rest, ice, compression, and elevation) for the first 24 to 48 hours.
   - REST the injured part for 24 hours. You may return to normal activity after 24 hours of rest if the activity does not cause pain.
   - Continue to apply crushed ICE packs for 10-20 minutes every hour for the first 4 hours. Then apply ice for 10-20 minutes 4 times a day for the first 2 days.
   - Apply COMPRESSION by wrapping the injured part with a snug, elastic bandage for 48 hours. If you experience numbness, tingling, or increased pain in the injured part, the bandage may be too tight. Loosen the bandage wrap.
   - Keep injured hand or wrist ELEVATED and at rest for 24 hours. Put your hand and wrist on a pillow positioned above heart level.
3. **Pain Medicines:**
   - For pain relief, take acetaminophen, ibuprofen, or naproxen.

   Acetaminophen (e.g., Tylenol):
   - Take 650 mg by mouth every 4-6 hours as needed. Each Regular Strength Tylenol pill has 325 mg of acetaminophen. The most you should take each day is 3,250 mg (10 pills a day).
   - Another choice is to take 1,000 mg every 8 hours. Each Extra Strength Tylenol pill has 500 mg of acetaminophen. The most you should take each day is 3,000 mg (6 pills a day).

   Ibuprofen (e.g., Motrin, Advil):
   - Take 400 mg by mouth every 6 hours.
   - Another choice is to take 600 mg by mouth every 8 hours.

   Naproxen (e.g., Aleve):
   - Take 250-500 mg by mouth every 12 hours.

   Extra Notes:
   - Acetaminophen is thought to be safer than ibuprofen or naproxen in people over 65 years old. Acetaminophen is in many OTC and prescription medicines. It might be in more than one medicine that you are taking. You need to be careful and not take an overdose. An acetaminophen overdose can hurt the liver.
   - **Caution:** Do not take acetaminophen if you have liver disease.
   - **Caution:** Do not take ibuprofen if you have stomach problems, kidney disease, are pregnant, or have been told by your doctor to avoid this type of anti-inflammatory drug. Do not take ibuprofen for more than 7 days without consulting your doctor.
   - Use the lowest amount of medicine that makes your pain feel better.
   - Before taking any medicine, read all the instructions on the package
4. **Expected Course:** Pain and swelling usually begin to improve 2 or 3 days after an injury. Swelling is usually gone in 7 days. Pain may take 2 weeks to completely resolve.
5. **Call Back If:**
   - Pain becomes severe.
   - Pain does not improve after 3 days.
   - Pain or swelling lasts more than 2 weeks.
   - You become worse.

FIRST AID

First Aid Advice for Bleeding:

Apply direct pressure to the entire wound with a clean cloth.

First Aid Advice for Severe Bleeding:

- Place 2 or 3 sterile dressings (or a clean towel or washcloth) over the wound immediately.
- Apply direct pressure to the wound, using your entire hand.
- If bleeding continues, apply pressure more forcefully or move the pressure to a slightly different spot.
- Act quickly because ongoing blood loss can cause shock.
- Do not use a tourniquet.

First Aid Advice for Penetrating Object:

If penetrating object still in place, don't remove it (Reason: removal could increase bleeding).

First Aid Advice for Shock:

Lie down with feet elevated.

First Aid Advice for a Sprain or Twisting Injury of Hand or Wrist:

- Apply a cold pack or an ice bag (wrapped in a moist towel) to the area for 20 minutes.
- Wrap area with an elastic bandage.

First Aid Advice for Suspected Fracture or Dislocation of Hand or Wrist:

- Immobilize the hand and wrist by placing them on a rigid splint (e.g., small board, magazine folded in half, folded-up newspaper).
- Tie several cloth strips around hand/wrist to keep the splint in place.
- Place injured arm in a sling. If no sling is available, victim can support the injured arm with the other non-injured hand.
- **Option—Soft Splint:** Immobilize the hand and wrist by wrapping them with a soft splint (e.g., a pillow, a rolled-up blanket, a towel). Use tape to keep this splint in place.

Transport of an Amputated Body Part:

- Briefly rinse amputated part with water (to remove any dirt).
- Place amputated part in plastic bag (to protect and keep clean).
- Place plastic bag containing part in a container of ice (to keep cool and preserve tissue).

BACKGROUND INFORMATION

Types of Injuries

- Fractures (broken bones)
- Dislocations (bone out of joint)
- **Sprains:** Stretches and tears of ligaments
- **Strains:** Stretches and tears of muscles (pulled muscle)
- **Contusion (Bruise):** A direct blow or crushing injury

TRAUMA, HEAD

DEFINITION

- Injuries to the head, including scalp, skull, and brain trauma

TRIAGE ASSESSMENT QUESTIONS

Call EMS 911 Now

- Acute neurologic symptom and symptom present now
  Definition: difficult to awaken OR confused thinking and talking OR slurred speech OR weakness of arms OR unsteady walking
  R/O: cerebral contusion, subdural or epidural hematoma
- Knocked out (unconscious) > 1 minute
  R/O: concussion, intracranial bleeding
- Seizure (convulsion) occurred
  Exception: prior history of seizures and now alert and without acute neurologic symptoms)
  Note: consider using Seizure protocol after triage with Trauma, Head protocol.
- Neck pain after dangerous injury (e.g., MVA, diving, trampoline, contact sports, fall > 10 feet, 305 cm)
  Exception: neck pain began > 1 hour after injury
  FIRST AID: Protect the neck from movement.
- Major bleeding (actively dripping or spurting) that can't be stopped
  FIRST AID: Apply direct pressure to the entire wound with a clean cloth.
- Penetrating head injury (e.g., knife, gunshot wound, metal object)
  FIRST AID: Don't remove penetrating object.
- Sounds like a life-threatening emergency to the triager

Go to ED Now

- Can't remember what happened (amnesia)
  Reason: probable concussion, needs neurologic examination
- Vomiting once or more
  R/O: concussion
- Watery or blood-tinged fluid dripping from the nose or ears
  R/O: basilar skull fracture

Go to ED Now (or to Office With PCP Approval)

- Acute neurologic symptom and now fine
- Knocked out (unconscious) < 1 minute and now fine
- Severe headache
- Dangerous injury (e.g., MVA, diving, trampoline, contact sports, fall > 10 feet or 3 meters) or severe blow from hard object (e.g., golf club or baseball bat)
  Reason: increased risk of injury
- Large swelling and size > palm of person's hand
  R/O: fracture, hematoma
- Skin is split open or gaping (or length > ½ inch or 12 mm)
  R/O: need for sutures
- Bleeding won't stop after 10 minutes of direct pressure (using correct technique)
- Black eyes on both sides and onset within 24 hours of head injury
  R/O: basilar skull fracture
- Taking Coumadin (warfarin), Pradaxa (dabigatran), or known bleeding disorder (e.g., thrombocytopenia)
  Reason: higher risk of cerebral bleed; may need for testing of INR, ProTime, or platelet count
- Sounds like a serious injury to the triager

See Today in Office

- Suspicious history for the injury
  R/O: domestic violence or elder abuse
- Patient wants to be seen

See Today or Tomorrow in Office

- After 3 days and headache persists
  R/O: fracture, concussion
- Wound and no tetanus booster in > 5 years (or greater than 10 years for clean cuts)

Home Care

- Minor head injury
  R/O: bruise, superficial cut or abrasion

HOME CARE ADVICE FOR MINOR HEAD INJURY

1. **Treatment of Minor Cuts, Scratches, and Scrapes (Abrasions):**
   - Apply direct pressure for 10 minutes to stop any bleeding.
   - Wash the wound with soap and water for 5 minutes.
   - For any dirt, scrub it gently with a washcloth.
   - Apply an antibiotic ointment daily.
2. **Treatment of Bruise or Hematoma ("Goose Egg"):**
   - Apply an ice bag or massage the area with ice for 20 minutes each hour for 4 consecutive hours (20 minutes of ice bag massage followed by 40 minutes of rest for 4 hours in a row).
   - 48 hours after the injury, use local heat for 10 minutes 3 times each day to help reabsorb the blood.
3. **Observation:**
   - The head-injured person should be observed closely during the first 2 hours following the injury.
   - The head-injured person should be awakened every 4 hours for the first 24 hours; check for the ability to walk and talk.
   - Mild headache, mild dizziness, and nausea are common.
4. **Diet:** Clear fluids to drink at first, in case of vomiting. May resume a regular diet after 2 hours.
5. **Pain Medicines:**
   - For pain relief, take acetaminophen, ibuprofen, or naproxen.

   Acetaminophen (e.g., Tylenol):
   - Take 650 mg by mouth every 4-6 hours as needed. Each Regular Strength Tylenol pill has 325 mg of acetaminophen. The most you should take each day is 3,250 mg (10 pills a day).
   - Another choice is to take 1,000 mg every 8 hours. Each Extra Strength Tylenol pill has 500 mg of acetaminophen. The most you should take each day is 3,000 mg (6 pills a day).

   Ibuprofen (e.g., Motrin, Advil):
   - Take 400 mg by mouth every 6 hours.
   - Another choice is to take 600 mg by mouth every 8 hours.

   Naproxen (e.g., Aleve):
   - Take 250-500 mg by mouth every 12 hours.

   Extra Notes:
   - Acetaminophen is thought to be safer than ibuprofen or naproxen in people over 65 years old. Acetaminophen is in many OTC and prescription medicines. It might be in more than one medicine that you are taking. You need to be careful and not take an overdose. An acetaminophen overdose can hurt the liver.
   - **Caution:** Do not take acetaminophen if you have liver disease.
   - **Caution:** Do not take ibuprofen if you have stomach problems, kidney disease, are pregnant, or have been told by your doctor to avoid this type of anti-inflammatory drug. Do not take ibuprofen for more than 7 days without consulting your doctor.
   - Use the lowest amount of medicine that makes your pain feel better.
   - Before taking any medicine, read all the instructions on the package
6. **Expected Course:**
   - Most head trauma only causes an injury to the scalp.
   - Pain and swelling usually begin to improve 2 or 3 days after an injury.
   - Swelling is usually gone in 7 days. Pain and tenderness at the site may take 1-2 weeks to completely resolve.
7. **Call Back If:**
   - Severe headache.
   - Extremity weakness or numbness occurs.
   - Slurred speech or blurred vision occurs.
   - Vomiting occurs.
   - You become worse.

FIRST AID

First Aid Advice for Bleeding:
Apply direct pressure to the entire wound with a clean cloth.

First Aid Advice for Penetrating Object:
If penetrating object still in place, don't remove it (Reason: removal could increase bleeding).

First Aid Advice for Shock:
Lie down with feet elevated.

First Aid Advice for Suspected Spinal Cord Injury:
Do not move until a spine board is applied.

First Aid Advice for Bruise:
Apply a cold pack or an ice bag (wrapped in a moist towel) to the area for 20 minutes.

BACKGROUND INFORMATION

Types of Head Injury
- **Skin Trauma:** Cut, scrape, bruise, or scalp hematoma (goose egg).
- **Skull Trauma:** Fracture.
- **Brain Trauma:** Concussion and other brain injuries can be recognized by the presence of loss of consciousness, amnesia, or other acute neurologic symptoms.

Acute Neurologic Symptoms—Requiring an EMS 911 Disposition
- The following acute neurologic symptoms after a head injury should receive an EMS 911 disposition:
  - Difficult to awaken OR
  - Confused or slow thinking and talking OR
  - Slurred speech OR
  - Weakness of arms or legs OR
  - Unsteady walking

What to Suture:
- Any cut that is split open or gaping probably needs sutures. Cuts longer than ½ inch (1 cm) usually need sutures. Any open wound that may need sutures should be evaluated by a physician regardless of the time that has passed since the initial injury.

Tetanus Booster
- **Clean Cuts and Scrapes: Every 10 Years:** Patients with clean MINOR wounds AND who have previously had 3 or more tetanus shots (full series), need a booster every 10 years. Examples of minor wounds include a superficial abrasion or a small cut sustained from standing up suddenly and hitting a clean metal cabinet. Obtain booster within 72 hours.
- **Dirty Wounds: Every 5 Years:** Patients with dirty wounds need a booster every 5 years. Examples of dirty wounds include any cut contaminated with soil, feces, saliva, and more serious wounds from deep punctures, crushing, and burns. Obtain booster within 72 hours.

Raccoon Eyes (Bilateral Black Eyes) Following Head Trauma
- The cause of bilateral black eyes can be determined by the timing of their onset.
- Forehead hematomas cause most of them. The black eyes appear 2 to 3 days after the initial minor forehead injury. Mechanism is the seepage of blood downward through the tissue planes with the help of gravity.
- Basilar skull fracture is occasionally the cause. A fracture of the frontal part of the base of skull can cause blood to seep anteriorly into the orbits. The black eyes usually appear within 12 hours of the initial injury. Also, there is no forehead bruise. Basilar skull fractures usually only follow major head trauma. Acute neurologic findings (e.g., altered mental status) are usually present.

Concussion
- **Definition:** A temporary impairment in neurologic function following a traumatic injury to the brain. A concussion is a functional disturbance in brain activity, not a structural injury. Loss of consciousness is not required.
- **Symptoms:** Headache, nausea, and feeling irritable and sleepy are common, especially during the first couple days after a concussion. Other symptoms of a concussion include amnesia (can't remember what happened), dizziness, difficulty concentrating or "foggy" feeling, poor memory, feeling tired, feeling dazed or not your normal self, and decreased coordination.

- **Diagnosis:** The diagnosis is made by a doctor based upon the clinical examination of the injured person. The CT scan of a patient with a concussion (and no other brain injuries) is normal. Often a head CT scan does not need to be performed.
- **Expected Course:** The majority (80-90%) of concussions resolve in 7-10 days.
- **Classification:** See American Academy of Neurology (AAN) classification below.
- **Return to Sports:** See the AAN recommendations below.
- **Prognosis:** Most people who sustain a concussion recover completely and there are no signs of permanent damage. Sometimes a person can have concussion symptoms that last for weeks or months afterwards.

AAN Concussion Classification

(American Academy of Neurology, 1997)

- **Grade 1:** Transient confusion; no loss of consciousness; concussion symptoms or mental status abnormalities on examination RESOLVE IN LESS THAN 15 MINUTES.
- **Grade 2:** Transient confusion; no loss of consciousness; concussion symptoms or mental status abnormalities on examination LAST MORE THAN 15 MINUTES.
- **Grade 3:** Any LOC, either brief (seconds) or prolonged (minutes).
- **Note:** All individuals with concussions need a neurologic examination by a health care provider.

Sports-Related Concussion and Sideline Evaluation

(*Clin J Sport Med.* 2009;19[3]:185–200)

- The player should be medically evaluated onsite using standard emergency management principles, and particular attention should be given to excluding a cervical spine injury.
- The appropriate disposition of the player must be determined by the treating health care provider in a timely manner. If no health care provider is available, the player should be safely removed from practice or play and urgent referral to a physician arranged.
- Once the first aid issues are addressed, then an assessment of the concussive injury should be made using the SCAT2 or other similar tool.
- The player should not be left alone following the injury, and serial monitoring for deterioration is essential over the initial few hours following injury.
- A player with diagnosed concussion should not be allowed to return to play on the day of injury.

Sports-Related Concussion and When to Return to Play

(*Clin J Sport Med.* 2009;19[3]:185–200)

- Return to play protocol following a concussion follows a stepwise process as outlined in bullets below. Generally, each step should take 24 hours; an athlete would typically take approximately 1 week to proceed through the full rehabilitation protocol assuming that patient has no post-concussion symptoms. If any post-concussion symptoms occur while in the stepwise program, then the patient should drop back to the previous asymptomatic level and try to progress again after a further 24-hour period of rest has passed.
- **Stage 1:** No activity.
- **Stage 2:** Light aerobic activity (walking, swimming, stationary cycling).
- **Stage 3:** Sports-specific exercise.
- **Stage 4:** Noncontact training drills.
- **Stage 5:** Full-contact practice.
- **Stage 6:** Return to play.
- **Note:** Multiple concussions require longer periods of recovery before returning to sports. The reason we sideline athletes who have a concussion is to prevent the "second impact injury." This is a second concussion that occurs within 1 or 2 weeks after the first one. The outcome can be catastrophic or even death.

Unilateral Dilated Pupil (Anisocoria)

- Anisocoria is the medical term for unequal pupil sizes.
- **Normal Variant:** Most commonly unequal pupils are a normal variant. Approximately 10% of the population has anisocoria. This is almost always the reason in alert individuals without other serious neurologic symptoms. One way to check to see if someone always has anisocoria is to look at a good-resolution (image size/detail) photo that shows the pupils; a driver's license photo is handy but the resolution is often to poor to be of use.
- **Local Eye Trauma (Traumatic Mydriasis):** Blunt trauma to one eye can cause unilateral dilation of the pupil (traumatic mydriasis). Associated symptoms will include eye pain, eye redness, blurred vision, and photophobia.
- **As a Sign of Brain Stem Herniation:** A unilaterally dilated pupil in the setting of head trauma always raises the concern about brain hemorrhage (intracranial hematoma, swelling, and herniation). A dilated pupil from brain herniation is always accompanied by altered mental status, severe headache, and other neurologic symptoms. Thus, if a patient is comatose AND has a unilateral widely dilated pupil, brain stem herniation should be suspected.

Air Bag Deployment

- Air bags inflate within 50 milliseconds of impact and at a speed of 100 miles per hour.
- The gas produced to inflate the air bag is harmless. The CDC reports no poisoning from air bag deployment (2009).
- In adults, air bag injuries are mainly minor abrasions or bruises. The areas most commonly affected are the face, arms, and hands; the skin may look red or abraded from being "slapped" by the air bag as it deployed.

Caution: Associated Neck Trauma

- Neck trauma should also be considered in all patients with a head injury. Concerning findings include: numbness, weakness, and neck pain.

TRAUMA, HIP

DEFINITION

- Injuries to a bone, muscle, joint, or ligament of the hip.
- Associated skin and soft tissue injuries are also included.

TRIAGE ASSESSMENT QUESTIONS

Call EMS 911 Now

- Major bleeding (actively dripping or spurting) that can't be stopped
  FIRST AID: Apply direct pressure to the entire wound with a clean cloth.
- Bullet, stabbed by knife, or other serious penetrating wound
  FIRST AID: If penetrating object still in place, don't remove it.
- Injury looks like a dislocated joint (crooked or deformed)
  R/O: fracture
- Can't stand (bear weight) or walk
- Sounds like a life-threatening emergency to the triager

See More Appropriate Protocol

- Wound looks infected
  Go to Protocol: Wound Infection on page 344
- Puncture wound of hip area
  Go to Protocol: Puncture Wound on page 206

Go to ED Now (or to Office With PCP Approval)

- Severe pain
- Skin is split open or gaping (or length > ½ inch or 12 mm)
  R/O: need for sutures
- Bleeding won't stop after 10 minutes of direct pressure (using correct technique)
- Dirt in the wound and not removed after 15 minutes of scrubbing
  Reason: needs irrigation or debridement
- Sounds like a serious injury to the triager

Go to Office Now

- Looks infected (e.g., spreading redness, pus, red streak)
  R/O: cellulitis, lymphangitis

See Today in Office

- Suspicious history for the injury
  R/O: domestic violence or elder abuse
- Patient wants to be seen

See Today or Tomorrow in Office

- Injury interferes with work or school
- High-risk adult (e.g., age > 60, osteoporosis, chronic steroid use)
  Reason: greater risk of fracture in patients with osteoporosis
- Wound and no tetanus booster in > 5 years (or greater than 10 years for clean cuts)

See Within 3 Days in Office

- Injury and pain has not improved after 3 days
- Injury is still painful or swollen after 2 weeks

Home Care

- Minor hip injury
  R/O: minor bruise, strain, or sprain of hip

HOME CARE ADVICE FOR MINOR BRUISE, SPRAIN, OR STRAIN

1. **Treatment of Bruise (e.g., Direct Blow to Hip Area):**
   - Apply a cold pack or an ice bag (wrapped in a towel) for 20 minutes each hour for 4 consecutive hours (20 minutes of cold followed by 40 minutes of rest for 4 hours in a row).
   - 48 hours after the injury, use local heat for 10 minutes 3 times each day to help reabsorb the blood.
   - Rest the injured part as much as possible for 48 hours.

2. **Treatment of Sprains and Strains of Hip and Upper Thigh:**
   - **First Aid:** Apply an ice pack (crushed ice in a plastic bag covered with a towel) to reduce bleeding, swelling, and pain.
   - REST the injured leg for 24 hours. You may return to normal activity after 24 hours of rest if the activity does not cause pain.
   - Continue to apply crushed ICE packs for 10-20 minutes every hour for the first 4 hours. Then apply ice for 10-20 minutes 4 times a day for the first 2 days.
   - Keep injured leg ELEVATED and at rest for 24 hours. Put your leg up on a pillow and stay off your feet as much as possible.
3. **Pain Medicines:**
   - For pain relief, take acetaminophen, ibuprofen, or naproxen.

   Acetaminophen (e.g., Tylenol):
   - Take 650 mg by mouth every 4-6 hours as needed. Each Regular Strength Tylenol pill has 325 mg of acetaminophen. The most you should take each day is 3,250 mg (10 pills a day).
   - Another choice is to take 1,000 mg every 8 hours. Each Extra Strength Tylenol pill has 500 mg of acetaminophen. The most you should take each day is 3,000 mg (6 pills a day).

   Ibuprofen (e.g., Motrin, Advil):
   - Take 400 mg by mouth every 6 hours.
   - Another choice is to take 600 mg by mouth every 8 hours.

   Naproxen (e.g., Aleve):
   - Take 250-500 mg by mouth every 12 hours.

   Extra Notes:
   - Acetaminophen is thought to be safer than ibuprofen or naproxen in people over 65 years old. Acetaminophen is in many OTC and prescription medicines. It might be in more than one medicine that you are taking. You need to be careful and not take an overdose. An acetaminophen overdose can hurt the liver.
   - **Caution:** Do not take acetaminophen if you have liver disease.
   - **Caution:** Do not take ibuprofen if you have stomach problems, kidney disease, are pregnant, or have been told by your doctor to avoid this type of anti-inflammatory drug. Do not take ibuprofen for more than 7 days without consulting your doctor.
   - Use the lowest amount of medicine that makes your pain feel better.
   - Before taking any medicine, read all the instructions on the package
4. **Expected Course:** Pain and swelling usually begin to improve 2 or 3 days after an injury. Swelling is usually gone in 7 days. Pain may take 2 weeks to completely resolve.
5. **Call Back If:**
   - Pain becomes severe.
   - Pain does not improve after 3 days.
   - Pain or swelling lasts more than 2 weeks.
   - You become worse.

FIRST AID

First Aid Advice for Bleeding:
Apply direct pressure to the entire wound with a clean cloth.

First Aid Advice for Penetrating Object:
If penetrating object still in place, don't remove it (Reason: removal could increase bleeding).

First Aid Advice for Shock:
Lie down with feet elevated.

BACKGROUND INFORMATION

Types of Injuries
- Fractures (broken bones)
- Dislocations (bone out of joint)
- **Sprains:** Stretches and tears of ligaments
- **Strains:** Stretches and tears of muscles (pulled muscle)
- **Contusion (Bruise):** A direct blow or crushing injury resulting in bruising of the skin, muscle, and underlying bone

TRAUMA, KNEE

DEFINITION

- Injuries to a bone, muscle, joint, or ligament of the knee.
- Associated skin and soft tissue injuries are also included.

TRIAGE ASSESSMENT QUESTIONS

Call EMS 911 Now

- Major bleeding (actively dripping or spurting) that can't be stopped
  FIRST AID: Apply direct pressure to the entire wound with a clean cloth.
- Bullet, stabbed by knife, or other serious penetrating wound
  FIRST AID: If penetrating object still in place, don't remove it.
- Injury looks like a dislocated joint (crooked or deformed)
  R/O: fracture
- Sounds like a life-threatening emergency to the triager

See More Appropriate Protocol

- Wound looks infected
  Go to Protocol: Wound Infection on page 344

Go to ED Now (or to Office With PCP Approval)

- Can't stand (bear weight) or walk
- Skin is split open or gaping (or length > ½ inch or 12 mm)
  R/O: need for sutures
- Bleeding won't stop after 10 minutes of direct pressure (using correct technique)
- Dirt in the wound and not removed after 15 minutes of scrubbing
  Reason: needs irrigation or debridement
- Sounds like a serious injury to the triager

Go to Office Now

- Looks infected (e.g., spreading redness, pus, red streak)
  R/O: cellulitis, lymphangitis

See Today in Office

- Severe pain
  R/O: fracture, joint effusion, severe sprain
- Suspicious history for the injury
  R/O: domestic violence or elder abuse
- Patient wants to be seen

See Today or Tomorrow in Office

- A "snap" or "pop" was heard at the time of injury
  R/O: Cruciate ligament tear
- Large swelling or bruise (> 2 inches or 5 cm)
- Wound and no tetanus booster in > 5 years (or greater than 10 years for clean cuts)
- High-risk adult (e.g., age > 60, osteoporosis, chronic steroid use)
  Reason: greater risk of fracture in patients with osteoporosis

See Within 3 Days in Office

- Limping
- Knee giving way (or buckling) when walking
  R/O: tear of anterior or posterior cruciate ligament, quadriceps tendon tear
- Knee feels like it is locking (i.e., joint gets stuck, catching)
  R/O: meniscal tear
- Pain has not improved after 3 days
- Injury is still painful or swollen after 2 weeks

Home Care

- Minor knee injury
  R/O: minor bruise, strain, or sprain of knee

HOME CARE ADVICE FOR MINOR BRUISE, SPRAIN, OR STRAIN

1. **Treatment of Bruise (e.g., Direct Blow to Knee Area):**
    - Apply a cold pack or an ice bag (wrapped in a moist towel) for 20 minutes each hour for 4 consecutive hours. (20 minutes of cold followed by 40 minutes of rest for 4 hours in a row).
    - 48 hours after the injury, use local heat for 10 minutes 3 times each day to help reabsorb the blood.
    - Rest the injured part as much as possible for 48 hours.
2. **Treatment of Sprains and Strains of Knee:**
    - **First Aid:** Wrap with a snug elastic bandage. Apply an ice pack (crushed ice in a plastic bag covered with a moist towel) to reduce bleeding, swelling, and pain.
    - Treat with RICE (rest, ice, compression, and elevation) for the first 24 to 48 hours.
    - REST the injured leg for 24 hours. You may return to normal activity after 24 hours of rest if the activity does not cause pain.
    - Continue to apply crushed ICE packs for 10-20 minutes every hour for the first 4 hours. Then apply ice for 10-20 minutes 4 times a day for the first 2 days.
    - Apply COMPRESSION by wrapping the injured part with a snug, elastic bandage for 48 hours. If you experience numbness, tingling, or increased pain in the injured part, the bandage may be too tight. Loosen the bandage wrap.
    - Keep injured leg ELEVATED and at rest for 24 hours. Put your leg up on a pillow and stay off your feet as much as possible.
3. **Pain Medicines:**
    - For pain relief, take acetaminophen, ibuprofen, or naproxen.

    Acetaminophen (e.g., Tylenol):
    - Take 650 mg by mouth every 4-6 hours as needed. Each Regular Strength Tylenol pill has 325 mg of acetaminophen. The most you should take each day is 3,250 mg (10 pills a day).
    - Another choice is to take 1,000 mg every 8 hours. Each Extra Strength Tylenol pill has 500 mg of acetaminophen. The most you should take each day is 3,000 mg (6 pills a day).

    Ibuprofen (e.g., Motrin, Advil):
    - Take 400 mg by mouth every 6 hours.
    - Another choice is to take 600 mg by mouth every 8 hours.

    Naproxen (e.g., Aleve):
    - Take 250-500 mg by mouth every 12 hours.

    Extra Notes:
    - Acetaminophen is thought to be safer than ibuprofen or naproxen in people over 65 years old. Acetaminophen is in many OTC and prescription medicines. It might be in more than one medicine that you are taking. You need to be careful and not take an overdose. An acetaminophen overdose can hurt the liver.
    - **Caution:** Do not take acetaminophen if you have liver disease.
    - **Caution:** Do not take ibuprofen if you have stomach problems, kidney disease, are pregnant, or have been told by your doctor to avoid this type of anti-inflammatory drug. Do not take ibuprofen for more than 7 days without consulting your doctor.
    - Use the lowest amount of medicine that makes your pain feel better.
    - Before taking any medicine, read all the instructions on the package
4. **Expected Course:** Pain and swelling usually begin to improve 2 or 3 days after an injury. Swelling is usually gone in 7 days. Pain may take 2 weeks to completely resolve.
5. **Call Back If:**
    - Pain becomes severe.
    - Pain does not improve after 3 days.
    - Pain or swelling lasts more than 2 weeks.
    - You become worse.

FIRST AID

First Aid Advice for Bleeding:

Apply direct pressure to the entire wound with a clean cloth.

First Aid Advice for Penetrating Object:

If penetrating object still in place, don't remove it (Reason: removal could increase bleeding).

First Aid Advice for Shock:

Lie down with feet elevated.

First Aid Advice for Sprained Knee:

- Apply a cold pack or an ice bag (wrapped in a moist towel) to the area for 20 minutes.
- Wrap knee with an elastic bandage.

BACKGROUND INFORMATION

Types of Injuries

- Abrasions.
- **Contusion (Bruise):** A direct blow or crushing injury results in bruising of the skin, muscle, and underlying bone.
- Cuts (lacerations).
- Dislocation (bone out of joint).
- Dislocation of patella (kneecap out of joint).
- Fracture (broken bones).
- **Sprain:** Stretches and tears of ligaments.
- **Strain:** Stretches and tears of muscles (pulled muscle).
- **Quadriceps Tendon Rupture:** There is pain in the insertion of the quadriceps muscle into the patella (area just above kneecap). There is weakness or inability to extend the knee fully (e.g., while sitting down on chair can't straighten knee).

TRAUMA, MOUTH

DEFINITION

- Injuries to the lip, frenulum (flap under the upper lip), tongue, buccal mucosa (inner cheeks), floor of the mouth, roof of the mouth (hard and soft palate), or back of the mouth (tonsils, oropharynx).
- Infected mouth wounds are covered here because they may look different from wound infections of the skin.

TRIAGE ASSESSMENT QUESTIONS

Call EMS 911 Now

- Major bleeding (actively dripping or spurting) that can't be stopped
  FIRST AID: Apply direct pressure to the entire wound with a clean cloth.
- Fainted or too weak to stand following large blood loss
  R/O: impending shock
  FIRST AID: Lie down with feet elevated and apply pressure to the wound.
- Knocked out (unconscious) > 1 minute
  R/O: concussion
- Difficult to awaken or acting confused (e.g., disoriented, slurred speech)
  R/O: concussion, intoxication
- Difficulty breathing
  R/O: swelling occluding airway, aspiration of blood
- Severe neck pain
  R/O: cervical spine injury
  FIRST AID: Protect the neck from movement.
- Sounds like a life-threatening emergency to the triager

See More Appropriate Protocol

- Main injury is to the teeth
  Go to Protocol: Trauma, Tooth on page 317

Go to ED Now

- Can't open or close the mouth fully
  R/O: jaw fracture or TMJ dislocation
- Unable to swallow or new onset of drooling
  R/O: significant traumatic swelling, Ludwig angina

Go to ED Now (or to Office With PCP Approval)

- Gaping cut of outer lip
  R/O: need for sutures
- Gaping cut through border of the lip where it meets the skin
  Reason: cuts through vermillion border need precise approximation
- Gaping cut of tongue or inside the mouth and size > ½ inch (12 mm)
  R/O: need for sutures
- Bleeding won't stop after 10 minutes of direct pressure (using correct technique)
  R/O: need for sutures
- Injury to the back of the throat, tonsil, or soft palate (e.g., pencil or other sharp object placed in mouth)
  R/O: posterior pharynx injury needing close follow-up
- Bite does not feel normal
  R/O: tooth displacement, mandible or maxilla fracture
- Sounds like a serious injury to the triager

Go to Office Now

- Looks infected (fever, spreading redness, pus)
  Note: healing wound in mouth is NORMALLY WHITE for several days.

See Today in Office

- Severe pain
  R/O: severe injury
- Suspicious history for the injury
  R/O: domestic violence or elder abuse
- Patient wants to be seen

See Within 3 Days in Office

- Wound and no tetanus booster in > 5 years (or greater than 10 years for clean cuts)
- Pain has not improved after 3 days

Home Care

- ○ Minor mouth injury
  R/O: bruise, small cut or scrape
- ○ Minor mouth burn from hot food or drink (mouth pain or lip pain)

HOME CARE ADVICE

Minor Mouth Injury

1. **Reassurance:** It sounds like a minor injury that we can treat at home.
2. **Stop Any Bleeding:**
   - **For Bleeding of the Outer Lip:** Apply direct pressure to the entire wound with a clean cloth or gauze.
   - **For Bleeding of the Inner Lip:** Press bleeding site against teeth or jaw for 10 minutes.
   - **For Bleeding From the Tongue:** Squeeze or press the bleeding site with a sterile gauze or piece of clean cloth for 10 minutes.
   - **For Bleeding From the Tissue That Connects the Upper Lip to the Gum (i.e., Torn Frenulum):** Apply pressure for 10 minutes.
   - **Caution:** Once bleeding from inside the lip stops, don't pull the lip out again to look at it (Reason: the bleeding will start up again; minor tears of the frenulum do not require sutures).
3. **Treatment of Bruised Lip or Tongue:**
   - **Bruised Lip:** Apply a cold pack or an ice bag wrapped in a towel for 20 minutes each hour for 4 consecutive hours (20 minutes of cold followed by 40 minutes of rest for 4 hours in a row).
   - **Bruised Tongue:** Put a piece of ice or Popsicle on the area that was injured for 20 minutes.
   - This helps reduce the pain and swelling.
4. **Treatment of Minor Cuts or Scrapes (Abrasions) of Lip:**
   - Apply direct pressure for 10 minutes to stop any bleeding.
   - Wash the wound with soap and water for 5 minutes.
   - Gently scrub out any dirt with a washcloth.
   - Apply an antibiotic ointment twice daily.
5. **Treatment of Minor Cuts or Scrapes (Abrasions) of Tongue and Inner Cheek:**
   - Apply direct pressure for 10 minutes to stop any bleeding.
   - Rinse mouth or tongue wounds with warm water immediately after meals.
6. **Diet:**
   - Eat a soft diet.
   - Avoid any spicy, hot, salty, or citrus foods that might sting.
7. **Pain Medicines:**
   - For pain relief, take acetaminophen, ibuprofen, or naproxen.

Acetaminophen (e.g., Tylenol):
- Take 650 mg by mouth every 4-6 hours as needed. Each Regular Strength Tylenol pill has 325 mg of acetaminophen. The most you should take each day is 3,250 mg (10 pills a day).
- Another choice is to take 1,000 mg every 8 hours. Each Extra Strength Tylenol pill has 500 mg of acetaminophen. The most you should take each day is 3,000 mg (6 pills a day).

Ibuprofen (e.g., Motrin, Advil):
- Take 400 mg by mouth every 6 hours.
- Another choice is to take 600 mg by mouth every 8 hours.

Naproxen (e.g., Aleve):
- Take 250-500 mg by mouth every 12 hours.

Extra Notes:
- Acetaminophen is thought to be safer than ibuprofen or naproxen in people over 65 years old. Acetaminophen is in many OTC and prescription medicines. It might be in more than one medicine that you are taking. You need to be careful and not take an overdose. An acetaminophen overdose can hurt the liver.
- **Caution:** Do not take acetaminophen if you have liver disease.
- **Caution:** Do not take ibuprofen if you have stomach problems, kidney disease, are pregnant, or have been told by your doctor to avoid this type of anti-inflammatory drug. Do not take ibuprofen for more than 7 days without consulting your doctor.
- Use the lowest amount of medicine that makes your pain feel better.
- Before taking any medicine, read all the instructions on the package.

8. **Expected Course:**
    - Small cuts of the inner cheeks, inner lip, and tongue generally heal quickly and do not require suturing. They usually heal up in 3 to 7 days.
    - Bruised lips slowly get better over about a week.
    - Infections of mouth injuries are rare.
9. **Call Back If:**
    - Severe pain persists longer than 2 hours after pain medicine and ice.
    - Area looks infected (mainly increasing pain or swelling after 48 hours) (Caution: any healing wound in the mouth is normally white for several days).
    - Fever occurs.
    - You become worse.

Minor Mouth Burn From Hot Food or Drink

1. **Reassurance:**
    - Burns of the mouth from hot food usually are painful for 2 days.
    - They heal quickly because the lining of the mouth heals twice as fast as the skin.
2. **Local Ice:**
    - Put a piece of ice in the mouth immediately for 10 minutes (Reason: reduce swelling and pain).
    - Rinse the mouth with ice water every hour for 4 hours.
3. **Call Back If:**
    - Difficulty with swallowing occurs.
    - Difficulty with breathing occurs.
    - Pain becomes severe.
    - You become worse.

FIRST AID

First Aid Advice for Bleeding:

Apply direct pressure to the entire wound with a clean cloth.

First Aid Advice for Penetrating Object:

If penetrating object still in place, don't remove it (Reason: removal could increase bleeding).

First Aid Advice for Shock:

Lie down with feet elevated.

BACKGROUND INFORMATION

Types of Mouth Injuries

- Cuts and bruises of the lips.
- Cuts inside of the cheeks.
- Cuts and bruises of the tongue.
- **Wounds of Posterior Pharynx:** Wounds can sometimes occur in the posterior pharynx. Usually this is the result of running and falling while having a sharp object in the mouth (e.g., a pencil, fork). This occurs more commonly in children than in adults. Such wounds are potentially serious and nearly all require evaluation by a physician.

Causes

- **Altercations:** Direct blow from punch, kick, or object.
- Contact sports.
- Falls.
- Motor vehicle accidents.
- **Seizure:** After a generalized tonic-clonic (grand mal) seizure approximately 20-30% of patients will awaken with bruising or a laceration of the tongue. These wounds nearly always occur on the side of the tongue.
- **Syncope:** Tongue lacerations occur only rarely from a syncopal (fainting) episode. When a cut does occur, it is usually a bite wound from suddenly falling and striking the chin on the ground.

What Cuts Need to Be Sutured?

- **Outer Lip Lacerations:** Any wound of the lip that crosses the vermillion border (border of the lip where it meets the skin) needs to be sutured to ensure healing and for cosmetic reasons. A cut longer than ¼ inch (6 mm) of the outer lip or face may need sutures, especially if it is gaping.
- **Inner Lip and Cheek Lacerations:** Small cuts of the inner cheeks or inner lip generally heal quickly and do not require suturing. A gaping wound that is > ½ inch (12 mm) long may require sutures.
- **Tongue Lacerations:** Small cuts of the tongue generally heal quickly and do not require suturing. A gaping wound that is > ½ inch (12 mm) long may require sutures.
- Any open wound that may need sutures should be evaluated by a physician regardless of the time that has passed since the initial injury.

Tetanus Booster

- **Clean Cuts and Scrapes: Every 10 Years:** Patients with clean MINOR wounds AND who have previously had 3 or more tetanus shots (full series) need a booster every 10 years. Examples of minor wounds include a superficial abrasion or a paper cut. Obtain booster within 72 hours.
- **Dirty Wound: Every 5 Years:** Patients with dirty wounds need a booster every 5 years. Examples of dirty wounds include any cut contaminated with soil, feces, saliva, and more serious wounds from deep punctures, crushing, and burns. Obtain booster within 72 hours.

Hot Food Burns of the Mouth

- **Definition:** Hot food or drink causes burn of the mouth's lining (mucous membrane).
- **Symptoms:** Immediate pain and redness. Sometimes causes small second-degree burn with area of white mucosa.
- **Causes:** Hot pizza burn is common because melted cheese sticks to roof of mouth. Hot chocolate or tea, hot soups or stews, etc. Microwaved foods also have increased risk.
- **Complications:** Mainly severe localized pain. Inability to swallow fluids (or drooling) and dehydration are very rare.
- **Treatment:** Immediate application of cold water or ice for 5 to 10 minutes. Then analgesics and soft diet for 2 days.

Caution—Associated Head and Neck Trauma

- Head trauma should be considered in all patients with a mouth injury. Signs of significant head injury include loss of consciousness, amnesia, unsteady walking, confusion, and slurred speech.
- Neck trauma should also be considered in all patients with a facial injury. Concerning findings include: numbness, weakness, and neck pain.
- After using the Trauma, Mouth protocol, if the triager or caller has remaining concerns about head or neck trauma, then the patient also should be triaged using the Trauma, Head protocol on page 290.

TRAUMA, NOSE

DEFINITION

- Injuries to the inside or outside of the nose

TRIAGE ASSESSMENT QUESTIONS

Call EMS 911 Now

- Knocked unconscious > 1 minute
  R/O: concussion
- Major bleeding (actively dripping or spurting) that can't be stopped
  FIRST AID: Apply direct pressure to the nose, lean forward.
- Sounds like a life-threatening emergency to the triager

See More Appropriate Protocol

- Wound looks infected
  Go to Protocol: Wound Infection on page 344
- Nosebleed not from trauma
  Go to Protocol: Nosebleed on page 193

Go to ED Now (or to Office With PCP Approval)

- Nosebleed won't stop after 10 minutes of pinching the nostrils closed (applied twice)
- Black-and-blue skin around both eyes (bilateral periorbital ecchymosis)
  R/O: nasal fracture, ethmoid fracture, or raccoon eyes from basilar skull fracture
- Clear fluid is dripping from the nose
- Skin is split open or gaping (or length > ¼ inch or 6 mm)
  R/O: need for sutures
- Sounds like a serious injury to the triager

Go to Office Now

- Very deformed or crooked nose
  R/O: fracture
- Breathing through the nose is blocked on one side or both sides
  R/O: nasal septal hematoma, significant fracture
- Fever and increasing nose pain, 2 or more days after injury
  R/O: nasal septal abscess

See Today in Office

- Severe pain
- Tip of nose is very tender
- Suspicious history for the injury
  R/O: domestic violence or elder abuse
- Nosebleed and taking Coumadin or known bleeding disorder (e.g., thrombocytopenia)
  Reason: INR level needed
- Patient wants to be seen

See Today or Tomorrow in Office

- Wound and no tetanus booster in > 5 years (or greater than 10 years for clean cuts)

See Within 3 Days in Office

- After 5 days and shape of the nose has not returned to normal
  R/O: fracture with deformity

Home Care

- Minor nose injury
  R/O: bruise, superficial cut or abrasion
  R/O: non-displaced fracture

HOME CARE ADVICE FOR MINOR INJURY OF THE NOSE

1. **Treatment of Superficial Cuts and Scrapes (Abrasions):**
   - Apply direct pressure with a sterile gauze or clean cloth for 10 minutes to stop any bleeding.
   - Wash the wound with soap and water for 5 minutes.
   - Apply an antibiotic ointment. Cover large scrapes with a Band-Aid or gauze dressing. Change daily.
2. **Treatment of Swelling or Bruise With Intact Skin:**
   - Apply a cold pack or an ice pack (wrapped in a moist towel) to the area for 20 minutes each hour for 4 consecutive hours.
   - 48 hours after the injury, use local heat for 10 minutes 3 times each day to help reabsorb the blood.

3. **Nosebleed:**
   - Place your thumb and index finger over each side of the soft lower portion of the nose.
   - Firmly pinch the nostrils together for 10-15 minutes.
4. **Concerns About a Broken (Fractured) Nose:**
   - Not all swollen noses have a fracture.
   - Even if the nose is broken, in most cases, the only treatment that is needed is cold packs and pain medications.
   - Surgery to fix the nose is only needed when the nose is very deformed. Swelling interferes with diagnosis and treatment. It is common practice is to delay fixing nose fractures until the swelling has decreased.
   - Looking at the nose after the swelling is gone (day 5 to 7) is the best way to tell if it is really fractured.
   - X-rays are often not helpful because 1) minor fractures are treated the same as a bruise, and 2) injuries to the cartilage do not show up on x-ray.
5. **Pain Medicine:**
   - For pain or fever relief, take acetaminophen.
   - Do not use aspirin for pain relief. Aspirin can interfere with normal blood clotting. Thus, it can increase the likelihood of nose bleeding

   Acetaminophen (e.g., Tylenol):
   - Take 650 mg by mouth every 4-6 hours as needed. Each Regular Strength Tylenol pill has 325 mg of acetaminophen. The most you should take each day is 3,250 mg (10 pills a day).
   - Another choice is to take 1,000 mg every 8 hours. Each Extra Strength Tylenol pill has 500 mg of acetaminophen. The most you should take each day is 3,000 mg (6 pills a day).

   Extra Notes:
   - Acetaminophen is in many OTC and prescription medicines. It might be in more than one medicine that you are taking. You need to be careful and not take an overdose. An acetaminophen overdose can hurt the liver.
   - **Caution:** Do not take acetaminophen if you have liver disease.
   - Use the lowest amount of medicine that makes your pain feel better.
   - Before taking any medicine, read all the instructions on the package.
6. **Call Back If:**
   - Pain becomes severe.
   - Shape of the nose has not returned to normal after 5 days.
   - Signs of infection occur (a yellow discharge, increasing tenderness, or fever).
   - You become worse.

FIRST AID

First Aid Advice for Bleeding:

Apply direct pressure to the entire wound with a clean cloth.

First Aid Advice for Nosebleed:

- Placing your thumb and index finger over each side of the soft lower portion of the nose, firmly pinch the nostrils together. Pinch the nostrils together for 10-15 minutes.
- Lean slightly forward; this keeps the blood from trickling down the back of your throat.

First Aid Advice for Penetrating Object:

If penetrating object still in place, don't remove it (Reason: removal could increase bleeding).

First Aid Advice for Shock:

Lie down with feet elevated.

BACKGROUND INFORMATION

General

- Due to the prominence of the nose in the midface, it is commonly injured in individuals with facial trauma.
- Patients with more than one site of injury may require you to use 2 or more Trauma protocols to ensure that you have recommended the safest disposition. Use your nursing judgment.

Types of Nose Injuries

- Bloody nose without a fracture
- Swelling and bruising of the nose without a fracture
- Nasal septal hematoma
- **Fracture of the Nose:** Severe fractures of the nose (e.g., crooked nose) are usually reset the same day in the operating room. Most surgeons don't repair mild fractures until day 5 to 7 post-injury.

Nasal Septal Hematoma

- **Definition:** A blood clot that develops between the cartilage of the nasal septum and the perichondrium. It can be unilateral or bilateral. This is a rare but urgent ENT problem.
- **Symptoms:** Blockage of nasal passage on one side (or both sides) with inability to breathe through that side. Another clue is severe tenderness of the tip of the nose, especially when it is pressed upward.
- **Treatment:** Drainage using a needle or an incision, followed by nasal packing.
- **Complications:** A septal hematoma can cause pressure necrosis of the nasal cartilage resulting in nasal deformity or perforated septum. This can occur if it is untreated for a period of days. A nasal septal abscess is a very rare complication; it is a superinfection of a septal hematoma. Symptoms are fever and increasing pain. This is an emergent ENT problem (See Within 4 Hours).
- **Time After Presentation of Injury:** Immediately to 14 days (mean 5.9 days) (Savage 2006). Therefore, the triage nurse needs to tell the caller to watch for symptoms of delayed onset of septal hematoma.

TRAUMA, SHOULDER

DEFINITION

- Injuries to a bone, muscle, joint, or ligament in the shoulder.
- Associated skin and soft tissue injuries are also included.

TRIAGE ASSESSMENT QUESTIONS

Call EMS 911 Now

- Major bleeding (actively dripping or spurting) that can't be stopped
  FIRST AID: Apply direct pressure to the entire wound with a clean cloth.
- Amputation or bone sticking through the skin
- Bullet, stabbed by knife, or other serious penetrating wound
  FIRST AID: If penetrating object still in place, don't remove it.
- Sounds like a life-threatening emergency to the triager

See More Appropriate Protocol

- Wound looks infected
  Go to Protocol: Wound Infection on page 344

Go to ED Now

- Injury looks like a broken bone or dislocated joint (crooked or deformed)

Go to ED Now (or to Office With PCP Approval)

- Can't move injured shoulder at all
- Collarbone is painful or tender to touch
  R/O: clavicle fracture
- Skin is split open or gaping (or length > ½ inch or 12 mm)
  R/O: need for sutures
- Bleeding won't stop after 10 minutes of direct pressure (using correct technique)
- Dirt in the wound and not removed after 15 minutes of scrubbing
  Reason: needs irrigation or debridement
- Sounds like a serious injury to the triager

See Today in Office

- Severe pain
  R/O: fracture, strain, rotator cuff tear
- Can't move injured shoulder normally (e.g., full range of motion, able to touch top of head)
  R/O: strain, sprain, rotator cuff tear
- Large swelling or bruise (> 2 inches or 5 cm)
- Suspicious history for the injury
  R/O: domestic violence or elder abuse
- Patient wants to be seen

See Today or Tomorrow in Office

- Injury interferes with work or school
- High-risk adult (e.g., age > 60, osteoporosis, chronic steroid use)
  Reason: greater risk of fracture in patients with osteoporosis
- Wound and no tetanus booster in > 5 years (or greater than 10 years for clean cuts)

See Within 3 Days in Office

- Pain has not improved after 3 days
- Injury is still painful or swollen after 2 weeks

Home Care

- Minor shoulder injury
  R/O: bruise, strain, or sprain

HOME CARE ADVICE FOR TRAUMA, SHOULDER

1. **Treatment of a Bruise (e.g., Direct Blow to Shoulder):**
   - Apply a cold pack or an ice pack (wrapped in a moist towel) to the area with ice for 20 minutes each hour for 4 consecutive hours (i.e., 20 minutes of cooling followed by 40 minutes of rest for 4 hours in a row).
   - Rest the injured part as much as possible for 48 hours.
   - 48 hours after the injury, use local heat for 10 minutes 3 times each day to help reabsorb the blood.

2. **Treatment of Sprains and Strains:**
   - **First Aid:** Apply an ice pack (crushed ice in a plastic bag covered with a moist towel) to reduce bleeding, swelling, and pain.
   - Continue to apply crushed ICE packs for 10-20 minutes every hour for the first 4 hours. Then apply ice for 10-20 minutes 4 times a day for the first 2 days.
   - REST the injured shoulder for 24 hours. You may return to normal activity after 24 hours of rest if the activity does not cause pain.
3. **Pain Medicines:**
   - For pain relief, take acetaminophen, ibuprofen, or naproxen.

   Acetaminophen (e.g., Tylenol):
   - Take 650 mg by mouth every 4-6 hours as needed. Each Regular Strength Tylenol pill has 325 mg of acetaminophen. The most you should take each day is 3,250 mg (10 pills a day).
   - Another choice is to take 1,000 mg every 8 hours. Each Extra Strength Tylenol pill has 500 mg of acetaminophen. The most you should take each day is 3,000 mg (6 pills a day).

   Ibuprofen (e.g., Motrin, Advil):
   - Take 400 mg by mouth every 6 hours.
   - Another choice is to take 600 mg by mouth every 8 hours.

   Naproxen (e.g., Aleve):
   - Take 250-500 mg by mouth every 12 hours.

   Extra Notes:
   - Acetaminophen is thought to be safer than ibuprofen or naproxen in people over 65 years old. Acetaminophen is in many OTC and prescription medicines. It might be in more than one medicine that you are taking. You need to be careful and not take an overdose. An acetaminophen overdose can hurt the liver.
   - **Caution:** Do not take acetaminophen if you have liver disease.
   - **Caution:** Do not take ibuprofen if you have stomach problems, kidney disease, are pregnant, or have been told by your doctor to avoid this type of anti-inflammatory drug. Do not take ibuprofen for more than 7 days without consulting your doctor.
   - Use the lowest amount of medicine that makes your pain feel better.
   - Before taking any medicine, read all the instructions on the package
4. **Expected Course:** Pain and swelling usually begin to improve 2 or 3 days after an injury. Swelling is usually gone in 7 days. Pain may take 2 weeks to completely resolve.
5. **Call Back If:**
   - Pain becomes severe.
   - Pain does not improve after 3 days.
   - Pain or swelling lasts more than 2 weeks.
   - You become worse.

FIRST AID

First Aid Advice for Bleeding:

Apply direct pressure to the entire wound with a clean cloth.

First Aid Advice for Penetrating Object:

If penetrating object still in place, don't remove it (Reason: removal could increase bleeding).

First Aid Advice for Shock:

Lie down with feet elevated.

First Aid Advice for Suspected Fracture or Dislocation of the Shoulder:

- Use a sling to support the arm. Make the sling with a triangular piece of cloth.
- Or, at the very least, the patient can support the injured arm with the other hand or a pillow.

BACKGROUND INFORMATION

Types of Shoulder Injuries

- Fractures (broken bones)
- Dislocations (bone out of joint)
- **Sprains:** Stretches and tears of ligaments
- **Strains:** Stretches and tears of muscles (e.g., pulled muscle)
- Muscle overuse injuries from sports or exercise (e.g., strain, bursitis, tendonitis)
- Muscle bruise from a direct blow (e.g., contusion)
- **Causes Extrinsic to Shoulder (Referred Pain):** Examples include neck pain, cardiac disease, abdominal disorders, spleen injury

What to Suture

- Any cut that is split open or gaping probably needs sutures. Cuts longer than ½ inch (1 cm) usually need sutures. Any open wound that may need sutures should be evaluated by a physician regardless of the time that has passed since the initial injury.

Tetanus Booster

- **Clean Cuts and Scrapes: Every 10 Years:** Patients with clean MINOR wounds AND who have previously had 3 or more tetanus shots (full series) need a booster every 10 years. Examples of minor wounds include a superficial abrasion or a small cut from a clean knife blade. Obtain booster within 72 hours.
- **Dirty Wounds: Every 5 Years:** Patients with dirty wounds need a booster every 5 years. Examples of dirty wounds include any cut or scrape contaminated with soil, feces, or saliva. Other examples are minor puncture wounds and small burns. Obtain booster within 72 hours.

TRAUMA, SKIN

DEFINITION

- Cuts, lacerations, gashes, and tears

TRIAGE ASSESSMENT QUESTIONS

Call EMS 911 Now

- Shock suspected (e.g., cold/pale/clammy skin, too weak to stand)
  R/O: shock
  FIRST AID: Lie down with the feet elevated.
- Cut on the neck, chest, back, or abdomen that may go deep (e.g., stab wound or other suspicious penetrating injury)
- Major bleeding (actively dripping or spurting) that can't be stopped
  FIRST AID: Apply direct pressure to the entire wound with a clean cloth.
- Amputation
  FIRST AID: Apply direct pressure to the entire wound with a clean cloth.
- Sounds like a life-threatening emergency to the triager

See More Appropriate Protocol

- Animal bite and broken skin
  Go to Protocol: Animal Bite on page 13
- Injury is a puncture wound
  Go to Protocol: Puncture Wound on page 206
- Splinter in the skin
  Go to Protocol: Skin, Foreign Body on page 236
- Wound looks infected
  Go to Protocol: Wound Infection on page 344
- Chemical burn
  Go to Protocol: Burns on page 40

Go to ED Now

- High-pressure injection injury (e.g., from paint gun, usually work-related)
  Reason: deep tissue damage may exceed superficial injury
- Skin loss involves more than 10% of surface area
  Note: the palm of the hand = 1%
  R/O: need for burn care

Go to ED Now (or to Office With PCP Approval)

- Skin is split open or gaping (length > ½ inch or 12 mm on the skin, ¼ inch or 6 mm on the face)
  R/O: need for sutures
- Bleeding won't stop after 10 minutes of direct pressure (using correct technique)
- Cut or scrape is very deep (e.g., can see bone or tendons)
  R/O: tendon injury
- Dirt in the wound and not removed after 15 minutes of scrubbing
  Reason: needs irrigation or debridement
- Wound causes numbness (i.e., loss of sensation)
  R/O: nerve injury
- Wound causes weakness (i.e., decreased ability to move hand, finger, toe)
  R/O: nerve injury
- Sounds like a serious injury to the triager

Go to Office Now

- Looks infected (fever, spreading redness, pus, or red streak)
  R/O: cellulitis, lymphangitis
- Expanding raised bruise with size > 2 inches (5 cm)
  R/O: progressive hematoma

See Today in Office

- Severe pain
- Suspicious history for the injury
  R/O: domestic violence or elder abuse
- Patient wants to be seen

See Today or Tomorrow in Office

- Last tetanus shot > 5 years and dirty cut or scrape (or greater than 10 years for clean cuts)
- Diabetic (diabetes mellitus) and has minor cut or scratch on foot
  Reason: increased risk of foot infection or ulcer

See Within 3 Days in Office

- After 14 days and wound isn't healed
  R/O: low-grade infection

Home Care

- Minor skin injury
  R/O: scratch, abrasion, bruise

HOME CARE ADVICE FOR MINOR CUT, SCRAPE, OR BRUISE

1. **Treatment of Minor Cuts, Scratches, and Scrapes (Abrasions):**
   - Apply direct pressure for 10 minutes to stop any bleeding.
   - Wash the wound with soap and water for 5 minutes.
   - Gently scrub out any dirt with a washcloth.
   - Cut off any pieces of dead loose skin using a fine scissors (cleaned with rubbing alcohol before and after use).
   - Apply an antibiotic ointment, covered by a Band-Aid or dressing. Change daily.
   - Another option is to use a liquid skin bandage that only needs to be applied once. Do not use antibioitic ointments if you use liquid skin bandage.
2. **Treatment of Minor Bruise:**
   - Apply a cold pack or an ice bag wrapped in a towel for 20 minutes each hour for 4 consecutive hours (20 minutes of cold followed by 40 minutes of rest for 4 hours in a row).
   - 48 hours after the injury, use local heat for 10 minutes 3 times each day to help reabsorb the blood.
   - Rest the injured part as much as possible for 48 hours.
3. **Pain Medicines:**
   - For pain relief, take acetaminophen, ibuprofen, or naproxen.

   Acetaminophen (e.g., Tylenol):
   - Take 650 mg by mouth every 4-6 hours as needed. Each Regular Strength Tylenol pill has 325 mg of acetaminophen. The most you should take each day is 3,250 mg (10 pills a day).
   - Another choice is to take 1,000 mg every 8 hours. Each Extra Strength Tylenol pill has 500 mg of acetaminophen. The most you should take each day is 3,000 mg (6 pills a day).

   Ibuprofen (e.g., Motrin, Advil):
   - Take 400 mg by mouth every 6 hours.
   - Another choice is to take 600 mg by mouth every 8 hours.

   Naproxen (e.g., Aleve):
   - Take 250-500 mg by mouth every 12 hours.

   Extra Notes:
   - Acetaminophen is thought to be safer than ibuprofen or naproxen in people over 65 years old. Acetaminophen is in many OTC and prescription medicines. It might be in more than one medicine that you are taking. You need to be careful and not take an overdose. An acetaminophen overdose can hurt the liver.
   - **Caution:** Do not take acetaminophen if you have liver disease.
   - **Caution:** Do not take ibuprofen if you have stomach problems, kidney disease, are pregnant, or have been told by your doctor to avoid this type of anti-inflammatory drug. Do not take ibuprofen for more than 7 days without consulting your doctor.
   - Use the lowest amount of medicine that makes your pain feel better.
   - Before taking any medicine, read all the instructions on the package
4. **Expected Course:** Pain and swelling usually begin to improve 2 or 3 days after an injury. Swelling is usually gone in 7 days. Pain may take 2 weeks to completely resolve.
5. **Call Back If:**
   - Looks infected (pus, redness, increasing tenderness).
   - Doesn't heal within 10 days.
   - You become worse.

FIRST AID

First Aid Advice for Bleeding:
Apply direct pressure to the entire wound with a clean cloth.

First Aid Advice for Severe Bleeding:
- Place 2 or 3 sterile dressings (or a clean towel or washcloth) over the wound immediately.
- Apply direct pressure to the wound, using your entire hand.
- If bleeding continues, apply pressure more forcefully or move the pressure to a slightly different spot.
- Act quickly because ongoing blood loss can cause shock.
- Do not use a tourniquet.

First Aid Advice for Penetrating Object:

If penetrating object still in place, don't remove it (Reason: removal could increase bleeding).

First Aid Advice for Shock:

Lie down with feet elevated.

First Aid Advice for Transport of an Amputated Finger or Toe:

- Briefly rinse amputated part with water (to remove any dirt).
- Place amputated part in plastic bag (to protect and keep clean).
- Place plastic bag containing part in a cup of ice water (to keep cool and preserve tissue).

BACKGROUND INFORMATION

Types of Skin Injury

- **Abrasions:** An abrasion (scrape) is an area of superficial skin that has been scraped off. They commonly occur on the knees, elbows, and palms.
- **Bruise:** A bruise (contusion) usually is the result of a direct blow from a blunt object. There is bleeding under the skin from damaged blood vessels.
- **Cut—Superficial:** Superficial cuts (scratches) only extend partially through the skin and rarely become infected.
- **Cut—Deep:** Deep cuts (lacerations) go through the skin (dermis). Cuts longer than ½ inch (6 mm) usually need sutures. Cuts on the face longer than ¼ inch (3 mm) usually need sutures.
- **Hematoma:** A hematoma is a collection of blood in the soft tissues.
- **Puncture Wound:** A puncture wound is the result of the skin being penetrated by a sharp, pointed object.
- **Skin Tear:** A skin tear is a separation of the epidermis from the underlying dermis. It is primarily seen in the elderly and in chronically-ill individuals. The most common location is the arms.

Lacerations—Methods of Repairing (Closing)

- **Suturing (Stitches):** This is the most common method for closing lacerations.
- **Stapling (Staples):** Wound staples work best in uncomplicated lacerations overlying flat areas of the body surface; for this reason, they are mostly used in cuts on the scalp, torso, arms, and legs.
- **Skin Glue (Tissue Adhesives):** Skin glue works well on small straight lacerations where there is little skin tension. Skin glue is often used to close small cuts on the face. Dermabond (2-octylcyanoacrylate, Ethicon) is the name of the skin glue used by doctors in the United States and Canada.
- **Tissue Tapes (e.g., 3M, Steri-Strips):** Tissue tapes can be used for very superficial cuts. They are available over-the-counter and can be applied at home. They do not work well over joints and tend to fall off if they become wet.

Lacerations—What to Repair

- Cuts that are gaping open and longer than ½ inch (12 mm) usually need repair (e.g. sutures).
- On the face, cuts longer than ¼ inch (6 mm) need repair.
- Any open wound that may need sutures should be evaluated by a physician regardless of the time that has passed since the initial injury.

Lacerations—Timing of Repair

- **Primary closure** is the repair of a new wound. The sooner a wound is closed, the lower the infection rate. Generally, lacerations on most parts of the body should be repaired (e.g., sutured) within 12 hours; lacerations of the face and scalp should be repaired within 24 hours (Reason: highly vascular area, less prone to infection). Clean wounds can wait longer than dirty wounds.
- **Secondary closure** is having a wound heal over without suturing it or using another method of repair. This leaves a wider scar. Secondary closure is needed for infected wounds and abscesses.
- **Delayed primary closure** is suturing a wound on day 4 or 5, after watching it to make certain it is not infected. This approach is used for contaminated wounds, many animal bites, and wounds that are brought in after 12 to 24 hours. All of these individuals need to be seen initially, however, for wound irrigation, debridement, and possibly antibiotics.

Liquid Skin Bandage for Minor Cuts and Scrapes

- Liquid skin bandage has several benefits when compared to a regular bandage (e.g., a dressing or a Band-Aid). Liquid bandage only needs to be applied once to minor cuts and scrapes. It helps stop minor bleeding. It seals the wound and may promote faster healing and lower infection rates. However, it is also more expensive.
- After the wound is washed and dried, the liquid is applied by spray or with a swab. It dries in less than a minute and usually lasts a week. Liquid skin bandage is resistant to bathing.
- Examples include: Band-Aid Liquid Bandage, New-Skin, Curad Spray Bandage, and 3M No Sting Liquid Bandage Spray.

What Is Tetanus?

- **Definition:** Tetanus is a rare infection caused by bacteria that are found in many places, especially in dirt and soil. The tetanus bacteria enter through a break in the skin and then spread through the body.
- **Symptoms:** Tetanus is commonly called lockjaw because the first symptom is a tightening of the muscles of the face. However, the final stage of the infection is much more serious. All of the muscles of the body go into severe spasm, including the muscles that control breathing. Eventually a person with a tetanus infection loses the ability to breath, and may die in spite of intensive treatment in the hospital.
- **Prevention:** A tetanus booster protects you from getting a tetanus infection. It does not prevent other kinds of wound infection.

Tetanus Booster—When Does an Adult Need a Tetanus Shot?

- **Clean Cuts and Scrapes: Booster Needed Every 10 Years:** Patients with clean MINOR wounds AND who have previously had 3 or more tetanus shots (full series) need a booster every 10 years. Examples of minor wounds include a superficial knee abrasion, a small cut from a clean knife blade, or a glass cut sustained while washing dishes. Obtain tetanus booster within 72 hours.
- **Dirty Wounds: Booster Needed Every 5 Years:** Patients with dirty wounds need a booster every 5 years. Examples of dirty wounds include any cut contaminated with soil, feces, saliva, and more serious wounds from deep punctures, crushing, and burns. Obtain tetanus booster within 72 hours.
- Contaminated major wounds (e.g., crush injuries, amputations, avulsions, gaping cuts, larger burns, or any other wound that needs debridement or irrigation) are all referred in immediately for wound care. For these patients, if a tetanus booster is required, it will be given on the day of the injury.

TRAUMA, TOE

DEFINITION

- Injuries to toe(s).
- Toe injuries include cuts, abrasions, stubbed toe, smashed toe, toenail injuries, subungual hematoma, dislocations, and fractures.

TRIAGE ASSESSMENT QUESTIONS

Call EMS 911 Now

- Major bleeding (actively dripping or spurting) that can't be stopped
  FIRST AID: Apply direct pressure to the entire wound with a clean cloth.
- Amputation of toe
  FIRST AID: Apply direct pressure to the entire wound with a clean cloth.
- Sounds like a serious injury to the triager

See More Appropriate Protocol

- Looks infected
  Go to Protocol: Wound Infection on page 344

Go to ED Now

- High-pressure injection injury (e.g., from paint gun, usually work-related)
  Reason: deep tissue damage may exceed superficial injury

Go to ED Now (or to Office With PCP Approval)

- Looks like a broken bone (e.g., crooked or deformed)
- Looks like a dislocated joint (e.g., crooked or deformed)
- Skin is split open or gaping (or length > ½ inch or 12 mm)
  R/O: need for sutures
- Bleeding won't stop after 10 minutes of direct pressure (using correct technique)
- Dirt in the wound and not removed after 15 minutes of scrubbing
  Reason: needs irrigation or debridement
- Sounds like a serious injury to the triager

Go to Office Now

- Looks infected (e.g., spreading redness, pus, red streak)
  R/O: cellulitis, lymphangitis
- Toenail is completely torn off
- Base of toenail has popped out from under skin fold
  Reason: needs to be reinserted

See Today in Office

- Severe pain
  R/O: dislocation or displaced fracture
- Moderate-Severe pain and blood present under the nail (usually > 50% of nail bed)
  R/O: severe subungual hematoma needing drainage

See Today or Tomorrow in Office

- Wound and no tetanus booster in > 5 years (Or greater than 10 years for clean cuts)
- Bad limp or can't wear shoes/sandals
  R/O: toe fracture
- Patient wants to be seen

See Within 3 Days in Office

- Injury interferes with work or school
- Small cut or scrape and has diabetes mellitus
  Reason: wounds heal slower in diabetics
- Pain has not improved after 3 days
- Injury is still painful or swollen after 2 weeks

Home Care

- Minor toe injury
  R/O: minor bruise or sprain, scrapes, small subungual hematoma

HOME CARE ADVICE FOR MINOR INJURIES OF TOE

1. **Treatment of Cuts, Scratches, and Scrapes (Abrasions):**
   - Apply direct pressure for 10 minutes to stop any bleeding.
   - Wash the wound with soap and water for 5 minutes.
   - Scrub out any dirt gently with a washcloth.
   - Cut off any pieces of dead loose skin using a fine scissors (cleaned with rubbing alcohol).
   - Apply an antibiotic ointment, covered by a Band-Aid or dressing. Change daily.
2. **Treatment of Bruised Toe:** Soak the toe in cold water for 20 minutes.
3. **Treatment of Jammed Toe:**
   - **Caution:** Be certain that there is no deformity (the toe lines up normally with the other toes).
   - Soak the toe in cold water for 20 minutes.
   - If the pain is more than mild, protect it by buddy-taping it to the next toe.
4. **Treatment of Smashed or Crushed Toe:**
   - Apply an ice bag to the area for 20 minutes.
   - Wash the toe with soap and water for 5 minutes.
   - Trim any small pieces of torn dead skin with a scissors cleaned with rubbing alcohol.
   - Cover any cuts with an antibiotic ointment and Band-Aid. Change daily.
5. **Treatment of Subungual Hematoma (Blood Present Under Toenail):** Apply an ice bag to the area for 20 minutes.
6. **Torn Nail (From Catching It on Something):**
   - For a cracked nail without rough edges, leave it alone.
   - For a large flap of nail that is almost torn through, use a sterile scissors to cut it off along the line of the tear (Reason: pieces of nail will catch on objects and tear further).
   - Apply an antibiotic ointment and cover with a Band-Aid. Change daily.
   - After about 7 days, the nail bed should be covered by new skin and no longer hurt. It takes about 6-12 weeks for a toenail to grow back completely.
7. **Pain Medicines:**
   - For pain relief, take acetaminophen, ibuprofen, or naproxen.

   Acetaminophen (e.g., Tylenol):
   - Take 650 mg by mouth every 4-6 hours as needed. Each Regular Strength Tylenol pill has 325 mg of acetaminophen. The most you should take each day is 3,250 mg (10 pills a day).
   - Another choice is to take 1,000 mg every 8 hours. Each Extra Strength Tylenol pill has 500 mg of acetaminophen. The most you should take each day is 3,000 mg (6 pills a day).

   Ibuprofen (e.g., Motrin, Advil):
   - Take 400 mg by mouth every 6 hours.
   - Another choice is to take 600 mg by mouth every 8 hours.

   Naproxen (e.g., Aleve):
   - Take 250-500 mg by mouth every 12 hours.

   Extra Notes:
   - Acetaminophen is thought to be safer than ibuprofen or naproxen in people over 65 years old. Acetaminophen is in many OTC and prescription medicines. It might be in more than one medicine that you are taking. You need to be careful and not take an overdose. An acetaminophen overdose can hurt the liver.
   - **Caution:** Do not take acetaminophen if you have liver disease.
   - **Caution:** Do not take ibuprofen if you have stomach problems, kidney disease, are pregnant, or have been told by your doctor to avoid this type of anti-inflammatory drug. Do not take ibuprofen for more than 7 days without consulting your doctor.
   - Use the lowest amount of medicine that makes your pain feel better.
   - Before taking any medicine, read all the instructions on the package
8. **Call Back If:**
   - Cut or scrape looks infected (redness, red streak, or pus).
   - Pain becomes severe.
   - Pain does not improve after 3 days.
   - Pain or swelling lasts more than 2 weeks.
   - You become worse.

FIRST AID

First Aid Advice for Bleeding:

Apply direct pressure to the entire wound with a clean cloth.

First Aid Advice for Penetrating Object:

If penetrating object still in place, don't remove it (Reason: removal could increase bleeding).

First Aid Advice for Shock:

Lie down with feet elevated.

First Aid Advice for a Sprain of the Toe:

- Remove any rings or jewelry from the injured toe.
- Tape the injured toe to the toe next to it (this is called a buddy splint).
- Apply a cold pack or an ice bag (wrapped in a moist towel) to the area for 20 minutes.

First Aid Advice for Suspected Fracture or Dislocation of the Toe:

- Remove any rings or jewelry from the injured toe.
- Tape the injured toe to the toe next to it (this is called a buddy splint).
- Apply a cold pack or an ice bag (wrapped in a moist towel) to the area for 20 minutes.

First Aid Advice for Transport of an Amputated Toe:

- Briefly rinse amputated part with water (to remove any dirt).
- Place amputated part in plastic bag (to protect and keep clean).
- Place plastic bag containing part in a cup of ice water (to keep cool and preserve tissue).

BACKGROUND INFORMATION

Types of Injuries

- **Abrasions or Scrapes:** An area of superficial skin that has been scraped off. Commonly occurs on the knuckles.
- **Bruises:** Bruises (contusions) result from a direct blow or a crushing injury; there is bleeding into the skin from damaged blood vessels without an overlying cut or abrasion.
- **Cuts and Scratches:** Superficial cuts (scratches) only extend partially through the skin and rarely become infected. Deep cuts (lacerations) go through the skin (dermis).
- Fractures (broken bones)
- Dislocations (bone out of joint)
- **Jammed or Stubbed Toe:** The end of a straightened toe receives a blow (usually from kicking something). The ligaments and tendons of the toe are stretched and torn.
- **Smashed or Crushed Toe:** This injury most often results from a heavy object falling on the toe. Usually the end of the toe receives a few cuts, a blood blister, or a bruise. Sometimes the nail is damaged. A fracture of the bones inside the toe can occasionally occur.
- **Subungual Hematoma (Blood Under Toenail):** This medical term is applied when a blood clot forms under the toenail. It is caused by a crush injury to the tip of the toe. Some are only mildly painful and blood is typically less than 50% of nail bed. Others can be severely painful and throbbing, and these may need the pressure released to relieve pain. The pressure can be released by putting a small hole through the nail. With larger subungual hematomas, the toenail will usually fall off. A new nail will grow back in 6 to 12 weeks.
- **Torn Nail:** From catching it on something.

When Are Stitches Needed?

- Any cut that is split open or gaping probably needs sutures (stitches). Cuts longer than ½ inch (12 mm) usually need sutures.
- A physician should evaluate any open wound that may need sutures regardless of the time that has passed since the initial injury.

TRAUMA, TOOTH

DEFINITION

- Injury to tooth or teeth

Note: Other mouth injuries are covered in the Trauma, Mouth protocol on page 300.

TRIAGE ASSESSMENT QUESTIONS

Call EMS 911 Now

- Knocked out (unconscious) for more than 1 minute
  R/O: concussion
- Difficult to awaken or acting confused (e.g., disoriented, slurred speech)
  R/O: concussion, intoxication
- Severe neck pain
  R/O: cervical spine injury
  FIRST AID: Protect the neck from movement.
- Sounds like a life-threatening emergency to the triager

See More Appropriate Protocol

- Wound looks infected
  Go to Protocol: Wound Infection on page 344

Go to ED or Dentist Now

- Tooth knocked out
  FIRST AID: See First Aid for knocked-out tooth.
- Tooth is almost falling out
- Bleeding won't stop after 10 minutes of direct pressure (using correct technique)
  R/O: need for sutures
- Sounds like a serious injury to the triager

Call Dentist Now

- Severe pain
- Chipped tooth (piece missing)
  R/O: possible fracture into pulp or dentine
- Tooth pushed out of its normal position
  Reason: displaced tooth needs repositioning and stabilizing
- Tooth sensitive to cold fluids
  R/O: dentin exposure
- Can see a crack in the tooth
  R/O: tooth fracture

See Today in Office

- Suspicious history for the injury
  R/O: domestic violence or elder abuse

Call Dentist Today

- Caller tries to move the tooth and it feels very loose
- Tooth becomes darker
  R/O: pulp necrosis
- Patient wants to be seen

Home Care

- Minor tooth injury

HOME CARE ADVICE FOR MINOR TOOTH INJURIES

1. **Local Cold:** For pain, apply a piece of ice or a Popsicle to the injured gum area for 20 minutes.
2. **Pain Medicines:**
   - For pain relief, take acetaminophen, ibuprofen, or naproxen.

   Acetaminophen (e.g., Tylenol):
   - Take 650 mg by mouth every 4-6 hours as needed. Each Regular Strength Tylenol pill has 325 mg of acetaminophen. The most you should take each day is 3,250 mg (10 pills a day).
   - Another choice is to take 1,000 mg every 8 hours. Each Extra Strength Tylenol pill has 500 mg of acetaminophen. The most you should take each day is 3,000 mg (6 pills a day).

   Ibuprofen (e.g., Motrin, Advil):
   - Take 400 mg by mouth every 6 hours.
   - Another choice is to take 600 mg by mouth every 8 hours.

   Naproxen (e.g., Aleve):
   - Take 250-500 mg by mouth every 12 hours.

Extra Notes:

- Acetaminophen is thought to be safer than ibuprofen or naproxen in people over 65 years old. Acetaminophen is in many OTC and prescription medicines. It might be in more than one medicine that you are taking. You need to be careful and not take an overdose. An acetaminophen overdose can hurt the liver.
- **Caution:** Do not take acetaminophen if you have liver disease.
- **Caution:** Do not take ibuprofen if you have stomach problems, kidney disease, are pregnant, or have been told by your doctor to avoid this type of anti-inflammatory drug. Do not take ibuprofen for more than 7 days without consulting your doctor.
- Use the lowest amount of medicine that makes your pain feel better.
- Before taking any medicine, read all the instructions on the package

3. **Soft Diet:** If you have any loose teeth, eat a soft diet for 3 days. After 3 days, they should be tightening up.
4. **Call Your Dentist If:**
   - Pain becomes severe.
   - Tooth becomes sensitive to hot or cold fluids.
   - Tooth becomes a darker color.
   - You become worse.

FIRST AID

First Aid Advice for Knocked-Out Tooth:

To save the tooth, it must be put back in its socket as soon as possible (2 hours is the maximum limit for survival). Use the following technique:

- Rinse off the tooth with saliva or water. Do not scrub the tooth.
- Replace it in the socket facing the correct way.
- Press down on the tooth with your thumb until the crown is level with the adjacent tooth.
- Lastly, bite down on a wad of cloth to stabilize the tooth until you can be seen by a dentist.

Transporting a Knocked-Out Tooth:

Follow these instructions if you are not able to put the tooth back in its socket:

- It is very important to keep the tooth moist. Do not let it dry out.
- Transport the tooth in saliva or milk.

BACKGROUND INFORMATION

Types of Tooth Injuries

- **Avulsion of Tooth (Knocked-Out Tooth):** This is a dental emergency. The avulsed permanent tooth needs to be placed back in its socket as soon as possible, ideally within minutes, and certainly within 2 hours.
- **Concussion of Tooth (Tooth Was Bumped But Is Not Loose):** An injury to a tooth without displacement, loosening, or fracture. This is the most common dental injury. No immediate dental care is needed. A soft diet should be recommended. Rarely a concussed tooth can undergo pulpal necrosis (tooth death) days to weeks later; this can be recognized when the tooth becomes darker than the adjacent teeth.
- **Crown Fracture—Complicated (Enamel-Dentin Fracture With Pulp Exposure):** A fracture which enters into the pulp of a tooth is referred to as complicated. Typically it is quite painful and is very sensitive to air and cold liquids. The caller will usually describe that a large piece of the tooth is broken off. The caller may be also able to see a small red dot or pink blush (the pulp) in the fractured area. To reduce pain and prevent pulpal damage, fractures into the pulp need to be treated urgently. Treatment in an emergency department may consist of temporarily covering the fracture with a dental cement or calcium hydroxide. Subsequent dental care is mandatory; most of these fractures will require root canal therapy.
- **Crown Fracture—Uncomplicated (Enamel-Dentin Fracture; Chipped Tooth; No Pulp Exposure):** A small painless chipped tooth can wait 24-72 hours for evaluation by a dentist.

- **Cracked Tooth (Infraction):** This is a small hairline crack of a tooth. The caller will report a thin fracture line without any missing piece of tooth. Generally, this should be evaluated by a dentist in 24-72 hours.
- **Intruded Tooth (Pushed Into Gum):** The tooth is pushed deeper into the gum and tooth socket. Generally, this should be evaluated by a dentist in 24-72 hours.
- **Loosened Tooth (Subluxation):** If there is only mild looseness, the tooth usually tightens up on its own (may bleed a little from the gums).
- **Loosened and Displaced Tooth (Luxation):** All need to see a dentist to assess damage. Displaced teeth that interfere with biting, chewing, or closing the mouth need to be repositioned within 4 hours for reasons of comfort and function. Mild displacement deserves evaluation within 24 hours.

Causes

- Contact sports
- Falls
- **Fights:** Direct blow from punch, kick, or object
- Motor vehicle accidents

Caution—Associated Head and Neck Trauma

- Head trauma should be considered in all patients with a mouth and dental injury. Signs of significant head injury include loss of consciousness, amnesia, unsteady walking, confusion, and slurred speech.
- Neck trauma should also be considered in all patients with a facial injury. Concerning findings include: numbness, weakness, and neck pain.

URINALYSIS RESULTS (FOLLOW-UP CALL)

DEFINITION

- Urinalysis or urine dipstick done and results called to triage nurse by the lab, PCP, or adult caller.
- Patient has been previously triaged by triage nurse or examined by PCP.
- Patient has some symptom(s) of a urinary tract infection (e.g., dysuria, frequency, urgency, foul-smelling urine, or hematuria).
- In most cases, the triage nurse needs to call the patient.

TRIAGE ASSESSMENT QUESTIONS

See More Appropriate Protocol

- Female taking antibiotic for diagnosed urine infection
  Go to Protocol: Urination Pain (Female) on page 323
- Male taking antibiotic for diagnosed urine infection
  Go to Protocol: Urination Pain (Male) on page 326

Go to ED Now (or to Office With PCP Approval)

- Patient sounds very sick or weak to the triager

Call Transferred to PCP Now

- Positive urine test (i.e., LE + or WBC > 10) and any of the following:
  - Fever > 100.5° F (38.1° C)
  - Side (flank) or lower back pain present

  R/O: pyelonephritis

See Today or Tomorrow in Office

- Negative urine test (i.e., LE - and WBC < 10) and urine symptoms continue or are worsening
  Note: triager judgment regarding need for further triage
- Patient wants to be seen

Discuss With PCP and Callback by Nurse Today

- Positive urine test (i.e., LE + or WBC > 10) and NO standing order to call in prescription for antibiotic
  Reason: antibiotic prescription needed
- Positive urine test and any of the following:
  - Antibiotic treatment in past month for urine infection
  - Has urinary catheter (e.g., Foley)
  - Bedridden (e.g., nursing home patient, CVA, chronic illness, recovering from surgery)
  - Chronic urinary incontinence

  Reason: possible antibiotic resistance
- Positive urine test and any of the following:
  - Diabetes mellitus
  - Immunocompromised (e.g., HIV positive, cancer chemotherapy, transplant patient)
  - Pregnant
  - Male

  Reason: special circumstances
- Triager uncertain how to interpret urine test results

Home Care

- Positive urine test (i.e., LE + or WBC > 10) and standing order to call in prescription for antibiotic
  Reason: antibiotic prescription needed for nonpregnant female with cystitis
- Negative urine test (i.e., LE - and WBC < 10)

HOME CARE ADVICE FOR URINALYSIS RESULTS FOLLOW-UP CALL

General Care Advice for Urination Pain

1. **Fluids:** Drink extra fluids. Drink 8-10 glasses of liquids a day (Reason: to produce a dilute, non-irritating urine).
2. **Cranberry Juice:**
   - Some people think that drinking cranberry juice may help in fighting urinary tract infections. However, there is no good research that has ever proved this.
   - **Dosage Cranberry Juice Cocktail:** 8 oz (240 mL) twice a day.
   - **Dosage 100% Cranberry Juice:** 1 oz (30 mL) twice a day.
   - Do not drink more than 12 oz (360 mL). Here is the reason: too much cranberry juice can also be irritating to the bladder.

3. **Pain Medicines:**
   - For pain relief, take acetaminophen, ibuprofen, or naproxen.

   Acetaminophen (e.g., Tylenol):
   - Take 650 mg by mouth every 4-6 hours as needed. Each Regular Strength Tylenol pill has 325 mg of acetaminophen. The most you should take each day is 3,250 mg (10 pills a day).
   - Another choice is to take 1,000 mg every 8 hours. Each Extra Strength Tylenol pill has 500 mg of acetaminophen. The most you should take each day is 3,000 mg (6 pills a day).

   Ibuprofen (e.g., Motrin, Advil):
   - Take 400 mg by mouth every 6 hours.
   - Another choice is to take 600 mg by mouth every 8 hours.

   Naproxen (e.g., Aleve):
   - Take 250-500 mg by mouth every 12 hours.

   Extra Notes:
   - Acetaminophen is thought to be safer than ibuprofen or naproxen in people over 65 years old. Acetaminophen is in many OTC and prescription medicines. It might be in more than one medicine that you are taking. You need to be careful and not take an overdose. An acetaminophen overdose can hurt the liver.
   - **Caution:** Do not take acetaminophen if you have liver disease.
   - **Caution:** Do not take ibuprofen if you have stomach problems, kidney disease, are pregnant, or have been told by your doctor to avoid this type of anti-inflammatory drug. Do not take ibuprofen for more than 7 days without consulting your doctor.
   - Use the lowest amount of medicine that makes your pain feel better.
   - Before taking any medicine, read all the instructions on the package
4. **Call Back If:**
   - You become worse.

Positive Urine Test—Antibiotic Treatment for Urine Infection

1. **Urine Test Positive:** Your urine test showed that you have an infection of your urine (bladder infection).
2. **Recommended Antibiotic:** Follow call center policy and physician's practice rules. Call in a prescription for one of the following:
   - Trimethoprim-sulfamethoxazole (Bactrim DS or Septra DS; 1 PO BID for 7 days); or
   - Nitrofurantoin (MacroBid; 1 PO BID for 7 days); or
   - Ciprofloxacin (Cipro; 250 mg PO BID for 7 days).
   - **Note:** Duration of antibiotics can be 3 instead of 7 days in healthy nonpregnant females less than 50 years of age.
3. **Caution—Antibiotics:** Ask patient about allergies. Bactrim is a sulfa - type antibiotic.
4. **Warm Saline Sitz Baths to Reduce Pain:** Sit in a warm saline bath for 20 minutes to cleanse the area and to reduce pain. Add 2 oz (60 g) of table salt or baking soda to a tub of water.
5. **OTC Phenazopyridine for Severe Dysyuria and Frequency:**
   - Phenazopyridine (Uristat) is available OTC (in United States only). Dosage is 2 pills by mouth 3 times a day.
   - It is also available as a prescription medicine (Pyridium, Urogesic). It has a numbing effect on the lining of the bladder and urethra. It can help reduce burning during urination, urgency, and frequency until the antibiotics start working.
   - It does not have any antibacterial effect.
   - Read the package instructions thoroughly on all medications that you take.
6. **Caution—Phenazopyridine:**
   - It turns the urine bright orange. This can cause staining of underwear. It can also sometimes stain contact lenses.
   - Do not take this medicine if you have kidney disease.
   - Do not use if pregnant (Reason: class B, should discuss with PCP first).
   - Do not use if breastfeeding (Reason: safety unknown, should discuss with PCP first).
   - DO NOT USE MORE THAN 2 DAYS.

7. **Call Back If:**
   - Fever more than 100.5° F (38.1° C).
   - Urine symptoms do not improve by day 3 on antibiotics.
   - You become worse.

BACKGROUND INFORMATION

General:

- This protocol assumes that 1) the patient has one or more urinary symptoms, 2) the clinician who ordered the urine test has a moderate suspicion that the patient has a urine infection, and 3) that it is safer to err on the side of antibiotic treatment.
- Antibiotic therapy is recommended in this guideline if the patient has a positive urine test (as defined below).

Positive Urine Test (Abnormal Urinalysis; Findings Suggestive of UTI)

Either of the following results supports the presence of a urinary tract infection:

- **Leukocyte Esterase (LE):** Positive (LE +)
- **White Blood Cells Per High-Power Field:** More than 10 WBC/HPF (> 10 WBC)

Negative Urine Test (Normal Dipstick Urinalysis)

The normal results for the chemical tests on the urine dipstick are as follows:

- **pH:** 4.8 - 7.5
- **Protein:** None or trace
- **Glucose:** None or trace
- **Ketones:** None
- **Hemoglobin:** None
- **Bilirubin:** None
- **Urobilinogen:** None
- **Leukocyte Esterase (LE):** Negative (LE -)
- **Nitrite:** Negative

Negative Urine Test (Normal Microscopic Urinalysis)

The normal results for the microscopic analysis are as follows:

- **Red Blood Cells Per High-Power Field:** 0-3 RBC/HPF
- **White Blood Cells Per High-Power Field:** 0-5 WBC/HPF
- **Epithelial Cells:** May be present
- **Bacteria:** None
- **Crystals:** Small numbers are normal

Types of Urine Infections

A urinalysis test is used to diagnose 2 main types of urinary tract infections (UTIs):

- **Cystitis:** An infection of the bladder mucosa. Painful urination, urinary frequency, and urgency are typically present. Blood in the urine may also be seen. There may be an associated mild midline suprapubic discomfort in the area of the bladder. In the 20- to 50-year-old, cystitis is 30 times more common in women than men. This gender difference may reflect the much shorter length of the female urethra, which facilitates migration of bacteria up into the bladder. Risk factors for female cystitis in younger women include sexual intercourse, spermicidal usage, and pregnancy. Risk factors for cystitis in older females include institutionalization (i.e., nursing home), urinary catheterization (i.e., Foley), and recent urologic surgery.
- **Pyelonephritis:** An infection of the kidney. An untreated cystitis may progress into pyelonephritis. Commonly associated symptoms include flank pain, fever, and chills. Symptoms of cystitis (dysuria, frequency) may or may not be present.

UTI—Symptoms

- **Dysuria:** Discomfort (pain, burning, or stinging) when passing urine; the most common symptom of UTI.
- **Frequency and Urgency:** Frequency means urinating frequently and passing small amounts; urgency refers to the periodic sensation of needing to rush to the bathroom (can't wait). Both are common symptoms of UTI.
- **Hematuria:** Blood in the urine; sometimes seen in UTI.
- **Flank Pain:** Pain in the side between the lower ribs and the top of the pelvis (iliac crest). Flank pain is a symptom of pyelonephritis.

URINATION PAIN (FEMALE)

DEFINITION

- Discomfort (pain, burning, or stinging) when passing urine.
- Associated symptoms may include urgency (can't wait) and frequency (passing small amounts) of urination.

Pain Severity Is Defined As:

- **Mild (1-3):** Complains slightly about urination hurting
- **Moderate (4-7):** Interferes with normal activities
- **Severe (8-10):** Excruciating, unwilling or unable to urinate because of the pain

TRIAGE ASSESSMENT QUESTIONS

Call EMS 911 Now

- Shock suspected (e.g., cold/pale/clammy skin, too weak to stand)
  R/O: urosepsis, shock
  FIRST AID: Lie down with the feet elevated.
- Sounds like a life-threatening emergency to the triager

Go to ED Now (or to Office With PCP Approval)

- Unable to urinate (or only a few drops) and bladder feels very full
  R/O: urinary retention
- Patient sounds very sick or weak to the triager

Go to Office Now

- Severe pain with urination
- Fever > 100.5° F (38.1° C)
  R/O: pyelonephritis
- Side (flank) or lower back pain present

See Today in Office

- Taking antibiotic > 24 hours for UTI and fever persists
  R/O: complication, resistant organism, or need for IV antibiotics
- Taking antibiotic > 3 days for UTI and painful urination not improved
  R/O: resistant organism
- Unusual vaginal discharge
  R/O: vaginitis, urethritis (STD)
- > 2 UTIs in last year
  R/O: recurrent UTI
- Patient is worried about sexually transmitted disease (STD)
  R/O: UTI, urethritis (STD)
- Age > 50 years
  R/O: UTI
- Possibility of pregnancy
  Reason: needs pregnancy test and urinary testing
- Painful urination AND EITHER frequency or urgency
  R/O: uncomplicated cystitis
  Note: see antibiotic treatment option in home care advice.
- All other females with painful urination, or patient wants to be seen
  R/O: UTI, urethritis (STD)

Home Care

- Taking antibiotic < 24 hours for UTI and fever persists
  Reason: taking antibiotic and no complications
- Taking antibiotic < 3 days for UTI and painful urination not improved
  Reason: taking antibiotic and no complications

HOME CARE ADVICE

Home Care Advice for Urination Pain (Pending PCP Evaluation)

1. **Fluids:** Drink extra fluids. Drink 8-10 glasses of liquids a day (Reason: to produce a dilute, non-irritating urine).
2. **Cranberry Juice:**
   - Some people think that drinking cranberry juice may help in fighting urinary tract infections. However, there is no good research that has ever proved this.
   - **Dosage Cranberry Juice Cocktail:** 8 oz (240 mL) twice a day.
   - **Dosage 100% Cranberry Juice:** 1 oz (30 mL) twice a day.

3. **Warm Saline Sitz Baths to Reduce Pain:** Sit in a warm saline bath for 20 minutes to cleanse the area and to reduce pain. Add 2 oz of table salt or baking soda to a tub of water.
4. **Call Back If:**
   - You become worse.

Antibiotic Treatment Option for Uncomplicated Cystitis

1. Some physicians are willing to initiate antibiotic therapy for uncomplicated cystitis over the telephone. Follow policy and the physician's practice rules.
2. **Must Be Present:** Dysuria AND EITHER frequency or urgency. Not essential, but helpful: caller states that it feels just like prior "bladder/urine infection."
3. **Must Be Absent:** New/changed vaginal discharge, fever, flank pain, age more than 50, pregnancy, diabetes, or any other significant health problem.
4. **Recommended Antibiotic:** Bactrim DS (trimethoprim-sulfamethoxazole; 1 PO BID for 3 days), MacroBid (nitrofurantoin; 1 PO BID for 3 days), or Cipro (ciprofloxacin; 250 mg PO BID for 3 days).
5. **Caution—Antibiotics:** Ask patient about allergies. Bactrim is a sulfa-type antibiotic.

Home Care Advice if Already Receiving Antibiotic Treatment for UTI

1. **Fluids:** Drink extra fluids. Drink 8-10 glasses of liquids a day. (Reason: to produce a dilute, nonirritating urine).
2. **Cranberry Juice:**
   - Some people think that drinking cranberry juice may help in fighting urinary tract infections. However, there is no good research that has ever proved this.
   - **Dosage Cranberry Juice Cocktail:** 8 oz (240 mL) twice a day.
   - **Dosage 100% Cranberry Juice:** 1 oz (30 mL) twice a day.
3. **OTC Phenazopyrine for Severe Dysyuria and Frequency:**
   - Phenazopyridine (Uristat) is available OTC (in United States only). Dosage is 2 pills by mouth 3 times a day.
   - It is also available as a prescription medicine (Pyridium, Urogesic). It has a numbing effect on the lining of the bladder and urethra. It can help reduce burning during urination, urgency, and frequency until the antibiotics start working.
   - It does not have any antibacterial effect.
   - Read the package instructions thoroughly on all medications that you take.
4. **Caution—Phenazopyridine:**
   - It turns the urine bright orange. This can cause staining of underwear. It can also sometimes stain contact lenses.
   - Do not take this medicine if you have kidney disease.
   - Do not use if pregnant (Reason: class B, should discuss with PCP first).
   - Do not use if breastfeeding (Reason: safety unknown, should discuss with PCP first).
   - DO NOT USE MORE THAN 2 DAYS.
5. **Call Back If:**
   - Fever lasts more than 24 hours on antibiotics.
   - Pain does not improve by day 3 on antibiotics.
   - Urine symptoms do not improve by day 3 on antibiotics.
   - You become worse.

FIRST AID

First Aid Advice for Shock:

Lie down with the feet elevated.

BACKGROUND INFORMATION

General

- Dysuria is the medical term that describes burning or pain with urination.
- Anything that irritates the urethral mucosa can cause dysuria. Urinary tract infections (UTIs) are the number one cause of dysuria. The term UTI is nonspecific and encompasses a number of more specific diagnoses.
- Half of all women experience at least one UTI at some point in their lifetime.

UTI Causes of Dysuria

- **Cystitis:** An infection of the bladder mucosa. Urinary frequency and urgency are typically present. Blood in the urine may also be seen. There may be an associated mild midline suprapubic discomfort in the area of the bladder. In the 20- to 50-year-old, cystitis is 30 times more common in women than men. This gender difference may reflect the much shorter length of the female urethra, which facilitates migration of bacteria up into the bladder. Risk factors for female cystitis in younger women include sexual intercourse, spermicidal usage, and pregnancy. Risk factors for cystitis in older females include institutionalization (i.e., nursing home), urinary catheterization (i.e., Foley), and recent urologic surgery.
- **Pyelonephritis:** An infection of the kidney. An untreated cystitis may develop into pyelonephritis. Commonly associated symptoms include flank pain, fever, and chills. Symptoms of cystitis (dysuria, frequency) may or may not be present.
- **Urethritis:** Urethritis is a sexually transmitted disease (STD). The 2 principal organisms responsible for urethritis are *Gonnorhea* and *Chlamydia*. Suprapubic pain and hematuria are absent.

Other Causes of Dysuria

- **Labial Sores:** If a women has a scratch or any type of sore on the labia near the urethra, the exiting warm urine may cause some pain. Many women will note that it "hurts outside." And unlike a cystitis, there is no frequency or urgency.
- **Vaginitis:** Vaginitis is a general term which means "vaginal inflammation." Vaginitis can have chemical etiology (excessive douching, or excessive use of OTC yeast medication). Vaginitis may have an infectious etiology: trichomonas or yeast *(Candida)*.
- **Vaginitis, Atrophic:** In postmenopausal women, the vaginal mucosa thins because of lack of estrogen. Some women complain of mild dysuria, others experience itching, and others describe dyspareunia (painful intercourse).

URINATION PAIN (MALE)

DEFINITION

- Discomfort (pain, burning, or stinging) when passing urine.
- Associated symptoms may include urgency (can't wait) and frequency (passing small amounts) of urination.

Pain Severity Is Defined As:

- **Mild (1-3):** Complains slightly about urination hurting
- **Moderate (4-7):** Interferes with normal activities
- **Severe (8-10):** Excruciating, unwilling or unable to urinate because of the pain

TRIAGE ASSESSMENT QUESTIONS

Call EMS 911 Now

- Shock suspected (e.g., cold/pale/clammy skin, too weak to stand)
  R/O: urosepsis, shock
  FIRST AID: Lie down with the feet elevated.
- Sounds like a life-threatening emergency to the triager

Go to ED Now (or to Office With PCP Approval)

- Unable to urinate (or only a few drops) and bladder feels very full
  R/O: urinary retention
- Pain in scrotum or testicle that persists > 1 hour
  R/O: torsion of testis or appendix testis, epididymitis
- Swollen scrotum
  R/O: torsion of testis, strangulated hernia, orchitis, epididymitis
- Patient sounds very sick or weak to the triager

Go to Office Now

- Severe pain with urination
  R/O: severe urethritis or cystitis
- Fever > 100.5° F (38.1° C)
  R/O: pyelonephritis
- Side (flank) or lower back pain present
  R/O: pyelonephritis

See Today in Office

- Taking antibiotic > 24 hours for UTI and fever persists
  R/O: complication, resistant organism, or need for IV antibiotics
- Taking antibiotic > 3 days for UTI and painful urination not improved
  R/O: resistant organism
- Taking treatment > 3 days for STD (e.g., penile discharge from gonorrhea, chlamydia) and painful urination not improved
  R/O: resistant organism
- All other males with painful urination, or patient wants to be seen
  R/O: UTI, urethritis (STD)

Home Care

- Taking antibiotic < 24 hours for UTI and fever persists
  Reason: taking antibiotic and no complications
- Taking antibiotic < 3 days for UTI and painful urination not improved
  Reason: taking antibiotic and no complications
- Taking antibiotic < 3 days for STD and painful urination not improved
  Reason: taking antibiotic and no complications

HOME CARE ADVICE

Home Care Advice for Urination Pain (Pending PCP Evaluation)

1. **Fluids:** Drink extra fluids (Reason: to produce a dilute, nonirritating urine).
2. **Call Back If:**
   - You become worse.

Home Care Advice if Already Receiving Antibiotic Treatment for UTI

1. **Fluids:** Drink extra fluids (Reason: to produce a dilute, nonirritating urine).
2. **Call Back If:**
   - Fever lasts more than 24 hours on antibiotics.
   - Pain does not improve by day 3 on antibiotics.
   - Urine symptoms do not improve by day 3 on antibiotics.
   - You become worse.

FIRST AID

First Aid Advice for Shock:

Lie down with the feet elevated.

BACKGROUND INFORMATION

General

- Dysuria is the medical term that describes burning or pain with urination. Adult males with dysuria require examination and laboratory evaluation to determine if an infection is present.
- Anything that irritates the urethral mucosa can cause dysuria. Urinary tract infections (UTIs) are the most common cause of dysuria. The term UTI is nonspecific and encompasses a number of more specific diagnoses: cystitis, urethritis, prostatitis.
- In younger men, it is more likely that the dysuria is the result of urethritis from a sexually transmitted disease.
- In older men, cystitis becomes the more likely culprit and the infection is caused by coliform bacteria like *E coli*.

UTI Causes of Dysuria

- **Cystitis:** An infection of the bladder mucosa. Urinary frequency and urgency may be present. There may be an associated mild midline suprapubic discomfort in the area of the bladder. Cystitis is much less common in men than women. Cystitis is rare in healthy young to middle-aged males. Risk factors for male cystitis include age over 60, urinary catheterization (i.e., Foley), and recent urologic surgery.
- **Pyelonephritis:** An infection of the kidney. Untreated cystitis may develop into pyelonephritis. Commonly associated symptoms include flank pain, fever, and chills. Symptoms of cystitis (dysuria, frequency) may or may not be present.
- **Prostatitis:** An infection of the prostate. Dysuria and other urine symptoms may be mild or absent. Sometimes there is fever and a vague poorly localized lower abdominal or lower back pain.
- **Orchitis/Epididymitis:** An infection of the testicle or epididymis. The presenting complaint is usually pain and swelling in and around the testicle.
- **Urethritis:** Urethritis is a sexually transmitted disease (STD). The 2 principal organisms responsible for urethritis are *Gonnorhea* and *Chlamydia*. Most men with urethritis will describe a clear-white to light yellow discharge from the penis.

Other Causes of Dysuria

- **Trauma:** Injuries to the penis with urethral damage can cause dysuria; the urine irritates the injured section of the male urethra.
- **Urethral Lithiasis:** Secondary to passing a kidney stone. As the stone passes through the male urethra, transient discomfort occurs.
- **Urinary Retention:** Prostate enlargement or a urethral stricture can cause obstructive symptoms and discomfort. True dysuria is usually absent, unless there is a concomitant UTI.

VAGINAL BLEEDING, ABNORMAL

DEFINITION

Menstrual bleeding is abnormal or excessive when any of the following occur:

- More than 7 days (1 week) of bleeding
- More than 6 well-soaked pads or tampons per day
- More than 21 pads or tampons per menstrual period
- Large blood clots (e.g., large coin, golf ball)
- Periods occur more frequently than every 21 days
- Periods occur less frequently than every 35 days
- Any bleeding or spotting between regular periods
- Has been diagnosed with anemia

Includes: Health information for abnormal vaginal bleeding associated with DepoProvera, Norplant, birth control patches, and missed birth control pills

Vaginal Bleeding Severity Is Described As:

- **Spotting:** Spotting, or pinkish/brownish mucous discharge; does not fill panti-liner or pad
- **Mild:** Less than 1 pad/hour; less than patient's usual menstrual bleeding
- **Moderate:** 1-2 pads/hour; small-medium blood clots (e.g., pea, grape, small coin)
- **Severe:** Soaking 2 or more pads/hour for 2 or more hours; bleeding not contained by pads or continuous red blood from vagina; large blood clots (e.g., golf ball, large coin)

TRIAGE ASSESSMENT QUESTIONS

Call EMS 911 Now

- Passed out (i.e., fainted, collapsed and was not responding)
  R/O: shock
  FIRST AID: Lie down with the feet elevated.
- Difficult to awaken or acting confused (e.g., disoriented, slurred speech)
  R/O: shock
  FIRST AID: Lie down with the feet elevated.
- Shock suspected (e.g., cold/pale/clammy skin, too weak to stand)
  R/O: shock
  FIRST AID: Lie down with the feet elevated.
- Severe bleeding (e.g., continuous red blood from vagina, or large blood clots) and very weak (can't stand)
- Sounds like a life-threatening emergency to the triager

See More Appropriate Protocol

- Vaginal discharge is main symptom and small amount of blood
  Go to Protocol: Vaginal Discharge on page 332

Go to ED Now

- Severe dizziness (e.g., unable to stand, requires support to walk, feels like passing out now)
  R/O: anemia
- Severe abdominal pain
  R/O: ectopic pregnancy
- Passed tissue (e.g., gray-white)
  R/O: spontaneous abortion

Go to ED Now (or to Office With PCP Approval)

- SEVERE vaginal bleeding (i.e., soaking 2 pads or tampons per hour and present 2 or more hours)
  Reason: severe bleeding
- MODERATE vaginal bleeding (i.e., soaking pad or tampon per hour and present > 6 hours)
  Reason: prolonged moderate bleeding
- Pale skin (pallor) of new onset or worsening
- Constant abdominal pain lasting > 2 hours
  R/O: endometritis, ectopic
- Patient sounds very sick or weak to the triager

See Today in Office

- Taking Coumadin (warfarin), Pradaxa (dabigatran), or known bleeding disorder (e.g., thrombocytopenia)
  Reason: higher risk of serious bleeding; may need for testing of INR, ProTime, or platelet count
- Skin bruises or nosebleed and not caused by an injury
  R/O: bleeding disorder
- Bleeding/spotting after procedure (e.g., biopsy) or pelvic examination (e.g., Pap smear) that persists > 3 days
- Patient wants to be seen

See Within 2 Weeks in Office

- Periods with > 6 soaked pads or tampons per day
  Reason: excessive vaginal bleeding, check for anemia
- Periods last > 7 days
  Reason: excessive vaginal bleeding, check for anemia
- Missed period has occurred 2 or more times in the last year and the cause is not known
  Reason: may need further evaluation and testing
- Menstrual cycle < 21 days OR > 35 days, and occurs more than 2 cycles (2 months) this past year
  Reason: may need further evaluation and testing
- Bleeding or spotting between regular periods occurs more than 2 cycles (2 months),
  R/O: dysfunctional uterine bleeding, fibroids, secondary anemia
- Bleeding or spotting between regular periods occurs more than 2 cycles (2 months), and using birth control medicine (e.g., pills, patch, DepoProvera, Implanon, vaginal ring, Mirena IUD)
  Reason: evaluation and counseling; change in management may be needed.
- Bleeding or spotting occurs after hysterectomy
  Reason: no menses should occur after hysterectomy
- Age > 39 years with irregular or excessive bleeding
  R/O: anovulatory bleeding from endometrial carcinoma
  Reason: endometrial assessment may be needed

Home Care

- Normal menstrual flow
- MILD bleeding or SPOTTING and could be pregnant (e.g., missed last period)
  Reason: check home pregnancy test and call back if positive. All triage questions negative.
- MILD bleeding or SPOTTING after procedure (e.g., biopsy) or pelvic examination (e.g., Pap smear) persisting < 4 days
- MILD bleeding or SPOTTING and immediately follows first intercourse
- Taking birth control pills and hasn't missed taking any pills
  R/O: breakthrough bleeding
- Taking birth control pills and has missed one or more pills
  R/O: expected breakthrough bleeding or spotting
- Using DepoProvera subdermal implant
  R/O: hormone side effect
- Has Implanon subdermal implant
  Reason: bleeding is probably a common side effect of birth control hormone
- Using birth control patch (i.e., transdermal contraceptive system)
  R/O: breakthrough bleeding
- Using vaginal contraceptive ring (i.e., NuvaRing)
  R/O: breakthrough bleeding
- Using Mirena IUD (a special IUD that releases the hormone progestin)
  R/O: irregular bleeding or spotting from this hormonal IUD

HOME CARE ADVICE

Mild Vaginal Bleeding

1. **Pregnancy Test, When in Doubt:**
   - If there is any possibility of pregnancy, obtain and use a urine pregnancy test from the local drugstore.
   - Follow the instructions included in the package.
2. **Spotting After a Procedure or Pelvic Exam:** The cervix bleeds easily and even an internal exam, Pap smear, or biopsy of the cervix can cause some spotting. This spotting should subside within 24-72 hours.
3. **Spotting After First Intercourse:** Mild bleeding or spotting with first intercourse is common. It should stop within 48 hours and not recur.
4. **Iron and Anemia:** Heavy periods are the most common cause of iron deficiency anemia in women of childbearing age. Women with heavy periods should eat a diet rich in iron or take a daily multivitamin pill with iron.
5. **Call Back If:**
   - Pregnancy test is positive.
   - You have difficulties with the home pregnancy test.
   - Bleeding becomes worse.
   - You become worse.

Irregular Vaginal Bleeding While Using Birth Control Medicine

1. **Spotting Between Periods and Taking Birth Control Pills:** Breakthrough bleeding or spotting is common with most current birth control pills, especially during the first 3 pill pack cycles.
2. **Irregular Bleeding and You Are Using Implanon or DepoProvera:** Irregular bleeding is a common side effect. It may include heavier, lighter, more frequent, or less frequent bleeding than your normal periods.
3. **Irregular Bleeding and You Are Using the Birth Control Patch:** Breakthrough bleeding or spotting is common with current birth control patches, especially during the first 3 cycles (months).
4. **Irregular Bleeding and You Are Using the Vaginal Contraceptive Ring (i.e., NuvaRing):** Breakthrough bleeding or spotting is not common with the vaginal contraceptive ring (i.e., NuvaRing). However, it can occur especially during the first 1 or 2 months of use (first 2 cycles).
5. **Irregular Bleeding and You Are Using the Mirena IUD:**
   - Bleeding and spotting may increase during the first several months after you get a Mirena IUD and your periods may be irregular.
   - Over time your menstrual periods may become shorter or lighter.
   - At some point your menstrual periods may stop completely. Your period will return after the IUD is removed by your health care provider.
6. **Diary:** Keep a record of the days you have any bleeding or spotting.
7. **Call Back If:**
   - Irregular bleeding occurs more than 2 cycles (2 months).
   - Bleeding becomes worse.
   - You become worse.

Taking Birth Control Pills and Missed One or More Pills

1. **Spotting Between Periods and You Forgot to Take a Birth Control Pill:**
   - Missing a pill may cause breakthrough bleeding or spotting.
   - If you ever forget to take more than one pill during a month, then you should use a backup contraceptive method (e.g., condom) until you start the next pill pack.
2. **Birth Control Pills—Missed 1:**
   - If you forget to take a pill, take it as soon as you remember. Then take the next one on schedule. This may mean you take 2 pills in 1 day.
   - If you ever forget to take more than 1 pill for a month, then you should use a backup contraceptive method (condom and foam) until you start the next pill pack.
3. **Birth Control Pills—Missed 2:**
   - If you forget to take 2 pills, then take 2 pills the next 2 days. Then take the next one on schedule.
   - Never take more than 2 pills in 1 day (Reason: nausea and vomiting are side effects of too much hormone from the pills).
   - You must use a backup contraceptive method (condom and foam) until you start the next pill pack.
4. **Birth Control Pills—Lost 1 Pill:**
   - Take the next pill in the pack today.
   - As a result, you will finish the birth control pill pack 1 day sooner.
   - Even though you will finish your pack 1 day sooner, you will probably want to start your next pill pack on your usual day (many women start their pill packs on a Sunday).
5. **Pregnancy Test, When in Doubt:**
   - If there is any possibility of pregnancy, obtain and use a urine pregnancy test from the local drugstore.
   - Follow the instructions included in the package.

FIRST AID

First Aid Advice for Shock:

Lie down with the feet elevated.

BACKGROUND INFORMATION

General Information

- The first day of menstrual bleeding is considered the first day of a new menstrual cycle.
- Menstrual bleeding typically lasts 3-7 days. The heaviest flow usually occurs during the first 1-3 days.
- Ovulation generally occurs around day 14 of the cycle.
- The length of the menstrual cycle varies from woman to woman. The range is from 24 to 35 days. The average is 28 days.
- Excessive vaginal bleeding is the most common cause of iron deficiency anemia in women of childbearing age.

Caution—Pregnancy

- The possibility of pregnancy must be considered in all women in their childbearing years who have vaginal bleeding.
- In early pregnancy, vaginal bleeding can be a sign of serious problems like miscarriage or pregnancy in the tubes.

VAGINAL DISCHARGE

DEFINITION

- Vaginal discharge

TRIAGE ASSESSMENT QUESTIONS

See More Appropriate Protocol

- Pain or burning with urination is main symptom
  Go to Protocol: Urination Pain (Female) on page 323

Go to ED Now (or to Office With PCP Approval)

- SEVERE abdominal pain (e.g., excruciating)
  R/O: acute salpingitis, ectopic pregnancy, appendicitis
- Patient sounds very sick or weak to the triager

Go to Office Now

- Yellow or green vaginal discharge and fever
  R/O: acute salpingitis
- Constant abdominal pain lasting > 2 hours
  R/O: acute salpingitis, ectopic pregnancy, appendicitis

See Today in Office

- Mild lower abdominal pain comes and goes (cramps) that lasts > 24 hours
  R/O: salpingitis
- Genital area looks infected (e.g., draining sore, spreading redness)
  R/O: STD, cellulitis, Bartholin cyst
- Rash is tiny water blisters (3 or more)
  R/O: herpes simplex, pustules
- Patient wants to be seen

See Today or Tomorrow in Office

- Rash (e.g., redness, tiny bumps, sore) of genital area present > 24 hours
  R/O: herpes, pubic lice, genital warts, or other sexually transmitted infection (STD/STI)

See Within 3 Days in Office

- Bad-smelling vaginal discharge
  R/O: vulvovaginitis from Trichomonas *or bacterial vaginosis*
- Abnormal color vaginal discharge (i.e., yellow, green, gray)
  R/O: vulvovaginitis from Trichomonas *or bacterial vaginosis*
- Symptoms of a yeast infection (i.e., itchy, white discharge, not bad smelling) and not improved > 3 days following home care advice
- 4 or more episodes of vaginal infection in past year
  Reason: recurrent vulvovaginitis; consider diabetes or other medical disorder
- Diabetes mellitus or immunocompromised (e.g., HIV positive, cancer chemotherapy, transplant patient)
  R/O: complicated vulvovaginitis
- Patient is worried about a sexually transmitted disease (STD)
  Reason: to relieve fear or prevent spread of STD

See Within 2 Weeks in Office

- Pain with sexual intercourse (dyspareunia)
  Exception: vaginal yeast infection suspected
  R/O: salpingitis, STD

Home Care

- Normal vaginal discharge
  R/O: physiologic discharge
- Symptoms of a vaginal yeast infection (i.e., white, thick, cottage-cheese–like, itchy, not bad-smelling discharge)
  Reason: probable vaginal yeast infection

HOME CARE ADVICE FOR NORMAL VAGINAL DISCHARGE OR YEAST INFECTION

1. **Pregnancy Test, When in Doubt:**
   - If there is any possibility of pregnancy, obtain and use a urine pregnancy test from the local drugstore.
   - Follow the instructions included in the package.
2. **Antifungal Medication for Vaginal Yeast Infection:** There are a number of over-the-counter medications for the treatment of vaginal yeast infections.
   - **Available in the United States:** Miconazole (Monistat 3), clotrimazole (Gyne-Lotrimin 3, Mycelex-7), butoconazole (Femstat 3).
   - **Available in Canada:** Miconazole (Monistat 3) and clotrimazole (Canesten 3, Myclo-Gyne).
   - Do not use yeast medication during the 24 hours prior to a physician appointment (Reason: interferes with examination).
   - **Caution:** If you are pregnant, speak with your doctor before using.
   - Read the package instructions thoroughly on all medications that you take.
3. **Genital Hygiene:**
   - Keep your genital area clean. Wash daily.
   - Keep your genital area dry. Wear cotton underwear or underwear with a cotton crotch.
   - Do not douche.
   - Do not use feminine hygiene products.
4. **Call Back If:**
   - Pregnancy test is positive.
   - You have difficulties with the home pregnancy test.
   - There is no improvement after treating yourself for a vaginal yeast infection.
   - You become worse.

BACKGROUND INFORMATION

Normal Vaginal Discharge

- Normal vaginal discharge may be clear or white, thin or thick.
- It is not odorous and there is no itching.

Abnormal Vaginal Discharge

- **Color:** Yellow, green, or gray-colored vaginal discharge is usually abnormal. Vulvovaginitis from *Trichomonas* or bacterial vaginosis should be suspected.
- **Smell:** Bad or foul-smelling discharge is usually abnormal. Vulvovaginitis from *Trichomonas* or bacterial vaginosis should be suspected.
- **Consistency:** A thick, white cottage-cheese–like, non-odorous, itchy discharge is usually abnormal. A yeast infection (vulvovaginitis from *Candida)* should be suspected.

Causes of Vaginal Discharge

- **Atrophic Vaginitis:** Perimenopausal and post-menopausal women will often describe itching and dryness of the vulvovaginal area. This is the result of atrophic changes in this area from the lack of estrogen stimulation.
- **Cervicitis:** Gonnorrhea and chlamydia are sexually transmitted diseases (STDs) which can cause cervicitis. Symptoms can include vaginal discharge, dysuria, pelvic pain, and bleeding.
- **Contact Dermatitis and Irritation:** Douching, soaps, and other chemical products can sometimes cause symptoms of itching and irritation.
- **Pelvic Inflammatory Disease:** Pelvic inflammatory disease (PID) is an infection of the tubes connecting the ovaries to the uterus. PID is a serious illness which in some cases requires hospitalization and intravenous antibiotics. The clinical presentation of PID is variable, but symptoms classically include: lower abdominal/pelvic pain, fever, and vaginal discharge.

- **Vaginal Foreign Bodies:** Vaginal foreign bodies (FBs) must be removed to prevent a vaginal infection. Sometimes FBs are not discovered until after the patient comes in for a bad-smelling yellow vaginal discharge. Most vaginal FBs can be easily removed in the doctor's office.
- **Vulvovaginitis:** Vaginal discharge and vulvovaginal itching are the symptoms of vulvovaginitis. The 3 main types of vulvovaginitis are candidiasis (yeast infection; symptoms of thick, white, cottage-cheese–like, non-odorous discharge), *Trichomonas* (foamy, yellow-green, foul-smelling discharge) and bacterial vaginosis (white-gray discharge, fishy odor).

Caution—Pregnancy

- The possibility of pregnancy must be considered in all women in their childbearing years.
- In the second half of pregnancy, increasing vaginal discharge can be a subtle sign of preterm labor.

VOMITING

DEFINITION

- Vomiting ("throwing up") is the forceful emptying of a portion of the stomach's contents through the mouth.
- Retching ("dry heaves") describes rhythmic contractions of the abdominal and intercostal muscles against a closed glottis (no vomit).

Vomiting Severity Is Defined As:

- **Mild:** 1-5 times/day
- **Moderate:** 6-10 times/day
- **Severe:** More than 10 times/day, vomits everything or nearly everything

TRIAGE ASSESSMENT QUESTIONS

Call EMS 911 Now

- Shock suspected (e.g., cold/pale/clammy skin, too weak to stand)
  R/O: shock
  FIRST AID: Lie down with the feet elevated.
- Difficult to awaken or acting confused (e.g., disoriented, slurred speech)
  R/O: shock
  FIRST AID: Lie down with the feet elevated.
- Sounds like a life-threatening emergency to the triager

See More Appropriate Protocol

- Vomiting occurs only while coughing
  Go to Protocol: Cough on page 66
- Chest pain
  Go to Protocol: Chest Pain on page 48
- Severe headache and similar to prior migraines
  Go to Protocol: Headache on page 148

Go to ED Now

- Vomiting red blood or black (coffee ground) material
  R/O: gastritis, peptic ulcer
- Insulin-dependent diabetes and glucose > 400
  R/O: DKA
- Recent head injury (within 3 days)
  R/O: subdural hematoma
- Recent abdominal injury (within 7 days)
  R/O: traumatic pancreatitis

Go to ED Now (or to Office With PCP Approval)

- SEVERE vomiting (e.g., > 10 times/day)
  Reason: greater risk for dehydration
- Vomiting 3 or more times (in past 24 hours) and age > 60
- Vomiting contains bile (green color)
  R/O: intestinal obstruction
- Severe pain in one eye
  R/O: acute glaucoma
- High-risk adult (e.g., diabetes mellitus, brain tumor, V-P shunt, hernia)
- Drinking very little and has signs of dehydration (e.g., no urine > 12 hours, very dry mouth, very light-headed)
  Reason: IV therapy needed
- Constant abdominal pain lasting > 2 hours
  R/O: GI obstruction
- Patient sounds very sick or weak to the triager

Go to Office Now

- Abdomen looks much more swollen than usual
  R/O: intestinal obstruction
- Fever > 103° F (39.4° C)
- Fever > 100.5° F (38.1° C) and over 60 years of age
- Fever > 100.5° F (38.1° C) and has a weakened immune system (e.g., HIV positive, cancer chemotherapy, organ transplant, splenectomy, chronic steroids)
- Fever > 100.5° F (38.1° C) and bedridden (e.g., nursing home patient, stroke, chronic illness, recovering from surgery)
  R/O: bacterial infection
  Note: may need ambulance transport to ED.
- Taking any of the following medications: digoxin (Lanoxin), lithium, theophylline, phenytoin (Dilantin)
  R/O: drug toxicity

Callback by PCP or Subspecialist Within 1 Hour

- Severe headache and vomiting
  R/O: migraine, increased ICP

See Today in Office

- Vomiting lasts > 48 hours
- Fever present > 3 days (72 hours)
- Patient wants to be seen

Callback by PCP Today

- Vomiting a prescribed medication or recently started on a new medication

See Within 3 Days in Office

- Alcohol abuse, known or suspected

See Within 2 Weeks in Office

- Vomiting is a chronic symptom (recurrent or ongoing AND lasting > 4 weeks)

Home Care

- Vomiting
  R/O: "stomach flu"

HOME CARE ADVICE FOR MILD VOMITING

1. **For Continuous Vomiting, Try Sleeping:**
   - Try to go to sleep (Reason: sleep often empties the stomach and relieves the need to vomit).
   - When you awaken, resume drinking liquids. Water works best initially.
2. **Clear Liquids:** Try to sip small amounts (1 tablespoon) of liquid frequently (every 5 minutes) for 8 hours, rather than trying to drink a lot of liquid all at one time.
   - Sip water or a rehydration drink (e.g., Gatorade or Powerade).
   - **Other Options:** ½-strength flat lemon-lime soda or ginger ale.
   - After 4 hours without vomiting, increase the amount.
3. **Solid Food:**
   - You may begin eating bland foods after 8 hours without vomiting. Start with saltine crackers, white bread, rice, mashed potatoes, cereal, applesauce, etc.
   - After 48 hours on a bland diet, you may resume a normal diet.
4. **Avoid Medicines:**
   - Discontinue all nonprescription medicines for 24 hours (Reason: they may make vomiting worse).
   - Call if vomiting a prescription medicine.
5. **Contagiousness:** You can return to work or school after vomiting and fever are gone.
6. **Expected Course:** Vomiting from viral gastritis usually stops in 12 to 48 hours. If diarrhea is present, it usually continues for several days.
7. **Call Back If:**
   - Vomiting persists for 48 hours.
   - Signs of dehydration occur.
   - You become worse.

FIRST AID

First Aid Advice for Shock:

Lie down with the feet elevated.

BACKGROUND INFORMATION

General

- Vomiting can occur in many type of illnesses.
- Nausea and abdominal discomfort usually precede each bout of vomiting.
- Vomiting occurring with diarrhea is suggestive of gastroenteritis (stomach flu) or some type of food poisoning. Most such patients can be managed at home.
- Maintaining hydration is the cornerstone of treatment of adults with acute vomiting. Patients with moderate to severe dehydration will require medical evaluation, usually in an emergency department or urgent care setting.
- In general, an adult who is alert, feels well, and who is not thirsty or dizzy is NOT dehydrated.

Causes

- Appendicitis.
- Bowel obstruction.
- **CNS:** Increased intracranial pressure may lead to vomiting.
- **Diabetic Ketoacidosis (DKA):** This is seen in diabetics who are taking insulin. Vomiting in insulin-dependent diabetics should be taken seriously and usually requires an emergency department disposition.
- Emotional response to certain smells.
- Food allergy.

- **Food-borne Illness ("Food Poisoning"):** Food poisoning is caused by toxins produced by bacteria growing in poorly refrigerated foods (e.g., *Staphylococcus* toxin in egg salad or *Bacillus cereus* toxin in rice dishes). Food-borne illnesses usually present with gastrointestinal symptoms of vomiting, diarrhea, and/or abdominal pain. The symptoms and their duration depend on the type of infection.
- **Gastroenteritis ("Stomach Flu"):** There are many viral and bacterial causes.
- Hepatitis.
- **Labyrinthine Disorders:** This grouping includes labyrinthitis and motion sickness. Typical symptoms are episodes of vertigo with nausea and vomiting.
- **Medications:** This may be the most common cause in adults, and certainly should be considered in elderly adults. Some examples include digoxin, narcotics, erythromycin, NSAIDs, and anticancer drugs.
- **Migraine Headaches:** Vomiting occurs commonly in some patients with migraine or cluster headaches.
- **Neurologic Disease:** Meningitis, encephalitis, Reye syndrome, blocked V-P shunt, head trauma, and other causes of increased intracranial pressure.
- Postoperative vomiting.
- **Renal Colic (Kidney Stone Attack):** Nausea and vomiting commonly accompany the flank pain of a kidney stone attack.
- Vomiting in first trimester of pregnancy (i.e., morning sickness).

Dehydration: Estimation by Telephone

Mild Dehydration

- **Urine Production:** Slightly decreased
- **Mucous Membranes:** Normal
- Heart rate < 100 beats/minute
- Slightly thirsty
- **Capillary Refill:** < 2 sec
- **Treatment:** Can usually treat at home

Moderate Dehydration

- **Urine Production:** Minimal or absent
- **Mucous Membranes:** Dry inside of mouth
- Heart rate 100-130 beats/minute
- Thirsty, light-headed when standing
- **Capillary Refill:** > 2 sec
- **Treatment:** Must be seen; go to ED NOW (or PCP triage)

Severe Dehydration

- **Urine Production:** None > 12 hours
- **Mucous Membranes:** Very dry inside of mouth
- Heart rate > 130 beats/minute
- Very thirsty, very weak, and light-headed; fainting may occur
- **Capillary Refill:** > 2-4 sec
- **Treatment:** Must be seen immediately; go to ED NOW or call EMS 911 NOW

Signs of Shock

- Confused, difficult to awaken, or unresponsive.
- Heart rate (pulse) is rapid and weak.
- Extremities (especially hands and feet) are bluish or gray, and cold.
- Too weak to stand or very dizzy when tries to stand.
- **Capillary Refill:** > 4 seconds.
- **Treatment:** Lie down with the feet elevated; call EMS 911 NOW.

VULVAR SYMPTOMS

DEFINITION

- Itching or dryness of external female genital area (vulva)
- Rashes of external female genital area including: sores, redness, blisters, lumps

Note:

- If vaginal discharge is the main symptom, see Vaginal Discharge protocol on page 332.

TRIAGE ASSESSMENT QUESTIONS

See More Appropriate Protocol

- Pain or burning with urination is main symptom
  Go to Protocol: Urination Pain (Female) on page 323
- Vaginal discharge is main symptom
  Go to Protocol: Vaginal Discharge on page 332
- Pubic lice suspected
  Go to Protocol: Pubic Lice on page 203
- STD exposure and prevention, question about
  Go to Protocol: STD Exposure and Prevention on page 249

Go to ED Now (or to Office With PCP Approval)

- Patient sounds very sick or weak to the triager

Go to Office Now

- Severe pain
  R/O: Bartholin cyst, herpes simplex

See Today in Office

- Genital area looks infected (e.g., draining sore, spreading redness)
  R/O: STD, cellulitis, Bartholin cyst
- Rash with painful tiny water blisters
  R/O: herpes simplex
- Patient wants to be seen

See Today or Tomorrow in Office

- Moderate-severe itching (i.e., interferes with school, work, or sleep)
  R/O: contact dermatitis, poison ivy, pubic lice
- Rash (e.g., redness, tiny bumps, sore) of genital area present > 24 hours
  R/O: herpes, pubic lice, genital warts
- Tender lump (swelling or "ball") at vaginal opening
  R/O: Bartholin cyst
  Note: the cyst is located in the left or right labia.
- Vulvar itching and not improved > 3 days following home care advice
  R/O: contact dermatitis, lichen sclerosis, STD
- Symptoms of a yeast infection (i.e., itchy, white discharge, not bad smelling) and not improved > 3 days following home care advice

See Within 3 Days in Office

- Patient is worried about a sexually transmitted disease (STD)
  Reason: to relieve fear or prevent spread of STD

See Within 2 Weeks in Office

- Itching or dryness of genital area and nearing menopause or after menopause
  R/O: atrophic vaginitis, dermatoses
- Pain in genital area is a chronic symptom (recurrent or ongoing AND lasting > 4 weeks)
  R/O: vulvodynia
- ALL other vulvar symptoms
  Exception: feels like prior yeast infection, or rash < 24 hour duration
  R/O: skin dermatoses or cancer, atrophic changes, psoriasis

Home Care

- Symptoms of a yeast infection (i.e., itchy, white discharge, not bad smelling), which feels like prior vaginal yeast infections
  R/O: yeast vulvovaginitis
- Rash (e.g., redness, tiny bumps, sore) of genital area present < 24 hours
  R/O: minor abrasion, mild irritation or contact dermatitis
- Mild vulvar itching
  R/O: contact dermatitis, excess moisture

HOME CARE ADVICE FOR MILD VULVAR SYMPTOMS

General

1. **Pregnancy Test, When in Doubt:**
   - If there is any possibility of pregnancy, obtain and use a urine pregnancy test from the local drugstore.
   - Follow the instructions included in the package.
2. **Call Back If:**
   - Pregnancy test is positive or if you have difficulties with the home pregnancy test.
   - Rash lasts longer than 24 hours.
   - Rash spreads or becomes worse.
   - Fever occurs.
   - No improvement after 3 days.
   - You become worse.

Symptoms of a Vaginal Yeast Infection

1. **Genital Hygiene:**
   - Keep your genital area clean. Wash daily.
   - Keep your genital area dry. Wear cotton underwear or underwear with a cotton crotch.
   - Do not douche.
   - Do not use feminine hygiene products.
2. **Antifungal Medication for Yeast Infection:** There are a number of over-the-counter medications for the treatment of yeast infections.
   - **Available in the United States:** Miconazole (Monistat 3), clotrimazole (Gyne-Lotrimin 3, Mycelex-7), butoconazole (Femstat 3).
   - **Available in Canada:** Miconazole (Monistat 3) and clotrimazole (Canesten 3, Myclo-Gyne).
   - Do not use yeast medication during the 24 hours prior to a physician appointment (Reason: interferes with examination).
   - **Caution:** If you are pregnant, speak with your doctor before using.
   - Read the package instructions thoroughly on all medications that you take.
3. **Expected Course:** If there is no improvement within 3 days, then you will need to be examined.
4. **Call Back If:**
   - Any rash lasts longer than 24 hours.
   - Fever occurs.
   - Yellow or green vaginal discharge occurs.
   - No improvement in "yeast infection" within 3 days.
   - You become worse.

Mild Vulvar Itching

1. **Reassurance:** Common causes of mild vaginal itching are new soaps/detergent, perfumed toilet products, hormone changes, and excessive perspiration. Sometimes itching can be caused by a yeast infection.
2. **Genital Hygiene:**
   - Keep your genital area clean. Wash daily.
   - Keep your genital area dry. Wear cotton underwear or underwear with a cotton crotch.
   - Do not douche.
   - Do not use feminine hygiene products.
3. **Cleaning:** Wash the area once thoroughly with unscented soap and water to remove any irritants.
4. **Take a Sitz Bath:**
   - Take a 10-15 minute sitz bath once or twice a day. Sitting in the warm water will help soothe the irritated skin. You can make a sitz bath by adding 2 ounces (60 grams) of baking soda to a bathtub containing warm water.
   - Afterward dry the area by gently patting it with a towel.
   - Lastly, apply a small amount of ointment or cream to help seal in the moisture. Good choices for this are Vaseline ointment or Eucerin.
5. **Call Back If:**
   - Any rash lasts longer than 24 hours.
   - Fever occurs.
   - Yellow or green vaginal discharge occurs.
   - No improvement in "yeast infection' within 3 days.
   - You become worse.

BACKGROUND INFORMATION

Causes

- Any preexisting skin disorders/rashes can also occur on the vulva (e.g., psoriasis, eczema, drug rashes).
- Bartholin cyst.
- Candidal vulvovaginitis (aka yeast infection).
- Contact dermatitis (e.g., soaps, feminine hygiene products).
- Irritation after sexual intercourse (e.g., inadequate lubrication, latex-condom allergy).
- Poison ivy.
- Skin cancer.
- Skin dermatoses (e.g., lichen sclerosis, squamous hyperplasia).
- STDs (e.g., herpes simplex, syphilis, pubic lice, genital warts).

Common Causes of Vulvar Itching

- **Contact Dermatitis—Irritant:** There are 2 different types of vulvar contact dermatitis: irritant and allergic. Products like soaps, detergents, and douches can cause local irritation. Urinary incontinence can result in the vulva being irritated by constant moisture. The treatment for irritant contact dermatitis is to avoid irritating products and to keep the vulvar area clean and dry (maintain good genital hygiene).
- **Contact Dermatitis—Allergic:** Women can develop an allergic skin reaction to a number of different OTC products. These products include: benzocaine (in Vagisil anti-itch cream), neomycin (antibiotic ointment), latex condoms, nail polish, and perfumes. The treatment for allergic contact dermatitis is to avoid allergic products and to keep the vulvar area clean and dry (maintain good genital hygiene).
- **Menopause:** At menopause the ovaries stop functioning, and as result the body produces less estrogen. Without estrogen, the skin in the genital area can become thin and women notice increased dryness. There are estrogen-based vaginal crèmes or lubricants that the physician can prescribe to reduce this itching and dryness.
- **Yeast Vulvovaginitis (Yeast Infection):** Sometimes itching can be caused by a yeast infection *(Candida)*. Often there is a new or increased vaginal discharge (thick, white, cottage-cheese–like, non-odorous discharge). There are a number of over-the-counter medications for the treatment of vaginal yeast infections.

WEAKNESS (GENERALIZED) AND FATIGUE

DEFINITION

- Patient complains of generalized body weakness.
- Patient complains of fatigue (tiredness, lack of energy).

Weakness Severity Is Defined As:

- **Mild:** Feels weak or tired but does not interfere with work, school, or normal activities.
- **Moderate:** Able to stand and walk; weakness interferes with work, school, or normal activities.
- **Severe:** Unable to stand or walk.

TRIAGE ASSESSMENT QUESTIONS

Call EMS 911 Now

- Severe difficulty breathing (e.g., struggling for each breath, speaks in single words)
  R/O: hypoxia and need for oxygen
- Shock suspected (e.g., cold/pale/clammy skin, too weak to stand)
  R/O: shock
  FIRST AID: Lie down with the feet elevated.
- Difficult to awaken or acting confused (e.g., disoriented, slurred speech)
  R/O: shock
  FIRST AID: Lie down with the feet elevated.
- Fainted > 15 minutes ago and still feels too weak or dizzy to stand
  R/O: hypovolemia, arrhythmia
- SEVERE weakness (i.e., unable to walk or barely able to walk, requires support) and new onset or worsening
  Reason: severe weakness, acute
  R/O: anemia, cardiac problem, serious infection, volume depletion, metabolic abnormality
- Sounds like a life-threatening emergency to the triager

See More Appropriate Protocol

- Weakness of the face, arm, or leg on one side of the body
  Go to Protocol: Neurologic Deficit on page 190
- Known diabetic and weakness from low blood sugar (i.e., < 60 mg/dL or 3.5 mmol/L)
  Go to Protocol: Diabetes, Low Blood Sugar on page 83
- Recent heat exposure, suspected cause of weakness
  Go to Protocol: Heat Exposure (Heat Exhaustion and Heatstroke) on page 146
- Vomiting is main symptom
  Go to Protocol: Vomiting on page 335
- Diarrhea is main symptom
  Go to Protocol: Diarrhea on page 89

Go to ED Now

- Difficulty breathing
  R/O: hypoxia with need for oxygen, acidosis
- Heart beating < 50 beats per minute OR > 140 beats per minute
  Reason: symptomatic bradycardia or tachycardia
- Extra heartbeats OR irregular heartbeating (i.e., "palpitations")
  R/O: dysrrhythmia
- Follows bleeding (e.g., from vomiting, rectum, vagina)
  R/O: hypovolemic shock from major blood loss
  Exception: small transient weakness from sight of a small amount of blood
- Black or tarry bowel movements
  R/O: melena from UGI bleeding

Go to ED Now (or to Office With PCP Approval)

- MODERATE weakness from poor fluid intake with no improvement after 2 hours of rest and fluids
  Reason: may need IV hydration
- Drinking very little and dehydration suspected (e.g., no urine > 12 hours, very dry mouth, very light-headed)
  Reason: may need IV hydration
- Patient sounds very sick or weak to the triager
  R/O: severe illness

Go to Office Now

- MODERATE weakness (i.e., interferes with work, school, normal activities) and cause unknown
  Exceptions: weakness with acute minor illness, or weakness from poor fluid intake
- Fever > 103° F (39.4° C) and not able to get the fever down using home care advice
- Fever > 101° F (38.3° C) and bedridden (e.g., nursing home patient, CVA, chronic illness, recovering from surgery)
- Fever > 100.5° F (38.1° C) and diabetes mellitus or immunocompromised (e.g., HIV positive, cancer chemotherapy, splenectomy, organ transplant, chronic steroids)
- Pale skin (pallor)

See Today in Office

- MODERATE weakness (i.e., interferes with work, school, normal activities) and persists > 3 days
- Taking a medicine that could cause weakness (e.g., blood pressure medications, diuretics)

See Within 3 Days in Office

- MILD weakness (i.e., does not interfere with ability to work, go to school, normal activities) and persists > 1 week
  R/O: depression, stress, anemia, viral syndrome, broad range of other medical conditions
- Fatigue (i.e., tires easily, decreased energy) and persists > 1 week
  R/O: depression, stress, chronic fatigue syndrome, insufficient sleep, broad range of other medical conditions

See Within 2 Weeks in Office

- Weakness is a chronic symptom (recurrent or ongoing AND lasting > 4 weeks)
  Reason: reevaluation of chronic unchanged symptom

Home Care

- MILD weakness or fatigue with acute minor illness (e.g., colds)
- Weakness from poor fluid intake

HOME CARE ADVICE FOR WEAKNESS (GENERALIZED) AND FATIGUE

Weakness or Fatigue From Acute Minor Illness (e.g., Colds, Viral Syndrome)

1. **Reassurance:**
   - Weakness often accompanies viral illnesses (e.g., colds and flu).
   - The weakness is usually worse the first 3 days of the illness, then gets better.
   - A fever can make you feel weak.
2. **Fever Medicines:**
   - For fevers above 101° F (38.3° C) take acetaminophen or ibuprofen.
   - The goal of fever therapy is to bring the fever down to a comfortable level. Remember that fever medicine usually lowers fever 2 degrees F (1 - 1 ½ degrees C).

Acetaminophen (e.g., Tylenol):

- Take 650 mg by mouth every 4-6 hours. Each Regular Strength Tylenol pill has 325 mg of acetaminophen.
- Another choice is to take 1,000 mg every 8 hours. Each Extra Strength Tylenol pill has 500 mg of acetaminophen. The most you should take each day is 3,000 mg.

Ibuprofen (e.g., Motrin, Advil):

- Take 400 mg by mouth every 6 hours.
- Another choice is to take 600 mg by mouth every 8 hours.
- Use the lowest amount that makes your pain feel better.

Extra Notes:

- Acetaminophen is thought to be safer than ibuprofen in people over 65 years old. Acetaminophen is in many OTC and prescription medicines. It might be in more than one medicine that you are taking. You need to be careful and not take an overdose. An acetaminophen overdose can hurt the liver.
- **Caution:** Do not take acetaminophen if you have liver disease.
- **Caution:** Do not take ibuprofen if you have stomach problems, kidney disease, are pregnant, or have been told by your doctor to avoid

this type of anti-inflammatory drug. Do not take ibuprofen for more than 7 days without consulting your doctor.
- Before taking any medicine, read all the instructions on the package.

3. **For All Fevers:**
    - Drink cold fluids orally to prevent dehydration (Reason: good hydration replaces sweat and improves heat loss via skin). Adults should drink 6-8 glasses of water daily.
    - Dress in one layer of lightweight clothing and sleep with one light blanket.
    - For fevers 100-101° F (37.8-38.3° C) this is the only treatment and fever medicine is unnecessary.
4. **Call Back If**
    - Unable to stand or walk.
    - Passes out.
    - Breathing difficulty occurs.
    - You become worse.

Weakness From Poor Fluid Intake

1. **Reassurance:**
    - Not drinking enough fluids and being a little dehydrated is a common cause of mild weakness.
    - Vomiting and diarrhea can lead to dehydration.
    - During hot weather you sweat more and can become dehydrated more easily.
2. **Fluids:** Drink several glasses of fruit juice, other clear fluids, or water. This will improve hydration and blood glucose.
3. **Rest:** Lie down with feet elevated for 1 hour. This will improve circulation and increase blood flow to the brain.
4. **Cool Off:** If the weather is hot, apply a cold compress to the forehead or take a cool shower or bath.
5. **Call Back If**
    - Still feeling weak after 2 hours of rest and fluids.
    - Passes out (faints).
    - You become worse.

FIRST AID

First Aid Advice for Shock:

Lie down with the feet elevated.

BACKGROUND INFORMATION

General

- **Weakness:** Weakness is a very nonspecific symptom. It can be caused by a wide range of medical conditions. It can accompany minor viral illness (e.g., colds, flu) but can also accompany major illness (e,g, GI bleeding, myocardial infarction, pneumonia). Weakness may also be a symptom of depression. Real weakness means that there is a decrease in muscle strength; this is a more concerning finding.
- **Fatigue:** Fatigue is somewhat different from weakness. It's a feeling of being tired and having decreased energy. Endurance is decreased. On testing, however, muscle strength is normal (i.e., no true weakness). Fatigue is often caused by insufficient sleep, inadequate caloric intake, stress, and viral infections.

Causes of Generalized Weakness and Fatigue

- Acute blood loss (e.g., gastrointestinal bleeding, vaginal bleeding).
- Cardiac disorders with decreased cardiac output (e.g., MI, arrhythmias, valvular heart disease, cardiomyopathies).
- Depression.
- Fever.
- Heat exhaustion.
- Hypoglycemia.
- Inadequate caloric intake.
- Infections (e.g., pneumonia, UTI).
- Insufficient sleep.
- Medication side effect.
- Metabolic (e.g., hypoglycemia, hyponatremia, hypokalemia).
- Stress.
- **Viral Syndrome:** Patients with viral illnesses (e.g., colds, flu) often report some generalized weakness along with all the other symptoms that they are experiencing.
- **Volume Depletion and Dehydration:** From vomiting, diarrhea, sweating.

WOUND INFECTION

DEFINITION

- Traumatic wound (break in the skin) shows signs of infection. This includes sutured wounds, puncture wounds and scrapes.
- Use this protocol only if the patient has symptoms that match wound infection.

Symptoms of a Wound Infection Include:

- Pus or cloudy fluid is draining from the wound.
- Pimple or yellow crust has formed on the wound *(R/O impetigo).*
- Increasing redness occurs around the wound *(R/O cellulitis).*
- Red streak is spreading from the wound toward the heart *(R/O lymphangitis).*
- Wound has become extremely tender *(R/O abscess, cellulitis, necrotizing fasciitis).*
- Wound has developed blebs, crepitus, severe pain, or black necrotic tissue *(R/O gangrene and myonecrosis).*
- Pain or swelling is increasing 48 hours after the wound occurred *(R/O abscess, cellulitis).*
- Lymph node draining that area of skin may become large and tender *(R/O lymphadenitis).*
- Onset of widespread bright red rash *(R/O exotoxin from staph or strep wound infection).*
- Onset of fever.
- Wound hasn't healed within 10 days after the injury.

Guideline includes follow-up calls regarding patients taking antibiotics for wound infections.

TRIAGE ASSESSMENT QUESTIONS

See More Appropriate Protocol

- Stitches and not infected
  Go to Protocol: Suture or Staple Questions on page 266

Go to ED Now (or to Office With PCP Approval)

- Bright red, widespread, sunburn-like rash
  R/O: staph or strep exotoxin
- Black (necrotic) or blisters develop in wound
- Looks infected (spreading redness, red streak, pus) and fever
  R/O: cellulitis
- Patient sounds very sick or weak to the triager

Go to Office Now

- Severe pain in the wound
  R/O: abscess or invasive strep
- Red streak runs from the wound
  R/O: lymphangitis.
- Facial wound looks infected (spreading redness)
  Reason: cosmetic concerns
  Note: it may be difficult to determine the rash color in people with darker-colored skin.
- Finger wound and entire finger swollen
  R/O: tenosynovitis

See Today in Office

- Skin redness around the wound larger than 2 inches (5 cm)
  R/O: cellulitis
  Note: it may be difficult to determine the rash color in people with darker-colored skin.
- Pus or cloudy fluid draining from wound
  R/O: wound infection
- Taking antibiotic > 48 hours and fever persists
  R/O: complication, abscess, resistant organism, MRSA
- Taking antibiotic > 72 hours (3 days) and infected wound not improved (pain, pus, redness)
  R/O: complication, abscess, resistant organism, MRSA
- Patient wants to be seen

See Today or Tomorrow in Office

- Pimple where a stitch comes through the skin
  R/O: stitch abscess

See Within 3 Days in Office

- Wound hasn't healed within 10 days after the injury
  R/O: low-grade wound infection

Home Care

- ○ Taking antibiotic < 48 hours for wound infection and fever persists
  Reason: taking antibiotic and no complications
- ○ Taking antibiotic < 72 hours (3 days) and infected wound doesn't look better
  Reason: taking antibiotic and no complications
- ○ Wound doesn't sound infected, or only mild redness
  Reason: all triage questions negative

HOME CARE ADVICE FOR MILD REDNESS OF WOUND

1. **Warm Soaks or Local Heat:** If the wound is open, soak it in warm water or put a warm wet cloth on the wound for 20 minutes 3 times per day. Use a warm saltwater solution containing 2 teaspoons of table salt per quart of water. If the wound is closed, apply a heating pad or warm, moist washcloth to the reddened area for 20 minutes 3 times per day.
2. **Antibiotic Ointment:** Apply an antibiotic ointment 3 times a day. If the area could become dirty, cover with a Band-Aid or a clean gauze dressing.
3. **Pain Medicines:**
   - For pain relief, take acetaminophen, ibuprofen, or naproxen.

   Acetaminophen (e.g., Tylenol):
   - Take 650 mg by mouth every 4-6 hours as needed. Each Regular Strength Tylenol pill has 325 mg of acetaminophen. The most you should take each day is 3,250 mg (10 pills a day).
   - Another choice is to take 1,000 mg every 8 hours. Each Extra Strength Tylenol pill has 500 mg of acetaminophen. The most you should take each day is 3,000 mg (6 pills a day).

   Ibuprofen (e.g., Motrin, Advil):
   - Take 400 mg by mouth every 6 hours.
   - Another choice is to take 600 mg by mouth every 8 hours.

   Naproxen (e.g., Aleve):
   - Take 250-500 mg by mouth every 12 hours.

   Extra Notes:
   - Acetaminophen is thought to be safer than ibuprofen or naproxen in people over 65 years old. Acetaminophen is in many OTC and prescription medicines. It might be in more than one medicine that you are taking. You need to be careful and not take an overdose. An acetaminophen overdose can hurt the liver.
   - **Caution:** Do not take acetaminophen if you have liver disease.
   - **Caution:** Do not take ibuprofen if you have stomach problems, kidney disease, are pregnant, or have been told by your doctor to avoid this type of anti-inflammatory drug. Do not take ibuprofen for more than 7 days without consulting your doctor.
   - Use the lowest amount of medicine that makes your pain feel better.
   - Before taking any medicine, read all the instructions on the package
4. **Expected Course:** Pain and swelling normally peak on day 2. Any redness should go away by day 3 or 4. Complete healing should occur by day 10.
5. **Contagiousness:** For true wound infections, you can return to work or school after any fever is gone and you have received antibiotics for 24 hours.
6. **Call Back If:**
   - Wound becomes more tender.
   - Redness starts to spread.
   - Pus, drainage, or fever occurs.
   - You become worse.

BACKGROUND INFORMATION

General

- When wounds become infected, the infection usually develops 24 to 72 hours after the initial break in the skin.
- CA-MRSA must be considered as a possible cause in newly infected wounds and in wounds that are not improving despite antibiotic therapy.

CA-MRSA: Community-Acquired Methicillin-Resistant Staphylococcus aureus

- *Staphylococcus aureus* is a bacteria that can cause a variety of skin infections including pimples, boils, abscesses, cellulitis, wound infections, and impetigo. It can also cause more serious infections like staphylococcal pneumonia, sepsis, and toxic shock syndrome.
- In the 1960s strains of *S aureus* that were resistant to penicillin-type antibiotics started appearing in hospitals and health care settings. These were referred to as methicillin-resistant *S aureus* (MRSA) infections.
- More recently, strains of penicillin-resistant *S aureus* have increasingly become the cause of skin infections in healthy individuals in the community. These are now being referred to as community-acquired methicillin-resistant *S aureus* (CA-MRSA) infections. There have been outbreaks in athletes (e.g., wrestling teams) and in prison populations.
- CA-MRSA requires treatment with specific types of antibiotics.
- More information about CA-MRSA is available at www.cdc.gov/mrsa.

Appendix A: User's Guide: How to Use *Adult Telephone Protocols: Office Version*

Table of Contents

Introduction

This User's Guide is primarily written for those office personnel who perform telephone triage and provide health information over the phone.

The goals of this book are:

- To provide telephone triage protocols for use by the triage personnel in adult primary care offices.
- To provide adult health information and care advice for use by office telephone triage personnel.
- To serve as a training tool for office staff who are responsible for performing triage and communicating health care information to patients.

This book contains 104 protocols that cover more than 90% of adult telephone chief complaints. They are arranged alphabetically.

Using protocols is a key element in delivering safe and effective telephone triage in a primary care office. There are several reasons why they are important. Protocols make it possible for a primary care office to:

- Deliver consistent health information to callers, independent of which staff person is handling the call.
- Provide a structured decision-support tool to guide the triager through a standardized telephone interview.
- Develop a consensus among several different physicians within an office practice by giving them a document to review, amend as needed, and approve.
- Reduce risk-management challenges by including screening questions that the triager might not have otherwised considered.
- Reconstruct the interview of a past telephone triage call.

Medical Review – These protocols should not be used unless they have been reviewed, amended as necessary, and approved by a supervising physician or medical director responsible for overseeing their use.

Decision Support – These protocols are clinical guidelines that must be used in conjunction with critical thinking and clinical judgment. These protocols provide decision support but do not make the decision; the clinical decision of whether and when a patient needs to be seen must be made by the staff person performing the triage.

Therefore, these protocols are most suitable for use by physicians and clinically experienced nurses, nurse practitioners, and physician assistants. All licensed health professionals should receive special training before using these protocols. Non-licensed and non-health professionals (e.g., secretaries) should not use these protocols.

Principles of Triage Decision-Making

Triage is the decision process of sorting patients to the level of care that best meets their medical needs. This decision process must take into consideration the seriousness (medical acuity) of the patient's medical complaint, the types of resources required to provide effective care, the patient's expectations, and several other factors. See Figure 1.

Medical Acuity – Medical acuity refers to the severity of the patient's problem or symptom. Medical acuity is the foundation; it is the fundamental deciding factor you will use to decide whether, when, and where a patient needs to be seen. A patient who is having an anaphylactic reaction (life-threatening allergic reaction) with shortness of breath and wheezing after a bee sting has a problem of high acuity. Based solely on the high acuity of this problem, you would recommend that the caller immediately contact an emergency ambulance service (Call EMS 911 NOW). In contrast, a patient who states they feel completely well except for a low-grade fever and a constant moderate sore throat of 2 days' duration has a problem of low acuity. You would likely recommend an appointment in the office today or tomorrow for evaluation (See in Office Today or Tomorrow). A patient with mild sunburn who calls for care advice has a problem of very low acuity. For such a patient, no appointment would be needed and instead you would provide brief health information on how to reduce the sunburn pain (Home Care).

During your triage decision-making process you will always need to consider...

- **Is there an immediate threat to life or limb?** You should recommend an emergency medical services (EMS) transport team for patient problems for which there is a clear or high likelihood of life, limb, or organ threat. Such patients may require resuscitative efforts; treatment often can be initiated within minutes by EMS providers. Examples of symptoms that require you to call EMS 911 services include:
  - Amputation
  - Chest pain lasting longer than 10 minutes, not relieved by nitroglycerin
  - Stopped breathing or severe difficulty breathing
  - Unconscious, comatose, or confused

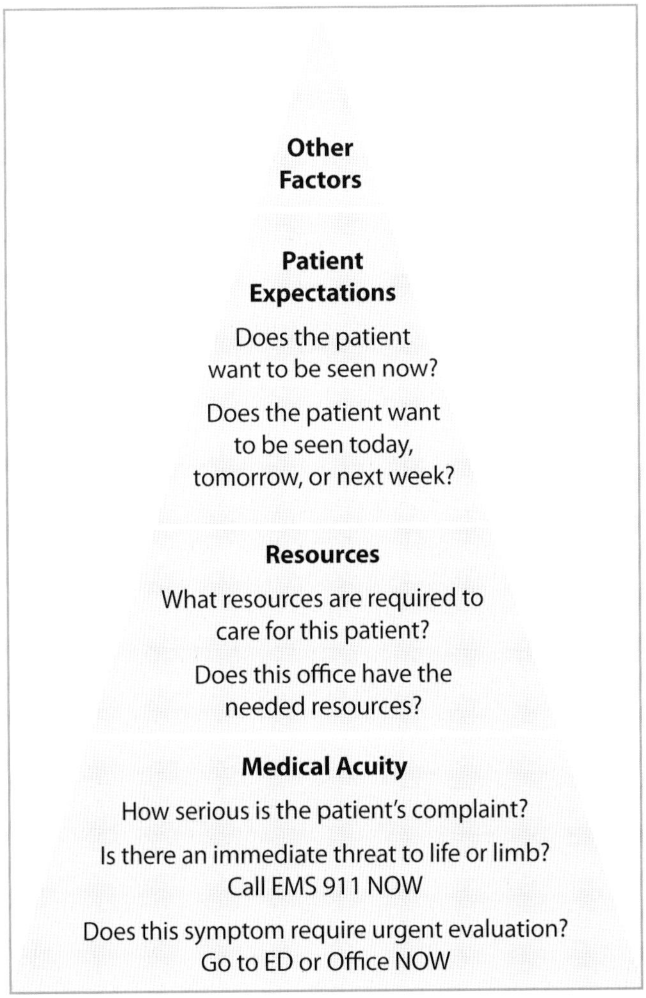

Other Factors

Patient Expectations

Does the patient want to be seen now?

Does the patient want to be seen today, tomorrow, or next week?

Resources

What resources are required to care for this patient?

Does this office have the needed resources?

Medical Acuity

How serious is the patient's complaint?

Is there an immediate threat to life or limb? Call EMS 911 NOW

Does this symptom require urgent evaluation? Go to ED or Office NOW

Figure 1. Factors Involved in the Telephone Triage Decision Process

You may wish to review Appendix C. It contains a table listing further examples of patient symptoms and problems that generally require activation of the EMS system.

- **Does the symptom require urgent evaluation?** Many symptoms are of such potentially high acuity that only through a complete medical evaluation can the diagnosis and necessary treatment be determined. Thus, you should recommend an immediate evaluation in the emergency department (ED) or office for patient problems for which there is an unclear or low to moderate likelihood of life, limb, or organ threat.

  Examples of symptoms that often require urgent evaluation include:
  - Chest pain
R/O: heart attack, etc.
  - Difficulty breathing
R/O: pneumonia, etc.
  - Abdominal pain persisting > 2 hours
R/O: appendicitis, etc.
  - Headache, fever, and stiff neck
R/O: meningitis, etc.

  You may wish to review Appendix D. It contains a table listing further examples of patient symptoms and problems that generally require an immediate visit to the office or emergency department for medical evaluation.

Resources – The resource needs of the patient's problem also impact your triage decision-making. "Resources" is a broad term describing the equipment, medications, supplies, and personnel skills needed for a specific patient problem.

During your triage decision-making process you will often need to consider...

- **What resources are required to care for this patient?** For example, a patient with a gaping 2-inch laceration on the hand needs treatment at a health care site that has the resources of suture material, a laceration repair tray, tetanus vaccine, and a provider skilled in performing laceration repair.

- **Does this office have the needed resources?**
  It is very helpful and improves your call efficiency if you know what resources your office has for provision of patient care. Try to avoid being in the situation of having to lean away from the phone and whisper, "Do we do ____ in this office? Do we have any tetanus shots left? Does Dr Smith remove insects from inside an ear?"

  You can tabulate the resources you have available in your office by using the forms in Appendix E. There are 3 basic categories of resources:

  - **Procedures –** e.g., foreign body removal, laceration repair, fracture reduction and casting, pelvic examination, intravenous fluid administration
  - **Tests –** e.g., electrocardiogram, chest radiograph, urine pregnancy, fingerstick glucose
  - **Medications –** e.g., tetanus vaccination, albuterol (metaproterenol) nebulizer treatment, acetaminophen (Tylenol)

Patient Expectations – A patient begins the telephone triage encounter with expectations about whether he or she needs to be seen in the office, and when an appointment would be convenient. From a customer service standpoint, the way to achieve patient satisfaction is to meet or exceed these expectations. If you are unable to meet the patient's expectations, to achieve patient satisfaction you will need to "manage" this expectation by successfully convincing the patient that an office visit is not needed or that it can be postponed.

- **Does the patient want to be seen in the office?**
  You should determine if the patient wants to be seen. Sometimes a patient calls with expectations to be seen in the office and other times the patient is just seeking health information for home care.
- **Does the patient want to be seen today, tomorrow, or next week?**
  What do you do if there are no office appointments available right now, today, tomorrow, or later this week? All too frequently office schedules are booked up with 2- to 8-week waits. If you have no appropriate open appointments, you may need to overbook the patient into the office schedule according to your scheduling policy or after discussion with the physician. Alternatively, sometimes you may have to recommend that the patient be seen in the local emergency department.

Some primary care offices have successfully implemented a new paradigm, called "open access" or "advanced access." Open access means that if a patient requests an appointment, you give an appointment today. The patient decides whether to come in today, tomorrow, or next week. The theme of open access scheduling is, do today's work—today!

Another office model is to dedicate a block of time for urgent care in the daily office schedule, and staff this clinic with an advanced practice nurse or physician assistant.

Other Factors – There are a number of other factors that you will need to take into consideration during the triage process.

- **What social factors affect the triage disposition?**
  There are a number of social factors that may affect the disposition you recommend to a patient. For example, a healthy ambulatory elderly patient with a cough and a fever of 102.5° F probably needs an urgent office visit; whereas a similar bedridden patient would likely need to be directed to the emergency department via ambulance solely because of the bedridden status. See Table 1 for a list of other important social factors.
- **Does the patient have any chronic medical problems?**
  You will need to be more cautious in your triage of patients with chronic illness. See Table 2 for a listing of important illnesses.
- **Is the patient pregnant?**
- **Is the patient taking any medications, especially new medications? Could the patient be experiencing an adverse reaction to the medications?**

Table 1. Social Factors: RATE the Patient

Reliability	• Barriers from language, intoxication, or limited education • Second-party callers • Truthfulness
Abuse	• Partner and elder abuse
Travel Distance and Access	• Distance from hospital and office • Access to car or other transportation • Ambulatory or bedridden
Emotional	• Anxiety, fear, hysteria

Table 2. Chronic Illness

Important Medical Conditions	Relevance to Triage Decision-Making
Common	
• AIDS and HIV positive, cancer chemotherapy, chronic steroids, transplant patients	Weakened immune system; more prone to infection.
• Asthma, emphysema	Increased risk of pneumonia, pneumothorax.
• Cardiac disease	Higher risk for further cardiac events (e.g., heart attack, congestive heart failure); cardiac medications can cause weakness, dizziness, and electrolyte problems.
• Central venous line (e.g. Port-a-Cath)	Increased risk of catheter-related infections.
• Diabetes	Weakened immune system, thus more prone to infection. Hyperglycemia and hypoglycemia may present with frequent urination, weakness, dizziness, altered mental status, or coma.
• Coagulopathy, Coumadin therapy	Increased tendency for bleeding; must be more cautious in these patients whenever they bleed or have a traumatic injury.
• Feeding tube	Increased risk of aspiration pneumonia, bowel obstruction, osmotic diarrhea.
• Hypertension	Prone to stroke; hypertension medications can cause weakness, dizziness, and electrolyte problems.
• Liver disease	Prone to bleeding problems.
• Urinary catheter (e.g., Foley)	Increased risk of urinary retention, urinary tract infection.
Geriatric Concerns	
• Dementia	Problems with getting an accurate history, safety issues.
• Osteoporosis	Loss of bone density increases likelihood of fracture from minor falls.
• Polypharmacy	Elderly patients frequently are taking multiple drugs. There are risks of drug-drug and drug-disease interactions.
Recent Injury	Possible undiagnosed injury, wound infection.
Recent Surgery	Surgical complications including urinary infection, bleeding, wound infection; increased risk of pulmonary embolism after major surgery.
Recent Infection	Antibiotics can frequently cause rashes; some antibiotics can cause *Clostridium difficile* diarrhea.

Structure of a Telephone Triage Encounter

The typical triage call has a structure that can be organized in the following manner. The call begins with a greeting followed by a short period of active listening. Brief demographic information is obtained, a protocol is selected, triage is performed using the triage assessment questions in the protocol, then a disposition is recommended to the caller. The call concludes with the triager providing relevant care advice, answering any final questions, and instructing the caller to call back if symptoms worsen. See Table 3.

Let's look at each of the components of a telephone triage encounter in more detail.

Greeting – The call begins with a greeting, during which you introduce yourself and apologize for any delays. The greeting ends with an invitation to the caller to describe their problem or symptom. Many successful office practices have a specific scripted approach to this first part of the encounter. Your greeting might contain the following scripted elements:

- Greeting *"Good morning."*
- Introduction *"This is Donna,"*
- Title *"the nurse working with Dr Smith."*
- Apology if indicated *"I am sorry that you had to wait on the phone."*
- Query *"How can I help you this morning?"*

Remember to smile. The caller easily can hear the smile in your voice even when they cannot see it.

Active Listening, the Chief Complaint – During the second part of the triage call you listen to the caller describe the problem in an open-ended manner with minimal interruptions. During this part of the call the triager is actively listening to the caller with the primary goal of identifying the caller's main complaint. Ideally this part of the call should last 30 to 60 seconds. This part of the call is often the most challenging for new triagers because callers may often present their concerns in a disjointed and rambling manner. If more than 30 to 60 seconds elapse and you remain unclear about the caller's main question, it is productive at this point to become more directive in your call. For example, asking clarifying questions is often helpful:

- "So while you have a sore throat and runny nose, the main reason you are calling is the bad cough. Is this right?"
- "Besides the cough and runny nose for the last 3 days, do you have any other symptoms that you are really worried about?"
- "When you fell and injured your ankle, did you hurt any other part of your body?"
- "It sounds like a lot of things are bothering you right now. What's the worst thing?"

Table 3. Structure of a Telephone Triage Encounter

Component	Description
Greeting	Greet caller. Introduce yourself as per approved office script. Apologize for any delays. Smile.
Active Listening, the Chief Complaint	Listen to the caller describe the problem or symptom. Try to avoid interrupting for the first 30 seconds. Determine the patient's main complaint or symptom. Select the correct protocol.
Demographic Information	Obtain or confirm patient identifying information: name, phone number, age, gender.
Chronic Illness, Social History, Pregnancy	Determine if there are chronic illnesses or social factors (RATE the patient) that may affect the disposition.
Triage Assessment Questions	Scan through the questions in the selected protocol. Ask questions in order provided. Assign a disposition level.
Home Care Advice	Provide care advice; give only First Aid advice to patients requiring immediate evaluation.
Closure	Confirm understanding and patient intent to follow recommendations. Provide Call Back If advice.

Demographic Information – During the third phase of the call, you should obtain brief identifying demographic information, if it was not provided previously. At the very least this usually consists of name, age, phone number, and gender. Obtaining several different phone numbers (e.g., home, mobile, pager) may save office time on callbacks. Some offices have a standard of obtaining demographic information before asking for any medical information. Some offices will only provide telephone advice to patients who have previously been seen in the office.

Chronic Illness, Social History, Pregnancy – During the fourth phase of the encounter it is important to inquire regarding the possibility of pregnancy, obtain any patient history of significant chronic illness, and identify any directly relevant social factors. See Tables 1 and 2.

Triage Assessment Questions – At this point in the telephone encounter, you will select the most relevant protocol and then systematically ask the triage assessment questions in the order presented in the protocol. You will be asking the highest acuity questions first. Be certain to ask the questions in the order presented until you obtain a positive response. The triage assessment questions in the protocol are organized under disposition categories.

Home Care Advice – You do not need to provide every piece of care advice listed for the protocol. Try to tailor the care advice to the patient's needs. Attempt to limit the care advice you provide to 2-3 instructions and keep your comments brief.

Closure – Closure is the end of the telephone triage encounter. The triager needs to confirm that the caller understands the care advice provided, has no further questions, and agrees with the recommended disposition. The triager and caller should be in agreement regarding the disposition before the call ends. The triager should conclude the conversation with a brief Call Back If statement. Suggested Call Back If statements are included at the bottom of the Home Care Advice section. Covering every worst-case scenario is impossible and will unduly alarm the caller. But at the least, the triager should instruct the patient to call back if *"you become worse."*

Structure of the Protocols in This Book

Each of the protocols in this book is organized identically and contain the following components.

- Title
- Definition
- Triage Assessment Questions
  - See More Appropriate Protocol
- Home Care Advice
- Background Information

Title – The title briefly describes the type of call for which the protocol is intended to be used. This is nearly always a symptom. For example, a patient might have "Sore Throat" or "Constipation." Some of the protocols have a diagnosis as a title; these are used in those limited clinical situations in which patients can reasonably diagnose themselves with a specific problem. For example, many patients will call up and state that they have "Poison Ivy/Oak/Sumac" or "Jock Itch."

Definition – From your review of the list of topics, you should find that most of the protocols are self-explanatory. The purpose of the symptom definition is to more specifically define the type of patient complaints for which a protocol is applicable. Read the symptom definition completely, especially the first time that you use a protocol. Make certain that your caller's complaint is specifically covered in this symptom definition. It is especially important to do this when using the protocols that have a diagnosis for a title (e.g. Jock Itch, Poison Ivy/Oak/Sumac, Pubic Lice).

Most of the protocols are symptom based. In general, symptoms mentioned by the patient can be accepted at face value (e.g., earache, headache, cough, head injury), but sometimes the definition requires clarification. For example, patients often diagnose themselves with hay fever; you should make certain that their symptoms match the Hay Fever (Nasal Allergies) definition.

As a general rule, neither the patient nor the triager should make diagnoses. However, there are exceptions such as adult illnesses that the average patient can easily recognize (e.g., Athlete's Foot, Pubic Lice, Asthma Attack). Patients may have had the illness previously or have friends or neighbors who suggest the diagnosis to them. For these patients, a diagnosis/disease-based protocol may be indicated. See Table 4.

The first safeguard in all of the disease-based protocols is that they start with a definition. The caller's description of the symptoms must match the definition before the protocol's triage assessment questions and care advice are used.

Table 4. Disease-Based Protocols

• Asthma Attack
• Athlete's Foot
• Colds
• Ear, Swimmer's (Otitis Externa)
• Hay Fever (Nasal Allergies)
• Hives
• Jock Itch
• Poison Ivy/Oak/Sumac
• Pubic Lice
• Sunburn

A second safeguard is that the triager can use the See More Appropriate Protocol section; this keeps the triager from overusing the disease-based guideline. If the criteria in the definition are not met, the triager can be redirected to a more appropriate protocol. For example, the triager might be directed from Hives to Rash, Widespread and Cause Unknown.

There are several advantages to using a disease-based protocol over a symptom-based protocol. First, the triage questions and care advice are more specific and targeted to the patient's complaint. Secondly, the call is faster and more effective.

Triage Assessment Questions – The triage questions are arranged in descending order of acuity. Restated, the questions are arranged so that the most serious causes of a symptom are considered first.

- You should ask the caller these questions in the order listed, continuing on until you get a "yes" (positive response) to a question.
- Stop asking questions as soon as you get a positive response.
- The remaining questions and other information can be asked by the physician in the emergency department or the office when the patient comes in for evaluation.

Often you will find that the caller has provided the answer to many of these Triage Assessment Questions in the first portion of the call, when he or she was first describing their problem or symptom. You do not need to re-ask the Triage Assessment Question if you already have been given the answer.

Disposition Category – The Triage Assessment Questions are grouped within different disposition categories. The disposition categories, like the Triage Assessment Questions, are arranged in descending order of acuity. (See Figure 2.) The standard disposition categories are:

- ***Call EMS 911 Now***
  Life-threatening emergencies.
- ***Go to ED Now***
  Emergent patients who need an ED for management.
- ***Go to ED Now (or to Office With PCP Approval)***
  Emergent patients. Discuss the best site with the primary care physician.
- ***Go to Office Now***
  Less emergent patients who can be evaluated in most adult primary care offices.
- ***See Today or Tomorrow in Office***
  (by appointment)
  Urgent or uncomfortable patients.
  Also included here are "Patient wants to be seen."
- ***See Today in Office***
  (by appointment)
  Nonurgent patients.
- ***See Within 3 Days in Office***
  (by appointment)
  Persisting symptoms or patients who are not getting better.
- ***See Within 2 Weeks in Office***
  (by appointment)
  Chronic or recurrent symptoms that are not becoming worse.
- ***Home Care***
  Do not see at all. All the triage questions are negative. Provide home treatment advice.

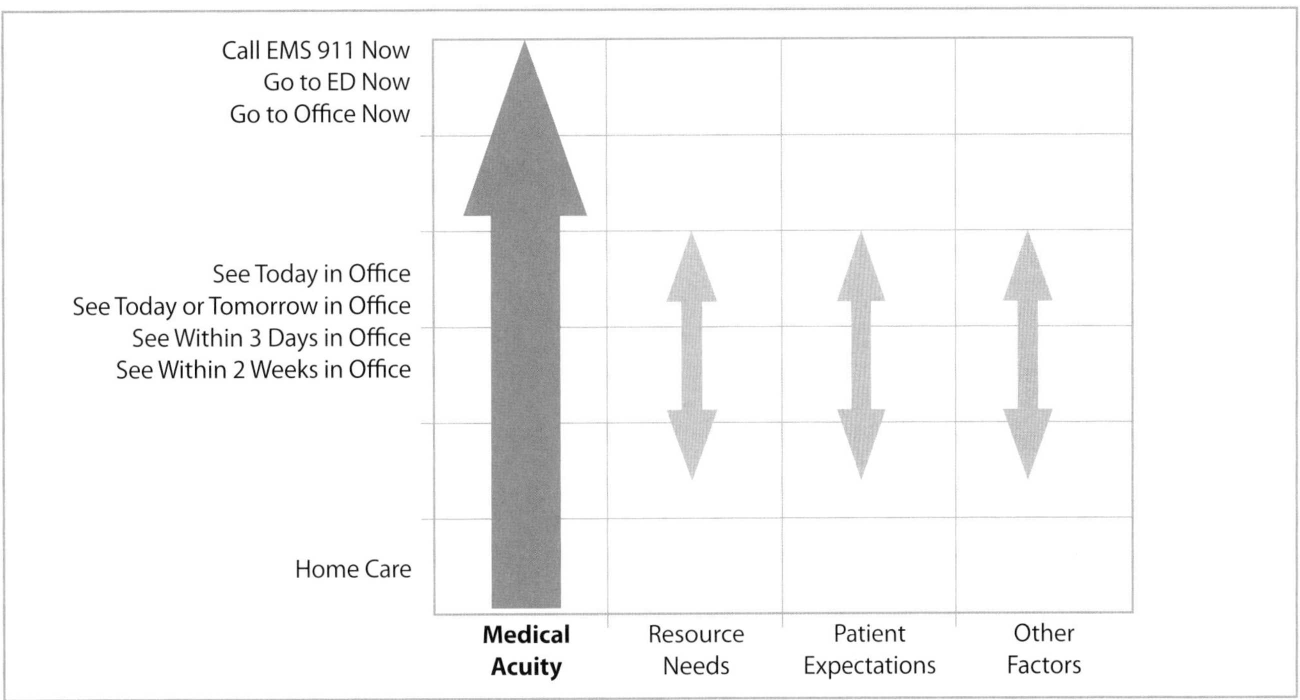

Figure 2. Disposition Categories

When it is seems medically safe, these protocols attempt to place the patient into the Home Care disposition category. Neither the patient nor the physician are interested in unnecessary visits. The triager can elect to move a patient to a higher disposition category (one of greater urgency and acuity). This is referred to as "upgrading" or overriding. Such upgrading of patients is medically harmless. Triagers should feel free to use their judgment and upgrade as they deem necessary.

The patient's desire to be seen should be respected. If the patient wants to be seen and the protocol recommends Home Care, the triager should make arrangements for the patient to be evaluated. In some cases this type of upgrade will turn out to be medically warranted, as the patient may have a medical illness that he or she was not able to communicate well or a medical illness with an atypical presentation. In other cases, this upgrade will turn out to be medically unwarranted, but the patient remains a customer of the office practice and meeting and exceeding the patient's expectations is important.

Downgrading is the term used to describe overriding the protocol disposition and giving the patient a home care or less urgent disposition. This should be done with great caution. Some office practices make it a policy to not downgrade; others allow downgrade only after discussing the patient with the physician. Of course, the patient may sometimes insist on a disposition lower than what the triager recommends. In such cases, the triager should document this. For example: *"Patient will not come into the office now as per my strong recommendation, instead the patient will come to the office at 5:00 pm."*

Home Care Advice – You do not need to provide every piece of care advice listed for the protocol. Try to tailor the care advice to the patient's needs. Attempt to limit the care advice you provide to 2-3 instructions and keep your comments brief. The reason for this is that the average caller cannot retain and act upon more than 2 or 3 key instructions.

Before giving advice, make sure that the caller has a paper and pen handy. This will serve as a memory aid for the caller, reduce callbacks, and ensure that medication dosages are correctly taken. It is often helpful to ask the caller, *"What treatment has the patient tried already?"* This keeps you from wasting the caller's and your time by going over familiar territory. A follow-up question to this is, *"How is this working?"*

Offer empathy, reassurance, and compliments. When a patient has injured himself or herself, it is appropriate to mirror the patient's own description of the pain. For example, the triager may wish to say: "That sounds like it hurts a lot." Callers are sometimes seeking reassurance that the symptoms they are experiencing are common (e.g., fever and muscle aches occur with a cold) and that the treatment they are using is correct (e.g., Tylenol dosing). A triager should provide reassurance whenever possible. Sometimes a sincere compliment is appreciated. Perhaps the patient has been following nearly all of the listed care advice already, in which case it may be appropriate for the triager to tell the caller that they are "doing everything just right." Such compliments provide the patient confidence to handle minor illness and injury on his or her own.

Background Information – Every protocol has some general background information that is provided for the patient's and your benefit. Some of this information is helpful when callers are simply seeking some health information. You should try to review all of the background information in this book as time permits.

Closure – Closure is the end of the telephone triage encounter. The triager will want to confirm that the caller understands the care advice provided, has no further questions, and is in agreement with the recommended disposition. The triager and the caller should be in alignment with the disposition before the call ends. The triager should conclude the conversation with a brief **Call Back If** statement. Suggested Call Back If statements are included at the bottom of the Home Care Advice section. Covering every worst-case scenario is impossible and will unduly alarm the caller. But at the least, the triager should instruct the patient to call back if *"you become worse."*

Selecting the Correct Protocol

Selecting the correct triage protocol is an important initial step in triaging calls.

What is the patient's main problem or symptom? Find the protocol that best matches that problem or symptom. In most circumstances the best protocol will be obvious. For example, a patient calling with a bad sore throat and minimal other symptoms would be triaged using the Sore Throat protocol.

Familiarize yourself with the alphabetic, anatomic, and category listings of protocols. By reviewing these lists you will be able quickly determine the best protocol.

If a caller has multiple symptoms, always select the most serious symptom. If none of the symptoms are serious, select the protocol that will result in the patient be seen the soonest. For most calls you should have to use only 1 protocol to triage a call. In approximately 5% of calls you will need to use 2 protocols.

Reason and Rule-Out Statements

Below many of the Triage Assessment Questions are rationale statements that provide useful information for the nurse triager.

"Rule-outs" (R/O) list the most likely conditions or diagnoses that could cause this symptom. "Reasons" provide the specific indications for a disposition. See Table 5.

Why Are These Reasons and Rule-Outs Provided?
The rationale statements allow physician reviewers to more easily critique the indications for seeing patients. Furthermore, the rationale statements allow the triager to:

- Understand the reasons behind each question.
- If unsure of patient's status, more easily create other questions to pursue relevant diagnoses.
- More easily memorize the questions (understanding increases recall).
- Increase triage nurse job satisfaction and improve nursing judgment.

Should the Caller Be Told the Listed Diagnosis?
Usually no. This should not be done for the following reasons:

- Generally, diagnoses should not be made without seeing the patient and performing a physical examination.
- Suggesting a diagnosis over the phone conveys to the patient that you know more than you actually do.
- A triager should not make a diagnosis over the phone.

If the caller asks you what he or she "might have," tell the caller, *"It's impossible to diagnose most conditions over the telephone, but from what you've told me, you need to be seen for a complete evaluation today."*

If the caller raises a diagnostic possibility, such as appendicitis, and you agree with it, tell the patient, *"It is a possibility and that's why you need to be evaluated today."*

Only as a last resort should you use "scare tactics" (i.e., telling potential diagnoses) to motivate a patient to comply with your recommendation to call an ambulance, go to the emergency department, or come to the office for an evaluation.

Table 5. Reason and Rule-Out Statements

Triage Assessment Question	Reasons and Rule-Outs
• Patient wants to be seen	
• Bleeding recurs 3 or more times in 24 hours despite direct pressure	
• Taking Coumadin or known bleeding disorder (e.g., thrombocytopenia)	*Reason: need for testing of INR, prothrombin time*
• Has skin bruises or bleeding gums, that are not caused by an injury	*R/O: bleeding disorder*
• Health care provider inserted a nasal packing to control bleeding and now has fever > 100.5° F (38.1° C)	*R/O: sinusitis*

Documentation

Every office should have a method for briefly documenting the telephone triage encounter. Often this takes the form of a telephone log with separate entries for each phone encounter. Some offices instead choose to use a memo pad, which they then tear off and place in the chart as a permanent record. Your office will need to decide on its own standard for documentation.

In Appendix F of this book you will find 3 sample telephone log sheets. Feel free to copy, modify, and use these samples. Simple, well-organized forms like these save you charting time and increase the number of calls you can take per hour.

Always record which protocol you used. If you used 2 protocols, write down the titles of both protocols.

If you decide to recommend EMS 911, direct the patient to the emergency department, or give the patient an appointment, then always list the reason for your decision. The reason is usually going to be the Triage Assessment Question to which you elicited a positive response. If you instead decide that the patient does not need to be seen and that home management is safe and appropriate, remember to document that "all triage questions are negative."

Be certain to document the name, dosage, and route of any medications that you instruct the patient to use. Callers commonly blame dosage errors on information that they received from the triager.

Because protocols are being used, documentation can be limited to pertinent positives.

You should write into the telephone log sheets while you are talking and listening to the caller. Do not try to write down the call afterward; such delayed documentation leads to errors and reduces your efficiency.

Prioritizing Calls

- Take **EMS 911 calls first.**
- Take or return **emergent/urgent** calls that may need to be **seen in the ED or office now next.**
- Take or return nonurgent calls last.

For busy signals or no answer: call back in 10 minutes and then again in 30 minutes.
If there is an answering machine, leave a message.
Document all of your attempts and any message that you leave in your telephone triage log.

May Need to Call EMS 911 Now

You should recommend an emergency medical services (EMS) transport team for patient problems for which there is a clear or high likelihood of life, limb, or organ threat. Such patients may require resuscitative efforts; treatment can often be initiated within minutes by EMS providers. You should immediately transfer the call to EMS. If your phone system cannot transfer a call in this manner, then you should instruct the patient to hang up and immediately call the local ambulance service. In most of the United States, emergency services are available by dialing 911.

Examples of symptoms that nearly always require EMS 911 services include:

- Stopped breathing or severe difficulty breathing
- Unconscious, comatose
- Chest pain lasting longer than 10 minutes, not relieved by nitroglycerin
- Amputation

You may wish to review Appendix C. It contains a table listing further examples of patient symptoms and problems that generally require activation of the EMS system.

In most circumstances the triager should provide no advice to the caller as this will delay the contacting of EMS 911. There are rare situations in which the triager might consider providing brief (10-15 seconds) life-saving advice to the caller. Examples might include:

- **Choking:** Heimlich maneuver.
- **Fainting:** Lay down with feet elevated.
- **Active Bleeding:** Apply direct pressure to the wound.

What are the exceptions to transferring callers directly to EMS 911? The main exception is the suicidal caller. Such a patient is better served by continuing the conversation and having another staff person in the office call EMS 911 to dispatch a rescue squad. Continue to provide support and understanding until the police or paramedics arrive.

May Need to Be Seen in ED or Office Now

You should recommend an immediate evaluation in the emergency department (ED) or office for patient problems for which there is an low to moderate likelihood of life, limb, or organ threat or if the likelihood is unclear after telephone triage. Many symptoms are of such potentially high seriousness that only through a complete face-to-face medical evaluation can the diagnosis and necessary treatment be determined. Examples of symptoms that often require urgent/emergent evaluation include:

- Chest pain — *R/O: heart attack, etc.*
- Difficulty breathing — *R/O: pneumonia, etc.*
- Abdominal pain persisting > 2 hours — *R/O: appendicitis, etc.*
- Headache, fever, and stiff neck — *R/O: meningitis, etc.*
- Unexplained purple spots — *R/O: meningococcemia*
- Fever higher than 103° F — *R/O: bacterial infection, etc.*
- Severe pain

You may wish to review Appendix D. It contains a table listing further examples of patient symptoms and problems that generally require an immediate visit to the office or emergency department for medical evaluation.

Nonurgent Calls

Return nonurgent calls last. Examples include cold and cough symptoms, most rashes, constipation, and minor injuries.

Training

1. The first step in training is to review this User's Guide. Ideally, you should read through it twice.
2. Make certain that you understand the structure of the typical telephone triage encounter.
3. Familiarize yourself with whatever documentation form your office uses for telephone triage calls.
4. Review your office's telephone care policies and procedures.
5. Study the Colds protocol. Read through and become acquainted with the different components of the protocol.
6. The next step is to review the following 22 protocols. Knowledge of these protocols will prepare you for the most common telephone triage complaints.

Abdominal Pain (Female)	Headache
Abdominal Pain (Male)	Neurologic Deficit
Asthma Attack	Rashes, Widespread and Cause Unknown
Back Pain	Rash or Redness, Localized and Cause Unknown
Bee Sting	Rectal Symptoms
Chest Pain	Sinus Pain andConges-tion
Colds	Sore Throat
Constipation	Trauma, Skin
Cough	Urination Pain (Female)
Diarrhea	Vaginal Bleeding, Abnormal
Earache	Vomiting

7. After studying these protocols, observe an experienced nurse or physician manage phone calls for a minimum of 16 hours.
   - Learn how to select the correct protocol.
   - Learn how to recognize serious symptoms (e.g., choking, chest pain).
   - Learn how to use the Triage Assessment Questions and reach a disposition that is appropriate for your office.
8. Lastly, triage calls yourself for a minimum of 24 hours with an experienced nurse or physician observing.
9. Learning is an ongoing process. Never hesitate to ask the physician in your office or another mentor questions. Your goal is to provide safe and efficacious medical advice to the patients in your office practice.

Risk Management

- The patient's safety and well-being are always the highest priority.
- Telephone triage is a point of entry into the health care system. Do not use triage as a method of limiting access; instead use it as a method of improving access to primary care.
- Prevent delayed visits of seriously ill patients by taking a proactive and cautious triage stance. When in doubt, see the patient or make arrangements for the patient to be seen. If the problem could be serious, see the patient immediately.
- If the patient sounds very sick or weak to you as the triager, have the patient come in immediately even if none of the other triage assessment questions are positive.
- Any patient that has become confused or too weak to stand needs immediate evaluation. Usually this patient will require EMS 911 activation.
- If the patient's condition sounds life-threatening or unstable, transfer the call to EMS 911 or call an ambulance yourself for the patient.
- A good exercise to improve your ability to recognize life-threatening or serious disease is to read the EMS 911 section of each protocol.
- After reviewing home care advice, ask the caller, "Do you feel comfortable with the plan?" Most will. If the caller does not, perform a callback in 1 hour or, even better, arrange for the patient to be seen. Always strive for "alignment" with the caller. If the caller insists that he or she needs to be seen, accommodate that request. From a risk management standpoint, it is challenging to defend a bad patient outcome when the patient insisted on being seen and the triager adamantly refused an appointment.
- The triager may override the protocol to suggest the patient goes to a higher level disposition. The triager should not override the protocol to a lower disposition, but instead should discuss with or refer such calls to the primary care physician.
- A nurse triager should not make a diagnosis over the phone. It may be appropriate in certain circumstances for a physician triager to provide a possible/probable diagnosis over the phone.
- Encourage all callers to call back if the condition worsens. Callers should be given specific reasons to call back. At the least, the triager should instruct the patient call back if "you become worse."
- Sometimes callers telephone seeking some brief health information and do not want to be triaged. When in doubt, perform a complete triage and document the call completely. For example, the 55-year-old male patient with "gas pressure" in his chest seeking information about the best antacid may actually be having a heart attack and should be triaged into the emergency department. The 22-year-old female who is calling with concerns about breastfeeding may actually have significant postpartum depression.
- Three calls equal a visit. If a patient calls seeking advice about the same problem 3 times, arrange an appointment. In fact, if the caller phones in 2 times in 12 hours, you usually should arrange an appointment. The reason you should see the patient is that either the caller was not reassured by the information provided over the phone or the patient is actually sicker than described. An exception to this rule is a patient calling in a second time to confirm a drug dosage.
- If a caller calls about a diagnosis (e.g., athlete's foot), do not accept the caller's diagnosis unless it meets the criteria listed in the definition at the beginning of the protocol.
- These protocols should be reviewed and amended as needed by the physicians in your medical practice.

References

Poole SR. *The Complete Guide: Providing Telephone Triage and Advice in a Family Practice.* Elk Grove Village, IL: American Academy of Pediatrics; 2004

Reisman AB, Stevens DL, eds. *Telephone Medicine: A Guide for the Practicing Physician.* Philadelphia, PA: American College of Physicians; 2002

Schmitt BD. *Pediatric Telephone Protocols: Office Version.* 14th ed. Elk Grove Village, IL: American Academy of Pediatrics; 2013

Wheeler S. *Telephone Triage: Theory, Practice and Protocol Development.* San Anselmo, CA: TeleTrage Systems Publishers; 1993

Appendix B

Red Flag Flowchart for Office Support Staff or Call Center Staff

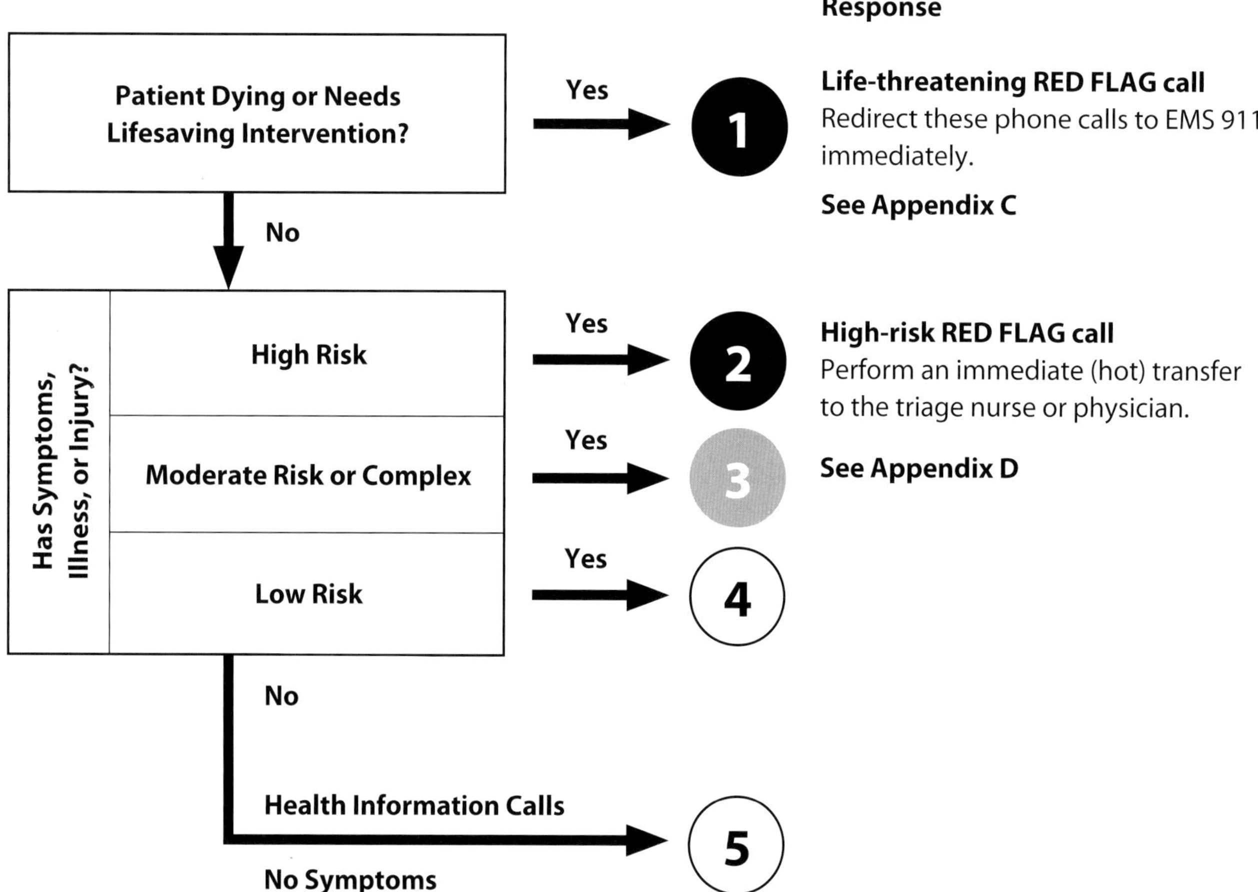

Appendix C

Prioritizing Calls

May Need to Call EMS 911 NOW

ABCs	Reason or Diagnosis
Airway	
● Choking	**Airway obstruction**
● Stopped breathing	**Respiratory arrest**
Breathing	
● Severe difficulty breathing (e.g., struggling for each breath, unable to speak)	**Respiratory failure**
● Lips or face are bluish	**Hypoxia**
● Rapid onset of cough, wheezing, or difficulty breathing after bee sting, insect bite, or other allergic exposure (e.g., medicine, food)	**Anaphylaxis**
Circulation	
● Signs of shock (e.g., cold/clammy, low blood pressure)	**Shock from cardiac, hypovolemic, or septic cause**
● Unconscious, coma	
● Lethargic	

Systems	Reason or Diagnosis
Allergic	
● Rapid onset of cough, wheezing, or difficulty breathing after bee sting, insect bite, or other allergic exposure (e.g., medicine, food)	**Anaphylaxis**
● Previous severe allergic reaction (anaphylaxis) to bees, yellow jackets, etc. (not just hives or swelling) and < 2 hours since sting	
Cardiovascular	
● Fainted and still feels dizzy or light-headed	**Arrhythmia, shock**
● Chest pain lasting longer than 5 minutes and any of the following:	**Myocardial infarction or unstable angina**
– Pain is crushing, pressure-like, or heavy	
– History of heart disease (e.g., angina, heart attack, bypass surgery, angioplasty)	
– Over 50 years old	
– Over 35 years old and one or more cardiac risk factors (i.e., high blood pressure, diabetes, high cholesterol, obesity, smoker, or strong family history of heart disease)	
– Took nitroglycerin and chest pain was not relieved	
Infectious	
● Too weak or sick to stand	**Sepsis**
● Fever and purple or blood-colored spots or dots	**Meningococcemia**
● Possible bioterrorism exposure	**Bioterrorism**
Neurologic	
● Difficult to awaken or acting confused (disoriented, slurred speech)	**Stroke (CVA)**
● Weakness of the face, arm, or leg on one side of the body (new onset)	
● Numbness of the face, arm, or leg on one side of the body (new onset)	
● Loss of speech or garbled speech (new onset)	
Psychiatric	
● Intentional overdose or poisoning (suicide attempt)	
● Suicide attempt	
● Suicidal or homicidal ideation	
Traumatic	
● Cut on the neck, chest, back, or abdomen that may go deep (e.g., stab wound)	**Penetrating trauma**
● Major bleeding (actively dripping or spurting) that can't be stopped	**Uncontrolled bleeding**
● Amputation	
● Head injury with loss of consciousness > 1 minute	**Epidural, subdural**
● Second- or third-degree burn involving > 10% of body surface area	

Appendix D

Prioritizing Calls — May Need to Be Seen in ED or Office NOW

General	Reason or Diagnosis
● Patient sounds very sick or weak to the triager	
● Sounds like a serious injury to the triager	
● Fever > 103° F (39.4° C)	**Bacterial infection**
● Fever > 100.4° F (38.0° C) and:	**Bacterial infection**
– Over 60 years of age	
– Diabetes mellitus or a weakened immune system (e.g., HIV positive, chemotherapy, chronic steroid treatment, splenectomy)	
– Bedridden (e.g., nursing home patient, stroke, chronic illness, recovering from surgery)	
– Transplant patient (e.g., liver, heart, kidney)	
● Drinking very little and signs of dehydration (e.g., no urine > 12 hours, very dry mouth, light-headed, etc.)	**Dehydration**
● Severe pain	**Severe pain should be treated**

Systems	Reason or Diagnosis
Cardiovascular	
● Heart beating irregularly or very rapidly	**Arrhythmia**
● Chest pain with any of the following:	**Acute myocardial infarction**
– Pain also present in the shoulder(s), arm(s), or jaw	
– Difficulty breathing or unusual sweating	
● Has known "angina" chest pain and pain has been increasing in severity or frequency	**Unstable angina**
Gastrointestinal	
● Constant abdominal pain persisting > 2 hours	**Surgical cause of pain**
● Vomiting red blood or black ("coffee ground") material	**GI bleed**
● Blood in bowel movements	
● Black or tarry bowel movements	
Infectious	
● Fever and rash	**Rocky Mountain spotted fever**
● Purple or blood-colored spots or dots	**Meningococcemia**
● Looks infected (spreading redness, pus, red streak)	**Cellulitis, lymphangitis**
Neurologic	
● Vision loss or change	
Respiratory	
● Coughing up blood	**Pneumonia, CHF, Pulmonary Embolus**
● Difficulty breathing (new or worsening)	
● Asthma and either:	**Significant asthma attack**
– Peak flow rate less than 50% of baseline level	
– Peak flow rate 50-80% of baseline level after nebulizer x 1 OR inhaler x 2 (2 puffs q 20 minutes)	
● Wheezing, audible	
Traumatic	
● Skin is split open or gaping	**Laceration needing sutures or staples**
● Minor bleeding won't stop after 10 minutes of direct pressure	
● Injury looks like a dislocated joint (crooked or deformed)	**Fracture or dislocation**
● Can't stand (bear weight) or walk	**Fracture or dislocation**
● Animal at risk for RABIES and any cut, puncture, or scratch	**Rabies vaccination**
● Burn blisters (open or closed) over area larger than palm of hand (>1% BSA)	**Large second-degree burn**
● Burn from acid or alkali (lye) burn	**Chemical burn**
Urologic	
● Unable to urinate and bladder feels very full	**Urinary retention**

Appendix E

Office Resources

Procedures

If this procedure is needed, how often would it be performed in this office (rather than referred to the ED or a surgeon's office)?	Always or Nearly Always	Sometimes (Ask PCP)	Never Refer to ED	Referral Notes
IV fluid for dehydration				
IM or IV antibiotics				
Phlebotomy (blood draw from vein)				
Extremity laceration repair using sutures				
Facial laceration repair using sutures				
Facial laceration repair using Dermabond (skin glue)				
Mouth laceration repair using sutures				
Animal bite wound care (vigorous irrigation)				
Reduction of angulated forearm fracture				
Reduction of finger dislocation (PIP or DIP)				
Reduction of shoulder dislocation				
Reduction of a nursemaid elbow				
Sling/strapping non-displaced clavicle fracture				
Splinting non-displaced finger fracture				
Foreign body removal from cornea				
Foreign body removal from conjunctiva				
Foreign body removal from ear canal				
Foreign body removal from nasal canal				
Foreign body removal from subcutaneous skin				
Fishhook removal from skin				
Fluorescein examination for corneal abrasion				
Incision and drainage of an abscess				
Drainage of a subungual hematoma				
Nasal packing for epistaxis				
Nasal cautery for epistaxis				
Pelvic exam and Pap smear				
Pelvic exam and foreign body removal				
Minor facial burn treatment and follow-up				
Minor extremity burn treatment and follow-up				
Sigmoidoscopy				
Urinary catheter insertion (Foley or coudé)				
Lumbar puncture				
Arthrocentesis (joint aspiration) of knee				

Office Resources — Tests

If this test is needed, can it be performed in this office?	Yes	No	Notes
Plain radiograph (i.e. CXR, extremity film)			
Urine dipstick			
Urine pregnancy test			
Fingerstick hemoglobin			
Fingerstick blood glucose			
Rapid strep test			
Pulse oximetry			
Peak flow rate			
EKG			

Office Resources — Medications

If this medication is needed, is it available in this office?	Route	Yes	No	Notes
Albuterol inhaler (or other beta-agonist)	Inhaler			
Albuterol for nebulization (or other beta-agonist)	Nebulizer			
Epinephrine 1:1000 for SQ administration	SQ			
Nitroglycerine SL pills or nasal spray	SL or Nasal			
Diphenhydramine pills or liquid (e.g., Benadryl or other oral antihistamine)	Oral			
Aspirin pills	Oral			
Acetaminophen suppositories (e.g., Tylenol)	Rectal			
Acetaminophen pills or liquid (e.g., Tylenol)	Oral			
Ibuprofen pills or liquid (e.g., Motrin, Advil)	Oral			
Influenza vaccine	IM			
Tetanus immunization (e.g., Td, Tdap)	IM			

Appendix F

Sample Telephone Triage Logs

Date & Times – Call Received – Call Back – Call Finished	**Patient's Name** – Age, Sex Phone Number **Social Factors** **Chronic Illness**	**Brief History of Illness/Injury** Document symptoms • Location, duration, severity List reason patient needs to be seen or mark "all triage questions negative"	**Disposition**	**Comments** – Special Advice – Drug Dosage – Follow-up Call **Triager**
		Protocol Reason to see ________ Or ☐ all triage questions negative	☐ EMS 911 ☐ ED Now ☐ Office Now ☐ See Today ☐ See Tomorrow ☐ See Later, protocol care advice given ☐ Home Care, protocol care advice given ☐ Patient agrees ☐ Refer call to PCP	
		Protocol Reason to see ________ Or ☐ all triage questions negative	☐ EMS 911 ☐ ED Now ☐ Office Now ☐ See Today ☐ See Tomorrow ☐ See Later, protocol care advice given ☐ Home Care, protocol care advice given ☐ Patient agrees ☐ Refer call to PCP	
		Protocol Reason to see ________ Or ☐ all triage questions negative	☐ EMS 911 ☐ ED Now ☐ Office Now ☐ See Today ☐ See Tomorrow ☐ See Later, protocol care advice given ☐ Home Care, protocol care advice given ☐ Patient agrees ☐ Refer call to PCP	

Time Phone Number	Patient Name Age/Sex	Problem/Symptom	Protocol Used	Disposition	Advice Per Protocol Drug Dosage

Date: ______________________ Triage Nurse: ______________________

<table>
<tr><td>Date</td><td>Time</td><td>Phone #</td><td>Patient</td></tr>
<tr><td colspan="2" rowspan="3">Age ______ Sex ☐ F ☐ M
Symptoms

Chronic Illness</td><td>Protocol</td><td>Disposition
☐ EMS 911 ☐ ED Now ☐ Office Now
☐ See Today
☐ See Tomorrow
☐ See Later, protocol care advice given
☐ Home Care, protocol care advice given</td></tr>
<tr><td rowspan="2">Reason to See

Or ☐ all triage questions negative</td></tr>
<tr><td>☐ Patient agrees
☐ Refer call to PCP</td></tr>
<tr><td colspan="3">☐ Advice Per Protocol</td><td>Triager</td></tr>
</table>

<table>
<tr><td>Date</td><td>Time</td><td>Phone #</td><td>Patient</td></tr>
<tr><td colspan="2" rowspan="3">Age ______ Sex ☐ F ☐ M
Symptoms

Chronic Illness</td><td>Protocol</td><td>Disposition
☐ EMS 911 ☐ ED Now ☐ Office Now
☐ See Today
☐ See Tomorrow
☐ See Later, protocol care advice given
☐ Home Care, protocol care advice given</td></tr>
<tr><td rowspan="2">Reason to See

Or ☐ all triage questions negative</td></tr>
<tr><td>☐ Patient agrees
☐ Refer call to PCP</td></tr>
<tr><td colspan="3">☐ Advice Per Protocol</td><td>Triager</td></tr>
</table>

<table>
<tr><td>Date</td><td>Time</td><td>Phone #</td><td>Patient</td></tr>
<tr><td colspan="2" rowspan="3">Age ______ Sex ☐ F ☐ M
Symptoms

Chronic Illness</td><td>Protocol</td><td>Disposition
☐ EMS 911 ☐ ED Now ☐ Office Now
☐ See Today
☐ See Tomorrow
☐ See Later, protocol care advice given
☐ Home Care, protocol care advice given</td></tr>
<tr><td rowspan="2">Reason to See

Or ☐ all triage questions negative</td></tr>
<tr><td>☐ Patient agrees
☐ Refer call to PCP</td></tr>
<tr><td colspan="3">☐ Advice Per Protocol</td><td>Triager</td></tr>
</table>

Appendix G

Reviewers

The author is grateful to the following individuals for their time and expertise in reviewing the triage content that has been incorporated into these guidelines.

Call Center Medical Directors

Lee-Anne Facey-Crowther, MD, Medical Advisor, Sykes, Toronto, Ontario, Canada

Susan MacLean, MD, Medical Advisor, Sykes, Toronto, Ontario, Canada

Barton Schmitt, MD, Professor of Pediatrics, Medical Director, After-Hours Call Center, Children's Hospital Colorado, Aurora, CO

Mark Rotty, MD, Medical Director, Medical Call Center, Children's Physician Network, Minneapolis, MN

Gary Setnik, MD, Chair, Emergency Medicine, Mount Auburn Hospital, Cambridge, MA; Codirector, Division of Emergency Medicine, Harvard Medical School; Medical Director, Sirona

Michael Wahl, MD, Medical Director, The Illinois Poison Center, Chicago, IL

Physicians

Charles Bareis, MD, General Internist, Chief Medical Officer, MacNeal Hospital and Health Network, Berwyn, IL

Gregor Blix, MD, Urologic Surgeon, Medical Director Healthcare Midwest Surgery Center, Bronson Methodist Hospital and Borgess Hospital, Kalamazoo MI

Carolyn B. Bridges, MD, CDR, USPHS, Associate Director for Science (acting), Influenza Division, NCIRD (proposed) Centers for Disease Control and Prevention

John Brofman, MD, Pulmonologist, Medical Director of Critical Care, MacNeal Hospital and Health Network, Berwyn IL

Dwayne Coad, MD, Emergency Physician and Hospice Physician, Yellowknife , Northwest Territories, Canada

Andrew Davis, MD, MPH, General Internist, Assistant Professor of Clinical Medicine, University of Chicago Hospitals, Chicago IL

Kellie Flood-Shaffer, MD, Assistant Professor, Division Director, Obstetrics and Gynecology, University of Cincinatti, Ohio

David Goldberg, MD, Director of Student Health, Assistant Professor of Medicine, Loyola University Medical Center, Maywood, IL

Joseph Grubenhoff, MD, Assistant Professor, Section of Emergency Medicine, The Children's Hospital, Denver, CO

Kenneth Heinrich, MD, Attending Emergency Physician, Emergency Consultants, Inc.

Inbar Kirson, MD, Attending, Obstetrics and Gynecology, Lutheran General Hospital, Park Ridge, IL

Tony Lang, MD, Intemist, Mercy Hospital and Medical Center, Chicago, IL

Matthew Levine, MD, Director of Trauma Services, Department of Emergency Medicine, Northwestern Memorial Hospital, Chicago, IL

Katherine Nolan-Watson, MD, Assistant Professor in Obstetrics and Gynecology, Loyola University Medical Center, Maywood, IL

Roger Kaldawy, MD, Assistant Professor in Ophthalmology and Visual Sciences, Boston University School of Medicine, Boston, MA

Samantha Mckelvey, Obstetrics and Gynecology, University of Arkansas for Medical Sciences; ANGELS program (Antenatal and Neonatal Guidelines, Education and Learning System), Little Rock, AR

Edward Otten, MD, Toxicologist, Professor of Emergency Medicine, University of Cincinatti Medical Center, Cincinatti, OH

Greg Ozark, MD, Director, Med-Peds Residency, Loyola University Medical Center, Maywood, IL

Paula Podrazik, MD, Geriatrician, General Internist and ED Physician, University of Chicago Hospitals, Chicago, IL

Anna B. Reisman, MD, Assistant Professor, Department of Internal Medicine, Yale University School of Medicine, New Haven, CT

Daniel Stone, MD, MBA, Attending Physician and Clinical Instructor, Northwestern University Emergency Medicine Residency, Chicago, IL

Physicians *(continued)*

Herb Sutherland, DO, Medical Director of Emergency Department and Medical Call Center, Central Dupage Hospital, Winfield, IL

Penny Tenzer, MD, Vice-Chair, Director of Family Medicine Residency, University of Miami Hospital and Medical School, FL

Diana Viravec, MD, Emergency Physician, Emergency Services, MacNeal Hospital and Health Network, Berwyn, IL

Gary Wainer, DO, Family Practice Attending, Chief Medical Officer, Chicago Health Systems, Chicago, IL

James Wilkerson, MD, Attending Pathologist, Merced Pathology Laboratory, Merced, CA

Nurses

Mary Alexander, CRNI, Chief Executive Officer, Infusion Nurses Society, Editor, *Journal of Infusion Nursing*, Norwood, MA

Tina Butler, WHNP-BC, MNSc, University of Arkansas for Medical Sciences ANGELS program (Antenatal and Neonatal Guidelines, Education and Learning System), Little Rock, AR

Joanne Dedowicz, RN, Director of Resource and Referral, Behavioral Health, Edwards-Linden Hospital, Naperville, IL

Jenny DuFresne, RN, Manager for Valley Connection Call Center, Santa Clara Valley Hospital, Santa Clara, CA

Jeanine Feirer, RN, Clinical Coordinator, Proactive Health, Marshfield Clinic, Unity, WI

Rebecca Gebhart, RN, MSN, Faculty, University of Phoenix AZ, Call Center Advisor, ExpertKnowledgeNetwork.com

Marlene Grasser, RN, LVM Systems, Phoenix A

Deborah Gresham, RNC, MSN, Clinical Nurse Specialist, Center for Women's Health Care, Miami Valley Hospital, Dayton, OH

Valerie Grossman, RN, BSN, CEN, Director of Medical-Surgical Services, Via Health Hospital, Rochester, NY

Teresa Hagarty, RN, Nurse Manager, Children's Hospital Colorado, Aurora, CO

Laura Mahlmeister, RN, PhD, Educational and Nurse Legal Consultant, L&D Nurse, Mahlmeister and Associates, San Francisco, CA

Kelli Massaro, RN, Telephone Triage Consultant, Call Center Nurse, After-Hours Call Center Children's Hospital Colorado, Aurora, CO

Melissa Masson, RN, BScN, MN(c), Clinical Practice Consultant, Sykes Telehealth Services, Ontario, Canada

Donna Matthews, RN, Newfoundland, Canada

Becky McGowan, RN, Call Center Nurse and Emergency Department Nurse, MacNeal Hospital and Health Network, Berwyn, IL

Kim McCormick, RN, Telephone Triage, Home Health and Hospice Nursing, MacNeal Home Health Care, Berwyn, IL

Cheryl Patterson, RNC, BSN, Educator Coordinator, Evergreen Healthline, Evergreen Hospital Medical Center, Kirkland, WA

Laurie Peachey, RN, Toronto, Ontario, Canada

Teresa Pounds, Nurse Manager and Clinical Content Coordinator, Sirona, Inc, Portland, MN

Joan Rucker, RN, Perinatal and Maternal Educator, MacNeal Hospital and Health Network, Berwyn, IL

Charlene Slaney, Director of Client and Clinical Services, FONEMED, Newfoundland, Canada

Susan Smith Dodson, MBA, BSN, RN, CCRC, Triage System Development Coordinator/Trainer, University of Arkansas for Medical Sciences ANGELS program (Antenatal and Neonatal Guidelines, Education and Learning System), Little Rock, AR

Beverley Tipsord-Klinkhammer, RN, MBA, Senior VP of Patient Services, Onslow Memorial Hospital, Jacksonville, NC

Michelle Violette, RN, BScN, MSc, Director of Chronic Disease Management, Sykes Telehealth Services, Toronto, Ontario, Canada

Donna Williams, RN, Nurse Manager, University of Arkansas for Medical Sciences ANGELS program (Antenatal and Neonatal Guidelines, Education and Learning System), Little Rock, AR

Dentist

James Discipio, DDS, LaGrange, IL

Behavioral Health Counselor

Jennifer Vitagliano, MC, CPC, Helpline Coordinator, Behavioral Health Services, Banner Health System Call Center

Appendix H

References for All Protocols

Abdominal Pain (Female)

1. Cappell MS, Friedel D. Abdominal pain during pregnancy. *Gastroenterol Clin North Am.* 2003;32(1):1–58
2. Cardall T, Glasser J, Guss DA. Clinical value of the total white blood cell count and temperature in the evaluation of patients with suspected appendicitis. *Acad Emerg Med.* 2004;11(10):1021–1027
3. Condous G. Ectopic pregnancy—risk factors and diagnosis. *Aust Fam Physician.* 2006;35(11):854–857
4. Flasar MH, Cross R, Goldberg E. Acute abdominal pain. *Prim Care.* 2006;33(3):659–684, vi
5. Hendrickson M, Naparst TR. Abdominal surgical emergencies in the elderly. *Emerg Med Clin North Am.* 2003;21(4):937–969
6. Kamin R. Nowicki TA, Courtney DS, Powers RD. Pearls and pitfalls in the emergency department evaluation of abdominal pain. *Emerg Med Clin North Am.* 2003;21(1):61–72, vi
7. Martinez JP, Hogan GJ. Mesenteric ischemia. *Emerg Med Clin North Am.* 2004;22(4):909–928
8. Martinez JP, Mattu A Abdominal pain in the elderly. *Emerg Med Clin North Am.* 2006;24(2):371–388, vii
9. North F, Odunukan O, Varkey P. The value of telephone triage for patients with appendicitis. *J Telemed Telecare.* 2011;17(8):417–420
10. Roy S, Weimersheimer P. Nonoperative cause of abdominal pain. *Surg Clin North Am.* 1997;77(6):1433–1454
11. Stewart C, Bosker G. Pelvic inflammatory disease. *Emerg Med Rep.* 1999;20(16):163–172
12. Yamamoto W, Kono H, Maekawa M, Fukui T. The relationship between abdominal pain regions and specific diseases: an epidemiologic approach to clinical practice. *J Epidemiol.* 1997;7(1):27–32

Abdominal Pain (Male)

1. Cardall T, Glasser J, Guss DA. Clinical value of the total white blood cell count and temperature in the evaluation of patients with suspected appendicitis. *Acad Emerg Med.* 2004;11(10):1021–1027
2. Flasar MH, Cross R, Goldberg E. Acute abdominal pain. *Prim Care.* 2006;33(3):659–684, vi
3. Hendrickson M, Naparst TR. Abdominal surgical emergencies in the elderly. *Emerg Med Clin North Am.* 2003;21(4):937–969
4. Kamin R. Nowicki TA, Courtney DS, Powers RD. Pearls and pitfalls in the emergency department evaluation of abdominal pain. *Emerg Med Clin North Am.* 2003;21(1):61–72, vi
5. Martinez JP, Hogan GJ. Mesenteric ischemia. *Emerg Med Clin North Am.* 2004;22(4):909–928
6. Martinez JP, Mattu A Abdominal pain in the elderly. *Emerg Med Clin North Am.* 2006;24(2):371–388, vii
7. North F, Odunukan O, Varkey P. The value of telephone triage for patients with appendicitis. *J Telemed Telecare.* 2011;17(8):417–420
8. Pearigen PD. Unusual causes of abdominal pain. *Emerg Med Clin North Am.* 1996;14(3):593–613
9. Roy S, Weimersheimer P. Nonoperative cause of abdominal pain. *Surg Clin North Am.* 1997;77(6):1433–1454
10. Yamamoto W, Kono H, Maekawa M, Fukui T. The relationship between abdominal pain regions and specific diseases: an epidemiologic approach to clinical practice. *J Epidemiol.* 1997;7(1):27–32

Abdominal Pain (Upper)

1. Canto JG, Shlipak MG, Rogers WJ, et al. Prevalence, clinical characteristics, and mortality among patients with myocardial infarction presenting without chest pain. *JAMA.* 2000;283(24): 3223–3229
2. Culic V, Eterovic D, Miric D, Silic N. Symptom presentation of acute myocardial infarction: influence of sex, age, and risk factors. *Am Heart J.* 2002;144(6):1012–1017
3. Flasar MH, Cross R, Goldberg E. Acute abdominal pain. *Prim Care.* 2006;33(3):659–684, vi
4. Lemire S. Assessment of clinical severity and investigation of uncomplicated gastroesophageal reflux disease and noncardiac angina-like chest pain. *Can J Gastroenterol.* 1997;11(suppl B):37B–40B
5. Martinez JP, Mattu A Abdominal pain in the elderly. *Emerg Med Clin North Am.* 2006;24(2):371–388, vii
6. North F, Odunukan O, Varkey P. The value of telephone triage for patients with appendicitis. *J Telemed Telecare.* 2011;17(8):417–420
7. Pearigen PD. Unusual causes of abdominal pain. *Emerg Med Clin North Am.* 1996;14(3):593–613
8. Roy S, Weimersheimer P. Nonoperative cause of abdominal pain. *Surg Clin North Am.* 1997;77(6):1433–1454
9. Sanson TG, O'Keefe KP. Evaluation of abdominal pain in the elderly. *Emerg Med Clin North Am.* 1996;14(3):615–627
10. Simrén M, Tack J. Functional dyspepsia: evaluation and treatment. *Gastroenterol Clin North Am.* 2003;32(2):577–599
11. Yamamoto W, Kono H, Maekawa M, Fukui T. The relationship between abdominal pain regions and specific diseases: an epidemiologic approach to clinical practice. *J Epidemiol.* 1997;7(1):27–32

Alcohol Use and Abuse and Dependence

1. Burge SK, Schneider FD. Alcohol-related problems: recognition and intervention. *Am Fam Physician.* 1999;59(2):361– 372
2. Cherpitel CJ. Screening for alcohol problems in the emergency department. *Ann Emerg Med.* 1995;26(2):158–166
3. Dart RC, Kuffner EK, Rumack BH. Treatment of pain or fever with paracetamol (acetaminophen) in the alcoholic patient: a systematic review. *Am J Ther.* 2000;7(2):123–134
4. Fiellin DA, Reid MC, O'Connor PG. Outpatient management of patients with alcohol problems. *Ann Intern Med.* 2000;133(10):815–827
5. Mayo-Smith MF, Beecher LH, Fischer TL, et al; and the American Society of Addiction Medicine Working Group on the Management of Alcohol Withdrawal Delirium, Practice Guidelines Committee. Management of alcohol withdrawal delirium. An evidence-based practice guideline. *Arch Intern Med.* 2004;164(13):1405–1412
6. Stein MD. Medical consequences of substance abuse. *Psychiatr Clin North Am.* 1999;22(2):351–370
7. National Institute on Alcohol Abuse and Alcoholism. *The Physicians' Guide to Helping Patients with Alcohol Problems.* Rockville, MD: US Dept of Health and Human Services, Public Health Service; 1995. NIH publication 95-3769
8. US Preventive Services Task Force. Screening for problem drinking. In: *Guide to Clinical Preventive Services.* 2nd ed. Alexandria, VA: International Medical Publishing, Inc; 1996:567–582

Animal Bite

1. Advisory Committee on Immunization Practices. Human rabies prevention—United States, 1999. Recommendations of the Advisory Committee on Immunization Practices (ACIP). *MMWR Recomm Rep.* 1999;48(RR-1):1–21
2. Dimick AR. Delayed wound closure: indications and techniques. *Ann Emerg Med.* 1988;17(12):1303–1304
3. Freer L. North American wild mammalian injuries. *Emerg Med Clin North Am.* 2004;22(2):445–473, ix
4. Glaser C, Lewis P, Wong S. Pet-, animal-, and vector-borne infections. *Pediatr Rev.* 2000;21(7):219–232
5. Griego RD, Rosen T, Orengo IF, Wolf JE. Dog, cat and human bites: a review. *J Am Acad Dermatol.* 1995;33(6):1019–1029
6. Harrison BP, Hillard MW. Emergency department evaluation and treatment of hand injuries. *Emerg Med Clin North Am.* 1999;17(4): 793–822, v
7. Jackson AC, Warrell MJ, Rupprecht CE, et al. Management of rabies in humans. *Clin Infect Dis.* 2003;36(1):60–63
8. MacBean CE, Taylor DM, Ashby K. Animal and human bite injuries in Victoria, 1998–2004. *Med J Aust.* 2007;186(1):38–40
9. Manning SE, Rupprecht CE, Fishbein D, et al; and the Advisory Committee on Immunization Practices, Centers for Disease Control and Prevention (CDC). Human rabies prevention—United States, 2008: recommendations of the Advisory Committee on Immunization Practices. *MMWR Recomm Rep.* 2008;57(RR-3):1–28
10. Medeiros I, Saconato H. Antibiotic prophylaxis for mammalian bites. *Cochrane Database Syst Rev.* 2001;(2):CD001738
11. Moran GJ, Talan DA, Abrahamian FM. Antimicrobial prophylaxis for wounds and procedures in the emergency department. *Infect Dis Clin North Am.* 2008;22(1):117–143, vii
12. National Association of State Public Health Veterinarians, Inc. Compendium of animal rabies prevention and control, 2000. *MMWR Recomm Rep.* 2000;49(RR-8):21–30
13. Public Health Agency of Canada. Canadian Immunization Guide; Seventh Edition – 2006. http://www.phac-aspc.gc.ca/publicat/cig-gci/index-eng.php. Accessed July 25, 2012
14. Rapoport M, Adam HM. Animal bites: assessing risk for rabies and providing treatment. *Pediatr Rev.* 1997;18(4):142–143
15. Rupprecht CE, Briggs D, Brown CM, et al. Use of a reduced (4-dose) vaccine schedule for postexposure prophylaxis to prevent human rabies: recommendations of the Advisory Committee on Immunization Practices. *MMWR Recomm Rep.* 2010;59(RR-2):1–9
16. Steele MT, Ma OJ, Nakase J, et al; and the EMERGEncy ID NET Study Group. Epidemiology of animal exposures presenting to emergency departments. *Acad Emerg Med.* 2007;14(5):398–403
17. Swartz MN. Clinical practice. Cellulitis. *N Engl J Med.* 2004;350(9): 904–912
18. Turner TW. Do mammalian bites require antibiotic prophylaxis? *Ann Emerg Med.* 2004;44(3):274–276

Arm Pain

1. Barry NN, McGuire JL. Overuse syndromes in adult athletes. *Rheum Dis Clin North Am.* 1996;22(3):515–530
2. Canto JG, Shlipak MG, Rogers WJ, et al. Prevalence, clinical characteristics, and mortality among patients with myocardial infarction presenting without chest pain. *JAMA.* 2000;283(24): 3223–3229
3. Coronado BE, Pope JH, Griffith JL, Beshansky JR, Selker HP. Clinical features, triage, and outcome of patients presenting to the ED with suspected acute coronary syndromes but without pain: a multicenter study. *Am J Emerg Med.* 2004;22(7):568–574
4. Culic V, Eterovic D, Miric D, Silic N. Symptom presentation of acute myocardial infarction: influence of sex, age, and risk factors. *Am Heart J.* 2002;144(6):1012–1017
5. Ling SM, Bathon JM. Osteoarthritis in older adults. *J Am Geriatr Soc.* 1998;46(2):216–225

Asthma Attack

1. American Heart Association. 2005 Guidelines for Cardiopulmonary Resuscitation and Emergency Cardiovascular Care. Part 10.5: Near-Fatal Asthma. *Circulation.* 2005;112(24)(suppl):IV-139–IV-142
2. American Heart Association. 2005 Guidelines for Cardiopulmonary Resuscitation and Emergency Cardiovascular Care. Part 14: First aid. *Circulation.* 2005;112(24)(suppl):IV-196–IV-203
3. Cates CJ, Crilly JA, Rowe BH. Holding chambers (spacers) versus nebulisers for beta-agonist treatment of acute asthma. *Cochrane Database Syst Rev.* 2006;(2):CD000052
4. Gibbs MA, Camargo CA, Rowe BH, Silverman RA. State of the art: therapeutic controversies in severe acute asthma. *Acad Emerg Med.* 2000;7(7):800–815
5. Hanson L. Telephone advice and triage. *Immunol Allergy Clin North Am.* 1999;19(1):171–176
6. Fiore AE, Fry A, Shay D, Gubareva L, Bresee JS, Uyeki TM. Antiviral agents for the treatment and chemoprophylaxis of influenza—recommendations of the Advisory Committee on Immunization Practices (ACIP). *MMWR Recomm Rep.* 2011;60(1):1–24
7. American Academy of Allergy, Asthma and Immunology Joint Task Force on Practice Parameters; American College of Allergy, Asthma, and Immunology; Joint Council of Allergy, Asthma, and Immunology. Attaining optimal asthma control: a practice parameter. *J Allergy Clin Immunol.* 2005;116(5):S3–S11
8. National Asthma Education and Prevention Program. Expert Panel Report 3 (EPR-3): Guidelines for the Diagnosis and Management of Asthma – Summary Report 2007. *J Allergy Clin Immunol.* 2007;120(5 suppl):S94–S138
9. National Asthma Education and Prevention Program. Expert Panel Report 2 (EPR-2). Guidelines for the Diagnosis and Management of Asthma Update on Selected Topics—2002. *J Allergy Clin Immunol.* 2002;110(5 suppl):S141–S219
10. National Asthma Education and Prevention Program. *Expert Panel Report 2: Guidelines for the Diagnosis and Management of Asthma.* Bethesda, MD: National Heart Lung and Blood Institute; 1997
11. Silverman R. Treatment of acute asthma. A new look at the old and the new. *Clin Chest Med.* 2000;21(2):361–379
12. Tilles SA, Nelson HS. Differential diagnosis of adult asthma. *Immunol Allergy Clin North Am.* 1996;16(1):19–34

Athlete's Foot

1. Bedinghaus JM, Niedfeldt MW. Over-the-counter foot remedies. *Am Fam Physician.* 2001;64(5):791–796
2. Gupta AK, Chow M, Daniel CR, Aly R. Treatments of tinea pedis. *Dermatol Clin.* 2003;21(3):431–462
3. Noble SL, Forbes RC, Stamm PL. Diagnosis and management of common tinea infections. *Am Fam Physician.* 1998;58(1):163–178
4. Rand S. Overview: the treatment of dermatophytosis. *J Am Acad Dermatol.* 2000;43(5 suppl):S104–S112
5. Rich P. Onychomycosis and tinea pedis in patients with diabetes. *J Am Acad Dermatol.* 2000;43(5 suppl):S130–S134
6. Rogers D, Kilkenny M, Marks R. The descriptive epidemiology of tinea pedis in the community. *Australas J Dermatol.* 1996;37(4): 178–184

Athlete's Foot (continued)

7. Rupke SJ. Fungal skin disorders. *Prim Care.* 2000;27(2):407–421
8. Stein DH. Tineas—superficial dermatophyte infections. *Pediatr Rev.* 1998;19(11):368–372
9. Young CC, Niedfeldt MW, Morris GA, Eerkes KJ. Clinical examination of the foot and ankle. *Prim Care.* 2005;32(1):105–132

Back Pain

1. Argoff CA, Wheeler AH. Spinal and radicular pain disorders. *Neurol Clin.* 1998;16(4):833–850
2. Atlas SJ, Nardin RA. Evaluation and treatment of low back pain: an evidenced-based approach to clinical care. *Muscle Nerve.* 2003;27(3):265–284
3. Chou R, Huffman LH; and the American Pain Society; American College of Physicians. Nonpharmacologic therapies for acute and chronic low back pain: a review of the evidence for an American Pain Society/American College of Physicians. clinical practice guideline. *Ann Intern Med.* 2007;147(7):492–504
4. Dart RC, Kuffner EK, Rumack BH. Treatment of pain or fever with paracetamol (acetaminophen) in the alcoholic patient: a systematic review. *Am J Ther.* 2000;7(2):123–134
5. Devereaux MW. Low back pain. *Prim Care.* 2004;31(1):33–51
6. Deyo RA, Weinstein JN. Low back pain. *N Eng J Med.* 2001;344(5): 363–370
7. Divoll M, Abernethy DR, Ameer B, Greenblatt DJ. Acetaminophen kinetics in the elderly. *Clin Pharmacol Ther.* 1982;31(2):151–156
8. French SD, Cameron M, Walker BF, Reggars JW, Esterman AJ. Superficial heat or cold for low back pain. *Cochrane Database Syst Rev.* 2006;(1):CD004750
9. Griffin G, Tudiver F, Grant WD. Do NSAIDs help in acute or chronic low back pain? *Am Fam Physician.* 2002;65(7):1319–1321
10. Dahm KT, Brurberg KG, Jamtvedt G, Hagen KB. Advice to rest in bed versus advice to stay active for acute low-back pain and sciatica. *Cochrane Database Syst Rev.* 2010;(6):CD007612
11. Hróbjartsson A, Gøtzsche PC. Placebo interventions for all clinical conditions. *Cochrane Database Syst Rev.* 2010;(1):CD003974
12. Kovacs FM, Abraira V, Pena A, et al. Effect of firmness of mattress on chronic non-specific low-back pain: randomized, double-blind, controlled, multicentre trial. *Lancet.* 2003;362(9396):1599–1604
13. Malmivaara A, Hakkinen U, Aro T, et al. The treatment of acute low back pain: bed rest, exercises, or ordinary activity? *N Engl J Med.* 1995;332(6):351–355
14. Rainsford KD. Ibuprofen: pharmacology, efficacy and safety. *Inflammopharmacology.* 2009;17(6):275–342
15. Roelofs PD, Deyo RA, Koes BW, Scholten RJ, van Tulder MW. Non-steroidal anti-inflammatory drugs for low back pain. *Cochrane Database Syst Rev.* 2008;(1):CD000396
16. Swenson R. Differential diagnosis: a reasonable clinical approach. *Neurol Clin.* 1999;17(1):43–63
17. Takala E. Immediate referral from general practice for lumbar spine X-ray does not improve quality of life or pain for people with lower back pain. *Evid Based Healthc.* 2002;6(2);91–92

Bee Sting

1. American Academy of Allergy, Asthma and Immunology (AAAAI). The use of epinephrine in the treatment of anaphylaxis. Position statement. http://www.aaaai.org/Aaaai/media/MediaLibrary/PDF%20Documents/Practice%20and%20Parameters/Epinephrine-in-treating-anaphylaxis-2002.pdf. Accessed July 25, 2012
2. Anchor J, Settipane RA. Appropriate use of epinephrine in anaphylaxis. *Am J Emerg Med.* 2004;22(6):488–490
3. Betten DP, Richardson WH, Tong TC, Clark RF. Massive honey bee envenomation-induced rhabdomyolysis in an adolescent. *Pediatrics.* 2006;117(1):231–235
4. Brown SG. Clinical features and severity grading of anaphylaxis. *J Allergy Clin Immunol.* 2004;114(2):371–376
5. Derlet RW, Richards JR. Cellulitis from insect bites: a case series. *Cal J Emerg Med.* 2003;4(2):27–30
6. Jerrard DA. ED management of insect stings. *Am J Emerg Med.* 1996;14(4):429–433
7. American Academy of Allergy, Asthma and Immunology Joint Task Force on Practice Parameters; American College of Allergy, Asthma and Immunology; Joint Council of Allergy, Asthma and Immunology. The diagnosis and management of anaphylaxis: an updated practice parameter. *J Allergy Clin Immunol.* 2005;115(3 suppl 2):S483–S523
8. Moffitt JE, Golden DB, Reisman RE, et al. Stinging insect hypersensitivity: a practice parameter update. *J Allergy Clin Immunol.* 2004;114(4): 869–886
9. Reisman RE. Insect stings. *N Engl J Med.* 1994;331(8):523–527
10. Sampson HA, Muñoz-Furlong A, Campbell RL, et al. Second symposium on the definition and management of anaphylaxis: summary report—Second National Institute of Allergy and Infectious Disease/Food Allergy and Anaphylaxis Network symposium. *J Allergy Clin Immunol.* 2006;117(2):391–397
11. Sherman RA. What physicians should know about Africanized honeybees. *West J Med.* 1995;163(6):541–546
12. Steen CJ, Carbonaro PA, Schwartz RA. Arthropods in dermatology. *J Am Acad Dermatol.* 2004;50(6):819–844
13. Teoh SC, Lee JJ, Fam HB. Corneal honeybee sting. *Can J Ophthalmol.* 2005;40(4):469–471
14. Visscher PK, Vetter RS, Camazine S. Removing bee stings. *Lancet.* 1996;348(9023):301–302

Breathing Difficulty

1. American Heart Association. 2005 Guidelines for Cardiopulmonary Resuscitation and Emergency Cardiovascular Care. Part 14: First aid. *Circulation.* 2005;112(24 suppl):IV-196–IV-203
2. Gallus AS. Travel, venous thromboembolism, and thrombophilia. *Semin Thromb Hemost.* 2005;31(1):90–96
3. Goldman L, Kirtane AJ. Triage of patients with acute chest pain and possible cardiac ischemia: the elusive search for diagnostic perfection. *Ann Intern Med.* 2003;139(12):987–995
4. Han J, Zhu Y, Li S, et al. The language of medically unexplained dyspnea. *Chest.* 2008;133(4):961–968
5. Hardie GE, Janson S, Gold WM, Carrieri-Kohlman V, Boushey HA. Ethnic differences: word descriptors used by African-American and white asthma patients during induced bronchoconstriction. *Chest.* 2000;117(4):935–943
6. Mahler DA, Harver A. Do you speak the language of dyspnea? *Chest.* 2000;117(4):928–929
7. Mateo J, Oliver A, Borrell M, Sala N, Fontcuberta J. Laboratory evaluation and clinical characteristics of 2,132 consecutive unselected patients with venous thromboembolism—results of the Spanish Multicentric Study on Thrombophilia (EMET Study). *Thromb Haemost.* 1997;77(3):444–451
8. McRae S. Pulmonary embolism. *Aust Fam Physician.* 2010;39(6): 462–466
9. McSweeney JC, Cody M, O'Sullivan P, Elberson K, Moser DK, Garvin BJ. Women's early warning symptoms of acute myocardial infarction. *Circulation.* 2003;108(21):2619–2623
10. Michelson E, Hollrah S. Evaluation of the patient with shortness of breath: an evidence based approach. *Emerg Med Clin North Am.* 1999;17(1):221–237, x

11. Philbrick JT, Shumate R, Siadaty MS, Becker DM. Air travel and venous thromboembolism: a systematic review. *J Gen Intern Med.* 2007;22(1):107–114
12. Sayre MR, Koster RW, Botha M, et al. Part 5: Adult basic life support: 2010 International Consensus on Cardiopulmonary Resuscitation and Emergency Cardiovascular Care Science With Treatment Recommendations. *Circulation.* 2010;122(16 suppl 2):S298–S324
13. Stein PD, Henry JW. Clinical characteristics of patients with acute pulmonary embolism stratified according to their presenting syndromes. *Chest.* 1997;112(4):974–979
14. Travers AH, Rea TD, Bobrow BJ, et al. Part 4: CPR overview: 2010 American Heart Association Guidelines for Cardiopulmonary Resuscitation and Emergency Cardiovascular Care. *Circulation.* 2010;122(18 suppl 3):S676–S684
15. Wang CS, FitzGerald JM, Schulzer M, Mak E, Ayas NT. Does this dyspneic patient in the emergency department have congestive heart failure? *JAMA.* 2005;294(15):1944–1956
16. Zoorob RJ, Campbell JS. Acute dyspnea in the office. *Am Fam Physician.* 2003;68(9):1803–1810

Burns

1. American Burn Association. Hospital and prehospital resources for optimal care of patients with burn injury: guidelines for development and operation of burn centers. *J Burn Care Rehabil.* 1990;11(2):98–104
2. Centers for Disease Control and Prevention (CDC). Updated recommendations for use of tetanus toxoid, reduced diphtheria toxoid and acellular pertussis (Tdap) vaccine from the Advisory Committee on Immunization Practices, 2010. *MMWR Morb Mortal Wkly Rep.* 2011;60(1):13–15
3. Davies JW. Prompt cooling of burned areas: a review of benefits and the effector mechanisms. *Burns Incl Therm Inj.* 1982;9(1):1–6
4. Demling RH, Mazess RB, Wolberg W. The effect of immediate and delayed cold immersion on burn edema formation and resorption. *J Trauma.* 1979;19(1):56–60
5. Hendricks WM. The classification of burns. *J Am Acad Dermatol.* 1990;22(5):838–839
6. Jull AB, Rodgers A, Walker N. Honey as a topical treatment for wounds. *Cochrane Database Syst Rev.* 2008;(4):CD005083
7. Kretsinger K, Broder KR, Cortese MM, et al. Preventing tetanus, diphtheria, and pertussis among adults: use of tetanus toxoid, reduced diphtheria toxoid and acellular pertussis vaccine recommendations of the Advisory Committee on Immunization Practices (ACIP) and recommendations of ACIP, supported by the Healthcare Infection Control Practices Advisory Committee (HICPAC), for the use of Tdap among health-care personnel. *MMWR Recomm Rep.* 2006;55(RR-17):1–37
8. Lawrence JC. British Burn Association recommended first aid for burns and scalds. *Burns Incl Therm Inj.* 1987;13(2):153
9. McCullough JE, Henderson AK, Kaufman JD. Occupational burns in Washington State, 1989–1993. *J Occup Environ Med.* 1998;40(12): 1083–1089
10. Morgan ED, Bledsoe SC, Barker J. Ambulatory management of burns. *Am Fam Physician.* 2000;62(9):2015–2032
11. Pearson AS, Wolford RW. Management of skin trauma. *Prim Care.* 2000;27(2):475–492
12. Ramzy PI, Barret JP, Herndon DN. Thermal injury. *Crit Care Clin.* 1999;15(2):333–352, ix
13. Rea S, Kuthubutheen J, Fowler B, Wood F. Burn first aid in Western Australia—do healthcare workers have the knowledge? *Burns.* 2005;31(8):1029–1034
14. Spector J, Fernandez WG. Chemical, thermal, and biological ocular exposures. *Emerg Med Clin North Am.* 2008;26(1):125–136, vii
15. Swain AH, Azadian BS, Wakeley CJ, Shakespeare PG. Management of blisters in minor burns. *Br Med J (Clin Res Ed).* 1987;295(6591):181
16. Venter TH, Karpelowsky JS, Rode H. Cooling of the burn wound: the ideal temperature of the coolant. *Burns.* 2007;33(7):917–922

Cast Symptoms and Questions

1. Pimentel L. Orthopedic trauma: office management of major joint injury. *Med Clin North Am.* 2006;90(2):355–382
2. Smith GD, Hart RG, Tsai TM. Fiberglass cast application. *Am J Emerg Med.* 2005;23(3):347–350

Chest Pain

1. American Heart Association. 2005 Guidelines for Cardiopulmonary Resuscitation and Emergency Cardiovascular Care. Part 8: Stabilization of the patient with acute coronary syndromes. *Circulation.* 2005;112(24 suppl):IV-89–IV-110
2. Antman EM, Anbe DT, Armstrong PW, et al. ACC/AHA guidelines for the management of patients with ST-elevation myocardial infarction – executive summary: a report of the American College of Cardiology/American Heart Association Task Force on Practice Guidelines (Writing Committee to Revise the 1999 Guidelines for the Management of Patients With Acute Myocardial Infarction). *Circulation.* 2004;110(5):588–636
3. Canto JG, Shlipak MG, Rogers WJ, et al. Prevalence, clinical characteristics, and mortality among patients with myocardial infarction presenting without chest pain. *JAMA.* 2000;283(24):3223–3229
4. Eisenberg MJ, Topal EJ. Prehospital administration of aspirin in patients with unstable angina and acute myocardial infarction. *Arch Int Med.* 1996;156(14):1506–1510
5. Gallus AS. Travel, venous thromboembolism, and thrombophilia. *Semin Thromb Hemost.* 2005;31(1):90–96
6. Goldman L, Kirtane AJ. Triage of patients with acute chest pain and possible cardiac ischemia: the elusive search for diagnostic perfection. *Ann Intern Med.* 2003;139(12):987–995
7. Goodacre S, Locker T, Morris F, Campbell S. How useful are clinical features in the diagnosis of acute undifferentiated chest pain? *Acad Emerg Med.* 2002;9(3):203–208
8. Han JH, Lindsell CJ, Storrow AB, et al; and the EMCREG i*trACS Investigators. The role of cardiac risk factor burden in diagnosing acute coronary syndromes in the emergency department setting. *Ann Emerg Med.* 2007;49(2):145–152
9. Jaffy MB, Meischke H, Eisenberg MS. Prevalence of aspirin use among patients calling 9-1-1 for chest pain. *Acad Emerg Med.* 1998;5(12):1146–1149
10. Kline JA, Courtney DM, Kabrhel C, et al. Prospective multicenter evaluation of the pulmonary embolism rule-out criteria. *J Thromb Haemost.* 2008;6(5):772–780
11. Lee TH, Goldman L. Evaluation of the patient with acute chest pain. *N Engl J Med.* 2000;342(16):1187–1195
12. Marsan RJ, Shaver KJ, Sease KL, Shofer FS, Sites FD, Hollander JE. Evaluation of a clinical decision rule for young adult patients with chest pain. *Acad Emerg Med.* 2005;12(1):26–31
13. McRae S. Pulmonary embolism. *Aust Fam Physician.* 2010;39(6): 462–466
14. McSweeney JC, Cody M, O'Sullivan P, Elberson K, Moser DK, Garvin BJ. Women's early warning symptoms of acute myocardial infarction. *Circulation.* 2003;108(21):2619–2623

Chest Pain (continued)

15. Pope JH, Aufderheide TP, Rughazer R, et al. Missed diagnoses of acute cardiac ischemia in the emergency department. *N Engl J Med.* 2000;342(16):1163–1170
16. Sayre MR, Koster RW, Botha M, et al. Part 5: Adult basic life support: 2010 International Consensus on Cardiopulmonary Resuscitation and Emergency Cardiovascular Care Science With Treatment Recommendations. *Circulation.* 2010;122(16 suppl 2):S298–S324
17. Swap CJ, Nagurney JT. Value and limitations of chest pain history in the evaluation of patients with suspected coronary syndromes. *JAMA.* 2005;294(20):2623–2629
18. Weber JE, Chudnofsky CR, Boczar M, Boyer EW, Wilkerson MD, Hollander JE. Cocaine associated chest pain: how common is myocardial infarction? *Acad Emerg Med.* 2000;7(8):873–877
19. Welch RD, Zalenski RJ, Frederick PD, et al. Prognostic value of a normal or nonspecific initial electrocardiogram in acute myoacardial infarction. *JAMA.* 2001;286(16):1977–1984

Cold Sores (Fever Blisters of Lip)

1. Emmert DH. Treatment of common cutaneous herpes simplex virus infections. *Am Fam Physician.* 2000;61(6):1697–1708
2. Gonsalves WC, Chi AC, Neville BW. Common oral lesions: Part I. Superficial mucosal lesions. *Am Fam Physician.* 2007;75(4):501–507
3. Sacks SL, Thisted RA, Jones TM, et al. Clinical efficacy of topical docosanol 10% cream for herpes simplex labialis: a multicenter, randomized, placebo-controlled trial. *J Am Acad Dermatol.* 2001;45(2):222–230
4. Spruance SL, Bodsworth N, Resnick H, et al. Single-dose, patient-initiated famciclovir: a randomized, double-blind, placebo-controlled trial for episodic treatment of herpes labialis. *J Am Acad Dermatol.* 2006;55(1):47–53
5. Spruance SL, Rea TL, Thoming C, Tucker R, Saltzman R, Boon R. Penciclovir cream for the treatment of herpes simplex labialis. A randomized, multicenter, double-blind, placebo-controlled trial. *JAMA.* 1997;277(17):1374–1379
6. Whitley R. New approaches to the therapy of HSV infections. *Herpes.* 2006;13(2):53–55

Colds

1. American Academy of Family Physicians. Patient information. Saline nasal irrigation for sinus problems. *Am Fam Physician.* 2009;80(10):1121
2. Bachert C, Chuchalin AG, Eisebitt R, Netayzhenko VZ, Voelker M. Aspirin compared with acetaminophen in the treatment of fever and other symptoms of upper respiratory tract infection in adults: a multicenter, randomized, double-blind, double-dummy, placebo-controlled, parallel-group, single-dose, 6-hour dose-ranging study. *Clin Ther.* 2005;27(7):993–1003
3. Barrett B, Brown, R, Rakel, et al. Echinacea for treating the common cold: a randomized trial. *Ann Intern Med.* 2010;153(12):769–777
4. Black RA, Hill DA. Over-the-counter medications in pregnancy. *Am Fam Physician.* 2003;67(12):2517–2524
5. Caruso TJ, Gwaltney JM Jr. Treatment of the common cold with echinacea: a structured review. *Clin Infect Dis.* 2005;40(6):807–810
6. Curley FJ, Irwin RS, Pratter MR, et al. Cough and the common cold. *Am Rev Respir Dis.* 1988;138(2):305–311
7. Douglas RM, Hemilä H, Chalker E, Treacy B. Vitamin C for preventing and treating the common cold. *Cochrane Database Syst Rev.* 2007;(3):CD000980
8. Eccles R. Understanding the symptoms of the common cold and influenza. *Lancet Infect Dis.* 2005;5(11):718–725
9. Erebara A, Bozzo P, Einarson A, Koren G. Treating the common cold during pregnancy. *Can Fam Physician.* 2008;54(5):687–689
10. Falsey AR, McCann RM, Hall WJ, et al. The "common cold" in frail older persons: impact of rhinovirus and coronavirus in a senior daycare center. *J Am Geriatr Soc.* 1997;45(6):706–711
11. Grimm W, Muller HH. A randomized controlled trial of the effect of fluid extract of Echinacea purpurea on the incidence and severity of colds and respiratory infections. *Am J Med.* 1999;106(2):138–143
12. Harvey R, Hannan SA, Badia L, Scadding G. Nasal saline irrigations for the symptoms of chronic rhinosinusitis. *Cochrane Database Syst Rev.* 2007;(3):CD006394
13. Jackson JL, Peterson C, Lesho E. A meta-analysis of zinc salts lozenges and the common cold. *Arch Intern Med.* 1997;157(20):2373–2376
14. Kim SY, Chang YJ, Cho HM, Hwang YW, Moon YS. Non-steroidal anti-inflammatory drugs for the common cold. *Cochrane Database Syst Rev.* 2009;(3):CD006362
15. Maltinski G. Nasal disorders and sinusitis. *Prim Care.* 1998;25(3):663–683
16. Mossad SB, Macknin ML, Medendorp SV, Mason P. Zinc gluconate lozenges for treating the common cold. A randomized, double-blind, placebo-controlled study. *Ann Intern Med.* 1996;125(2):81–88
17. Paul IM, Beiler JS, King TS, Clapp ER, Vallati J, Berlin CM Jr. Vapor rub, petrolatum, and no treatment for children with nocturnal cough and cold symptoms. *Pediatrics.* 2010;126(6):1092–1099
18. Paul IM, Yoder KE, Crowell KR, et al. Effect of dextromethorphan, diphenhydramine, and placebo on nocturnal cough and sleep quality for coughing children and their parents. *Pediatrics.* 2004;114(1):e85–e90
19. Prasad AS, Fitzgerald JT, Bao B, Beck FW, Chandrasekar PH. Duration of symptoms and plasma cytokine levels in patients with the common cold treated with zinc acetate. A randomized, double-blind, placebo-controlled trial. *Ann Intern Med.* 2000;133(4):245–252
20. Rabago D, Barrett B, Marchand L, Maberry R, Mundt M. Qualitative aspects of nasal irrigation use by patients with chronic sinus disease in a multimethod study. *Ann Fam Med.* 2006;4(4):295–301
21. Rosenfeld RM, Andes D, Bhattacharyya N, et al. Clinical practice guideline: adult sinusitis. *Otolaryngol Head Neck Surg.* 2007;137(3)(suppl):S1–S31
22. Schroeder K, Fahey T. Over-the-counter medications for acute cough in children and adults in ambulatory settings. *Cochrane Database Syst Rev.* 2004;(4):CD001831
23. Simasek M, Blandino DA. Treatment of the common cold. *Am Fam Physician.* 2007;75(4):515–520
24. Singh M. Heated, humidified air for the common cold. *Cochrane Database Syst Rev.* 2011;(5):CD001728
25. Slapak I, Skoupá J, Strnad P, Horník P. Efficacy of isotonic nasal wash (seawater) in the treatment and prevention of rhinitis in children. Arch *Otolaryngol Head Neck Surg.* 2008;134(1):67–74
26. Sperber, SJ, Hendley, JO, Hayden, FG, Riker DK, Sorrentino JV, Gwaltney JM Jr. Effects of naproxen on experimental rhinovirus colds. A randomized, double-blind, controlled trial. *Ann Intern Med.* 1992;117(1):37–41
27. Taverner D, Latte J. Nasal decongestants for the common cold. *Cochrane Database Syst Rev.* 2007;(1):CD001953
28. Wallace DV, Dykewicz MS, Bernstein DI, et al. The diagnosis and management of rhinitis: an updated practice parameter. *J Allergy Clin Immunol.* 2008;122(2 suppl):S1–S84
29. Yale SH, Liu K. Echinacea purpurea therapy for the treatment of the common cold: a randomized, double-blind, placebo-controlled clinical trial. *Arch Intern Med.* 2004;164(11):1237–1241

Confusion (Delirium)

1. Feske SK. Coma and confusional states: emergency diagnosis and management. *Neurol Clin.* 1998;16(2):237–256
2. Freedman R. Schizophrenia. *N Engl J Med.* 2003;349(18):1738–1749
3. Jacobson SA. Delirium in the elderly. *Psychiatr Clin North Am.* 1997;20(1):91–110
4. Lukens TW, Wolf SJ, Edlow JA, et al. Clinical policy: critical issues in the diagnosis and management of the adult psychiatric patient in the emergency department. *Ann Emerg Med.* 2006;47(1):79–99
5. Mayo-Smith MF, Beecher LH, Fischer TL, et al. Management of alcohol withdrawal delirium. An evidence-based practice guideline. *Arch Intern Med.* 2004;164(13):1405–1412
6. Meagher DJ. Delirium: optimising management. *BMJ.* 2001; 322(7279): 144–149
7. Murphy BA. Delirium. *Emerg Med Clin North Am.* 2000;18(2): 243–252
8. O'Brien RF, Kifuji K, Summergrad P. Medical conditions with psychiatric manifestations. *Adolesc Med Clin.* 2006;17(1):49–77
9. Piechniczek-Buczek J. Psychiatric emergencies in the elderly population. *Emerg Med Clin North Am.* 2006;24(2): 467–490, viii
10. Teasdale G, Jennett B. Assessment of coma and impaired consciousness. A practical scale. *Lancet.* 1974;2(7872):81–84

Constipation

1. American College of Gastroenterology Chronic Constipation Task Force. An evidence-based approach to the management of chronic constipation in North America. *Am J Gastroenterol.* 2005;100(suppl 1):S1–S4
2. Bonapace ES Jr., Fisher RS. Constipation and diarrhea in pregnancy. *Gastroenterol Clin North Am.* 1998;27(1):197–211
3. Brandt LJ, Prather CM, Quigley EM, Schiller LR, Schoenfeld P, Talley NJ. Systematic review on the management of chronic constipation in North America. *Am J Gastroenterol.* 2005;100(suppl 1): S5–S21
4. DiPalma JA, DeRidder PH, Orlando RC, Kolts BE, Cleveland MB. A randomized, placebo-controlled, multicenter study of the safety and efficacy of a new polyethylene glycol laxative. *Am J Gastroenterol.* 2000;95(2):446–450
5. Hsieh C. Treatment of constipation in older adults. *Am Fam Physician.* 2005;72(11):2277–2284
6. Ramkumar D, Rao SS. Efficacy and safety of traditional medical therapies for chronic constipation: systematic review. *Am J Gastroenterol.* 2005;100(4):936–971
7. Rao SSC. Constipation: evaluation and treatment. *Gastroenterol Clin North Am.* 2003;32(2):659–683
8. Wald A. Constipation. *Med Clin North Am.* 2000;84(5):1231–1246, ix

Cough

1. Aagaard E, Gonzales R. Management of acute bronchitis in healthy adults. *Infect Dis Clin North Am.* 2004;18(4):919–937, x
2. American College of Chest Physicians. Cough as a symptom. *Chest.* 1998;114:133S–181S
3. Irwin RS, Boulet LP, Cloutier MM, et al. Managing cough as a defense mechanism and as a symptom. A consensus panel report of the American College of Chest Physicians. *Chest.* 1998;114(2 suppl): 133S–181S
4. Black RA, Hill DA. Over-the-counter medications in pregnancy. *Am Fam Physician.* 2003;67(12):2517–2524
5. Cornia PB, Hersh AL, Lipsky BA, Newman TB, Gonzales R. Does this coughing adolescent or adult patient have pertussis? *JAMA.* 2010;304(8):890–896
6. Curley FJ, Irwin RS, Pratter MR, et al. Cough and the common cold. *Am Rev Respir Dis.* 1988;138(2):305–311
7. Eccles R. Understanding the symptoms of the common cold and influenza. *Lancet Infect Dis.* 2005;5(11):718–725
8. Fabbri L, Pauwels RA, Hurd SS; and the Gold Scientific Committee. Global strategy for the diagnosis, management, and prevention of chronic obstructive pulmonary disease: GOLD Executive Summary updated 2003. *COPD.* 2004;1(1):103–141
9. Irwin RS, Baumann MH, Bolser DC, et al. Diagnosis and management of cough executive summary: ACCP evidence-based clinical practice guidelines. *Chest.* 2006;129(1 suppl):1S–23S
10. Little P, Rumsby K, Kelly J, et al. Information leaflet and antibiotic prescribing strategies for acute lower respiratory tract infection: a randomized controlled trial. *JAMA.* 2005;293(24):3029–3035
11. Morice AH, McGarvey L, Pavord I; and the British Thoracic Society Cough Guideline Group. Recommendations for the management of cough in adults. *Thorax.* 2006;61(suppl 1):i1–i24
12. O'Connell EJ, Li JT. Chronic cough. *Immunol Allergy Clin North Am.* 1996;16(1):1–17
13. Paul IM, Beiler J, McMonagle A, Shaffer ML, Duda L, Berlin CM Jr. Effect of honey, dextromethorphan, and no treatment on nocturnal cough and sleep quality for coughing children and their parents. *Arch Pediatr Adolesc Med.* 2007;161(12):1140–1146
14. Paul IM, Beiler JS, King TS, Clapp ER, Vallati J, Berlin CM Jr. Vapor rub, petrolatum, and no treatment for children with nocturnal cough and cold symptoms. *Pediatrics.* 2010;126(6):1092–1099
15. Paul IM, Yoder KE, Crowell KR, et al. Effect of dextromethorphan, diphenhydramine, and placebo on nocturnal cough and sleep quality for coughing children and their parents. *Pediatrics.* 2004;114(1): e85–e90
16. Quon BS, Gan WQ, Sin DD. Contemporary management of acute exacerbations of COPD: a systematic review and metaanalysis. *Chest.* 2008;133(3):756–766
17. Rubin BK. Mucolytics, expectorants, and mucokinetic medications. *Respir Care.* 2007;52(7):859–865
18. Schroeder K, Fahey T. Over-the-counter medications for acute cough in children and adults in ambulatory settings. *Cochrane Database Syst Rev.* 2004;(4):CD001831
19. Simasek M, Blandino DA. Treatment of the common cold. *Am Fam Physician.* 2007;75(4):515–520
20. Smucny J, Fahey T, Becker L, Glazier R. Antibiotics for acute bronchitis. *Cochrane Database Syst Rev.* 2004;(4):CD000245
21. Sperber, SJ, Hendley, JO, Hayden, FG, Riker DK, Sorrentino JV, Gwaltney JM Jr. Effects of naproxen on experimental rhinovirus colds: a randomized, double-blind, controlled trial. *Ann Intern Med.* 1992;117(1):37–41
22. Wenzel RP, Fowler AA 3rd. Clinical practice. Acute bronchitis. *N Engl J Med.* 2006;355(20):2125–2130

Dental Procedure Antibiotic Prophylaxis

1. American Dental Association, American Academy of Orthopedic Surgeons. Antibiotic prophylaxis for dental patients with total joint replacements. *J Am Dent Assoc.* 2003;134(7):895–899
2. Baddour LM, Wilson WR, Bayer AS, et al. Infective endocarditis: diagnosis, antimicrobial therapy, and management of complications: a statement for healthcare professionals from the Committee on Rheumatic Fever, Endocarditis, and Kawasaki Disease, Council on Cardiovascular Disease in the Young, and the Councils on Clinical Cardiology, Stroke, and Cardiovascular Surgery and Anesthesia, American Heart Association: endorsed by the Infectious Diseases Society of America. *Circulation.* 2005;111(23):e394–e434

Dental Procedure Antibiotic Prophylaxis (continued)

3. Canadian Dental Association. Antibiotic Prophylaxis for Dental Patients with Total Joint Replacement. http://www.cda-adc.ca/_files/position_statements/antiobiotic_prophylaxis_joint.pdf. Accessed July 26, 2012
4. Durack DT. Prevention of infective endocarditis. *N Engl J Med.* 1995;332(1):38–44
5. Greenberg JD, Bonwit AM, Roddy MG. Subacute bacterial endocarditis prophylaxis: a succinct review for pediatric emergency physicians and nurses. *Clin Pediatr Emerg Med.* 2005;6(4):266–272
6. Tong DC, Rothwell BR. Antibiotic prophylaxis in dentistry: a review and practice recommendations. *J Am Dent Assoc.* 2000;131(3): 366–374
7. Wilson W, Taubert KA, Gewitz M, et al. Prevention of infective endocarditis: guidelines from the American Heart Association. *J Am Dent Assoc.* 2007;138(6):739–760
8. Wilson W, Taubert KA, Gewitz M, et al. Prevention of infective endocarditis: guidelines from the American Heart Association. *Circulation.* 2007:116(15):1736–1754

Depression

1. Lukens TW, Wolf SJ, Edlow JA, et al. Clinical policy: critical issues in the diagnosis and management of the adult psychiatric patient in the emergency department. *Ann Emerg Med.* 2006;47(1):79–99
2. O'Brien RF, Kifuji K, Summergrad P. Medical conditions with psychiatric manifestations. *Adolesc Med Clin.* 2006;17(1):49–77
3. Sowers W, George C, Thompson K. Level of care utilization system for psychiatric and addiction services (LOCUS): a preliminary assessment of reliability and validity. *Community Ment Health J.* 1999;35(6):545–563
4. Szewczyk M, Chennault SA. Women's health. Depression and related disorders. *Prim Care.* 1997;24(1):83–101
5. US Preventive Services Task Force. Screening for depression: recommendations and rationale. *Ann Intern Med.* 2002;136(10): 760–764

Diabetes, High Blood Sugar

1. American Diabetes Association. Standards of medical care in diabetes—2008. *Diabetes Care.* 2008;31(suppl 1):S12–S54
2. American Diabetes Association. Standards of medical care in diabetes—2009. *Diabetes Care.* 2009;32(suppl 1):S13–S61
3. Cheng AY, Fantus IG. Oral antihyperglycemic therapy for type 2 diabetes mellitus. *CMAJ.* 2005;172(2):213–226
4. DeWitt DE, Hirsch IB. Outpatient insulin therapy in type 1 and type 2 diabetes mellitus: scientific review. *JAMA.* 2003;289(17):2254–2264
5. Feinglos MN, Bethel MA. Treatment of type 2 diabetes mellitus. *Med Clin North Am.* 1998;82(4):757–790
6. Harrigan RA, Nathan MS, Beattie P. Oral agents for the treatment of type 2 diabetes mellitus: pharmacology, toxicity, and treatment. *Ann Emerg Med.* 2001;38(1):68–78
7. Harris SB, Lank CN. Recommendations from the Canadian Diabetes Association. 2003 guidelines for prevention and management of diabetes and related cardiovascular risk factors. *Can Fam Physician.* 2004;50(3):425–433
8. Herbel G, Boyle PJ. Hypoglycemia. Pathophysiology and treatment. *Endocrinol Metab Clin North Am.* 2000;29(4):725–743
9. Herbst KL, Hirsch IB. Insulin strategies for primary care providers. *Clin Diabetes.* 2002;20(1):11–17
10. Jani R, Triplitt C, Reasner C, Defronzo RA. First approved inhaled insulin therapy for diabetes mellitus. *Expert Opin Drug Deliv.* 2007;4(1):63–76
11. Kamboj MK, Draznin MB. Office management of the adolescent with diabetes mellitus. *Prim Care.* 2006;33(2):581–602
12. Laffel L. Sick day management in type 1 diabetes. *Endocrinol Metab Clin North Am.* 2000;29(4):707–723
13. Norwood P, Dumas R, Cefalu W, et al. Randomized study to characterize glycemic control and short-term pulmonary function in patients with type 1 diabetes receiving inhaled human insulin (Exubera). *J Clin Endocrinol Metab.* 2007;92(6):2211–2244
14. Siebenhofer A, Plank J, Berghold A, et al. Short acting insulin analogues versus regular human insulin in patients with diabetes mellitus. *Cochrane Database Syst Rev.* 2006;(2):CD003287
15. Singh SR, Ahmad F, Lal A, Yu C, Bai Z, Bennett H. Efficacy and safety of insulin analogues for the management of diabetes mellitus: a meta-analysis. *CMAJ.* 2009;180(4):385–397
16. Tibaldi J. Initiating and intensifying insulin therapy in type 2 diabetes mellitus. *Am J Med.* 2008;121(6 suppl):S20–S29
17. Lewis C. Diabetes: a growing public health concern. *FDA Consumer.* 2002;36(1):26–33

Diabetes, Low Blood Sugar

1. American Diabetes Association. Standards of medical care in diabetes—2008. *Diabetes Care.* 2008;31(suppl 1):S12–S54
2. American Diabetes Association. Standards of medical care in diabetes—2009. *Diabetes Care.* 2009;32(suppl 1):S13–S61
3. Cheng AY, Fantus IG. Oral antihyperglycemic therapy for type 2 diabetes mellitus. *CMAJ.* 2005;172(2):213–226
4. Cryer PE, Davis SN, Shamoon H. Hypoglycemia in diabetes. *Diabetes Care.* 2003;26(6):1902–1912
5. DeWitt DE, Hirsch IB. Outpatient insulin therapy in type 1 and type 2 diabetes mellitus: scientific review. *JAMA.* 2003;289(17):2254–2264
6. Feinglos MN, Bethel MA. Treatment of type 2 diabetes mellitus. *Med Clin North Am* 1998;82(4):757–790
7. Harrigan RA, Nathan MS, Beattie P. Oral agents for type 2 diabetes mellitus: pharmacology, toxicity, and treatment. *Ann Emerg Med.* 2001;38(1):68–78
8. Harris SB, Lank CN. Recommendations from the Canadian Diabetes Association. 2003 guidelines for prevention and management of diabetes and related cardiovascular risk factors. *Can Fam Physician.* 2004;50(3):425–433
9. Herbel G, Boyle PJ. Hypoglycemia. Pathophysiology and treatment. *Endocrinol Metab Clin North Am.* 2000;29(4):725–743
10. Herbst KL, Hirsch IB. Insulin strategies for primary care providers. *Clin Diabetes.* 2002;20(1):11–17
11. Kamboj MK, Draznin MB. Office management of the adolescent with diabetes mellitus. *Prim Care.* 2006;33(2):581–602
12. Laffel L. Sick day management in type 1 diabetes. *Endocrinol Metab Clin North Am.* 2000;29(4):707–723
13. Ragone M, Lando HM. Errors of insulin commission? *Clin Diabetes.* 2002;20(4):221–222
14. Singh SR, Ahmad F, Lal A, Yu C, Bai Z, Bennett H. Efficacy and safety of insulin analogues for the management of diabetes mellitus: a meta-analysis. *CMAJ.* 2009;180(4):385–397
15. Tibaldi J. Initiating and intensifying insulin therapy in type 2 diabetes mellitus. *Am J Med.* 2008;121(6 suppl):S20–S29
16. Lewis C. Diabetes: a growing public health concern. *FDA Consumer.* 2002;36(1):26–33
17. American Diabetes Association Workgroup on Hypoglycemia. Defining and reporting hypoglycemia in diabetes: a report from the American Diabetes Association Workgroup on Hypoglycemia. *Diabetes Care.* 2005;28(5):1245–1249

Diarrhea

1. Acheson DW, Fiore AE. Preventing foodborne disease—what clinicians can do. *N Engl J Med.* 2004;350(5):437–440
2. Black RA, Hill DA. Over-the-counter medications in pregnancy. *Am Fam Physician.* 2003;67(12):2517–2524
3. Centers for Disease Control and Prevention (CDC). Diagnosis and management of foodborne illnesses: a primer for physicians and other health care professionals. *MMWR Recomm Rep.* 2004;53(RR-4):1–33
4. DuPont HL. New insights and directions in travelers' diarrhea. *Gastroenterol Clin North Am.* 2006;35(2):337–353, viii–ix
5. DuPont HL. Guidelines on acute infectious diarrhea in adults. The Practice Parameters Committee of the American College of Gastroenterology. *Am J Gastroenterol.* 1997;92(11):1962–1975
6. Fekety R. Guidelines for the diagnosis and management of Clostridium difficile-associated diarrhea and colitis. American College of Gastroenterology Practice Parameters Committee. *Am J Gastroenterol.* 1997;92(5):739–750
7. Goodgame R. A Bayesian approach to acute infectious diarrhea in adults. *Gastroenterol Clin North Am.* 2006;35(2):249–273
8. Gore JI, Surawicz C. Severe acute diarrhea. *Gastroenterol Clin North Am.* 2003;32(4):1249–1267
9. Guerrant RL, Van Gilder TV, Steiner TS, et al. Practice guidelines for the management of infectious diarrhea. *Clin Infect Dis.* 2001;32(3):331–351
10. Kamat D, Mathur A. Prevention and management of travelers' diarrhea. *Dis Mon.* 2006;52(7):289–302
11. McGee S, Abernethy WB 3rd, Simel DL. The rational clinical examination. Is this patient hypovolemic? *JAMA.* 1999;281(11): 1022–1029
12. Ryan ET, Wilson ME, Kain KC. Illness after international travel. *N Eng J Med.* 2002;347(7):505–516
13. Schiller LR. Diarrhea. *Med Clin North Am.* 2000;84(5):1259–1274, x
14. Sinert R, Spektor M. Evidence-based emergency medicine/rational clinical examination abstract. Clinical assessment of hypovolemia. *Ann Emerg Med.* 2005;45(3):327–329
15. Thielman NM. Guerrant RL. Acute infectious diarrhea. *N Eng J Med.* 2004;350(1):38–47
16. Trinh C, Prabhakar K. Diarrheal diseases in the elderly. *Clin Geriatr Med. 2007*;23(4):833–856, vii

Dizziness

1. Baloh RW. Dizziness: neurologic emergencies. *Neurol Clin.* 1998; 16(2):305–321
2. Goldman L, Kirtane AJ. Triage of patients with acute chest pain and possible cardiac ischemia: the elusive search for diagnostic perfection. *Ann Intern Med.* 2003;139(12):987–995
3. Gommans J, Barber PA, Fink J. Preventing strokes: the assessment and management of people with transient ischaemic attack. *N Z Med J.* 2009;122(1293):3556
4. Kim AS, Fullerton HJ, Johnston SC. Risk of vascular events in emergency department patients discharged home with diagnosis of dizziness or vertigo. *Ann Emerg Med.* 2011;57(1):34–41
5. Newman-Toker DE, Hsieh YH, Camargo CA Jr, Pelletier AJ, Butchy GT, Edlow JA. Spectrum of dizziness visits to US emergency departments: cross-sectional analysis from a nationally representative sample. *Mayo Clin Proc.* 2008;83(7):765–775
6. Sinert R, Spektor M. Evidence-based emergency medicine/rational clinical examination abstract. Clinical assessment of hypovolemia. *Ann Emerg Med.* 2005;45(3):327–329
7. Tusa RJ. Dizziness. *Med Clin North Am.* 2003;87(3):609–641, vii
8. Walker JS, Barnes SB. Dizziness. *Emerg Med Clin North Am.* 1998; 16(4):845–875, vii
9. Wasserman J, Perry J, Dowlatshahi D, et al. Stratified, urgent care for transient ischemic attack results in low stroke rates. *Stroke.* 2010;41(11):2601–2605

Ear, Swimmer's (Otitis Externa)

1. Belleza WG, Kalman S. Otolaryngologic emergencies in the outpatient setting. *Med Clin North Am.* 2006;90(2):329–353
2. Cantor RM. Otitis externa and otitis media. A new look at old problems. *Emerg Med Clin North Am.* 1995;13(2):445–455
3. Hosey RG, Rodenberg RE. Training room management of medical conditions: infectious diseases. *Clin Sports Med.* 2005;24(3): 477–506, vii
4. Hughes E, Lee JH. Otitis externa. *Pediatr Rev.* 2001;22(6):191–197
5. Mellman MF, Podesta L. Common medical problems in sports. *Clin Sports Med.* 1997;16(4):635–662
6. Nichols AW. Nonorthopedic problems in the aquatic athlete. *Clin Sports Med.* 1999;18(2):395–411, viii
7. Nussinovitch M, Rimon A, Volovitz B, Raveh E, Prais D, Amir J. Cotton-tip applicators as a leading cause of otitis externa. *Int J Pediatr Otorhinolaryngol.* 2004;68(4):433–435
8. Osguthorpe JD, Nielsen DR. Otitis externa: review and clinical update. *Am Fam Physician.* 2006;74(9):1510–1516
9. Rosenfeld RM, Brown L, Cannon CR, et al. Clinical practice guideline: acute otitis externa. *Otolaryngol Head Neck Surg.* 2006; 134(4 suppl):S4–S23
10. Rosenfeld RM, Singer M, Wasserman JM, Stinnett SS. Systematic review of topical antimicrobial therapy for acute otitis externa. *Otolaryngol Head Neck Surg.* 2006;134(4 suppl):S24–S48
11. van Balen FA, Smit WM, Zuithoff NP, Verheij TJ. Clinical efficacy of three common treatments in acute otitis externa in primary care: randomized controlled trial. *BMJ.* 2003;327(7425):1201–1205

Ear Piercing

1. Association of Professional Piercers (APP) Procedure Manual 2005. http://www.safepiercing.org/wp-content/uploads/2010/05/2005_Manual.pdf. Accessed July 26, 2012
2. Belleza WG, Kalman S. Otolaryngologic emergencies in the outpatient setting. *Med Clin North Am.* 2006;90(2):329–353
3. Cohen HA, Nussinovitch M, Straussberg R. Embedded earrings. *Cutis.* 1994;53(2):82
4. Ferguson H. Body piercing. *BMJ.* 1999;319(7225):1627–1629
5. Fernandez Ade P, Castro Neto I, Anias CR, Pinto PC, Castro Jde C, Carpes AF. Post-piercing perichondritis. *Braz J Otorhinolaryngol.* 2008;74(6):933–937
6. Garner LA. Contact dermatitis to metals. *Dermatol Ther.* 2004;17(4):321–327
7. Gauglitz GG, Korting HC, Pavicic T, Ruzicka T, Jeschke MG. Hypertrophic scarring and keloids: pathomechanisms and current and emerging treatment strategies. *Mol Med.* 2011;17(1-2):113–125
8. Hanif J, Frosh A, Marnane C, Ghufoor K, Rivron R, Sandhu G. Lesson of the week: "high" ear piercing and the rising incidence of perichondritis of the pinna. *BMJ.* 2001;322(7291):906–907
9. Hendricks WM. Complications of ear piercing: treatment and prevention. *Cutis.* 1991;48(5):386–394
10. Hogan D, Ledet JJ. Impact of regulation on contact dermatitis. *Dermatol Clin.* 2009;27(3):385–394, viii
11. Laumann AE, Derick AJ. Tattoos and body piercings in the United States: a national data set. *J Am Acad Dermatol.* 2006;55(3):413–421

Ear Piercing (continued)

12. Lehman EJ, Huy J, Levy E, Viet SM, Mobley A, McCleery TZ. Bloodborne pathogen risk reduction activities in the body piercing and tattooing industry. *Am J Infect Control.* 2010;38(2):130–138
13. Mark BJ, Slavin RG. Allergic contact dermatitis. *Med Clin North Am.* 2006;90(1):169–185
14. Mayers LB, Chiffriller SH. Body art (body piercing and tattooing) among undergraduate university students: "then and now." *J Adolesc Health.* 2008;42(2):201–203
15. Meltzer DI. Complications of body piercing. *Am Fam Physician.* 2005;72(10):2029–2034
16. Mortz CG, Andersen KE. New aspects in allergic contact dermatitis. *Curr Opin Allergy Clin Immunol.* 2008;8(5):428–432
17. Reiter D, Alford EL. Torn earlobe: a new approach to management with a review of 68 cases. *Ann Otol Rhinol Laryngol.* 1994;103(11):879–884
18. Swartz MN. Clinical Practice. Cellulitis. *N Engl J Med.* 2004;350(9): 904–912

Earache

1. Belleza WG, Kalman S. Otolaryngologic emergencies in the outpatient setting. *Med Clin North Am.* 2006;90(2):329–353
2. Brown TP. Middle ear symptoms while flying. Ways to prevent a severe outcome. *Postgrad Med.* 1994;96(2):135–142
3. Foxlee R, Johansson A, Wejfalk J, Dawkins J, Dooley L, Del Mar C. Topical analgesia for acute otitis media. *Cochrane Database Syst Rev.* 2006;(3):CD005657
4. Hoberman A, Paradise JL, Reynolds EA, Urkin J. Efficacy of Auralgan for treating ear pain in children with acute otitis media. *Arch Pediatr Adolesc Med.* 1997;151(7):675–678
5. Kreisberg MK, Turner J. Dental causes of referred otalgia. *Ear Nose Throat J.* 1987;66(10):398–408
6. Rosenfeld RM, Brown L, Cannon CR, et al. Clinical practice guideline: acute otitis externa. *Otolaryngol Head Neck Surg.* 2006;134(4 suppl):S4–S23
7. Stewart MH, Siff JE, Cydulka RK. Evaluation of the patient with sore throat, earache, and sinusitis: an evidence based approach. *Emerg Med Clin North Am.* 1999;17(1):153–187, ix
8. Thaller SR, Desilva A. Otalgia with normal ear. *Am Fam Physician.* 1987;36(4):129–136

Elbow Pain

1. Barry NN, McGuire JL. Overuse syndromes in adult athletes. *Rheum Dis Clin North Am.* 1996;22(3):515–530
2. Canto JG, Shlipak MG, Rogers WJ, et al. Prevalence, clinical characteristics, and mortality among patients with myocardial infarction presenting without chest pain. *JAMA.* 2000;283(24): 3223–3229
3. Coakley G, Mathews C, Field M, et al; and the British Society for Rheumatology Standards, Guidelines and Audit Working Group. BSR & BHPR, BOA, RCGP and BSAC guidelines for management of the hot swollen joint in adults. *Rheumatology (Oxford).* 2006;45(8):1039–1041
4. Colman WW, Strauch RJ. Physical examination of the elbow. *Orthop Clin North Am.* 1999;30(1):15–20
5. Coronado B, Pope JH, Griffith JL, Beshansky JR, Selker HP. Clinical features, triage, and outcome of patients presenting to the ED with suspected acute coronary syndromes but without pain: a multicenter study. *Am J Emerg Med.* 2004;22(7):568–574
6. Culic V, Eterovic D, Miric D, Silic N. Symptom presentation of acute myocardial infarction: influence of sex, age, and risk factors. *Am Heart J.* 2002;144(6):1012–1017
7. Pioro MH, Mandell BF. Septic arthritis. *Rheum Dis Clin North Am.* 1997;23(2):239–258
8. Rainsford KD. Ibuprofen: pharmacology, efficacy and safety. *Inflammopharmacology.* 2009;17(6):275–342
9. Weston V, Coakley G; and the British Society for Rheumatology (BSR) Standards, Guidelines and Audit Working Group; et al. Guideline for the management of the hot swollen joint in adults with a particular focus on septic arthritis. *J Antimicrob Chemother.* 2006;58(3):492–493

Eye, Chemical In

1. Bronstein AC, Spyker DA, Cantilena LR Jr, Green JL, Rumack BH, Heard SE; and the American Association of Poison Control Centers. 2007 Annual Report of the American Association of Poison Control Centers' National Poison Data System (NPDS): 25th Annual Report. *Clin Toxicol (Phila).* 2008;46(10):927–1057
2. Brown L, Takeuchi D, Challoner K. Corneal abrasions associated with pepper spray exposure. *Am J Emerg Med.* 2000;18(3):271–272
3. Crumpton KL, Shockley LW. Ocular trauma: a quick illustrated guide to treatment, triage, and medicolegal implications. *Emerg Med Rep.* 1997;18(23):223–234
4. Harlan JB Jr, Pieramici DJ. Evaluation of patients with ocular trauma. *Ophthalmol Clin North Am.* 2002;15(2):153–161
5. Kuckelhorn R, Schrage N, Keller G, Redbrake C. Emergency treatment of chemical and thermal eye burns. *Acta Ophthalmol Scand.* 2002;80(1):4–10
6. Naradzay J, Barish RA. Approach to ophthalmologic emergencies. *Med Clin North Am.* 2006;90(2):305–328, vii–viii
7. Pokhrel PK, Loftus SA. Ocular emergencies. *Am Fam Physician.* 2007;76(6):829–836
8. Spector J, Fernandez WG. Chemical, thermal, and biological ocular exposures. *Emerg Med Clin North Am.* 2008;26(1):125–136, vii

Eye, Foreign Body

1. Crumpton KL, Shockley LW. Ocular trauma: a quick illustrated guide to treatment, triage, and medicolegal implications. *Emerg Med Rep.* 1997;18(23):223–234
2. Harlan JB Jr, Pieramici DJ. Evaluation of patients with ocular trauma. *Ophthalmol Clin North Am.* 2002;15(2):153–161
3. Hulbert MF. Efficacy of eyepad in corneal healing after corneal foreign body removal. *Lancet.* 1991;337(8742):643
4. Jayamanne DG. Do patients presenting to accident and emergency departments with the sensation of a foreign body in the eye (gritty eye) have significant ocular disease? *J Accid Emerg Med.* 1995;12(4):286–287
5. Naradzay J, Barish RA. Approach to ophthalmologic emergencies. *Med Clin North Am.* 2006;90(2):305–328, vii–viii
6. Pokhrel PK, Loftus SA. Ocular emergencies. *Am Fam Physician.* 2007;76(6):829–836
7. Wilson SA, Last A. Management of corneal abrasions. *Am Fam Physician.* 2004;70(1):123–128

Eye, Pus or Discharge

1. Bielory L, Friedlaender MH, Fujishima H. Allergic conjunctivitis. *Immunol Allergy Clin North Am.* 1997;17(1):19–31
2. Cronau H, Kankanala RR, Mauger T. Diagnosis and management of red eye in primary care. *Am Fam Physician.* 2010;81(2):137–144
3. Diamant JI, Hwang DG. Therapy for bacterial conjunctivitis. *Ophthalmol Clin North Am.* 1999;12(1):15–20
4. Patel PB, Diaz MC, Bennett JE, Attia MW. Clinical features of bacterial conjunctivitis in children. *Acad Emerg Med.* 2007;14(1):1–5

5. Pokhrel PK, Loftus SA. Ocular emergencies. *Am Fam Physician.* 2007;76(6):829–836
6. Rietveld RP, van Weert HC, ter Riet G, Sloos JH, Bindels PJ. Predicting bacterial cause in infectious conjunctivitis: cohort study on informativeness of combinations of signs and symptoms. *BMJ.* 2004;329(7459):206–210
7. Sheikh A, Hurwitz B. Topical antibiotics for acute bacterial conjunctivitis: Cochrane systematic review and meta-analysis update. *Br J Gen Pract.* 2005;55(521):962–964
8. Steinert RF. Current therapy for bacterial keratitis and bacterial conjunctivitis. *Am J Ophthalmol.* 1991;112(4 suppl):10S–14S
9. Weiss A, Brinser JH, Nazar-Stewart V. Acute conjunctivitis in childhood. *J Pediatr.* 1993;122(1):10–14
10. Wirbelauer C. Management of the red eye for the primary care physician. *Am J Med.* 2006;119(4):302–306

Eye, Red Without Pus

1. Cronau H, Kankanala RR, Mauger T. Diagnosis and management of red eye in primary care. *Am Fam Physician.* 2010;81(2):137–144
2. Leibowitz HM. The red eye. *N Engl J Med.* 2000;343(5):345–351
3. Morgan A, Hemphill RR. Acute visual change. *Emerg Med Clin North Am.* 1998;16(4):825–843, vii
4. Naradzay J, Barish RA. Approach to ophthalmologic emergencies. *Med Clin North Am.* 2006;90(2):305–328, vii–viii
5. Pokhrel PK, Loftus SA. Ocular emergencies. *Am Fam Physician.* 2007;76(6):829–836
6. Wirbelauer C. Management of the red eye for the primary care physician. *Am J Med.* 2006;119(4):302–306

Fainting

1. Calkins H, Shyr Y, Frumin H, Schork A, Morady F. The value of the clinical history in the differentiation of syncope due to ventricular tachycardia, atrioventricular block, and neurocardiogenic syncope. *Am J Med.* 1995;98(4):365–373
2. Centers for Disease Control and Prevention (CDC). Syncope after vaccination—United States, January 2005–July 2007. *MMWR Morb Mortal Wkly Rep.* 2008;57(17):457–460
3. Forman DE, Lipsitz LA. Syncope in the elderly. *Cardiol Clin.* 1997;15(2):295–311
4. Huff JS, Decker WW, Quinn JV, et al; and the American College of Emergency Physicians. Clinical policy: critical issues in the evaluation and management of adult patients presenting to the emergency department with syncope. *Ann Emerg Med.* 2007;49(4):431–444
5. Kapoor WN. Syncope. *N Engl J Med.* 2000;343(25):1856–1862
6. Martin GJ, Adams SL, Martin HG, Mathews J, Zull D, Scanlon PJ. Prospective evaluation of syncope. *Ann Emerg Med.* 1984;13(7): 499–504
7. Martin TP, Hanusa BH, Kapoor WN. Risk stratification of patients with syncope. *Ann Emerg Med.* 1997;29(4):459–466
8. Meyer MD, Handler J. Evaluation of the patient with syncope: an evidence based approach. *Emerg Med Clin North Am.* 1999;17(1): 189–201, ix
9. Perry JJ, Stiell IG, Sivilotti ML, et al. High risk clinical characteristics for subarachnoid haemorrhage in patients with acute headache: prospective cohort study. *BMJ.* 2010;341:c5204
10. Quinn J, McDermott D, Kramer N, et al. Death after emergency department visits for syncope: how common and can it be predicted? *Ann Emerg Med.* 2008;51(5):585–590
11. Quinn J, McDermott D, Stiell I, Kohn M, Wells G. Prospective validation of the San Francisco Syncope Rule to predict patients with serious outcomes. *Ann Emerg Med.* 2006;47(5):448–454
12. Sarasin FP, Hanusa BH, Perneger T, Louis-Simonet M, Rajeswaran A, Kapoor WN. A risk score to predict arrhythmias in patients with unexplained syncope. *Acad Emerg Med.* 2003;10(12):1312–1317
13. Sinert R, Spektor M. Evidence-based emergency medicine/rational clinical examination abstract. Clinical assessment of hypovolemia. *Ann Emerg Med.* 2005;45(3):327–329
14. Sotiriades ES, Evans JC, Larson MG, et al. Incidence and prognosis of syncope. *N Engl J Med.* 2002;347(12):878–885
15. Stewart JM. Postural tachycardia syndrome and reflex syncope: similarities and differences. *J Pediatr.* 2009;154(4):481–485
16. Strickberger SA, Benson DW, Biaggioni I, et al. AHA/ACCF scientific statement on the evaluation of syncope. *Circulation.* 2006;113(2): 316–327

Fever

1. Bachert C, Chuchalin AG, Eisebitt R, Netayzhenko VZ, Voelker M. Aspirin compared with acetaminophen in the treatment of fever and other symptoms of upper respiratory tract infection in adults: a multicenter, randomized, double-blind, double-dummy, placebo-controlled, parallel-group, single-dose, 6-hour dose-ranging study. *Clin Ther.* 2005;27(7):993–1003
2. Bottieau E, Clerinx J, Schrooten W, et al. Etiology and outcome of fever after a stay in the tropics. *Arch Intern Med.* 2006;166(15):1642–1648
3. Chamberlain JM, Terndrup TE, Alexander DT, et al. Determination of normal ear temperature with an infrared emission detection thermometer. *Ann Emerg Med.* 1995;25(1):15–20
4. Dart RC, Kuffner EK, Rumack BH. Treatment of pain or fever with paracetamol (acetaminophen) in the alcoholic patient: a systematic review. *Am J Ther.* 2000;7(2):123–134
5. de La Torre SH, Mandel L, Goff BA. Evaluation of postoperative fever: usefulness and cost-effectiveness of routine workup. *Am J Obstet Gynecol.* 2003;188(6):1642–1647
6. Divoll M, Abernethy DR, Ameer B, Greenblatt DJ. Acetaminophen kinetics in the elderly. *Clin Pharmacol Ther.* 1982;31(2):151–156
7. Donowitz GR. Fever in the compromised host. *Infect Dis Clin North Am.* 1996;10(1):129–148
8. Johnson DH, Cunha BA. Drug fever. *Infect Dis Clin North Am.* 1996;10(1):85–91
9. Klein NC, Cunha BA. Treatment of fever. *Infect Dis Clin North Am.* 1996;10(1):211–216
10. Mackowiak PA, Wasserman SS, Levine MM. A critical appraisal of 98.6°F, the upper limit of the normal body temperature, and other legacies of Carl Reinhold August Wunderlich. *JAMA.* 1992;268(12):1578–1580
11. McGee DC, Gould MK. Preventing complications of central venous catheterization. *N Engl J Med.* 2003;348(12):1123–1133
12. Norman DC, Yoshikawa TT. Fever in the elderly. *Infect Dis Clin North Am.* 1996;10(1):93–99
13. Prescott LF. Paracetamol: past, present, and future. *Am J Ther.* 2000;7(2):143–147
14. Ryan ET, Wilson ME, Kain KC. Illness after international travel. *N Eng J Med.* 2002;347(7):505–516
15. Scholssberg D. Fever and rash. *Infect Dis Clin North Am.* 1996;10(1):101–110
16. Suh KN, Kain KC, Keystone JS Malaria. *CMAJ.* 2004;170(11):1693–1702
17. Andersen AM, Vastrup P, Wohlfahrt J, Andersen PK, Olsen J, Melbye M. Fever in pregnancy and risk of fetal death: a cohort study. *Lancet.* 2002;360(9345):1552–1556

Foot Pain

1. Aldridge T. Diagnosing heel pain in adults. *Am Fam Physician.* 2004;70(2):332–338
2. Bedinghaus J, Niedfeldt MW. Over-the-counter foot remedies. *Am Fam Physician.* 2001;64(5):791–796
3. Coakley G, Mathews C, Field M, et al; and the British Society for Rheumatology Standards, Guidelines and Audit Working Group. BSR & BHPR, BOA, RCGP and BSAC guidelines for management of the hot swollen joint in adults. *Rheumatology (Oxford).* 2006;45(8):1039–1041
4. Cole C, Seto C, Gazewood J. Plantar fasciitis: evidence-based review of diagnosis and therapy. *Am Fam Physician.* 2005;72(11): 2237–2242
5. Glazer JL, Hosey RG. Soft-tissue injuries of the lower extremity. *Prim Care.* 2004;31(4):1005–1024
6. Schroeder BM; and the American College of Foot and Ankle Surgeons. Diagnosis and treatment of heel pain. *Am Fam Physician.* 2002;65(8):1686–1688
7. Shapiro BE, Preston DC. Entrapment and compressive neuropathies. *Med Clin North Am.* 2003;87(3):663–696, viii
8. Weston V, Coakley G; and the British Society for Rheumatology (BSR) Standards, Guidelines and Audit Working Group; et al. Guideline for the management of the hot swollen joint in adults with a particular focus on septic arthritis. *J Antimicrob Chemother.* 2006;58(3):492–493
9. Young CC, Niedfeldt MW, Morris GA, Eerkes KJ. Clinical examination of the foot and ankle. *Prim Care.* 2005;32(1):105–132

Frostbite

1. American Heart Association. 2005 Guidelines for Cardiopulmonary Resuscitation and Emergency Cardiovascular Care. Part 14: First aid. *Circulation.* 2005;112(24)(suppl):IV-196–IV-203
2. Centers for Disease Control and Prevention (CDC). Acute illness from dry ice exposure during hurricane Ivan—Alabama, 2004. *MMWR Morb Mortal Wkly Rep.* 2004;53(50):1182–1183
3. Murphy TV, Slade BA, Broder KR, et al. Prevention of pertussis, tetanus, and diphtheria among pregnant and postpartum women and their infants recommendations of the Advisory Committee on Immunization Practices (ACIP). *MMWR Recomm Rep.* 2008;57 (RR-4):1–51
4. Centers for Disease Control and Prevention (CDC). Diptheria, tetanus, and pertussis: recommendations for vaccine use and other preventive measures. Recommendations of the Immunization Practices Advisory Committee (ACIP). *MMWR Recomm Rep.* 1991;40(RR-10):1–28
5. Heggers JP, Robson MC, Manavalen K, et al. Experimental and clinical observations on frostbite. *Ann Emerg Med.* 1987;16(9):1056–1062
6. Jurkovich GJ. Environmental cold-induced injury. *Surg Clin North Am.* 2007;87(1):247–267, viii
7. Miller MB, Koltai PJ. Treatment of experimental frostbite with pentoxifylline and aloe vera cream. Arch *Otolaryngol Head Neck Surg.* 1995;121(6):678–680
8. O'Toole G, Rayatt S. Frostbite at the gym: a case report of an ice pack burn. *Br J Sports Med.* 1999;33(4):278–279
9. Patel NN, Patel DN. Frostbite. *Am J Med.* 2008;121(9):765–766
10. Weiss EA. Medical considerations for wilderness and adventure travelers. *Med Clin North Am.* 1999;83(4):885–902, v–vi

Hand and Wrist Pain

1. Barry NN, McGuire JL. Overuse syndromes in adult athletes. *Rheum Dis Clin North Ame.* 1996;22(3):515–530
2. Campbell WW. Diagnosis and management of common compression and entrapment neuropathies. *Neurol Clin.* 1997;15(3):549–567
3. Canto JG, Shlipak MG, Rogers WJ, et al. Prevalence, clinical characteristics, and mortality among patients with myocardial infarction presenting without chest pain. *JAMA.* 2000;283(24):3223–3229
4. Coakley G, Mathews C, Field M, et al; and the British Society for Rheumatology Standards, Guidelines and Audit Working Group. BSR & BHPR, BOA, RCGP and BSAC guidelines for management of the hot swollen joint in adults. *Rheumatology (Oxford).* 2006;45(8):1039–1041
5. Coronado BE, Pope JH, Griffith JL, Beshansky JR, Selker HP. Clinical features, triage, and outcome of patients presenting to the ED with suspected acute coronary syndromes but without pain: a multicenter study. *Am J Emerg Med.* 2004;22(7):568–574
6. Culic V, Eterovic D, Miric D, Silic N. Symptom presentation of acute myocardial infarction: influence of sex, age, and risk factors. *Am Heart J.* 2002;144(6):1012–1017
7. Izzi J, Dennison D, Noerdlinger M, Dasilva M, Akelman E. Nerve injuries of the elbow, wrist, and hand in athletes. *Clin Sports Med.* 2001;20(1):203–217
8. Ling SM, Bathon JM. Osteoarthritis in older adults. *J Am Geriatr Soc.* 1998;46(2):216–225
9. Rainsford KD. Ibuprofen: pharmacology, efficacy and safety. *Inflammopharmacology.* 2009;17(6):275–342
10. Weston V, Coakley G; and the British Society for Rheumatology (BSR) Standards, Guidelines and Audit Working Group; et al. Guideline for the management of the hot swollen joint in adults with a particular focus on septic arthritis. *J Antimicrob Chemother.* 2006;58(3):492–493

Hay Fever (Nasal Allergies)

1. Bousquet J, Van Cauwenberge P, Khaltaev N; and the Aria Workshop Group; World Health Organization. Allergic rhinitis and its impact on asthma. *J Allergy Clin Immunol.* 2001;108(5 suppl):S147–S334
2. Eapen RJ, Ebert CS Jr, Pillsbury HC 3rd. Allergic rhinitis—history and presentation. *Otolaryngol Clin North Am.* 2008;41(2):325–30, vi–vii
3. Hadley JA. Evaluation and management of allergic rhitis. *Med Clin North Am.* 1999;83(1):13–25
4. Incaudo GA, Takach P. The diagnosis and treatment of allergic rhinitis during pregnancy and lactation. *Immunol Allergy Clin North Am.* 2006;26(1):137–154
5. Léger D, Annesi-Maesano I, Carat F, et al. Allergic rhinitis and its consequences on quality of sleep: an unexplored area. *Arch Intern Med.* 2006;166(16):1744–1748
6. Rabago D, Barrett B, Marchand L, Maberry R, Mundt M. Qualitative aspects of nasal irrigation use by patients with chronic sinus disease in a multimethod study. *Ann Fam Med.* 2006;4(4):295–301
7. Rabago D, Zgierska A. Saline nasal irrigation for upper respiratory conditions. *Am Fam Physician.* 2009;80(10):1121
8. Rosenfeld RM, Andes D, Bhattacharyya N, et al. Clinical practice guideline: adult sinusitis. *Otolaryngol Head Neck Surg.* 2007; 137(3 suppl):S1–S31
9. Skoner DP. Allergic rhinitis: definition, epidemiology, pathophysiology, detection and diagnosis. *J Allergy Clin Immunol.* 2001;108 (1 suppl):S2–S8
10. Wallace DV, Dykewicz MS, Bernstein DI, et al. The diagnosis and management of rhinitis: an updated practice parameter. *J Allergy Clin Immunol.* 2008;122(2 suppl):S1–S84

Headache

1. Edlow JA, Panagos PD, Godwin SA, Thomas TL, Decker WW; and the American College of Emergency Physicians. Clinical policy: critical issues in the evaluation and management of adult patients presenting to the emergency department with acute headache. *Ann Emerg Med.* 2008;52(4):407–436
2. American College of Emergency Physicians. Clinical policy: critical issues in the evaluation and management of patients presenting to the emergency department with acute headache. *Ann Emerg Med.* 2002;39(1):108–122
3. Attia J, Hatala R, Cook DJ, Wong JG. Does this adult patient have acute meningitis? *JAMA.* 1999;282(2):175–181
4. Edlow JA Diagnosis of subarachnoid hemorrhage in the emergency department. Emerg *Med Clin North Am.* 2003;21(1):73–87
5. Friedman DI. The eye and headache. *Ophthalmol Clin North Am.* 2004;17(3):357–369, vi
6. Gus M, Fuchs FD, Pimentel M, Rosa D, Melo AG, Moreira LB. Behavior of ambulatory blood pressure surrounding episodes of headache in mildly hypertensive patients. *Arch Intern Med.* 2001;161(2):252–255
7. Headache Classification Committee of the International Headache Society. The International Classification of Headache Disorders. 2nd ed. *Cephalalgia.* 2004;24(1 suppl):1–160
8. Lipton RB, Stewart WF, Liberman JN. Self-awareness of migraine: interpreting the labels that headache sufferers apply to their headaches. *Neurology.* 2002;58(9 suppl 6):S21–S26
9. Martin-Schild S, Albright KC, Tanksley J, et al. Zero on the NIHSS does not equal the absence of stroke. *Ann Emerg Med.* 2011;57(1): 42–45
10. Muiesan ML, Padovani A, Salvetti M, et al. Headache: prevalence and relationship with office or ambulatory blood pressure in a general population sample (the Vobarno Study). *Blood Press.* 2006;15(1): 14–19
11. Perry JJ, Stiell IG, Sivilotti ML, et al. High risk clinical characteristics for subarachnoid haemorrhage in patients with acute headache: prospective cohort study. *BMJ.* 2010;341:c5204
12. Purdy RA, Kirby S. Headaches and brain tumors. *Neurol Clin.* 2004;22(1):39–53
13. Rainsford KD. Ibuprofen: pharmacology, efficacy and safety. *Inflammopharmacology.* 2009;17(6):275–342
14. Saper JR. Medicolegal issues: headache. *Neurol Clin.* 1999;17(2): 197–214
15. Segard J, Montassier E, Trewick D, Le Conte P, Guillon B, Berrut G. Urgent computed tomography brain scan for elderly patients: can we improve its diagnostic yield? *Eur J Emerg Med.* 2011 Dec 18. [Epub ahead of print]
16. Sheftell FD. Role and impact of over-the-counter medications in the management of headache. *Neurol Clin.* 1997;15(1):187–198
17. Silberstein SD. Drug-induced headache. *Neurol Clin.* 1998;16(1): 107–123
18. Walker RA, Wadman MC. Headache in the elderly. *Clin Geriatr Med.* 2007;23(2):291–305, v–vi

Heart Rate and Heartbeat Questions

1. American Heart Association. 2005 Guidelines for Cardiopulmonary Resuscitation and Emergency Cardiovascular Care. Part 7.3: Management of symptomatic bradycardia and tachycardia. *Circulation.* 2005;112(24 suppl):IV-67–IV-77
2. Hood RE, Shorofsky SR. Management of arrhythmias in the emergency department. *Cardiol Clin.* 2006;24(1):125–133, vii
3. Leaman TL. Anxiety disorders. *Prim Care.* 1999;26(2):197–210
4. Pinski SL, Trohman RG. Implantable cardioverter-defibrillators: implications for the nonelectrophysiologist. *Ann Intern Med.* 1995;122(10):770–777
5. Sarasin FP, Hanusa BH, Perneger T, Louis-Simonet M, Rajeswaran A, Kapoor WN. A risk score to predict arrhythmias in patients with unexplained syncope. *Acad Emerg Med.* 2003;10(12):1312–1317
6. Schnipper JL, Kapoor WN. Diagnostic evaluation and management of patients with syncope. *Med Clin North Am.* 2001;85(2):423–456, xi
7. Sears SF Jr, Shea JB, Conti JB. How to respond to an implantable cardioverter-defibrillator shock. *Circulation.* 2005;111(23):e380–e382

Heat Exposure (Heat Exhaustion and Heatstroke)

1. Armstrong LE, Casa DJ, Millard-Stafford M, Moran DS, Pyne SW, Roberts WO. Exertional heat illness during training and competition. *Med Sci Sports Exerc.* 2007;39(3):556–572
2. Armstrong LE, Epstein Y, Greenleaf JE, et al. American College of Sports Medicine position stand. Heat and cold illnesses during distance running. *Med Sci Sports Exerc.* 1996;28(12): i–x
3. Backer HD, Shopes E, Collins SL, Barkan H. Exertional heat illness and hyponatremia in hikers. *Am J Emerg Med.* 1999;17(6):532–539
4. Bouchama A, Knochel JP. Heat stroke. *N Eng J Med.* 2002;346(25): 1978–1988
5. Casa DJ, Armstrong LE, Hillman SK, et al. National Athletic Trainers' Association position statement: fluid replacement for athletes. *J Athl Train.* 2000;35(2):212–224
6. Glazer JL. Heat exhaustion and heatstroke: what you should know. *Am Fam Physician.* 2005;71(11):2141–2142
7. Grubenhoff JA, du Ford K, Roosevelt GE. Heat-related illness. *Clin Pediatr Emerg Med.* 2007;8(1):59–64
8. Khosla R, Guntupalli KK. Heat-related illness. *Crit Care Clin.* 1999;15(2):251–263
9. Lugo-Amador NM, Rothenhaus T, Moyer P. Heat-related illness. *Emerg Med Clin North Am.* 2004;22(2):315–327, viii

High Blood Pressure

1. Acelajado MC, Oparil S. Hypertension in the elderly. *Clin Geriatr Med.* 2009;25(3):391–412
2. Chiang WK, Jamshahi B. Asymptomatic hypertension in the ED. *Am J Emerg Med.* 1998;16(7):701–704
3. Chobanian AV, Bakris GL, Black HR, et al. The Seventh Report of the Joint National Committee on Prevention, Detection, Evaluation, and Treatment of High Blood Pressure: the JNC 7 report. *JAMA.* 2003;289(19):2560–2572
4. Drager LF, Lotufo PA, Bensenor IM. Letter regarding article by Law et al, "headaches and the treatment of blood pressure: results from a meta-analysis of 94 randomized placebo-controlled trials with 24,000 participants." *Circulation.* 2006;113(7):e164
5. Fung TT, Chiuve SE, McCullough ML, Rexrode KM, Logroscino G, Hu FB. Adherence to a DASH-style diet and risk of coronary heart disease and stroke in women. *Arch Intern Med.* 2008;168(7):713–720
6. Goldstein LB, Adams R, Alberts MJ, et al. Primary prevention of ischemic stroke: a guideline from the American Heart Association/ American Stroke Association Stroke Council. *Circulation.* 2006;113(24): e873–e923
7. Gus M, Fuchs FD, Pimentel M, Rosa D, Melo AG, Moreira LB. Behavior of ambulatory blood pressure surrounding episodes of headache in mildly hypertensive patients. *Arch Intern Med.* 2001;161(2):252–255

High Blood Pressure (continued)

8. Lima SG, Nascimento LS, Santos Filho CN, Albuquerque Mde F, Victor EG. Systemic hypertension at emergency units. The use of symptomatic drugs as choice for management [Portuguese]. *Arq Bras Cardiol.* 2005;85(2):115–123
9. Ma G, Sabin N, Dawes M. A comparison of blood pressure measurement over a sleeved arm versus a bare arm. *CMAJ.* 2008;178(5): 585–589
10. Muiesan ML, Padovani A, Salvetti M, et al. Headache: prevalence and relationship with office or ambulatory blood pressure in a general population sample (the Vobarno Study). *Blood Press.* 2006;15(1): 14–19
11. Joint National Committee on Prevention, Detection, Evaluation, and Treatment of High Blood Pressure; National High Blood Pressure Education Program Coordinating Committee. The Sixth Report of the Joint National Committee on Prevention, Detection, Evaluation, and Treatment of High Blood Pressure. *Arch Intern Med.* 1997; 157(21):2413–2446
12. Pickering TG. Principles and techniques of blood pressure measurement. *Cardiol Clin.* 2002;20(2):207–223
13. Smulyan H, Safar ME. The diastolic blood pressure in systolic hypertension. *Ann Intern Med.* 2000;132(3):233–237
14. Varon J, Marik PE. The diagnosis and management of hypertensive crises. *Chest.* 2000;18(1):214–227
15. Whelton PK, He J, Appel LJ, et al. Primary prevention of hypertension: clinical and public health advisory from the National High Blood Pressure Education Program. *JAMA.* 2002;288(15):1882–1888

Hives

1. Agency for Toxic Substances and Disease Registry. Contact dermatitis and urticaria from environmental exposures. *Am Fam Physician.* 1993;48(5):773–780
2. Braganza SC, Acworth JP, Mckinnon DR, Peake JE, Brown AF. Paediatric emergency department anaphylaxis: different patterns from adults. *Arch Dis Child.* 2006;91(2):159–163
3. Kennedy MS. Evaluation of chronic eczema and urticaria and angioedema. *Immunol Allergy Clin North Am.* 1999;19(1):19–33
4. American Academy of Allergy, Asthma and Immunology Joint Task Force on Practice Parameters; American College of Allergy, Asthma and Immunology Joint Council of Allergy, Asthma and Immunology. The diagnosis and management of anaphylaxis: an updated practice parameter. *J Allergy Clin Immunol.* 2005;115(3 suppl 2):S483–S523
5. Pollack CV Jr, Romano TJ. Outpatient management of acute uriticaria. *Ann Emerg Med.*1995;26(5):547–551
6. Sampson HA, Muñoz-Furlong A, Campbell RL, et al. Second symposium on the definition and management of anaphylaxis: summary report–Second National Institute of Allergy and Infectious Disease/ Food Allergy and Anaphylaxis Network symposium. *J Allergy Clin Immunol.* 2006;117(2):391–397
7. Sampson HA. Anaphylaxis and emergency treatment. *Pediatrics.* 2003;111(6 suppl 3):1601–1608

Immunization Reactions

1. Advisory Committee on Immunization Practices. Recommended adult immunization schedule: United States, 2011. *Ann Intern Med.* 2011;154(3):168–173
2. Atkinson WL, Pickering LK, Schwartz B, et al. General recommendations on immunization. Recommendations of the Advisory Committee on Immunization Practices (ACIP) and the American Academy of Family Physicians (AAFP). *MMWR Recomm Rep.* 2002;51(RR-2):1–35
3. Centers for Disease Control and Prevention (CDC). Syncope after vaccination—United States, January 2005–July 2007. *MMWR Morb Mortal Wkly Rep.* 2008;57(17):457–460
4. Centers for Disease Control and Prevention (CDC). Updated recommendations for use of tetanus toxoid, reduced diphtheria toxoid and acellular pertussis (Tdap) vaccine from the Advisory Committee on Immunization Practices, 2010. *MMWR Morb Mortal Wkly Rep.* 2011;60(1):13–15
5. Centers for Disease Control and Prevention (CDC). Recommended adult immunization schedule—United States, 2011. *MMWR Morb Mortal Wkly Rep.* 20114;60(4):1–4
6. Centers for Disease Control and Prevention (CDC). Diptheria, tetanus, and pertussis: recommendations for vaccine use and other preventive measures. Recommendations of the Immunization Practices Advisory Committee (ACIP). *MMWR Recomm Rep.* 1991;40:(RR-10):1–28
7. Fiore AE, Uyeki TM, Broder K, et al. Prevention and control of influenza with vaccines: recommendations of The Advisory Committee on Immunization Practices (ACIP), 2010. *MMWR Recomm Rep.* 2010;59(RR-8):1–62
8. Kretsinger K, Broder KR, Cortese MM, et al. Preventing tetanus, diphtheria, and pertussis among adults: use of tetanus toxoid, reduced diphtheria toxoid and acellular pertussis vaccine recommendations of the Advisory Committee on Immunization Practices (ACIP) and recommendation of ACIP, supported by the Healthcare Infection Control Practices Advisory Committee (HICPAC), for use of Tdap among health-care personnel. *MMWR Recomm Rep.* 2006;55(RR-17):1–37
9. Centers for Disease Control and Prevention (CDC); Advisory Committee on Immunization Practices (ACIP). Immunization of health-care personnel: recommendations of the Advisory Committee on Immunization Practices (ACIP). *MMWR Recomm Rep.* 2011;60(RR-7):1–45
10. Prymula R, Siegrist CA, Chlibek R, et al. Effect of prophylactic paracetamol administration at time of vaccination on febrile reactions and antibody responses in children: two open-label, randomized controlled trials. *Lancet.* 2009;374(9698):1339–1350
11. Public Health Agency of Canada. Canadian Immunization Guide; Seventh Edition - 2006. http://www.phac-aspc.gc.ca/publicat/cig-gci/ index-eng.php. Accessed July 27, 2012
12. Vaughn JA, Miller RA. Update on immunizations in adults. *Am Fam Physician.* 2011;84(9):1015–1020
13. Workowski KA, Berman S; and the Centers for Disease Control and Prevention (CDC). Sexually transmitted diseases treatment guidelines 2010 [published correction appears in *MMWR Recomm Rep.* 2011 Jan 14;60(1):18]. *MMWR Recomm Rep.* 2010;59(RR-12): 1–110
14. World Health Organization Department of Vaccines and Biologicals. Supplementary information on vaccine safety. Part 2: Background rates of adverse events following immunization. http://www.who.int/ vaccines-documents/DocsPDF00/www562.pdf. Accessed July 27, 2012

Influenza

1. Fiore AE, Shay DK, Broder K, et al. Prevention and control of influenza: recommendations of the Advisory Committee on Immunization Practices (ACIP), 2008. *MMWR Recomm Rep.* 2008;57(RR-7):1–60
2. Advisory Committee on Immunization Practices. Recommended adult immunization schedule: United States, 2011. *Ann Intern Med.* 2011;154(3):168–173

3. Bachert C, Chuchalin AG, Eisebitt R, Netayzhenko VZ, Voelker M. Aspirin compared with acetaminophen in the treatment of fever and other symptoms of upper respiratory tract infection in adults: a multicenter, randomized, double-blind, double-dummy, placebo-controlled, parallel-group, single-dose, 6-hour dose-ranging study. *Clin Ther.* 2005;27(7):993–1003
4. Eccles R. Understanding the symptoms of the common cold and influenza. *Lancet Infect Dis.* 2005;5(11):718–725
5. Fagbuyi DB, Brown KM, Mathison DJ, et al. A rapid medical screening process improves emergency department patient flow during surge associated with novel H1N1 influenza virus. *Ann Emerg Med.* 2011;57(1):52–59
6. Fiore AE, Uyeki TM, Broder K, et al. Prevention and control of influenza with vaccines: recommendations of the Advisory Committee on Immunization Practices (ACIP), 2010. *MMWR Recomm Rep.* 2010;59(RR-8):1–62
7. Guo R, Pittler MH, Ernst E. Complementary medicine for treating or preventing influenza or influenza-like illness. *Am J Med.* 2007;120(11):923–929
8. Fiore AE, Fry A, Shay D, et al. Antiviral agents for the treatment and chemoprophylaxis of influenza—recommendations of the Advisory Committee on Immunization Practices (ACIP). *MMWR Recomm Rep.* 2011;60(1):1–24
9. Jain S, Kamimoto L, Bramley AM, et al; and the 2009 Pandemic Influenza A (H1N1) Virus Hospitalizations Investigation Team. Hospitalized patients with 2009 H1N1 influenza in the United States, April–June 2009. *N Engl J Med.* 2009;361(20):1935–1944
10. Kim SY, Chang YJ, Cho HM, Hwang YW, Moon YS. Non-steroidal anti-inflammatory drugs for the common cold. *Cochrane Database Syst Rev.* 2009;(3):CD006362
11. Paul IM, Beiler JS, King TS, Clapp ER, Vallati J, Berlin CM Jr. Vapor rub, petrolatum, and no treatment for children with nocturnal cough and cold symptoms. *Pediatrics.* 2010;126(6):1092–1099
12. Public Health Agency of Canada. Canadian Immunization Guide; Seventh Edition - 2006. http://www.phac-aspc.gc.ca/publicat/cig-gci/index-eng.php. Accessed July 27, 2012
13. Rothberg MB, Haessler SD, Brown RB. Complications of viral influenza. *Am J Med. 2008*;121(4):258–264
14. Stamboulian D, Bonvehi PE, Nacinovich FM, Cox N. Influenza. *Infect Dis Clin North Am.* 2000;14(1):141–166
15. US Preventive Services Task Force. Postexposure prophylaxis for selected infectious diseases. In: *Guide to Clinical Preventive Services.* 2nd ed. Alexandria, VA: International Medical Publishing, Inc; 1996:815–827

Insect Bite

1. American Academy of Allergy, Asthma and Immunology (AAAAI). The use of epinephrine in the treatment of anaphylaxis. Position statement. http://www.aaaai.org/Aaaai/media/MediaLibrary/PDF%20Documents/Practice%20and%20Parameters/Epinephrine-in-treating-anaphylaxis-2002.pdf. Accessed July 27, 2012
2. Brown M, Hebert AA. Insect repellents: an overview. *J Am Acad Dermatol.* 1997;36(2):243–249
3. Derlet RW, Richards JR. Cellulitis from insect bites: a case series. *Cal J Emerg Med.* 2003;4(2):27–30
4. Fradin MS. Mosquitoes and mosquito repellents: a clinician's guide. *Ann Int Med.* 1998;128(11):931–940
5. Hwang SW, Svoboda TJ, De Jong IJ, Kabasele KJ, Gogosis E. Bed bug infestations in an urban environment. *Emerg Infect Dis.* 2005;11(4):533–538
6. Koren G, Matsui D, Bailey B. DEET–based insect repellants: safety implications for children and pregnant and lactating women. *CMAJ.* 2003;169(3):209–212
7. American Academy of Allergy, Asthma and Immunology Joint Task Force on Practice Parameters; American College of Allergy, Asthma and Immunology Joint Council of Allergy, Asthma and Immunology. The diagnosis and management of anaphylaxis: an updated practice parameter. *J Allergy Clin Immunol.* 2005;115(3 suppl 2):S483–S523
8. US Environmental Protection Agency. Using insect repellents safely. http://epa.gov/pesticides/insect/safe.htm. Accessed July 27, 2012
9. Sampson HA, Muñoz-Furlong A, Campbell RL, et al. Second symposium on the definition and management of anaphylaxis: summary report—Second National Institute of Allergy and Infectious Disease/Food Allergy and Anaphylaxis Network symposium. *J Allergy Clin Immunol.* 2006;117(2):391–397
10. Steen CJ, Carbonaro PA, Schwartz RA. Arthropods in dermatology. *J Am Acad Dermatol.* 2004;50(6):819–844
11. Thomas I, Kihiczak GG, Schwartz RA. Bedbug bites: a review. *Int J Dermatol.* 2004;43(6):430–433

Jock Itch

1. Cordoro KM, Ganz JE. Training room management of medical conditions: sports dermatology. *Clin Sports Med.* 2005;24(3):565–598, viii–ix
2. Loo DS. Cutaneous fungal infections in the elderly. *Dermatol Clin.* 2004;22(1):33–50
3. Noble SL, Forbes RC, Stamm PL. Diagnosis and management of common tinea infections. *Am Fam Physician.* 1998;58(1):163–178
4. Rupke SJ. Fungal skin disorders. *Prim Care.* 2000;27(2):407–421

Knee Pain

1. Bjordal JM, Ljunggren AE, Klovning A, Slordal L. Non-steroidal anti-inflammatory drugs, including cyclo-oxygenase-2 inhibitors, in osteoarthritic knee pain: meta-analysis of randomized placebo controlled trials. *BMJ.* 2004;329(7478):1317
2. Calmbach WL, Hutchens M. Evaluation of patients presenting with knee pain: part I. History, physical examination, radiographs, and laboratory tests. *Am Fam Physician.* 2003;68(5):907–912
3. Calmbach WL, Hutchens M. Evaluation of patients presenting with knee pain: Part II. Differential diagnosis. *Am Fam Physician.* 2003;68(5):917–922
4. Coakley G, Mathews C, Field M, et al; and the British Society for Rheumatology Standards, Guidelines and Audit Working Group. BSR & BHPR, BOA, RCGP and BSAC guidelines for management of the hot swollen joint in adults. *Rheumatology (Oxford).* 2006;45(8):1039–1041
5. Dearborn JT, Jergesen HE. The evaluation and initial management of arthritis. *Prim Care.* 1996;23(2):215–240
6. Divoll M, Abernethy DR, Ameer B, Greenblatt DJ. Acetaminophen kinetics in the elderly. *Clin Pharmacol Ther.* 1982;31(2):151–156
7. Pioro MH, Mandell BF. Septic arthritis. *Rheum Dis Clin North Am.* 1997;23(2):239–258
8. Rainsford KD. Ibuprofen: pharmacology, efficacy and safety. *Inflammopharmacology.* 2009;17(6):275–342
9. Roberts DM, Stallard TC. Emergency department evaluation and treatment of knee and leg injuries. *Emerg Med Clin North Am.* 2000;18(1):67–84, v–vi
10. Solomon DH, Simel DL, Bates DW, Katz JN, Schaffer JL. Does this patient have a torn meniscus or ligament of the knee? Value of the physical examination. *JAMA.* 2001;286(13):1610–1620

Knee Pain (continued)

11. Weston V, Coakley G; and the British Society for Rheumatology (BSR) Standards, Guidelines and Audit Working Group; et al. Guideline for the management of the hot swollen joint in adults with a particular focus on septic arthritis. *J Antimicrob Chemother.* 2006;58(3):492–493

Leg Pain

1. Andreou ER, Koru-Sengul T, Linkins L, Bates SM, Ginsberg JS, Kearon C. Differences in clinical presentation of deep vein thrombosis in men and women. *J Thromb Haemost.* 2008;6(10):1713–1719
2. Baker WF Jr. Diagnosis of deep venous thrombosis and pulmonary embolism. *Med Clin North Am.* 1998;82(3):459–476
3. Bartholomew JR, Schaffer JL, McCormick GF. Air travel and venous thromboembolism: minimizing the risk. *Cleve Clin J Med.* 2011;78(2): 111–120
4. Bates SM, Ginsberg JS. Clinical practice. Treatment of deep-vein thrombosis. *N Eng J Med.* 2004;351(3):268–277
5. Butler JV, Mukerrin EC, O'Keefe ST. Nocturnal leg cramps in older people. *Postgrad Med J.* 2002;78(924):596–598
6. Gallus AS. Travel, venous thromboembolism, and thrombophilia. *Semin Thromb Hemost.* 2005;31(1):90–96
7. Glazer JL, Hosey RG. Soft-tissue injuries of the lower extremity. *Prim Care.* 2004;31(4):1005–1024
8. Kline JA, Courtney DM, Kabrhel C, et al. Prospective multicenter evaluation of the pulmonary embolism rule-out criteria. *J Thromb Haemost.* 2008;6(5):772–780
9. Maitra RS, Johnson DL. Stress fractures. Clinical history and physical examination. *Clin Sports Med.* 1997;16(2):259–274
10. Mateo J, Oliver A, Borrell M, Sala N, Fontcuberta J. Laboratory evaluation and clinical characteristics of 2,132 consecutive unselected patients with venous thromboembolism—results of the Spanish Multicentric Study on Thrombophilia (EMET-Study). *Thromb Haemost.* 1997;77(3):444–451
11. McRae S. Pulmonary embolism. *Aust Fam Physician.* 2010;39(6): 462–466
12. Newman AB. Peripheral arterial disease: insights from population studies of older adults. *J Am Geriatr Soc.* 2000;48(9):1157–1162
13. Philbrick JT, Shumate R, Siadaty MS, Becker DM. Air travel and venous thromboembolism: a systematic review. *J Gen Intern Med.* 2007;22(1):107–114
14. Rosendaal FR. Venous thrombosis: a multicausal disease. *Lancet.* 1999;353(9159):1167–1173
15. Wells PS, Anderson DR, Bormanis J, et al. Value of assessment of pretest probability of deep-vein thrombosis in clinical management. *Lancet.* 1997;350(9094):1795–1798
16. Wells PS, Hirsh J, Anderson DR, et al. Accuracy of clinical assessment of deep-vein-thrombosis. *Lancet.* 1995;345(8961):1326–1330

Leg Swelling and Edema

1. Andreou ER, Koru-Sengul T, Linkins L, Bates SM, Ginsberg JS, Kearon C. Differences in clinical presentation of deep vein thrombosis in men and women. *J Thromb Haemost.* 2008;6(10):1713–1719
2. Baker WF Jr. Diagnosis of deep venous thrombosis and pulmonary embolism. *Med Clin North Am.* 1998;82(3):459–476
3. Bartholomew JR, Schaffer JL, McCormick GF. Air travel and venous thromboembolism: minimizing the risk. *Cleve Clin J Med.* 2011;78(2): 111–120
4. Bates SM, Ginsberg JS. Clinical practice. Treatment of deep-vein thrombosis. *N Eng J Med.* 2004;351(3):268–277
5. Gallus AS. Travel, venous thromboembolism, and thrombophilia. *Semin Thromb Hemost.* 2005;31(1):90–96
6. Kline JA, Courtney DM, Kabrhel C, et al. Prospective multicenter evaluation of the pulmonary embolism rule-out criteria. *J Thromb Haemost.* 2008;6(5):772–780
7. McRae S. Pulmonary embolism. *Aust Fam Physician.* 2010;39(6): 462–466
8. Newman AB. Peripheral arterial disease: insights from population studies of older adults. *J Am Geriatr Soc.* 2000;48(9):1157–1162
9. Philbrick JT, Shumate R, Siadaty MS, Becker DM. Air travel and venous thromboembolism: a systematic review. *J Gen Intern Med.* 2007;22(1):107–114
10. Rosendaal FR. Venous thrombosis: a multicausal disease. *Lancet.* 1999;353(9159):1167–1173
11. Wang CS, FitzGerald JM, Schulzer M, Mak E, Ayas NT. Does this dyspneic patient in the emergency department have congestive heart failure? *JAMA.* 2005;294(15):1944–1956
12. Wells PS, Anderson DR, Bormanis J, et al. Value of assessment of pretest probability of deep-vein thrombosis in clinical management. *Lancet.* 1997;350(9094):1795–1798
13. Wells PS, Hirsh J, Anderson DR, et al. Accuracy of clinical assessment of deep-vein-thrombosis. *Lancet.* 1995;345(8961):1326–1330

Lymph Nodes, Swollen

1. Ferrer R. Lymphadenopathy: differential diagnosis and evaluation. *Am Fam Physician.* 1998;58(6):1313–1320
2. Habermann TM, Steensma DP. Lymphadenopathy. *Mayo Clin Proc.* 2000;75(7):723–732
3. Peter J, Ray CG. Infectious mononucleosis. *Pediatr Rev.* 1998;19(8): 276–279
4. Peters TR, Edwards KM. Cervical lymphadenopathy and adenitis. *Pediatr Rev.* 2000;21(12):399–405

Menstrual Period, Missed or Late

1. Brill SR, Rosenfeld WD. Contraception. *Med Clin North Am.* 2000;84(4):907–925
2. Kothari S, Thacker HL. Risk assessment of the menopausal patient. *Med Clin North Am.* 1999;83(6):1489–1502
3. Mitan LA, Slap GB. Adolescent menstrual disorders. Update. *Med Clin North Am.* 2000;84(4):851–868
4. Murray H, Baakdah H, Bardell T, Tulandi T. Diagnosis and treatment of ectopic pregnancy. *CMAJ.* 2005;173(8):905–912

Neck Pain or Stiffness

1. Argoff CA, Wheeler AH. Spinal and radicular pain disorders. *Neurol Clin.* 1998;16(4):833–850
2. Attia J, Hatala R, Cook DJ, Wong JG. Does this adult patient have acute meningitis? *JAMA.* 1999;282(2):175–181
3. Devereaux MW. Neck pain. *Prim Care.* 2004;31(1):19–31
4. Haldeman S. Diagnostic tests for the evaluation of back and neck pain. *Neurol Clin.* 1996;14(1):103–117
5. Perry JJ, Stiell IG, Sivilotti ML, et al. High risk clinical characteristics for subarachnoid haemorrhage in patients with acute headache: prospective cohort study. *BMJ.* 2010;341:c5204
6. Rainsford KD. Ibuprofen: pharmacology, efficacy and safety. *Inflammopharmacology.* 2009;17(6):275–342
7. Swezey RL. Chronic neck pain. *Rheum Dis Clin North Am.* 1996;22(3):411–437

Neurologic Deficit

1. Baumlin KM, Richardson LD. Stroke syndromes. *Emerg Med Clin North Am.* 1997;15(3):551–561
2. Chalela JA, Kidwell CS, Nentwich LM, et al. Magnetic resonance imaging and computed tomography in emergency assessment of patients with suspected acute stroke: a prospective comparison. *Lancet.* 2007;369(9558):293–298
3. Goldstein LB, Adams R, Alberts MJ, et al; and the American Heart Association; American Stroke Association Stroke Council. Primary prevention of ischemic stroke: a guideline from the American Heart Association/American Stroke Association Stroke Council. *Circulation.* 2006;113(24):e873–e923
4. Gommans J, Barber PA, Fink J. Preventing strokes: the assessment and management of people with transient ischaemic attack. *N Z Med J.* 2009;122(1293):3556
5. Johnston SC, Rothwell PM, Nguyen-Huynh MN, et al. Validation and refinement of scores to predict very early stroke risk after transient ischaemic attack. *Lancet.* 2007;369(9558):283–292
6. Kidwell CS, Chalela JA, Saver JL, et al. Comparison of MRI and CT for detection of acute intracerebral hemorrhage. *JAMA.* 2004;292(15):1823–1830
7. Kidwell CS, Starkman S, Eckstein M, Weems K, Saver JL. Identifying stroke in the field. prospective validation of the Los Angeles Prehospital Stroke Screen (LAPSS). *Stroke.* 2000;31(1):71–76
8. Kothari R, Hall K, Brott T, Broderick J. Early stroke recognition: developing an out-of-hospital NIH stroke scale. *Acad Emerg Med.* 1997;4(10):986–990
9. Lockhart P, Daly F, Pitkethly M, Comerford N, Sullivan F. Antiviral treatment for Bell's palsy (idiopathic facial paralysis). *Cochrane Database Syst Rev.* 2009;(4):CD001869
10. Martin-Schild S, Albright KC, Tanksley J, et al. Zero on the NIHSS does not equal the absence of stroke. *Ann Emerg Med.* 2011;57(1): 42–45
11. Nor AM, Davis J, Sen B, et al. The Recognition of Stroke in the Emergency Room (ROSIER) scale: development and validation of a stroke recognition instrument. *Lancet Neurol.* 2005;4(11):727–734
12. Numthavaj P, Thakkinstian A, Dejthevaporn C, Attia J. Corticosteroid and antiviral therapy for Bell's palsy: a network meta-analysis. *BMC Neurol.* 2011;11:1
13. Perry JJ, Stiell IG, Sivilotti ML, et al. High risk clinical characteristics for subarachnoid haemorrhage in patients with acute headache: prospective cohort study. *BMJ.* 2010;341:c5204
14. Schwamm LH, Pancioli A, Acker JE III, et al. Recommendations for the establishment of stroke systems of care: recommendations from the American Stroke Association's Task Force on the Development of Stroke Systems. *Stroke.* 2005;36(3):690–703
15. Selman WR, Tarr R, Landis DM. Brain attack: emergency treatment of ischemic stroke. *Am Fam Physician.* 1997;55(8):2655–2666
16. Stead LG, Suravaram S, Bellolio MF, et al. An assessment of the incremental value of the ABCD2 score in the emergency department evaluation of transient ischemic attack. *Ann Emerg Med.* 2011;57(1):46–51
17. Tiemstra JD, Khatkhate N. Bell's palsy: diagnosis and management. *Am Fam Physician.* 2007;76(7):997–1002
18. Wasserman J, Perry J, Dowlatshahi D, et al. Stratified, urgent care for transient ischemic attack results in low stroke rates. *Stroke.* 2010;41(11):2601–2605

Nosebleed

1. Pantanowitz L. Epistaxis in the older hypertensive patient. *J Am Geriatr Soc.* 1999;47(5):631
2. Tan LK, Calhoun KH. Epistaxis. *Med Clin North Am.* 1999;83(1): 43–56

Penis and Scrotum Symptoms

1. Burgher SW. Acute scrotal pain. *Emerg Med Clin North Am.* 1998;16(4):781–809, vi
2. English JC III, Laws RA, Keough GC, Wilde JL, Foley JP, Elston DM. Dermatoses of the glans penis and prepuce. *J Am Acad Dermatol.* 1997;37(1):1–26
3. Fazio L, Brock G. Erectile dysfunction: management update. *CMAJ.* 2004;170(9):1429–1437
4. Gresser U, Gleiter CH. Erectile dysfunction: comparison of efficacy and side effects of the PDE-5 inhibitors sildenafil, vardenafil and tadalafil—review of the literature. *Eur J Med Res.* 2002;7(10):435–446
5. Kodner C. Sexually transmitted infections in men. *Prim Care.* 2003;30(1):173–191
6. Montague DK, Jarow J, Broderick GA, et al. American Urological Association guideline on the management of priapism. *J Urol.* 2003;170(4):1318–1324
7. Montorsi F, Kuritzky L, Sadovsky R, Fredlund P, Cordell WH. Frequently asked questions about tadalafil for treating men with erectile dysfunction. *J Mens Health Gend.* 2005;2(1):141–157
8. Public Health Agency of Canada. Primary care and sexually transmitted infections. In: Canadian Guidelines on Sexually Transmitted Infections 2006 Edition. Ottawa, Ontario: Public Health Agency of Canada; 2006:7–29. http://pubs.cpha.ca/PDF/P37/23384.pdf. Accessed July 27, 2012
9. Roberts RG, Hartlaub PP. Evaluation of dysuria in men. *Am Fam Physician.* 1999;60(3):865–872
10. Rogers ZR. Priapism in sickle cell disease. *Hematol Oncol Clin North Am.* 2005;19(5):917–928, viii
11. Rupke SJ. Fungal skin disorders. *Prim Care.* 2000;27(2):407–421
12. Workowski KA, Berman S; and the Centers for Disease Control and Prevention (CDC). Sexually transmitted diseases treatment guidelines 2010 [published correction appears in MMWR Recomm Rep. 2011;60(1):18]. *MMWR Recomm Rep.* 2010;59(RR-12):1–110

Poison Ivy/Oak/Sumac

1. Beltrani VS. Allergic dermatoses. *Med Clin North Am.* 1998;82(5): 1105–1133, vi
2. Mark BJ, Slavin RG. Allergic contact dermatitis. *Med Clin North Am.* 2006;90(1):169–185
3. Marks JG Jr, Fowler JF Jr, Sheretz EF, Rietschel RL. Prevention of poison ivy and poison oak allergic contact dermatitis by quaternium-18 bentonite. *J Am Acad Dermatol.* 1995;33(2):212–216
4. Tanner TL. Rhus (Toxicodendron) dermatitis. *Prim Care.* 2000;27(2): 493–502

Poisoning

1. American College of Emergency Physicians. Clinical policy for the initial approach to patients presenting with acute toxic ingestion or dermal or inhalation exposure. *Ann Emerg Med.* 1999;33(6):735–761
2. American College of Emergency Physicians. Poison information and treatment systems. *Ann Emerg Med.* 1996;27(5):686
3. American Heart Association. 2005 Guidelines for Cardiopulmonary Resuscitation and Emergency Cardiovascular Care. Part 14: First aid. *Circulation.* 2005;112(24 suppl):IV-196–IV-203

Poisoning (continued)

4. Beck DA, Frohberg NR. Coprophagia in an elderly man: a case report and review of the literature. *Int J Psychiatry Med.* 2005;35(4):417–427
5. Bond GR. The role of activated charcoal and gastric emptying in gastrointestinal decontanimation: a state-of-the-art review. *Ann Emerg Med.* 2002;39(3):273–286
6. Bronstein AC, Spyker DA, Cantilena LR Jr, Green JL, Rumack BH, Heard SE; and the American Association of Poison Control Centers. 2007 Annual Report of the American Association of Poison Control Centers' National Poison Data System (NPDS): 25th Annual Report. *Clin Toxicol (Phila).* 2008;46(10):927–1057
7. Crouch BI, Caravati EM, Mitchell A, Martin AC. Poisoning in older adults: a 5-year experience of US poison control centers. *Ann Pharmacother.* 2004;38(12):2005–2011
8. Manoguerra AS, Cobaugh DJ; and the Guidelines for the Management of Poisoning Consensus Panel. Guideline on the use of ipecac syrup in the out-of-hospital management of ingested poisons. *Clin Toxicol (Phila).* 2005;43(1):1–10
9. McGuigan MA; and the Guideline Consensus Panel. Guideline for the out-of-hospital management of human exposures to minimally toxic substances. *J Toxicol Clin Toxicol.* 2003;41(7):907–917
10. US Preventive Services Task Force. Counseling to prevent household and recreational injuries. In: *Guide to Clinical Preventive Services.* 2nd ed. Alexandria,VA: International Medical Publishing, Inc; 1996:659–685

Pubic Lice

1. Brown TJ, Yen-Moore A, Tyring SK. An overview of sexually transmitted diseases. Part II. *J Am Acad Dermatol.* 1999;41(5):661–680
2. Centers for Disease Control and Prevention (CDC). Parasites – Lice – Pubic "Crab" Lice Web site. http://www.cdc.gov/parasites/lice/pubic/index.html. Accessed July 27, 2012
3. Flinders DC, De Schweinitz P. Pediculosis and scabies. *Am Fam Physician.* 2004;69(2):341–348
4. Larimore WL, Petrie KA. Drug use during pregnancy and lactation. *Prim Care.* 2000;27(1):35–53
5. Maunder JW. Lice and scabies. Myths and reality. *Dermatol Clin.* 1998;16(4):843–845, xv
6. Public Health Agency of Canada. Primary care and sexually transmitted infections. In: *Canadian Guidelines on Sexually Transmitted Infections.* 2006 Edition. Ottawa, Ontario: Public Health Agency of Canada; 2006:7–29. http://pubs.cpha.ca/PDF/P37/23384.pdf. Accessed July 27, 2012
7. Workowski KA, Berman S; and the Centers for Disease Control and Prevention (CDC). Sexually transmitted diseases treatment guidelines 2010 [published correction appears in *MMWR Recomm Rep.* 2011;60(1):18]. *MMWR Recomm Rep.* 2010 Dec 17;59(RR-12):1–110

Puncture Wound

1. American Heart Association. 2005 Guidelines for Cardiopulmonary Resuscitation and Emergency Cardiovascular Care. Part 14: First aid. *Circulation.* 2005;112(24 suppl):IV-196–IV-203
2. Baldwin G, Colbourne M. Puncture wounds. *Pediatr Rev.* 1999;20(1):21–23
3. Centers for Disease Control and Prevention (CDC). Updated recommendations for use of tetanus toxoid, reduced diphtheria toxoid and acellular pertussis (Tdap) vaccine from the Advisory Committee on Immunization Practices, 2010. *MMWR Morb Mortal Wkly Rep.* 2011;60(1):13–15
4. Murphy TV, Slade BA, Broder KR, et al. Prevention of pertussis, tetanus, and diphtheria among pregnant and postpartum women and their infants recommendations of the Advisory Committee on Immunization Practices (ACIP). *MMWR Recomm Rep.* 2008;5(RR-4):1–51
5. Centers for Disease Control and Prevention (CDC). Diptheria, tetanus, and pertussis: recommendations for vaccine use and other preventive measures. Recommendations of the Immunization Practices Advisory Committee (ACIP) *MMWR Recomm Rep.* 1991;40(RR-10):1–28
6. Gonzalez R, Kasdan ML. High pressure injection injuries of the hand. *Clin Occup Environ Med.* 2006;5(2):407–411, ix
7. Hogan CJ, Ruland RT. High-pressure injection injuries to the upper extremity: a review of the literature. *J Orthop Trauma.* 2006;20(7):503–511
8. Kretsinger K, Broder KR, Cortese MM, et al. Preventing tetanus, diphtheria, and pertussis among adults: use of tetanus toxoid, reduced diphtheria toxoid and acellular pertussis vaccine recommendations of the Advisory Committee on Immunization Practices (ACIP) and recommendation of ACIP, supported by the Healthcare Infection Control Practices Advisory Committee (HICPAC), for use of Tdap among health-care personnel. *MMWR Recomm Rep.* 2006;55(RR-17):1–37
9. Lavery LA, Armstrong DG, Wunderlich RP, Mohler MJ, Wendel CS, Lipsky BA. Risk factors for foot infections in individuals with diabetes. *Diabetes Care.* 2006;29(6):1288–1293
10. Moran GJ, Talan DA, Abrahamian FM. Antimicrobial prophylaxis for wounds and procedures in the emergency department. *Infect Dis Clin North Am.* 2008;22(1);117–143, vii
11. Moscati RM, Mayrose J, Reardon RF, Janicke DM, Jehle DV. A multicenter comparison of tap water versus sterile saline for wound irrigation. *Acad Emerg Med.* 2007;14(5):404–409
12. Pearson AS, Wolford RW. Management of skin trauma. *Prim Care.* 2000;27(2):475–492
13. Talan DA, Abrahamian FM, Moran GJ, et al. Tetanus immunity and physician compliance with tetanus prophylaxis practices among emergency department patients presenting with wounds. *Ann Emerg Med.* 2004;43(3):305–314
14. Wedmore IS, Charette J. Emergency department evaluation and treatment of ankle and foot injuries. *Emerg Med Clin North Am.* 2000;18(1):85–113, vi

Rash, Widespread and Cause Unknown

1. Edwards FJ. Dermatologic ED presentations: from the mundane to the life-threatening. *Emerg Med Rep.* 1996;17(17):173–180
2. Roberts WE. Dermatologic problems of older women. *Dermatol Clin.* 2006;24(2):271–280, viii
3. Salzman MB, Rubin LG. Meningococcemia. *Infect Dis Clin North Am.* 1996;10(4):709–725
4. Schlossberg D. Fever and rash. *Infect Dis Clin North Am.* 1996;10(1):101–110

Rash, Widespread on Drugs (Drug Reaction)

1. Beltrani VS. Cutaneous manifestations of adverse drug reactions. *Immunol Allergy Clin North Am.* 1998;18(4):867–895
2. Bigby M, Jick S, Jick H, Arndt K. Drug-induced cutaneous reactions. A report from the Boston Collaborative Drug Surveillance Program on 15,438 consecutive inpatients, 1975 to 1982. *JAMA.* 1986;256(24):3358–3363
3. Bigby M. Rates of cutaneous reactions to drugs. *Arch Dermatol.* 2001;137(6):765–770

4. Davidson MH. Niacin use and cutaneous flushing: mechanisms and strategies for prevention. *Am J Cardiol.* 2008;101(8A):14B–19B
5. Drake LA, Dinehart SM, Farmer Er, et al. Guidelines of care for cutaneous adverse drug reactions. American Academy of Dermatology. *J Am Acad Dermatol.* 1996;35(3):458–461
6. Gruchalla RS. Drug allergies. *Prim Care.* 1998;25(4):791–807
7. Kacalak-Rzepka A, Klimowicz A, Bielecka-Grzela S, Zaluga E, Maleszka R, Fabiaczyk H. Retrospective analysis of adverse cutaneous drug reactions in patients hospitalized in Department of Dermatology and Venereology of Pomeranian Medical University in 1996–2006 [Polish]. *Ann Acad Med Stetin.* 2008;54(2):52–58
8. Paolini JF, Bays HE, Ballantyne CM, et al. Extended–release niacin/laropiprant: reducing niacin-induced flushing to better realize the benefit of niacin in improving cardiovascular risk factors. *Cardiol Clin.* 2008;26(4):547–560
9. Patel LM, Lambert PJ, Gagna CE, Maghari A, Lambert WC. Cutaneous signs of systemic disease. *Clin Dermatol.* 2011;29(5): 511–522
10. Revuz J. New advances in severe adverse drug reactions. *Dermatol Clin.* 2001;19(4):697–709, ix
11. Riedl MA, Casillas AM. Adverse drug reactions: types and treatment options. *Am Fam Physician.* 2003;68(9):1781–1790

Rash or Redness, Localized and Cause Unknown

1. Callahan EF, Adal KA, Tomecki KJ. Cutaneous (non-HIV) infections. *Dermatol Clin.* 2000;18(3);497–508, x
2. Edwards FJ. Dermatologic ED presentations: from the mundane to the life-threatening. *Emerg Med Rep.* 1996;17(17):173–180
3. Frazee BW, Lynn J, Charlebois ED, Lambert L, Lowery D, Perdreau-Remington F. High prevalence of methicillin-resistant Staphylococcus aureus in emergency department skin and soft tissue infections. *Ann Emerg Med.* 2005;45(3):311–320
4. Fridkin SK, Hageman JC, Morrison M, et al. Methicillin-resistant Staphylococcus aureus disease in three communities. *N Eng J Med.* 2005;352(14):1436–1444
5. Garner LA. Contact dermatitis to metals. *Dermatol Ther.* 2004;17(4): 321–327
6. Gorwitz RJ, Jernigan DB, Powers JH, Jernigan JA; and the Participants in the CDC-Convened Experts' Meeting on Management of MRSA in the Community. Strategies for clinical management of MRSA in the community: summary of an experts' meeting convened by the Centers for Disease Control and Prevention. 2006. http://www.cdc.gov/mrsa/pdf/MRSA-Strategies-ExpMtgSummary-2006.pdf. Accessed July 31, 2012
7. Hogan D, Ledet JJ. Impact of regulation on contact dermatitis. *Dermatol Clin.* 2009;27(3):385–394, viii
8. Mark BJ, Slavin RG. Allergic contact dermatitis. *Med Clin North Am.* 2006; 90(1):169–185
9. Mortz CG, Andersen KE. New aspects in allergic contact dermatitis. *Curr Opin Allergy Clin Immunol.* 2008;8(5):428–432
10. Mounsey AL, Matthew LG, Slawson DC. Herpes zoster and post-herpetic neuralgia: prevention and management. *Am Fam Physician.* 2005;72(6):1075–1080
11. Odell ML. Skin and wound infections: an overview. *Am Fam Physician.* 1998;57(10):2424–2432
12. Patel LM, Lambert PJ, Gagna CE, Maghari A, Lambert WC. Cutaneous signs of systemic disease. *Clin Dermatol.* 2011;29(5): 511–522
13. Rhody C. Bacterial infections of the skin. *Prim Care.* 2000;27(2): 459–473
14. Roberts WE. Dermatologic problems of older women. *Dermatol Clin.* 2006;24(2):271–280, viii
15. Schlossberg D. Fever and rash. *Infect Dis Clin North Am.* 1996;10(1): 101–110
16. Swartz MN. Clinical practice. Cellulitis. *N Engl J Med.* 2004;350(9): 904–912
17. Tibbles CD, Edlow JA. Does this patient have erythema migrans? *JAMA.* 2007;297(23):2617–2627

Rectal Bleeding

1. Eikelboom JW, Wallentin L, Connolly SJ, et al. Risk of bleeding with 2 doses of dabigatran compared with warfarin in older and younger patients with atrial fibrillation: an analysis of the randomized evaluation of long-term anticoagulant therapy (RE-LY) trial. *Circulation.* 2011;123(21):2363–2372
2. Fallah MA, Prakash C, Edmundowicz S. Acute gastrointestinal bleeding. *Med Clin North Am.* 2000;84(5):1183–1208
3. Farrel JJ, Friedman LS. Gastrointestinal bleeding in older people. *Gastroenterol Clin North Am.* 2000;29(1):1–36, v
4. Fathi DJ. Common anorectal symptomatology. *Prim Care.* 1999;26(1): 1–13
5. Janicke DM, Pundt MR. Anorectal disorders. *Emerg Med Clin North Am.* 1996;14(4):757–788
6. Raje D, Scott M, Irvine T, et al. Telephonic management of rectal bleeding in young adults: a prospective randomized controlled trial. *Colorectal Dis.* 2007;9(1):86–89
7. Sinert R, Spektor M. Evidence-based emergency medicine/rational clinical examination abstract. Clinical assessment of hypovolemia. *Ann Emerg Med.* 2005;45(3):327–329
8. Stapley S, Peters TJ, Sharp D, Hamilton W. The mortality of colorectal cancer in relation to the initial symptom at presentation to primary care and to the duration of symptoms: a cohort study using medical records. *Br J Cancer.* 2006;95(10):1321–1325
9. Strate LL, Orav EJ, Syngal S. Early predictors of severity in acute lower intestinal tract bleeding. *Arch Inter Med.* 2003;163(7):838–843
10. Wald A. Constipation. *Med Clin North Am.* 2000;84(5):1231–1246

Rectal Symptoms

1. Fathi DJ. Common anorectal symptomatology. *Prim Care.* 1999;26(1): 1–13
2. Janicke DM, Pundt MR. Anorectal disorders. *Emerg Med Clin North Am.* 1996;14(4):757–788
3. MacLean J, Russell D. Pruritus ani. *Aust Fam Physician.* 2010;39(6): 366–370
4. Vincent C. Anorectal pain and irritation: anal fissure, levator syndrome, proctalgia fugax, and pruritus ani. *Prim Care.* 1999;26(1):53–68

Seizure

1. American Academy of Neurology. Consensus statements: medical management of epilepsy. *Neurology.* 1998;51(5 suppl 4):S39–S43
2. American College of Emergency Physicians. Clinical policy for the initial approach to patients presenting with a chief complaint of seizure who are not in status epilepticus. *Ann Emerg Med.* 1997;29(5): 706–724
3. American Heart Association. 2005 Guidelines for Cardiopulmonary Resuscitation and Emergency Cardiovascular Care. Part 14: First aid. *Circulation.* 2005;112(24 suppl):IV-196–IV-203
4. Clawson J, Olola C, Scott G, Heward A, Patterson B. Effect of a medical priority dispatch system key question addition in the seizure/convulsion/fitting protocol to improve recognition of ineffective (agonal) breathing. *Resuscitation.* 2008;79(2):257–264

Seizure (continued)

5. American Academy of Neurology Quality Standards Subcommittee. Practice parameter: management issues for women with epilepsy (summary statement). *Neurology.* 1998;51(4):944–948
6. Willmore LJ. Epilepsy emergencies; the first seizure and status epilepticus. *Neurology.* 1998;51(5 suppl):S34–S38

Sexual Assault or Rape

1. Amercan College of Emergency Physicians. Clinical policy for the management and risk stratification of community-acquired pneumonia in adults in the emergency department. *Ann Emerg Med.* 2001;38(1):107–113
2. American College of Emergency Physicians. Selective triage for victims of sexual assault to designated exam facilities. *Ann Emerg Med.* 2007;49(5):725
3. American College of Obstetricians and Gynecologists. Sexual assault. Number 242, November 1997. *Int J Gynaecol Obstet.* 1998;60(3): 297–304
4. Bechtel LK, Holstege CP. Criminal poisoning: drug-facilitated sexual assault. *Emerg Med Clin North Am.* 2007;25(2):499–525, x
5. Linden JA. Sexual assault. *Emerg Med Clin North Am.* 1999;17(3): 685–697, vii
6. Merritt DF. Genital trauma in the pediatric and adolescent female. *Obstet Gynecol Clin North Am.* 2009;36(1):85–98
7. Public Health Agency of Canada. Primary care and sexually transmitted infections. In: *Canadian Guidelines on Sexually Transmitted Infections.* 2006 Edition. Ottawa, Ontario: Public Health Agency of Canada; 2006:7–29. http://pubs.cpha.ca/PDF/P37/23384.pdf. Accessed July 31, 2012
8. Public Health Agency of Canada. Sexual assault in postpubertal adolescents and adults. In: *Canadian Guidelines on Sexually Transmitted Infections.* 2006 Edition. Ottawa, Ontario: Public Health Agency of Canada; 2006:305–314. http://pubs.cpha.ca/PDF/P37/23384.pdf. Accessed July 31, 2012
9. Riggs N. Analysis of 1,076 cases of sexual assault. *Ann Emerg Med.* 2000;35(4):358–362
10. Sugar NF, Fine DN, Eckert LO. Physical injury after sexual assault: findings of a large case series. *Am J Obstet Gynecol.* 2004;190(1):71–76
11. US Department of Justice. A National Protocol for Sexual Assault Medical Forensic Examinations: Adults/Adolescents. 2004. http://www.ncjrs.gov/pdffiles1/ovw/206554.pdf. Accessed July 31, 2012
12. Wessells H, Long L. Penile and genital injuries. *Urol Clin North Am.* 2006;33(1):117–126, vii
13. Workowski KA, Berman S; and the Centers for Disease Control and Prevention. Sexually transmitted diseases treatment guidelines, 2010 [published correction appears in *MMWR Recomm Rep.* 2011;60(1):18]. *MMWR Recomm Rep.* 2010;59(RR-12):1–110

Sinus Pain and Congestion

1. American Academy of Family Physicians. Patient information. Saline nasal irrigation for sinus problems. *Am Fam Physician.* 2009;80(10):1121
2. Bachert C, Chuchalin AG, Eisebitt R, Netayzhenko VZ, Voelker M. Aspirin compared with acetaminophen in the treatment of fever and other symptoms of upper respiratory tract infection in adults: a multicenter, randomized, double-blind, double-dummy, placebo-controlled, parallel-group, single-dose, 6-hour dose-ranging study. *Clin Ther.* 2005;27(7):993–1003
3. Bucher HC, Tschudi P, Young J, et al. Effect of amoxicillin-clavulanate in clinically diagnosed acute rhinosinusitis: a placebo-controlled, double-blind, randomized trial in general practice. *Arch Intern Med.* 2003;163(15):1793–1798
4. Cady RK, Schreiber CP. Sinus headache: a clinical conundrum. *Otolaryngol Clin North Am.* 2004;37(2):267–288
5. Eapen RJ, Ebert CS Jr, Pillsbury HC III. Allergic rhinitis—history and presentation. *Otolaryngol Clin North Am.* 2008;41(2):325–330, vi–vii
6. Eccles R. Understanding the symptoms of the common cold and influenza. *Lancet Infect Dis.* 2005;5(11):718–725
7. Erebara A, Bozzo P, Einarson A, Koren G. Treating the common cold during pregnancy. *Can Fam Physician.* 2008;54(5):687–689
8. Harvey R, Hannan SA, Badia L, Scadding G. Nasal saline irrigations for the symptoms of chronic rhinosinusitis. *Cochrane Database Syst Rev.* 2007;(3):CD006394
9. Incaudo GA, Takach P. The diagnosis and treatment of allergic rhinitis during pregnancy and lactation. *Immunol Allergy Clin North Am.* 2006;26(1):137–154
10. Kirkpatrick GL. The common cold. *Prim Care.* 1996;23(4):657–675
11. Leung RS, Katial R. The diagnosis and management of acute and chronic sinusitis. *Prim Care.* 2008;35(1):11–24, v–vi
12. Maltinski G. Nasal disorders and sinusitis. *Prim Care.* 1998;25(3): 663–683
13. Rabago D, Barrett B, Marchand L, Maberry R, Mundt M. Qualitative aspects of nasal irrigation use by patients with chronic sinus disease in a multimethod study. *Ann Fam Med.* 2006;4(4):295–301
14. Rabago D, Zgierska A. Saline nasal irrigation for upper respiratory conditions. *Am Fam Physician.* 2009;80(10):1117–1119
15. Rosenfeld RM, Andes D, Bhattacharyya N, et al. Clinical practice guideline: adult sinusitis. *Otolaryngol Head Neck Surg.* 2007; 137(3 suppl):S1–S31
16. Simasek M, Blandino DA. Treatment of the common cold. *Am Fam Physician.* 2007;75(4):515–520
17. Spector SL, Bernstein IL, Li JT, et al. Parameters for the diagnosis and management of sinusitis. *J Allergy Clin Immunol.* 1998; 102(6 suppl 2):S107–S144
18. Wallace DV, Dykewicz MS, Bernstein DI, et al. The diagnosis and management of rhinitis: an updated practice parameter. *J Allergy Clin Immunol.* 2008;122(2 suppl):S1–S84

Skin, Foreign Body

1. Baldwin G, Colbourne M. Puncture wounds. *Pediatr Rev.* 1999;20(1): 21–23
2. Blankenship RB, Baker T. Imaging modalities in wounds and superficial skin infections. *Emerg Med Clin North Am.* 2007;25(1):223–234
3. Chan C, Salam GA. Splinter removal. *Am Fam Physician.* 2003;67(12):2557–2562
4. Halaas GW. Management of foreign bodies in the skin. *Am Fam Physician.* 2007;76(5):683–688
5. Hollander JE, Singer AJ, Valentine SM, Shofer FS. Risk factors for infection in patients with traumatic lacerations. *Acad Emerg Med.* 2001;8(7):716–720
6. Kaye ET. Topical antibacterial agents. *Infect Dis Clin North Am.* 2000;14(2):321–339
7. Moran GJ, Talan DA, Abrahamian FM. Antimicrobial prophylaxis for wounds and procedures in the emergency department. *Infect Dis Clin North Am.* 2008;22(1);117–143, vii
8. Pearson AS, Wolford RW. Management of skin trauma. *Prim Care.* 2000;27(2):475–492
9. Wedmore IS, Charette J. Emergency department evaluation and treatment of ankle and foot injuries. *Emerg Med Clin North Am.* 2000;18(1):85–113, vi

Skin Lesion (Moles or Growths)

1. Cokkinides V, Weinstock M, Lazovich D, Ward E, Thun M. Indoor tanning use among adolescents in the US, 1998 to 2004. *Cancer.* 2009;115(1):190–198
2. Dewberry C, Norman RA. Skin cancer in elderly patients. *Dermatol Clin.* 2004; 22(1): 93–96, vii
3. Jerant AF, Johnson JT, Sheridan CD, Caffrey TJ. Early detection and treatment of skin cancer. *Am Fam Physician.* 2000;62(2):357–382
4. US Preventive Services Task Force. Screening for skin cancer—including counseling to prevent skin cancer. In: *Guide to Clinical Preventive Services.* 2nd ed. Alexandria, VA: International Medical Publishing, Inc; 1996:141–152

Sore Throat

1. Belleza WG, Kalman S. Otolaryngologic emergencies in the outpatient setting. *Med Clin North Am.* 2006;90(2):329–353
2. Bisno AL, Gerber MA, Gwaltney JM Jr, Kaplan EL, Schwartz RH; and the Infectious Diseases Society of America. Practice guidelines for the diagnosis and management of group A streptococcal pharyngitis. *Clin Infect Dis.* 2002;35(2):113–125
3. Clancy CM, Centor RM, Campbell MS, Dalton HP. Rational decision making based on history: adult sore throats. *J Gen Intern Med.* 1988;3(3):213–217
4. Cooper RJ, Hoffman JR, Bartlett JG, et al. Principles of appropriate antibiotic use for acute pharyngitis in adults: background. *Ann Intern Med.* 2001;134(6):509–517
5. Eccles R. Understanding the symptoms of the common cold and influenza. *Lancet Infect Dis.* 2005;5(11):718–725
6. Gerber MA, Baltimore RS, Eaton CB, et al. Prevention of rheumatic fever and diagnosis and treatment of acute streptococcal pharyngitis: a scientific statement from the American Heart Association. *Circulation.* 2009;119(11):1541–1551
7. Green SM. Acute pharyngitis: the case for empiric antimicrobial therapy. *Ann Emerg Med.* 1995;25(3):404–406
8. Kerdemelidis M, Lennon D, Arroll B, Peat B. Guidelines for sore throat management in New Zealand. *N Z Med J.* 2009;122(1301): 10–18
9. Kljakovic M, Crampton P. Sore throat management in New Zealand general practice. *N Z Med J.* 2005;118(1220):U1609
10. Komaroff AL, Pass TM, Aronson MD, et al. The prediction of streptococcal pharyngitis in adults. *J Gen Intern Med.* 1986;1(1):1–7
11. Del Mar CB, Glasziou PP, Spinks AB. Antibiotics for sore throat. *Cochrane Database Syst Rev.* 2004;(4):CD000023
12. Matsuda A, Tanaka H, Kanaya T, Kamata K, Hasegawa M. Peritonsillar abscess: a study of 724 cases in Japan. *Ear Nose Throat J.* 2002;81(6):384–389
13. McIsaac WJ, Kellner JD, Aufricht P, Vanjaka A, Low DE. Empirical validation of guidelines for the management of pharyngitis in children and adults [published correction appears in *JAMA.* 2005;294(21): 2700]. *JAMA.* 2004;291(13):1587–1595
14. Peter J, Ray CG. Infectious mononucleosis. *Pediatr Rev.* 1998;19(8): 276–279
15. van Driel ML, De Sutter A, Deveugele M, et al. Are sore throat patients who hope for antibiotics actually asking for pain relief? *Ann Fam Med.* 2006;4(6):494–499

Spider Bite

1. Anderson PC. Spider bites in the United States. *Dermatol Clin.* 1997;15(2):307–311
2. Blaikie AJ, Ellis J, Sanders R, MacEwen CJ. Eye disease associated with handling pet tarantulas: three case reports. *BMJ.* 1997;314(7093): 1524–1525
3. Clark RF, Wethern-Kestner S, Vance MV, Gerkin R. Clinical presentation and treatment of black widow spider envenomation: a review of 163 cases. *Ann Emerg Med.* 1992;21(7):782–787
4. Derlet RW, Richards JR. Cellulitis from insect bites: a case series. *Cal J Emerg Med.* 2003;4(2):27–30
5. Diaz JH, Leblanc KE. Common spider bites. *Am Fam Physician.* 2007;75(6):869–873
6. Glavas SN Necrotic wound on the hand. *Am Fam Physician.* 2008;78(10):1209–1210
7. Goddard J, Upshaw S, Held D, Johnnson K. Severe reaction from envenomation by the brown widow spider, Latrodectus geometricus (Araneae: Theridiidae). *South Med J.* 2008;101(12):1269–1270
8. Gorwitz RJ, Jernigan DB, Powers JH, Jernigan JA; and the Participants in the CDC-Convened Experts' Meeting on Management of MRSA in the Community. Strategies for clinical management of MRSA in the community: summary of an experts' meeting convened by the Centers for Disease Control and Prevention. 2006. http://www.cdc.gov/mrsa/pdf/MRSA-Strategies-ExpMtgSummary-2006.pdf. Accessed July 31, 2012
9. Sams HH, Dunnick CA, Smith ML, King LE Jr. Necrotic arachnidism. *J Am Acad Dermatol.* 2001;44(4):561–576
10. Singletary EM, Rochman AS, Bodmer JC, Holstege CP. Envenomations. *Med Clin North Am.* 2005;89(6); 1195–1224
11. Steen CJ, Carbonaro PA, Schwartz RA. Arthropods in dermatology. *J Am Acad Dermatol.* 2004;50(6):819–844
12. Suchard JR. Diagnosis and treatment of cutaneous anthrax. *JAMA.* 2002;288(1):43–44
13. Suchard JR. Spider bite. *Ann Emerg Med.* 2009;54(1):8, 11
14. Swanson DL, Vetter RS. Bites of brown recluse spiders and suspected necrotic arachnidism. *N Eng J Med.* 2005;352(7):700–707
15. Wright SW, Wrenn KD, Murray L, Seger D. Clinical presentation and outcome of brown recluse spider bite. *Ann Emerg Med.* 1997;30(1): 28–32

STD Exposure and Prevention

1. Advisory Committee on Immunization Practices. Recommended adult immunization schedule: United States, 2011. *Ann Intern Med.* 2011;154(3):168–173
2. Braverman PK. Sexually transmitted diseases in adolescents. *Med Clin North Am.* 2000;84(4):869–889, vi–vii
3. Kodner C. Sexually transmitted infections in men. *Prim Care.* 2003;30(1):173–191
4. Miller KE. Women's health. Sexually transmitted diseases. *Prim Care.* 1997;24(1):179–193
5. Public Health Agency of Canada. Primary care and sexually transmitted infections. In: *Canadian Guidelines on Sexually Transmitted Infections.* 2006 Edition. Ottawa, Ontario: Public Health Agency of Canada; 2006:7–29. http://pubs.cpha.ca/PDF/P37/23384.pdf. Accessed July 31, 2012
6. Workowski KA, Berman S; and the Centers for Disease Control and Prevention. Sexually transmitted diseases treatment guidelines, 2010 [published correction appears in *MMWR Recomm Rep.* 2011;60(1):18]. *MMWR Recomm Rep.* 2010;59(RR-12):1–110

Strep Throat Test (Follow-up Call)

1. Bisno AL, Gerber MA, Gwaltney JM Jr, Kaplan EL, Schwartz RH. Diagnosis and management of group A streptococcal pharyngitis: a practice guideline. *Clin Infect Dis.* 1997;25(3):574–583
2. Bisno AL, Gerber MA, Gwaltney JM Jr, Kaplan EL, Schwartz RH; and the Infectious Diseases Society of America. Practice guidelines for the diagnosis and management of group A streptococcal pharyngitis. *Clin Infect Dis.* 2002;35(2):113–125
3. Clancy CM, Centor RM, Campbell MS, Dalton HP. Rational decision making based on history: adult sore throats. *J Gen Intern Med.* 1988;3(3):213–217
4. Cooper RJ, Hoffman JR, Bartlett JG, et al. Principles of appropriate antibiotic use for acute pharyngitis in adults: background. *Ann Intern Med.* 2001;134(6):509–517
5. Gerber MA, Baltimore RS, Eaton CB, et al. Prevention of rheumatic fever and diagnosis and treatment of acute Streptococcal pharyngitis: a scientific statement from the American Heart Association. *Circulation.* 2009;119(11):1541–1551
6. Green SM. Acute pharyngitis: the case for empiric antimicrobial therapy. *Ann Emerg Med.* 1995;25(3):404–406
7. Kerdemelidis M, Lennon D, Arroll B, Peat B. Guidelines for sore throat management in New Zealand. *N Z Med J.* 2009;122(1301): 10–18
8. Kljakovic M, Crampton P. Sore throat management in New Zealand general practice. *N Z Med J.* 2005;118(1220):U1609
9. Komaroff AL, Pass TM, Aronson MD, et al. The prediction of streptococcal pharyngitis in adults. *J Gen Intern Med.* 1986;1(1): 1–7
10. McIsaac WJ, Kellner JD, Aufricht P, Vanjaka A, Low DE. Empirical validation of guidelines for the management of pharyngitis in children and adults [published correction appears in *JAMA.* 2005;294(21):2700]. *JAMA.* 2004;291(13):1587–1595
11. van Driel ML, De Sutter A, Deveugele M, et al. Are sore throat patients who hope for antibiotics actually asking for pain relief? *Ann Fam Med.* 2006;4(6):494–499

Substance Abuse and Dependence

1. Camí J, Farré M. Drug addiction. *N Engl J Med.* 2003;349(10):975–986
2. Cleary M, Hunt G, Matheson S, Siegfried N, Walter G. Psychosocial interventions for people with both severe mental illness and substance misuse. *Cochrane Database Syst Rev.* 2008;(1):CD001088
3. Giannini AJ. An approach to drug abuse, intoxication, and withdrawal. *Am Fam Physician.* 2000;61(9):2763–2774
4. Knight JR. A 35-year-old physician with opioid dependence. *JAMA.* 2004;292(11):1351–1357
5. McRae AL. Alcohol and substance abuse. *Med Clin North Am.* 2001;85(3):779–801
6. Sowers W, George C, Thompson K. Level of care utilization system for psychiatric and addiction services (LOCUS): a preliminary assessment of reliability and validity. *Community Ment Health J.* 1999;35(6):545–563
7. Stein MD. Medical consequences of substance abuse. *Psychiatr Clin North Am.* 1999;22(2):351–370
8. Williams JF, Kokotailo PK. Abuse of proprietary (over-the-counter) drugs. *Adolesc Med Clin.* 2006;17(3):733–750, xiii
9. Williams JF, Storck M; and the American Academy of Pediatrics Committee on Substance Abuse, Committee on Native American Child Health. Inhalant abuse. *Pediatrics.* 2007;119(5):1009–1017
10. Zealberg JJ, Brady KT. Substance abuse and emergency psychiatry. *Psychiatr Clin North Am.* 1999;22(4):803–817

Suicide Concerns

1. American Psychiatric Association. Practice guideline for the assessment and treatment of patients with suicidal behaviors. http://www.renepca.com/docs1/pg_suicidalbehaviors.pdf. Accessed July 31, 2012
2. Conwell Y, Lyness JM, Duberstein P, et al. Completed suicide among older patients in primary care practices: a controlled study. *J Am Geriatr Soc.* 2000;48(1):23–29
3. Doshi A, Boudreaux ED, Wang N, Pelletier AJ, Camargo CA Jr. National study of US emergency department visits for attempted suicide and self-inflicted injury, 1997–2001. *Ann Emerg Med.* 2005;46(4):369–375
4. Gibb SJ, Beautrais AL, Fergusson DM. Mortality and further suicidal behaviour after an index suicide attempt: a 10-year study. *Aust N Z J Psychiatry.* 2005;39(1-2):95–100
5. Harwitz D, Ravizza L. Suicide and depression. *Emerg Med Clin North Am.* 2000;18(2):263–271, ix
6. Suominen K, Isometsa E, Haukka J, Lonnqvist J. Substance use and male gender as risk factors for deaths and suicide—a 5-year follow-up study after deliberate self-harm. *Soc Psychiatry Psychiatr Epidemiol.* 2004;39(9):720–724
7. Suominen K, Isometsa E, Ostamo A, Lonnqvist J. Level of suicidal intent predicts overall mortality and suicide after attempted suicide: a 12-year follow-up study. *BMC Psychiatry.* 2004;4:11
8. Szewczyk M, Chennault SA. Women's health. Depression and related disorders. *Prim Care.* 1997;24(1):83–101
9. US Preventive Services Task Force. Screening for suicide risk. In: *Guide to Clinical Preventive Services.* 2nd ed. Alexandria, VA: International Medical Publishing, Inc; 1996:547–554
10. Wiebe DJ. Homicide and suicide risks associated with firearms in the home: a national case-control study. *Ann Emerg Med.* 2003;41(6):771–782

Sunburn

1. Cokkinides V, Weinstock M, Lazovich D, Ward E, Thun M. Indoor tanning use among adolescents in the US, 1998 to 2004. *Cancer.* 2009;115(1):190–198
2. Debuys HV, Levy SB, Murray JC, Madey DL, Pinnell SR. Modern approaches to photoprotection. *Dermatol Clin.* 2000;18(4):577–590
3. Duteil L, Queille-Roussel C, Lorenz B, Thieroff-Ekerdt R, Ortonne JP. A randomized, controlled trial of the safety and efficacy of topical corticosteroid treatments of sunburn in healthy volunteers. *Clin Exp Dermatol.* 2002;27(4):314–318
4. Eberlein-Konig B, Placzek M, Przybilla B. Protective effect against sunburn of combined systemic ascorbic acid (vitamin C) and d-alpha-tocopherol (vitamin E). *J Am Acad Dermatol.* 1998;38(1): 45–48
5. Elliott B, Silverman PR. Keratoconjunctivitis caused by a broken high-intensity mercury-vapor lamp. *Del Med J.* 1986;58(10):665–667
6. Hatch KL, Osterwalder U. Garments as solar ultraviolet radiation screening materials. *Dermatol Clin.* 2006;24(1):85–100
7. Kirschke DL, Jones TF, Smith NM, Schaffner W. Photokeratitis and UV-radiation burns associated with damaged metal halide lamps. *Arch Pediatr Adolesc Med.* 2004;158(4):372–376
8. Kullavanijaya P, Lim HW. Photoprotection. *J Am Acad Dermatol.* 2005;52(6):937–962
9. Lim HW, Cooper K. The health impact of solar radiation and prevention strategies: report of the Environment Council, American Academy of Dermatology. *J Am Acad Dermatol.* 1999;41(1):81–99
10. Lincoln EA. Sun-induced skin changes. *Prim Care.* 2000;27(2): 435–445

11. Lowe NJ. An overview of ultraviolet radiation, sunscreens, and photo-induced dermatoses. *Dermatol Clin.* 2006;24(1):9–17
12. Prevention and treatment of sunburn. *Med Lett Drugs Ther.* 2004;46(1184):45–46
13. Morgan ED, Bledsoe SC, Barker J. Ambulatory management of burns. *Am Fam Physician.* 2000;62(9):2015–2032
14. Olson AL, Starr P. The challenge of intentional tanning in teens and young adults. *Dermatol Clin.* 2006;24(2):131–136, v
15. Thun MJ, Altman R, Ellingson O, Mills LF, Talansky ML. Ocular complications of malfunctioning mercury vapor lamps. *Ann Ophthalmol.* 1982;14(11):1017–1020
16. World Health Organization. Ultraviolet radiation and human health. Fact sheet No. 305. 2009. July 2006. http://www.who.int/mediacentre/factsheets/fs305/en/index.html. Accessed July 31, 2012

Suture or Staple Questions

1. Dire DJ, Coppola M, Dwyer DA, Lorette JJ, Karr JL. Prospective evaluation of topical antibiotics for preventing infections in uncomplicated soft-tissue wounds repaired in the ED. *Acad Emerg Med.* 1995;2(1):4–10
2. Hollander JE, Singer AJ, Valentine SM, Shofer FS. Risk factors for infection in patients with traumatic lacerations. *Acad Emerg Med.* 2001;8(7):716–720
3. Hollander JE, Singer AJ. Laceration management. *Ann Emerg Med.* 1999;34(3):356–367
4. Kaye ET. Topical antibacterial agents. *Infect Dis Clin North Am.* 2000;14(2):321–339
5. Khoosal D, Goldman RD. Vitamin E for treating children's scars. Does it help reduce scarring? *Can Fam Physician.* 2006;52(7):855–856
6. Pearson AS, Wolford RW. Management of skin trauma. *Prim Care.* 2000;27(2):475–492
7. Thomsen TW, Barclay DA, Setnik GS. Videos in clinical medicine. Basic laceration repair. *N Engl J Med.* 2006;355(17):e18

Tick Bite

1. Edlow JA. Lyme disease and related tick-borne illnesses. *Ann Emerg Med.* 1999;33(6):680–693
2. Koren G, Matsui D, Bailey B. DEET-based insect repellants: safety implications for children and pregnant and lactating women. *CMAJ.* 2003;169(3):209–212
3. Nadelman RB, Nowakowski J, Fish D, et al. Prophylaxis with single-dose doxycycline for the prevention of Lyme disease after an ixodes scapularis tick bite. *N Engl J Med.* 2001;345(2):79–84
4. Needham GR. Evaluation of five popular methods for tick removal. *Pediatrics.* 1985;75(6):997–1002
5. US Environmental Protection Agency. Using insect repellents safely. http://epa.gov/pesticides/insect/safe.htm. Accessed July 31, 2012
6. Ozuah PO. Tick removal. *Pediatr Rev.* 1998;19(8):280
7. Shapiro ED. Doxycycline for tick bites – not for everyone. *N Engl J Med.* 2001;345(2):133–134
8. Steere AC. Lyme disease. *N Engl J Med.* 2001;345(2):115–125
9. Tibbles CD, Edlow JA. Does this patient have erythema migrans? *JAMA.* 2007;297(23):2617–2627
10. Warshafsky S, Nowakowski J, Nadelman RB, Kamer RS, Peterson SJ, Wormser GP. Efficacy of antibiotic prophylaxis for prevention of Lyme disease. *J Gen Intern Med.* 1996;11(6):329–333
11. Wormser GP, Nadelman RB, Dattwyler RJ, et al. Practice guidelines for the treatment of Lyme disease. *Clin Infect Dis.* 2000;31(1 suppl): 1–14

Toothache

1. Annino DJ Jr, Goguen LA. Pain from the oral cavity. *Otolaryngol Clin North Am.* 2003;36(6):1127–1135, vi–vii
2. Douglass AB, Douglass JM. Common dental emergencies. *Am Fam Physician.* 2003;67(3):511–516
3. Flynn TR. The swollen face. Severe odontogenic infections. *Emerg Med Clin North Am.* 2000;18(3):481–519
4. Ma M, Lindsell CJ, Jauch ED, Pancioli AM. Effect of education and guidelines for treatment of uncomplicated dental pain on patient provider behavior. *Ann Emerg Med.* 2004;44(4):323–329
5. MacDonald DE. Principles of geriatric dentistry and their application to the older adult with a physical disability. *Clin Geriatr Med.* 2006;22(2):413–434, x
6. Nguyen DH, Martin JT. Common dental infections in the primary care setting. *Am Fam Physician.* 2008;77(6):797–802

Trauma, Ankle and Foot

1. American Heart Association. 2005 Guidelines for Cardiopulmonary Resuscitation and Emergency Cardiovascular Care. Part 14: First aid. *Circulation.* 2005;112(24 suppl):IV-196–IV-203
2. Bachmann LM, Kolb E, Koller MT, Steurer J, ter Riet G. Accuracy of Ottawa ankle rules to exclude fractures of the ankle and mid-foot: a systematic review. *BMJ.* 2003;326(7386):417
3. Bleakley C, McDonough S, MacAuley D. The use of ice in the treatment of acute soft-tissue injury: a systematic review of randomized controlled trials. *Am J Sports Med.* 2004;32(1):251–261
4. Boyce SH, Quigley MA, Campbell S. Management of ankle sprains: a randomized controlled trial of the treatment of inversion injuries using an elastic support bandage or an Aircast ankle brace. *Br J Sports Med.* 2005;39(2):91–96
5. Clanton TO, Porter DA. Primary care of foot and ankle injuries in the athlete. *Clin Sports Med.* 1997;16(3):435–466
6. Collins NC. Is ice right? Does cryotherapy improve outcome for acute soft tissue injury? *Emerg Med J.* 2008;25(2):65–68
7. Dake AD, Stack L. Penetrating trauma to the extremities: systematic assessment and targeted management of weapons-related injuries. *Emerg Med Rep.* 1997;18(7):65–74
8. Dalton JD Jr, Schweinle JE. Randomized controlled noninferiority trial to compare extended release acetaminophen and ibuprofen for the treatment of ankle sprains. *Ann Emerg Med.* 2006;48(5):615–623
9. Hocutt JE Jr, Jaffe R, Rylander CR, Beebe JK. Cryotherapy in ankle sprains. *Am J Sports Med.* 1982;10(5):316–319
10. Kellett J. Acute soft tissue injuries—a review of the literature. *Med Sci Sports Exerc.* 1986;18(5):489–500
11. Kerkhoffs GM, Struijs PA, Marti RK, Assendelft WJ, Blankevoort L, van Dijk CN. Different functional treatment strategies for acute lateral ankle ligament injuries in adults. *Cochrane Database Syst Rev.* 2002;(3):CD002938
12. Kretsinger K, Broder KR, Cortese MM, et al. Preventing tetanus, diphtheria, and pertussis among adults: use of tetanus toxoid, reduced diphtheria toxoid and acellular pertussis vaccine recommendations of the Advisory Committee on Immunization Practices (ACIP) and recommendation of ACIP, supported by the Healthcare Infection Control Practices Advisory Committee (HICPAC), for use of Tdap among health-care personnel. *MMWR Recomm Rep.* 2006;55(RR-17):1–37
13. Lavery LA, Armstrong DG, Wunderlich RP, Mohler MJ, Wendel CS, Lipsky BA. Risk factors for foot infections in individuals with diabetes. *Diabetes Care.* 2006;29(6):1288–1293

Trauma, Ankle and Foot (continued)

14. Markert RJ, Walley ME, Guttman TG, Mehta R. A pooled analysis of the Ottawa ankle rules used on adults in the ED. *Am J Emerg Med.* 1998;16(6):564–567
15. McMaster WC, Liddle S, Waugh TR. Laboratory evaluation of various cold therapy modalities. *Am J Sports Med.* 1978;6(5):291–294
16. Moran GJ, Talan DA, Abrahamian FM. Antimicrobial prophylaxis for wounds and procedures in the emergency department. *Infect Dis Clin North Am.* 2008;22(1):117–143, vii
17. Stiell IG, McKnight RD, Greenberg GH, et al. Implementation of the Ottawa ankle rules. *JAMA.* 1994;271(11):827–832
18. Wedmore IS, Charette J. Emergency department evaluation and treatment of ankle and foot injuries. *Emerg Med Clin North Am.* 2000;18(1):85–113, vi

Trauma, Elbow

1. American Heart Association. 2005 Guidelines for Cardiopulmonary Resuscitation and Emergency Cardiovascular Care. Part 14: First aid. *Circulation.* 2005;112(24 suppl):IV-196–IV-203
2. Barry NN, McGuire JL. Acute injuries and specific problems in adult athletes. *Rheum Dis Clin North Am.* 1996;22(3):531–549
3. Brady WJ, Degnan GG, Buchanon LP, Schwartz S, Chhabra A. Challenging and elusive orthopedic injuries: diagnostic and treatment strategies for optimizing clinical outcomes. Part 1: upper extremity fractures and dislocations. *Emerg Med Rep.* 1999;20(9):87–98
4. Collins NC. Is ice right? Does cryotherapy improve outcome for acute soft tissue injury? *Emerg Med J.* 2008;25(2):65–68
5. Colman WW, Strauch RJ. Physical examination of the elbow. *Orthop Clin North Am.* 1999;30(1):15–20
6. Kellett J. Acute soft tissue injuries—a review of the literature. *Med Sci Sports Exerc.* 1986;18(5):489–500
7. McMaster WC, Liddle S, Waugh TR. Laboratory evaluation of various cold therapy modalities. *Am J Sports Med.* 1978;6(5):291–294
8. Pimentel L. Orthopedic trauma: office management of major joint injury. *Med Clin North Am.* 2006;90(2):355–382

Trauma, Eye

1. American Heart Association. 2005 Guidelines for Cardiopulmonary Resuscitation and Emergency Cardiovascular Care. Part 14: First aid. *Circulation.* 2005;112(24 suppl):IV-196–IV-203
2. Crumpton KL, Shockley LW. Ocular trauma: a quick illustrated guide to treatment, triage, and medicolegal implications. *Emerg Med Rep.* 1997;18(23):223–234
3. Harlan JB Jr, Pieramici DJ. Evaluation of patients with ocular trauma. *Ophthalmol Clin North Am.* 2002;15(2):153–161
4. Kaiser PK. A comparison of pressure patching versus no patching for corneal abrasions due to trauma or foreign body removal. *Ophthalmology.* 1995;102(12):1936–1942
5. Markoff DD, Chacko D. Common ophthalmologic emergencies: examination, differential diagnosis, and targeted management. *Emerg Med Rep.* 1999;20(1):1–12
6. Naradzay J, Barish RA. Approach to ophthalmologic emergencies. *Med Clin North Am.* 2006;90(2):305–328, vii–viii
7. Rubin S, Hallagan L. Lids, lacrimals, and lashes. *Emerg Med Clin North Am.* 1995;13(3):631–648
8. Wilson SA, Last A. Management of corneal abrasions. *Am Fam Physician.* 2004;70(1):123–128

Trauma, Finger

1. American Heart Association. 2005 Guidelines for Cardiopulmonary Resuscitation and Emergency Cardiovascular Care. Part 14: First aid. *Circulation.* 2005;112(24 suppl):IV-196–IV-203
2. Collins NC. Is ice right? Does cryotherapy improve outcome for acute soft tissue injury? *Emerg Med J.* 2008;25(2):65–68
3. Harrison BP, Hillard MW. Emergency department evaluation and treatment of hand injuries. *Emerg Med Clin North Am.* 1999;17(4): 793–822, v
4. Hogan CJ, Ruland RT. High-pressure injection injuries to the upper extremity: a review of the literature. *J Orthop Trauma.* 2006;20(7): 503–511
5. Kretsinger K, Broder KR, Cortese MM, et al. Preventing tetanus, diphtheria, and pertussis among adults: use of tetanus toxoid, reduced diphtheria toxoid and acellular pertussis vaccine recommendations of the Advisory Committee on Immunization Practices (ACIP) and recommendation of ACIP, supported by the Healthcare Infection Control Practices Advisory Committee (HICPAC), for use to Tdap among health-care personnel. *MMWR Recomm Rep.* 2006;55(RR-17):1–37
6. Leggit JC, Meko CJ. Acute finger injuries: part I. Tendons and ligaments. *Am Fam Physician.* 2006;73(5):810–816
7. Leggit JC, Meko CJ. Acute finger injuries: part II. Fractures, dislocations, and thumb injuries. *Am Fam Physician.* 2006;73(5): 827–834
8. Mastey RD, Weiss AP, Akelman E. Primary care of hand and wrist athletic injuries. *Clin Sports Med.* 1997;16(4):705–724
9. Wang QC, Johnson BA. Fingertip injuries. *Am Fam Physician.* 2001;63(10):1961–1966

Trauma, Hand and Wrist

1. American Heart Association. 2005 Guidelines for Cardiopulmonary Resuscitation and Emergency Cardiovascular Care. Part 14: First aid. *Circulation.* 2005;112(24 suppl):IV-196–IV-203
2. Brady WJ, Degnan GG, Buchanon LP, Schwartz S, Chhabra A. Challenging and elusive orthopedic injuries: diagnostic and treatment strategies for optimizing clinical outcomes. Part I: upper extremity fractures and dislocations. *Emerg Med Rep.* 1999;20(9):87–98
3. Collins NC. Is ice right? Does cryotherapy improve outcome for acute soft tissue injury? *Emerg Med J.* 2008;25(2):65–68
4. Gonzalez R, Kasdan ML. High pressure injection injuries of the hand. *Clin Occup Environ Med.* 2006;5(2):407–411, ix
5. Harrison BP, Hillard MW. Emergency department evaluation and treatment of hand injuries. *Emerg Med Clin North Am.* 1999;17(4):793–822, v
6. Hogan CJ, Ruland RT. High-pressure injection injuries to the upper extremity: a review of the literature. *J Orthop Trauma.* 2006;20(7): 503–511
7. Kretsinger K, Broder KR, Cortese MM, et al. Preventing tetanus, diphtheria, and pertussis among adults: use of tetanus toxoid, reduced diphtheria toxoid and acellular pertussis vaccine recommendations of the Advisory Committee on Immunization Practices (ACIP) and recommendation of ACIP, supported by the Healthcare Infection Control Practices Advisory Committee (HICPAC), for use of Tdap among health-care personnel. *MMWR Recomm Rep.* 2006;55(RR-17):1–37
8. Mastey RD, Weiss AP, Akelman E. Primary care of hand and wrist athletic injuries. *Clin Sports Med.* 1997;16(4):705–724
9. McMaster WC, Liddle S, Waugh TR. Laboratory evaluation of various cold therapy modalities. *Am J Sports Med.* 1978;6(5):291–294

10. Parmelee-Peters K, Eathorne SW. The wrist: common injuries and management. *Prim Care.* 2005;32(1):35–70
11. Pimentel L. Orthopedic trauma: office management of major joint injury. *Med Clin North Am.* 2006;90(2):355–382

Trauma, Head

1. American Academy of Neurology Quality Standards Subcommittee. Practice parameter: the management of concussion in sports (summary statement). *Neurology.* 1997;48(3):581–585
2. American Heart Association. 2005 Guidelines for Cardiopulmonary Resuscitation and Emergency Cardiovascular Care. Part 10: First aid. *Circulation.* 2005;112(24 suppl):IV-196–IV-203
3. Benson BW, Meeuwisse WH, Rizos J, Kang J, Burke CJ. A prospective study of concussions among National Hockey League players during regular season games: the NHL-NHLPA Concussion Program. *CMAJ.* 2011;183(8):905–911
4. Borczuk P. Mild head trauma. *Emerg Med Clin North Am.* 1997;15(3): 563–579
5. Borczuk P. Predictors of intracranial injury in patients with mild head trauma. *Ann Emerg Med.* 1995;25(6):731–736
6. Bracken ME, Medzon R, Rathlev NK, Mower WR, Hoffman JR. Effect of intoxication among blunt trauma patients selected for head computed tomography scanning. *Ann Emerg Med.* 2007;49(1):45–51
7. Roberts I, Yates D, Sandercock P, et al; and the CRASH Trial Collaborators. Effect of inravenous corticosteroids on death within 14 days in 10,008 adults wth clinically significant head injury (MRC CRASH trial): randomized placebo-controlled trial. *Lancet.* 2004;364(9442):1321–1328
8. Eikelboom JW, Wallentin L, Connolly SJ, et al. Risk of bleeding with 2 doses of dabigatran compared with warfarin in older and younger patients with atrial fibrillation: an analysis of the randomized evaluation of long-term anticoagulant therapy (RE-LY) trial. *Circulation.* 2011;123(21):2363–2372
9. Halstead ME, Walter KD; and the American Academy of Pediatrics Council on Sports Medicine and Fitness. Clinical report—sport-related concussion in children and adolescents. *Pediatrics.* 2010;126(3):597–615
10. Haydel MJ, Preston CA, Mills TJ, Luber S, Blaudeau E, DeBlieux PM. Indications for CT in patients with minor head injury. *N Engl J Med.* 2000;343(2):100–105
11. Jagoda AS, Cantrill SV, Wears RL, et al. Clinical policy: neuroimaging and decisionmaking in adult mild traumatic brain injury in the acute setting. *Ann Emerg Med.* 2002;40(2):231–249
12. Kuppermann N, Holmes JF, Dayan PS, et al. Identification of children at very low risk of clinically-important brain injuries after head trauma: a prospective cohort study. *Lancet.* 2009;374(9696): 1160–1170
13. McCrea M, Guskiewicz KM, Marshall SW, et al. Acute effects and recovery time following concussion in collegiate football players: the NCAA Concussion Study. *JAMA.* 2003;290(19):2556–2563
14. McCrory P, Meeuwisse W, Johnston K, et al. Consensus statement on concussion in sport. 3rd International Conference on Concussion in Sport held in Zurich, November 2008. *Clin J Sport Med.* 2009;19(3):185–200
15. Nee PA, Hadfield JM, Yates DW, Faragher EB. Significance of vomiting after head injury. *J Neurol Neurosurg Psychiatry.* 1999;66(4):470–473
16. Stiell IG, Wells GA, Vandemheen K, et al. The Canadian CT Head Rule for patients with minor head injury. *Lancet.* 2001;357(9266): 1391–1396
17. Teasdale G, Jennett B. Assessment of coma and impaired consciousness. A practical scale. *Lancet.* 1974;2(7872):81–84

Trauma, Hip

1. American Heart Association. 2005 Guidelines for Cardiopulmonary Resuscitation and Emergency Cardiovascular Care. Part 14: First aid. *Circulation.* 2005;112(24 suppl):IV-196–IV-203
2. Brunner LC, Eshilian-Oates, Kuo TY. Hip fractures. *Am Fam Physician.* 2003;67(3):537–542
3. Collins NC. Is ice right? Does cryotherapy improve outcome for acute soft tissue injury? *Emerg Med J.* 2008;25(2):65–68
4. Dake AD, Stack L. Penetrating trauma to the extremities: systematic assessment and targeted management of weapons-related injuries. *Emerg Med Rep.* 1997;18(7):65–74
5. Rudman N. Emergency department evaluation and treatment of hip and thigh injuries. *Emerg Med Clin North Am.* 2000;18(1):29–66, v

Trauma, Knee

1. American Heart Association. 2005 Guidelines for Cardiopulmonary Resuscitation and Emergency Cardiovascular Care. Part 14: First aid. *Circulation.* 2005;112(24 suppl):IV-196–IV-203
2. Collins NC. Is ice right? Does cryotherapy improve outcome for acute soft tissue injury? *Emerg Med J.* 2008;25(2):65–68
3. Dake AD, Stack L. Penetrating trauma to the extremities: systematic assessment and targeted management of weapons-related injuries. *Emerg Med Rep.* 1997;18(7):65–74
4. Fadale PD, Hulstyn MJ. Common athletic knee injuries. *Clin Sports Med.* 1997;16(3):479–499
5. Kellett J. Acute soft tissue injuries—a review of the literature. *Med Sci Sports Exerc.* 1986;18(5):489–500
6. Kretsinger K, Broder KR, Cortese MM, et al. Preventing tetanus, diphtheria, and pertussis among adults: use of tetanus toxoid, reduced diphtheria toxoid and acellular pertussis vaccine recommendations of the Advisory Committee on Immunization Practices (ACIP) and recommendation of ACIP, supported by the Healthcare Infection Control Practices Advisory Committee (HICPAC), for use of Tdap among health-care personnel. *MMWR Recomm Rep.* 2006;55(RR-17):1–37
7. McMaster WC, Liddle S, Waugh TR. Laboratory evaluation of various cold therapy modalities. *Am J Sports Med.* 1978;6(5):291–294
8. Pimentel L. Orthopedic trauma: office management of major joint injury. *Med Clin North Am.* 2006;90(2):355–382
9. Roberts DM, Stallard TC. Emergency department evaluation and treatment of knee and leg injuries. *Emerg Med Clin North Am.* 2000;18(1):67–84, v–vi
10. Seaberg DC, Yealy DM, Lukens T, Auble T, Mathias S. Multicenter comparison of two clinical decision rules for the use of radiography in acute, high-risk knee injuries. *Ann Emerg Med.* 1998;32(1):8–13
11. Solomon DH, Simel DL, Bates DW, Katz JN, Schaffer JL. Does this patient have a torn meniscus or ligament of the knee? Value of the physical examination. *JAMA.* 2001;286(13):1610–1620
12. Stewart C. Knee injuries: diagnosis and repair. *Emerg Med Rep.* 1997;18(1):1–12

Trauma, Mouth

1. American Heart Association. 2005 Guidelines for Cardiopulmonary Resuscitation and Emergency Cardiovascular Care. Part 14: First aid. *Circulation.* 2005;112(24 suppl):IV-196–IV-203
2. Armstrong BD. Lacerations of the mouth. *Emerg Med Clin North Am.* 2000;18(3):471–480, vi
3. Benbadis SR, Wolgamuth BR, Goren H, Brener S, Fouad-Tarazi F. Value of tongue biting in the diagnosis of seizures. *Arch Intern Med.* 1995;155(21):2346–2349

Trauma, Mouth (continued)

4. Benbadis SR. The value of tongue laceration in the diagnosis of blackouts. *Am Fam Physician.* 2004;70(9):1757–1758
5. Colucciello SA. The treacherous and complex spectrum of maxillofacial trauma: etiologies, evaluation, and emergency stabilization. *Emerg Med Rep.* 1995;16(7):59–70
6. Dale RA. Dentoalveolar trauma. *Emerg Med Clin North Am.* 2000;18(3)521–538
7. Howes DS, Dowling PJ. Triage and initial evaluation of the oral facial emergency. *Emerg Med Clin North Am.* 2000;18(3):371–378
8. Lamell CW, Fraone G, Casamassimo PS, Wilson S. Presenting characteristics and treatment outcomes for tongue lacerations in children. *Pediatr Dent.* 1999;21(1):34–38

Trauma, Nose

1. American Heart Association. 2005 Guidelines for Cardiopulmonary Resuscitation and Emergency Cardiovascular Care. Part 14: First aid. *Circulation.* 2005;112(24 suppl):IV-196–IV-203
2. Belleza WG, Kalman S. Otolaryngologic emergencies in the outpatient setting. *Med Clin North Am.* 2006;90(2):329–353
3. Collins NC. Is ice right? Does cryotherapy improve outcome for acute soft tissue injury? *Emerg Med J.* 2008;25(2):65–68
4. Coluciello SA. The treacherous and complex spectrum of maxillofacial trauma: etiologies, evaluation, and emergency stabilization. *Emerg Med Rep.* 1995;16(7):59–70
5. Junnila J. Swollen masses in the nose. *Am Fam Physician.* 2006;73(9): 1617–1618
6. Kaufman BR, Heckler FR. Sports-related facial injuries. *Clin Sports Med.* 1997;16(3):543–562
7. Kucik CJ, Clenney T, Phelan J. Management of acute nasal fractures. *Am Fam Physician.* 2004;70(7):1315–1320
8. Li S, Papsin B, Brown DH. Value of nasal radiographs in nasal trauma management. *J Otolaryngol.* 1996;25(3):162–164
9. Savage RR, Valvich C. Hematoma of the nasal septum. *Pediatr Rev.* 2006;(12):478–479
10. Tan LK, Calhoun KH. Epistaxis. *Med Clin North Am.* 1999;83(1): 43–56

Trauma, Shoulder

1. American Heart Association. 2005 Guidelines for Cardiopulmonary Resuscitation and Emergency Cardiovascular Care. Part 14: First aid. *Circulation.* 2005;112(24 suppl):IV-196–IV-203
2. Belzer JP, Durkin RC. Common disorders of the shoulder. *Prim Care.* 1996;23(2):365–388
3. Bleakley C, McDonough S, MacAuley D. The use of ice in the treatment of acute soft-tissue injury: a systematic review of randomized controlled trials. *Am J Sports Med.* 2004;32(1):251–261
4. Brady WJ, Degnan GG, Buchanon LP, Schwartz S, Chhabra A. Challenging and elusive orthopedic injuries: diagnostic and treatment strategies for optimizing clinical outcomes. Part I: upper extremity fractures and dislocations. *Emerg Med Rep.* 1999;20(9):87–98
5. Collins NC. Is ice right? Does cryotherapy improve outcome for acute soft tissue injury? *Emerg Med J.* 2008;25(2):65–68
6. Daigneault JK, Cooney LM Jr. Shoulder pain in older people. *J Am Geriatr Soc.* 1998;46(9):1144–1151
7. Kellett J. Acute soft tissue injuries—a review of the literature. *Med Sci Sports Exerc.* 1986;18(5):489–500
8. McMaster WC, Liddle S, Waugh TR. Laboratory evaluation of various cold therapy modalities. *Am J Sports Med.* 1978;6(5):291–294
9. Pimentel L. Orthopedic trauma: office management of major joint injury. *Med Clin North Am.* 2006;90(2);355–382

Trauma, Skin

1. American College of Emergency Physicians. Clinical policy for the initial approach to patients presenting with penetrating extremity trauma. *Ann Emerg Med.* 1999;33(5):612–636
2. American Heart Association. 2005 Guidelines for Cardiopulmonary Resuscitation and Emergency Cardiovascular Care. Part 14: First aid. *Circulation.* 2005;112(24 suppl):IV-196–IV-203
3. Bleakley C, McDonough S, MacAuley D. The use of ice in the treatment of acute soft-tissue injury: a systematic review of randomized controlled trials. *Am J Sports Med.* 2004;32(1):251–261
4. Centers for Disease Control and Prevention (CDC). Updated recommendations for use of tetanus toxoid, reduced diphtheria toxoid and acellular pertussis (Tdap) vaccine from the Advisory Committee on Immunization Practices, 2010. *MMWR Morb Mortal Wkly Rep.* 2011;60(1):13–15
5. Centers for Disease Control and Prevention. Diptheria, tetanus, and pertussis: recommendations for vaccine use and other preventive measures. Recommendations of the Immunization Practices Advisory Committee (ACIP). *MMWR Recomm Rep.* 1991;40:(RR-10):1–28
6. Centers for Disease Control and Prevention Advisory Committee on Immunization Practices. Prevention of pertussis, tetanus, and diphtheria among pregnant and postpartum women and their infants recommendations of the Advisory Committee on Immunization Practices (ACIP). *MMWR Recomm Rep.* 2008;57:(RR-4):1–51
7. Collins NC. Is ice right? Does cryotherapy improve outcome for acute soft tissue injury? *Emerg Med J.* 2008;25(2):65–68
8. Dimick AR. Delayed wound closure: indications and techniques. *Ann Emerg Med.* 1988;17(12):1303–1304
9. Eaglstein WH, Sullivan T. Cyanoacrylates for skin closure. *Dermatol Clin.* 2005;23(2); 193–198
10. Gergen PJ, McQuillan GM, Kiely M, Ezzati-Rice TM, Sutter RW, Virella G. A population-based serologic survey of immunity to tetanus in the United States. *N Engl J Med.* 1995;332(12):761–766
11. Hollander JE, Singer AJ, Valentine SM, Shofer FS. Risk factors for infection in patients with traumatic lacerations. *Acad Emerg Med.* 2001;8(7):716–720
12. Hubbard TJ, Denegar CR. Does cryotherapy improve outcomes with soft tissue injury? *J Athl Train.* 2004;39(3):278–279
13. Kellett J. Acute soft tissue injuries—a review of the literature. *Med Sci Sports Exerc.* 1986;18(5):489–500
14. Kretsinger K, Broder KR, Cortese MM, et al. Preventing tetanus, diphtheria, and pertussis among adults: use of tetanus toxoid, reduced diphtheria toxoid and acellular pertussis vaccine recommendations of the Advisory Committee on Immunization Practices (ACIP) and recommendation of ACIP, supported by the Healthcare Infection Control Practices Advisory Committee (HICPAC), for use of Tdap among health-care personnel. *MMWR Recomm Rep.* 2006;55(RR-17):1–37
15. McMaster WC, Liddle S, Waugh TR. Laboratory evaluation of various cold therapy modalities. *Am J Sports Med.* 1978;6(5):291–294
16. Merrick MA, Rankin JM, Andres FA, Hinman CL. A preliminary examination of cryotherapy and secondary injury in skeletal muscle. *Med Sci Sports Exerc.* 1999;31(11):1516–1521
17. Milne CT, Corbett LQ. A new option in the treatment of skin tears for the institutionalized resident: formulated 2-octylcyanoacrylate topical bandage. *Geriatr Nurs.* 2005;26(5):321–325
18. Moran GJ, Talan DA, Abrahamian FM. Antimicrobial prophylaxis for wounds and procedures in the emergency department. *Infect Dis Clin North Am.* 2008;22(1):117–143, vii

19. Moscati RM, Mayrose J, Reardon RF, Janicke DM, Jehle DV. A multicenter comparison of tap water versus sterile saline for wound irrigation. *Acad Emerg Med.* 2007;14(5):404–409
20. Pearson AS, Wolford RW. Management of skin trauma. *Prim Care.* 2000;27(2):475–492
21. Perelman VS, Francis GJ, Rutledge T, Foote J, Martino F, Dranitsaris G. Sterile versus nonsterile gloves for repair of uncomplicated lacerations in the emergency department: a randomized controlled trial. *Ann Emerg Med.* 2004;43(3):362–370
22. Ratliff CR, Fletcher KR. Skin tears: a review of the evidence to support prevention and treatment. *Ostomy Wound Manage.* 2007;53(3):32–40
23. Singer AJ, Quinn JV, Clark RE, Hollander JE; and the TraumaSeal Study Group. Closure of lacerations and incisions with octylcyanoacrylate: a multicenter randomized controlled trial. *Surgery.* 2002;131(3):270–276
24. Swartz MN. Clinical practice. Cellulitis. *N Engl J Med.* 2004;350(9): 904–912
25. US Preventive Services Task Force. Postexposure prophylaxis for selected infectious diseases. In: *Guide to Clinical Preventive Services.* 2nd ed. Alexandria, VA: International Medical Publishing, Inc; 1996:815–827
26. Xu X, Lau K, Taira BR, Singer AJ. The current management of skin tears. *Am J Emerg Med.* 2009;27(6):729–733

Trauma, Toe

1. American Heart Association. 2005 Guidelines for Cardiopulmonary Resuscitation and Emergency Cardiovascular Care. Part 14: First aid. *Circulation.* 2005;112(24 suppl):IV-196–IV-203
2. Clanton TO, Porter DA. Primary care of foot and ankle injuries in the athlete. *Clin Sports Med.* 1997;16(3):435–466
3. Collins NC. Is ice right? Does cryotherapy improve outcome for acute soft tissue injury? *Emerg Med J.* 2008;25(2):65–68
4. Kretsinger K, Broder KR, Cortese MM, et al. Preventing tetanus, diphtheria, and pertussis among adults: use of tetanus toxoid, reduced diphtheria toxoid and acellular pertussis vaccine recommendations of the Advisory Committee on Immunization Practices (ACIP) and recommendation of ACIP, supported by the Healthcare Infection Control Practices Advisory Committee (HICPAC), for use of Tdap among health-care personnel. *MMWR Recomm Rep.* 2006;55(RR-17):1–37
5. Lavery LA, Armstrong DG, Wunderlich RP, Mohler MJ, Wendel CS, Lipsky BA. Risk factors for foot infections in individuals with diabetes. *Diabetes Care.* 2006;29(6):1288–1293
6. Wedmore IS, Charette J. Emergency department evaluation and treatment of ankle and foot injuries. *Emerg Med Clin North Am.* 2000;18(1):85–113, vi

Trauma, Tooth

1. American Academy of Dentistry. Guideline on management of acute dental trauma. *Pediatr Dent.* 2011;33(6):220–228
2. American Heart Association. 2005 Guidelines for Cardiopulmonary Resuscitation and Emergency Cardiovascular Care. Part 14: First aid. *Circulation.* 2005;112(24 suppl):IV-196–IV-203
3. Andreasen JO, Andreasen FM, Skeie A, Hjorting-Hansen E, Schwartz O. Effect of treatment delay upon pulp and periodontal healing of traumatic dental injuries—a review article. *Dent Traumatol.* 2002;18(3):116–128
4. Andreasen JO, Borum MK, Jacobsen HL, Andreasen FM. Replantation of 400 avulsed permanent incisors. 4. Factors related to periodontal ligament healing. *Endod Dent Traumatol.* 1995;11(2):76–89
5. Camp JH, Stewart C. Dental trauma: diagnostic considerations, emergency procedures, and definitive management. *Emerg Med Rep.* 1995;16(9):79–86
6. Dale RA. Dentoalveolar trauma. *Emerg Med Clin North Am.* 2000;18(3)521–538
7. Douglass AB, Douglass JM. Common dental emergencies. *Am Fam Physician.* 2003;67(3):511–516
8. Layug ML, Barrett EJ, Kenny DJ. Interim storage of avulsed permanent teeth. *J Can Dent Assoc.* 1998;64(5):357–369
9. McTigue DJ. Diagnosis and management of dental injuries in children. *Pediatr Clin North Am.* 2000;47(5):1067–1084

Urinalysis Results (Follow-up Call)

1. Bent S, Nallamothu BK, Simel DL, Fihn SD, Saint S. Does this woman have an acute uncomplicated urinary tract infection? *JAMA.* 2002;287(20):2701–2710
2. Bent S, Saint S. The optimal use of diagnostic testing in women with acute uncomplicated cystitis. *Am J Med.* 2002;113(1 suppl 1):20S–28S
3. Campbell J, Felver M, Kamarei S. 'Telephone treatment' of uncomplicated acute cystitis. *Cleve Clin J Med.* 1999;66(8):495–501
4. Di Martino P, Agniel R, David K, et al. Reduction of Escherichia coli adherence to uroepithelial bladder cells after consumption of cranberry juice: a double-blind randomized placebo-controlled cross-over trial. *World J Urol.* 2006;24(1):21–27
5. Hooton TM, Winter C, Tiu F, Stamm WE. Randomized comparative trial and cost analysis of 3-day antimicrobial regimens for treatment of acute cystitis in women. *JAMA.* 1995;273(1):41–45
6. Huppert JS, Biro F, Lan D, Mortensen JE, Reed J, Slap GB. Urinary symptoms in adolescent females: STI or UTI? *J Adolesc Health.* 2007;40(5):418–424
7. Jepson RG, Mihaljevic L, Craig J. Cranberries for treating urinary tract infections. *Cochrane Database Syst Rev.* 2000;(2):CD001322
8. Jepson RG, Craig J. Cranberries for preventing urinary tract infections. *Cochrane Database Syst Rev.* 2008;(1):CD001321
9. Lammers RL, Gibson S, Kovacs D, Sears W, Strachan G. Comparison of test characteristics of urine dipstick and urinalysis at various test cutoff points. *Ann Emerg Med.* 2001;38(5):505–512
10. Patel HP. The abnormal urinalysis. *Pediatr Clin North Am.* 2006;53(3): 325–337, v
11. Saint S, Scholes D, Fihn SD, Farrell RG, Stamm WE. The effectiveness of a clinical practice guideline for the management of presumed uncomplicated urinary tract infection in women. *Am J Med.* 1999;106(6):636–641
12. Schauberger CW, Merkitch KW, Prell AM. Acute cystitis in women: experience with a telephone-based algorithm. *WMJ.* 2007;106(6): 326–329
13. Schwartz DS, Barone JE. Correlation of urinalysis and dipstick results with catheter-associated urinary tract infections in surgical ICU patients. *Intensive Care Med.* 2006;32(11):1797–1801
14. Simerville JA, Maxted WC, Pahira JJ. Urinalysis: a comprehensive review. *Am Fam Physician.* 2005;71(6):1153–1162
15. Warren JW, Abrutyn E, Hebel JR, Johnson JR, Schaeffer AJ, Stamm WE. Guidelines for antimicrobial treatment of uncomplicated acute bacterial cystitis and acute pyelonephritis in women. Infectious Diseases Society of America (IDSA). *Clin Infect Dis.* 1999;29(4): 745–758

Urination Pain (Female)

1. Avorn J, Monane M, Gurwitz JH, Glynn RJ, Choodnovskiy I, Lipsitz LA. Reduction of bacteruria and pyuria after ingestion of cranberry juice. *JAMA.*1994;71(10):751–754
2. Bass PF III, Jarvis JA, Mitchell CK. Urinary tract infections. *Prim Care.* 2003;30(1):41–61, v–vi
3. Bent S, Nallamothu BK, Simel DL, Fihn SD, Saint S. Does this woman have an acute uncomplicated urinary tract infection? *JAMA.* 2002;287(20):2701–2710
4. Bent S, Saint S. The optimal use of diagnostic testing in women with acute uncomplicated cystitis. *Am J Med.* 2002;113(1 suppl 1): 20S–28S
5. Di Martino P, Agniel R, David K, et al. Reduction of Escherichia coli adherence to uroepithelial bladder cells after consumption of cranberry juice: a double-blind randomized placebo-controlled cross-over trial. *World J Urol.* 2006;24(1):21–27
6. Gupta K, Scholes D, Stamm WE. Increasing prevalence of anti-microbial resistance among uropathogens causing uncomplicated cystitis in women. *JAMA.* 1999;281(8):736–738
7. Hooton TM, Winter C, Tiu F, Stamm WE. Randomized comparative trial and cost analysis of 3-day antimicrobial regimens for treatment of acute cystitis in women. *JAMA.* 1995;273(1):41–45
8. Huppert JS, Biro F, Lan D, Mortensen JE, Reed J, Slap GB. Urinary symptoms in adolescent females: STI or UTI? *J Adolesc Health.* 2007;40(5):418–424
9. Jepson RG, Mihaljevic L, Craig J. Cranberries for treating urinary tract infections. *Cochrane Database Syst Rev.* 2000;(2):CD001322
10. Jepson RG, Craig J. Cranberries for preventing urinary tract infections. *Cochrane Database Syst Rev.* 2008;(1):CD001321
11. Llenderrozos HJ. Urinary tract infections: management rationale for uncomplicated cystitis. *Clin Fam Pract.* 2004;6(1):157–173
12. McLaughlin SP, Carson CC. Urinary tract infections in women. *Med Clin North Am.* 2004;88(2):417–429
13. Patel HP. The abnormal urinalysis. *Pediatr Clin North Am.* 2006;53(3): 325–337, v
14. Simerville JA, Maxted WC, Pahira JJ. Urinalysis: a comprehensive review. *Am Fam Physician.* 2005;71(6):1153–1162
15. Stapleton A. Urinary tract infections in patients with diabetes. *Am J Med.* 2002;113(1 suppl 1): 80S–84S
16. Workowski KA, Berman S; and the Centers for Disease Control and Prevention. Sexually transmitted diseases treatment guidelines, 2010 [published correction appears in *MMWR Recomm Rep.* 2011;60(1):18]. *MMWR Recomm Rep.* 2010;59(RR-12):1–110
17. Yoshikawa TT, Nicolle LE, Norman DC. Management of complicated urinary tract infection in older patients. *J Am Geriatr Soc.* 1996;44(10):1235–1241

Urination Pain (Male)

1. Bass PF III, Jarvis JA, Mitchell CK. Urinary tract infections. *Prim Care.* 2003;30(1):41–61, v–vi
2. Burgher SW. Acute scrotal pain. *Emerg Med Clin North Am.* 1998;16(4):781–809, vi
3. Roberts RG, Hartlaub PP. Evaluation of dysuria in men. *Am Fam Physician.* 1999;60(3):865–872
4. Stapleton A. Urinary tract infections in patients with diabetes. *Am J Med.* 2002;113(1 suppl 1): 80S–84S
5. Workowski KA, Berman S; and the Centers for Disease Control and Prevention. Sexually transmitted diseases treatment guidelines, 2010 [published correction appears in *MMWR Recomm Rep.* 2011;60(1):18]. *MMWR Recomm Rep.* 2010;59(RR-12):1–110
6. Yoshikawa TT, Nicolle LE, Norman DC. Management of complicated urinary tract infection in older patients. *J Am Geriatr Soc.* 1996;44(10):1235–1241

Vaginal Bleeding, Abnormal

1. American College of Obstetricians and Gynecologists Committee on Practice Bulletins. ACOG practice bulletin: management of anovulatory bleeding. *Int J Gynaecol Obstet.* 2001;72(3):263–271
2. Albers JR, Hull SK, Wesley RM. Abnormal uterine bleeding. *Am Fam Physician.* 2004;69(8):1915–1926
3. American College of Emergency Physicians. Clinical policy for the initial approach to patients presenting with a chief complaint of vaginal bleeding. *Ann Emerg Med.* 1997;29(3):435–458
4. Brenner PF. Differential diagnosis of abnormal uterine bleeding. *Am J Obstet Gynecol.* 1996;175(3 suppl 2):766–769
5. Brill SR, Rosenfeld WD. Contraception. *Med Clin North Am.* 2000;84(4):907–925
6. Burkman RT. The transdermal contraceptive system. *Am J Obstet Gynecol.* 2004;190(4 suppl):S49–S53
7. Casablanca Y. Management of dysfunctional uterine bleeding. *Obstet Gynecol Clin North Am.* 2008;35(2):219–234, viii
8. Daniels RV, McCusky C. Abnormal vaginal bleeding in the non-pregnant patient. Emerg *Med Clin North Am.* 2003;21(3):751–772
9. Dawood MY. Primary dysmenorrhea: advances in pathogenesis and management. *Obstet Gynecol.* 2006;108(2):428–441
10. Eikelboom JW, Wallentin L, Connolly SJ, et al. Risk of bleeding with 2 doses of dabigatran compared with warfarin in older and younger patients with atrial fibrillation: an analysis of the randomized evaluation of long-term anticoagulant therapy (RE-LY) trial. *Circulation.* 2011;123(21):2363–2372
11. Espey E, Ogburn T, Fotieo D. Contraception: what every internist should know. Med Clin North Am. 2008;92(5):1037–1058, ix–x
12. Farrell E. Dysfunctional uterine bleeding. *Aust Fam Physician.* 2004;33(11):906–908
13. Lethaby A, Augood C, Duckitt K, Farquhar C. Nonsteroidal anti-inflammatory drugs for heavy menstrual bleeding. *Cochrane Database Syst Rev.* 2007;(4):CD000400
14. Mansfield PK, Voda A, Allison G. Validating a pencil-and-paper measure of perimenopausal menstrual blood loss. *Womens Health Issues.* 2004;14(6):242–247
15. McGee S, Abernethy WB III, Simel DL. The rational clinical examination. Is this patient hypovolemic? *JAMA.* 1999;281(11):1022–1029
16. Minjarez DA, Bradshaw KD. Abnormal uterine bleeding in adolescents. *Obstet Gynecol Clin North Am.* 2000;27(1):63–78
17. Mosher WD, Jones J. Use of contraception in the United States: 1982–2008. *Vital Health Stat 23.* 2010;(29):1–44
18. Santer M, Wyke S, Warner P. What aspects of periods are most bothersome for women reporting heavy menstrual bleeding? Community survey and qualitative study. *BMC Womens Health.* 2007;7:8
19. Shapley M, Jordan J, Croft PR. A systematic review of postcoital bleeding and risk of cervical cancer. *Br J Gen Pract.* 2006;56(527): 453–460
20. Sinert R, Spektor M. Evidence-based emergency medicine/rational clinical examination abstract. Clinical assessment of hypovolemia. *Ann Emerg Med.* 2005;45(3):327–329
21. Swica Y. The transdermal patch and the vaginal ring: two novel methods of combined hormonal contraception. *Obstet Gynecol Clin North Am.* 2007;34(1):31–42, viii
22. Telner DE, Jakubovicz D. Approach to diagnosis and management of abnormal uterine bleeding. *Can Fam Physician.* 2007;53(1):58–64
23. Victor I, Fink RA. Comparing patient telephone callback rates for different hormonal birth control delivery systems. *Am J Ther.* 2006;13(6):507–512

24. Warner PE, Critchley HO, Lumsden MA, Campbell-Brown M, Douglas A, Murray GD. Menorrhagia I: measured blood loss, clinical features, and outcome in women with heavy periods: a survey with follow-up data. *Am J Obstet Gynecol.* 2004;190(5):1216–1223
25. Warner PE, Critchley HO, Lumsden MA, Campbell-Brown M, Douglas A, Murray GD. Menorrhagia II: is the 80-mL blood loss criterion useful in management of complaint of menorrhagia? *Am J Obstet Gynecol.* 2004;190(5):1224–1229

Vaginal Discharge

1. Allen-Davis JT, Beck A, Parker R, Ellis JL, Polley D. Assessment of vulvovaginal complaints: accuracy of telephone triage and in-office diagnosis. *Obstet Gynecol.* 2002;99(1):18–22
2. ACOG Committee on Practice Bulletins—Gynecology. ACOG Practice Bulletin. Clinical management guidelines for obstetrician-gynecologists, Number 72, May 2006: Vaginitis. *Obstet Gynecol.* 2006;107(5):1195–1206
3. Eckert LO. Clinical practice. Acute vulvovaginitis. *N Engl J Med.* 2006;355(12):1244–1252
4. Egan ME, Lipsky MS. Diagnosis of vaginitis. *Am Fam Physician.* 2000;62(5):1095–1104
5. Forhan SE, Gottlieb SL, Sternberg MR, et al. Prevalence of sexually transmitted infections among female adolescents aged 14 to 19 in the United States. *Pediatrics.* 2009;124(6):1505–1512
6. Goldenberg RL, Andrews WW, Yuan AC, MacKay HT, St Louis ME. Sexually transmitted diseases and adverse outcomes of pregnancy. *Clin Perinatol.* 1997;24(1):23–41
7. Johnson E, Berwald N. Evidence-based emergency medicine/rational clinical examination abstract. Diagnostic utility of physical examination, history, and laboratory evaluation in emergency department patients with vaginal complaints. *Ann Emerg Med.* 2008;52(3):294–297
8. Miller KE. Women's health. Sexually transmitted diseases. *Prim Care.* 1997;24(1):179–193
9. Oduyebo OO, Anorlu RI, Ogunsola FT. The effects of antimicrobial therapy on bacterial vaginosis in non-pregnant women. *Cochrane Database Syst Rev.* 2009;(3):CD006055
10. Public Health Agency of Canada. Primary care and sexually transmitted infections. In: *Canadian Guidelines on Sexually Transmitted Infections.* 2006 Edition. Ottawa, Ontario: Public Health Agency of Canada; 2006:7–29. http://pubs.cpha.ca/PDF/P37/23384.pdf. Accessed July 31, 2012
11. Quan M. Vaginitis: diagnosis and management. *Postgrad Med.* 2010;122(6):117–127
12. Stewart C, Bosker G. Pelvic inflammatory disease (PID): diagnosis, disposition, and current antimicrobial guidelines. *Emerg Med Rep.* 1999;20(16):163–172
13. Van Vranken M. Prevention and treatment of sexually transmitted diseases: an update. *Am Fam Physician.* 2007;76(12):1827–1832
14. Workowski KA, Berman S; and the Centers for Disease Control and Prevention. Sexually transmitted diseases treatment guidelines, 2010 [published correction appears in *MMWR Recomm Rep.* 2011;60(1):18]. *MMWR Recomm Rep.* 2010;59(RR-12):1–110

Vomiting

1. Acheson DW, Fiore AE. Preventing foodborne disease—what clinicians can do. *N Engl J Med.* 2004;350(5):437–440
2. American Academy of Family Physicians. Information from your family doctor. Nausea and vomiting. *Am Fam Physician.* 2004;69(5):1176
3. Centers for Disease Control and Prevention. Diagnosis and management of foodborne illnesses: a primer for physicians. *MMWR Recomm Rep.* 2004;53(RR-4):1–33
4. Flasar MH, Cross R, Goldberg E. Acute abdominal pain. *Prim Care.* 2006;33(3):659–684, vi
5. Frese T, Klauss S, Herrmann K, Sandholzer H. Nausea and vomiting as the reasons for encounter in general practice. *J Clin Med Res.* 2011;3(1):23–29
6. Lichter I. Nausea and vomiting in patients with cancer. *Hematol Oncol Clin North Am.* 1996;10(1):207–220
7. Metz A, Hebbard G. Nausea and vomiting in adults—a diagnostic approach. *Aust Fam Physician.* 2007;36(9):688–692
8. Mines D, Stahmer S, Shepherd SM. Poisonings: food, fish, shellfish. *Emerg Med Clin North Am.* 1997;15(1):157–177
9. Montagnini ML, Moat ME. Non-pain symptom management in palliative care. *Clin Fam Pract.* 2004;6(2);395–422
10. Nee PA, Hadfield JM, Yates DW, Faragher EB. Significance of vomiting after head injury. *J Neurol Neurosurg Psychiatry.* 1999;66(4):470–473
11. Quigley EM, Hasler WL, Parkman HP. AGA technical review on nausea and vomiting. *Gastroenterology.* 2001;120(1):263–286
12. Sampson HA, Sicherer SH, Birnbaum AH. AGA technical review on the evaluation of food allergy in gastrointestinal disorders. *Gastroenterology.* 2001;120(4):1026–1040
13. Scorza K, Williams A, Phillips JD, Shaw J. Evaluation of nausea and vomiting. *Am Fam Physician.* 2007;76(1):76–84
14. Sinert R, Spektor M. Evidence-based emergency medicine/rational clinical examination abstract. Clinical assessment of hypovolemia. *Ann Emerg Med.* 2005;45(3):327–329
15. Williams KS. Postoperative nausea and vomiting. *Surg Clin North Am.* 2005;85(6):1229–1241, xi

Vulvar Symptoms

1. Allen-Davis JT, Beck A, Parker R, Ellis JL, Polley D. Assessment of vulvovaginal complaints: accuracy of telephone triage and in-office diagnosis. *Obstet Gynecol.* 2002;99(1):18–22
2. ACOG Committee on Practice Bulletins—Gynecology. ACOG Practice Bulletin. Clinical management guidelines for obstetrician-gynecologists, Number 72, May 2006: Vaginitis. *Obstet Gynecol.* 2006;107(5):1195–1206
3. Eckert LO. Clinical practice. Acute vulvovaginitis. *N Engl J Med.* 2006;355(12):1244–1252
4. Goldenberg RL, Andrews WW, Yuan AC, MacKay HT, St Louis ME. Sexually transmitted diseases and adverse outcomes of pregnancy. *Clin Perinatol.* 1997;24(1):23–41
5. Haider Z, Condous G, Kirk E, Mukri F, Bourne T. The simple outpatient management of Bartholin's abscess using the Word catheter: a preliminary study. *Aust N Z J Obstet Gynaecol.* 2007;47(2):137–140
6. MacNeill C. Dyspareunia. *Obstet Gynecol Clin North Am.* 2006;33(4):565–577, viii
7. Margesson LJ. Vulvar disease pearls. *Dermatol Clin.* 2006;24(2):145–155, v
8. Miller KE. Women's health. Sexually transmitted diseases. *Prim Care.*1997;24(1):179–193
9. Oduyebo OO, Anorlu RI, Ogunsola FT. The effects of antimicrobial therapy on bacterial vaginosis in non-pregnant women. *Cochrane Database Syst Rev.* 2009;(3):CD006055
10. Omole F, Simmons BJ, Hacker Y. Management of Bartholin's duct cyst and gland abscess. *Am Fam Physician.* 2003;68(1):135–140

Vulvar Symptoms (continued)

11. Quan M. Vaginitis: diagnosis and management. *Postgrad Med.* 2010;122(6):117–127
12. Van Vranken M. Prevention and treatment of sexually transmitted diseases: an update. *Am Fam Physician.* 2007;76(12):1827–1832
13. Workowski KA, Berman S; and the Centers for Disease Control and Prevention. Sexually transmitted diseases treatment guidelines, 2010 [published correction appears in *MMWR Recomm Rep.* 2011;60(1):18]. *MMWR Recomm Rep.* 2010;59(RR-12):1–110

Weakness (Generalized) and Fatigue

1. Goldman L, Kirtane AJ. Triage of patients with acute chest pain and possible cardiac ischemia: the elusive search for diagnostic perfection. *Ann Intern Med.* 2003;139(12):987–995
2. McGee S, Abernethy WB III, Simel DL. The rational clinical examination. Is this patient hypovolemic? *JAMA.* 1999;281(11):1022–1029
3. McSweeney JC, Cody M, O'Sullivan P, Elberson K, Moser DK, Garvin BJ. Women's early warning symptoms of acute myocardial infarction. *Circulation.* 2003;108(21):2619–2623
4. Morrison RE, Keating HJ III. Fatigue in primary care. *Obstet Gynecol Clin North Am.* 2001;28(2):225–240, v–vi
5. Sinert R, Spektor M. Evidence-based emergency medicine/rational clinical examination abstract. Clinical assessment of hypovolemia. *Ann Emerg Med.* 2005;45(3):327–329
6. Tusa RJ. Dizziness. *Med Clin North Am.* 2003;87(3):609–641, vii

Wound Infection

1. Nicolle L. Community-acquired MRSA: a practitioner's guide. *CMAJ.* 2006;175(2):145
2. American Heart Association. 2005 Guidelines for Cardiopulmonary Resuscitation and Emergency Cardiovascular Care. Part 14: First aid. *Circulation.* 2005;112(24 suppl):IV-196–IV-203
3. Berger RS, Pappert AS, Van Zile PS, Cetnarowski WE. A newly formulated topical triple-antibiotic ointment minimizes scarring. *Cutis.* 2000;65(6):401–404
4. Murphy TV, Slade BA, Broder KR, et al: and the Advisory Committee on Immunization Practices, Centers for Disease Control and Prevention. Prevention of pertussis, tetanus, and diphtheria among pregnant and postpartum women and their infants recommendations of the Advisory Committee on Immunization Practices (ACIP). *MMWR Recomm Rep.* 2008;57(RR-4):1–51
5. Cho CY, Lo JS. Dressing the part. *Dermatol Clin.* 1998;16(1):25–47
6. Degreef HJ. How to heal a wound fast. *Dermatol Clin.* 1998;16(2):365–375
7. Dire DJ, Coppola M, Dwyer DA, Lorette JJ, Karr JL. Prospective evaluation of topical antibiotics for preventing infections in uncomplicated soft-tissue wounds repaired in the ED. *Acad Emerg Med.* 1995;2(1):4–10
8. Frazee BW, Lynn J, Charlebois ED, Lambert L, Lowery D, Perdreau-Remington F. High prevalence of methicillin-resistant Staphylococcus aureus in emergency department skin and soft tissue infections. *Ann Emerg Med.* 2005;45(3):311–320
9. Fridkin SK, Hageman JC, Morrison M, et al. Methicillin-resistant Staphylococcus aureus disease in three communities. *N Eng J Med.* 2005;352(14):1436–1444
10. Gergen PJ, McQuillan GM, Kiely M, Ezzati-Rice TM, Sutter RW, Virella G. A population-based serologic survey of immunity to tetanus in the United States. *N Engl J Med.* 1995;332(12):761–766
11. Gorwitz RJ, Jernigan DB, Powers JH, Jernigan JA; and the Participants in the CDC-Convened Experts' Meeting on Management of MRSA in the Community. Strategies for clinical management of MRSA in the community: summary of an experts' meeting convened by the Centers for Disease Control and Prevention. 2006. http://www.cdc.gov/mrsa/pdf/MRSA-Strategies-ExpMtgSummary-2006.pdf. Accessed July 31, 2012
12. Hollander JE, Singer AJ, Valentine SM, Shofer FS. Risk factors for infection in patients with traumatic lacerations. *Acad Emerg Med.* 2001;8(7):716–720
13. Howell JM, Chisholm CD. Wound care. *Emerg Med Clin North Am.* 1997;15(2):417–425
14. Jones RN, Li Q, Kohut B, Biedenbach DJ, Bell J, Turnidge JD. Contemporary antimicrobial activity of triple antibiotic ointment: a multiphased study of recent clinical isolates in the United States and Australia. *Diagn Microbiol Infect Dis.* 2006;54(1):63–71
15. Kaye ET. Topical antibacterial agents. *Infect Dis Clin North Am.* 2000;14(2):321–339
16. Swartz MN. Clinical practice. Cellulitis. *N Engl J Med.* 2004;350(9):904–912

Appendix I

Over-the-Counter Medications

- Dosages for a number of commonly used over-the-counter (OTC) medications are included in this book.
- These OTC medications should not be recommended by the office triager unless this listing has been **reviewed, amended as necessary, and approved** by the supervising physician or office medical director.
- Concise and limited information for these OTC medications is provided in this book. The triager is strongly encouraged to read the *Physicians' Desk Reference for Nonprescription Drugs* or other trustworthy drug reference for all OTC medications that the triager recommends to patients.
- Patients should be instructed to **read the package warnings and instructions** on all OTC medications that they take.

Abrasions, Scratches, and Minor Cuts

Adult OTC Drug Dosage Table

Wound Care—Abrasions (Scrapes), Scratches, and Minor Cuts

Medication	Dosage	Notes
Antibiotic Ointment Bacitracin Neosporin Polysporin (bacitracin and polymyxin B) Triple Antibiotic (bacitracin, neomycin, and polymixin B)	Use after cleaning the wound. Apply ointment BID-TID.	**Caution:** Stop ointment if a rash or allergic reaction occurs.
Liquid Skin Bandage Band-Aid Liquid Bandage New-Skin Curad Spray Bandage 3M Nexcare No Sting Liquid Bandage Spray	Use after cleaning the wound. Needs to be applied only once.	This is an alternative to antibiotic ointment and a regular bandage (e.g., gauze dressing or Band-Aid).

Important Notice

- These OTC (over-the-counter) medications should not be recommended by the telephone triager unless this listing has been reviewed, amended as necessary, and approved by the supervising physician, office medical director, or call center medical director.
- Concise and limited information for these OTC medications is provided in these tables. The triager is strongly encouraged to read the *Physicians' Desk Reference for Nonprescription Drugs* or other trustworthy drug reference for all OTC medications that the triager recommends to patients. Extensive drug information is available at the National Library of Medicine drug information Web site (MedlinePlus).
- Patients should be instructed to read the package warnings and instructions on all OTC medications that they take.

Acid Indigestion, Heartburn, and Sour Stomach

Adult OTC Drug Dosage Table

Treatment of Acid Indigestion, Heartburn, and Sour Stomach

Medication	Dosage	Notes
Antacids Maalox Mylanta Rolaids Tums	**Liquid and Tablets** Read package instructions.	**Caution:** There are other serious causes of epigastric discomfort, including: myocardial infarction and gallstones.
H_2 Blocker—Ranitidine Zantac	75-mg tablets 75 mg once or twice daily	**Caution:** There are other serious causes of epigastric discomfort, including: myocardial infarction and gallstones.

Important Notice

- These OTC (over-the-counter) medications should not be recommended by the telephone triager unless this listing has been reviewed, amended as necessary, and approved by the supervising physician, office medical director, or call center medical director.
- Concise and limited information for these OTC medications is provided in these tables. The triager is strongly encouraged to read the *Physicians' Desk Reference for Nonprescription Drugs* or other trustworthy drug reference for all OTC medications that the triager recommends to patients. Extensive drug information is available at the National Library of Medicine drug information Web site (MedlinePlus).
- Patients should be instructed to read the package warnings and instructions on all OTC medications that they take.

Athlete's Foot

Adult OTC Drug Dosage Table

Treatment of Athlete's Foot (Tinea Pedis)

Medication	Dosage	Notes
Antifungal Cream—Terbinafine Lamisil AT **Antifungal Cream—Clotrimazole** Lotrimin **Antifungal Cream—Miconazole** Lotrimin AF Micatin Monistat-Derm	Apply cream 2 times per day to the affected areas of the feet. Continue the cream for at least 7 days after the rash is cleared.	**Keep the Feet Clean and Dry:** Wash the feet 2 times every day. Dry the feet completely, especially between the toes. You can use a blow dryer set on the cool setting or you can gently pat the area dry with a towel. After drying your feet, then apply the cream. Wear clean socks and change them twice daily. Terbinafine (Lamisil AT) is most recommended but is not available in Canada. **Expected Course:** With proper treatment, athlete's foot should decrease substantially within 1 week and disappear within 2-3 weeks.

Important Notice

- These OTC (over-the-counter) medications should not be recommended by the telephone triager unless this listing has been reviewed, amended as necessary, and approved by the supervising physician, office medical director, or call center medical director.
- Concise and limited information for these OTC medications is provided in these tables. The triager is strongly encouraged to read the *Physicians' Desk Reference for Nonprescription Drugs* or other trustworthy drug reference for all OTC medications that the triager recommends to patients. Extensive drug information is available at the National Library of Medicine drug information Web site (MedlinePlus).
- Patients should be instructed to read the package warnings and instructions on all OTC medications that they take.

Chapped Lips

Adult OTC Drug Dosage Table

Treatment of Chapped Lips

Medication	Dosage	Notes
Lip Moisturizers Carmex ChapStick		

Important Notice

- These OTC (over-the-counter) medications should not be recommended by the telephone triager unless this listing has been reviewed, amended as necessary, and approved by the supervising physician, office medical director, or call center medical director.
- Concise and limited information for these OTC medications is provided in these tables. The triager is strongly encouraged to read the *Physicians' Desk Reference for Nonprescription Drugs* or other trustworthy drug reference for all OTC medications that the triager recommends to patients. Extensive drug information is available at the National Library of Medicine drug information Web site (MedlinePlus).
- Patients should be instructed to read the package warnings and instructions on all OTC medications that they take.

Cold Symptoms (Upper Respiratory Infection)

Adult OTC Drug Dosage Table

Cold Symptoms

Medication	Dosage	Notes
Zinc Lozenge Cold-Eeze	Take 1 lozenge every 2-4 hours. Begin taking them within 48 hours of cold onset. Use for 3 days.	Some studies have reported that zinc gluconate lozenges may reduce the duration and severity of cold symptoms. Some people complain of nausea and a bad taste in their mouth when they take zinc.

Cold Symptoms—Treatment of Cough

Medication	Dosage	Notes
Cough Suppressant With Dextromethorphan Benylin Robitussin DM Vicks 44 Cough Medicine	Read package instructions.	Cough syrups containing the cough supppresant dextromethorphan (DM) may help decrease your cough. Cough syrups work best for coughs that keep you awake at night. They can also sometimes help in the late stages of a respiratory infection when the cough is dry and hacking. They can be used along with cough drops. **Special Notes About Dextromethorphan:** Some recent research suggests that dextromethorphan is no better than placebo at reducing a cough. However, there is no over-the-counter medicine that works better than DM and generally DM has no side effects. It should also be noted that dextromethorphan has become a drug of abuse. This problem has been seen most commonly in adolescents. Overdose symptoms can range from giggling and euphoria to hallucinations and coma.
Cough Expectorant With Guaifenesin Humibid Hytuss Robitussin	Read package instructions.	Guaifenesin thins and loosens the mucus in the airways, making it easier to cough up. Breathing in the mist from a steamy shower probably works even better than a cough expectorant. It moistens and helps loosen up the phlegm. Drinking plenty of liquids and staying well-hydrated is also important (Caution: unless patient has doctor-ordered fluid restriction).

Cold Symptoms (Upper Respiratory Infection) *(continued)*

Adult OTC Drug Dosage Table

Cold Symptoms—Treatment of Cough *(continued)*

Medication	Dosage	Notes
Cough Drops (Lozenges) Halls Halls Sugar-Free Robitussin Vicks	Read package instructions.	Cough drops can help a lot, especially for mild coughs. They reduce coughing by soothing your irritated throat and removing that tickle sensation in the back of the throat. Cough drops also have the advantage of portability. You can carry them with you. A piece of hard candy often works just as well as an over-the-counter cough drop.

Cold Symptoms—Treatment of Fever, Headache, and Muscle Aches

Medication	Dosage	Notes
Acetaminophen Tylenol Regular Strength Tylenol Extra Strength Tylenol Adult Liquid Pain Reliever Tylenol Arthritis Extended Relief	325-mg regular strength tablets or caplets: 650 mg (2 pills) every 4-6 hours 500-mg extra strength gelcaps, caplets, or tablets: 1,000 mg (2 pills) every 8 hours 500-mg liquid per tablespoon: 1,000 mg (2 tablespoons or 30 cc) every 8 hours	**Treatment of Fever:** Drink cold fluids orally to prevent dehydration. Good hydration replaces sweat and improves heat loss via skin. Adults should drink 6-8 glasses of water daily. Dress in one layer of lightweight clothing and sleep with one light blanket. **Acetaminophen for Fever:** For fevers 100-101° F (37.8-38.3° C), fever medicine is generally not needed. For fevers above 101° F (38.3° C) you can take acetaminophen. The goal of fever therapy is to bring the fever down to a comfortable level. Remember that fever medicine usually lowers fever 2 degrees F (1 - 1½ degrees C). **Acetaminophen for Headache and Muscle Aches:** You can take acetaminophen for headache and muscle aches. **Instructions for Taking Acetaminophen:** Take 650 mg by mouth every 4-6 hours. Each Regular Strength Tylenol pill has 325 mg of acetaminophen. Another choice is to take 1,000 mg every 8 hours. Each Extra Strength Tylenol pill has 500 mg of acetaminophen. The most you should take each day is 3,000 mg. **Extra Notes:** Acetaminophen is in many OTC and prescription medicines. It might be in more than one medicine that you are taking. You need to be careful and not take an overdose. An acetaminophen overdose can hurt the liver. **Caution:** Do not take acetaminophen if you have liver disease. ***Before taking any medicine, read all the instructions on the package.***

Cold Symptoms (Upper Respiratory Infection) *(continued)*

Adult OTC Drug Dosage Table

Cold Symptoms—Treatment of Fever, Headache, and Muscle Aches *(continued)*

Medication	Dosage	Notes
Ibuprofen Advil Motrin Nuprin	200-mg caplets or tablets: 200-400 mg every 6 hours	**Treatment of Fever:** Drink cold fluids orally to prevent dehydration. Good hydration replaces sweat and improves heat loss via skin. Adults should drink 6-8 glasses of water daily. Dress in one layer of lightweight clothing and sleep with one light blanket. **Ibuprofen for Fever:** For fevers 100-101° F (37.8-38.3° C), fever medicine is generally not needed. For fevers above 101° F (38.3° C) you can take ibuprofen. The goal of fever therapy is to bring the fever down to a comfortable level. Remember that fever medicine usually lowers fever 2 degrees F (1 - 1½ degrees C). **Ibuprofen for Headache and Muscle Aches:** You can take ibuprofen for headache and muscle aches. **Instructions for Taking Ibuprofen:** Take 400 mg by mouth every 6 hours. Another choice is to take 600 mg by mouth every 8 hours. Use the lowest amount that makes your pain feel better. **Extra Notes:** Acetaminophen is thought to be safer than ibuprofen in people over 65 years old. **Caution:** Do not take ibuprofen if you have stomach problems, kidney disease, are pregnant, or have been told by your doctor to avoid this type of anti-inflammatory drug. Do not take ibuprofen for more than 7 days without consulting your doctor. ***Before taking any medicine, read all the instructions on the package.***

Cold Symptoms (Upper Respiratory Infection) *(continued)*

Adult OTC Drug Dosage Table

Cold Symptoms—Treatment of a Very Runny Nose

Medication	Dosage	Notes
Nasal Decongestant Spray—Oxymetazoline Afrin	Clean out the nose before using. Spray each nostril once, wait 1 minute for absorption, and then spray a second time.	Decongestants shrink the swollen nasal mucosa and allow for easier breathing. If you have a very runny nose, they can reduce the amount of drainage. They can be taken as pills by mouth or as a nasal spray. ***Most people do NOT need to use these medicines.*** **Caution:** Do not use nasal sprays for more than 3 days (Reason: rebound nasal congestion can occur). **Caution:** Do not take these medications if you have high blood pressure, heart disease, prostate enlargement, or an overactive thyroid. **Caution:** Do not take these medications if you are pregnant. **Caution:** Do not take these medicatopms if you have used an MAO inhibitor such as isocarboxazid (Marplan), phenelzine (Nardil), rasagiline (Azilect), selegiline (Eldepryl, Emsam), or tranylcypromine (Parnate) in the past 2 weeks. Life-threatening side effects can occur.
Nasal Decongestant Spray—Phenylephrine Neo-Synephrine	Clean out the nose before using. Spray each nostril once, wait 1 minute for absorption, and then spray a second time.	Decongestants shrink the swollen nasal mucosa and allow for easier breathing. If you have a very runny nose, they can reduce the amount of drainage. They can be taken as pills by mouth or as a nasal spray. ***Most people do NOT need to use these medicines.*** **Caution:** Do not use nasal sprays for more than 3 days (Reason: rebound nasal congestion can occur). **Caution:** Do not take these medications if you have high blood pressure, heart disease, prostate enlargement, or an overactive thyroid. **Caution:** Do not take these medications if you are pregnant. **Caution:** Do not take these medicatopms if you have used an MAO inhibitor such as isocarboxazid (Marplan), phenelzine (Nardil), rasagiline (Azilect), selegiline (Eldepryl, Emsam), or tranylcypromine (Parnate) in the past 2 weeks. Life-threatening side effects can occur.
Nasal Decongestant Pills—Phenylephrine Sudafed PE	10-mg tablets 10 mg (1 tablet) every 4 hours	Decongestants shrink the swollen nasal mucosa and allow for easier breathing. If you have a very runny nose, they can reduce the amount of drainage. They can be taken as pills by mouth or as a nasal spray. ***Most people do NOT need to use these medicines.*** **Caution:** Do not use nasal sprays for more than 3 days (Reason: rebound nasal congestion can occur). **Caution:** Do not take these medications if you have high blood pressure, heart disease, prostate enlargement, or an overactive thyroid. **Caution:** Do not take these medications if you are pregnant. **Caution:** Do not take these medicatopms if you have used an MAO inhibitor such as isocarboxazid (Marplan), phenelzine (Nardil), rasagiline (Azilect), selegiline (Eldepryl, Emsam), or tranylcypromine (Parnate) in the past 2 weeks. Life-threatening side effects can occur.

Cold Symptoms (Upper Respiratory Infection) *(continued)*

Adult OTC Drug Dosage Table

Cold Symptoms—Treatment of a Very Runny Nose *(continued)*

Medication	Dosage	Notes
Nasal Decongestant Pills—Pseudoephedrine Sudafed Sudafed 12 Hour	30-mg tablets: 60 mg (2 tablets) every 6 hours 120-mg (12-hour) tablets: 120 mg (1 tablet) every 12 hours	Decongestants shrink the swollen nasal mucosa and allow for easier breathing. If you have a very runny nose, they can reduce the amount of drainage. They can be taken as pills by mouth or as a nasal spray. ***Most people do NOT need to use these medicines.*** **Caution:** Do not use nasal sprays for more than 3 days (Reason: rebound nasal congestion can occur). **Caution:** Do not take these medications if you have high blood pressure, heart disease, prostate enlargement, or an overactive thyroid. **Caution:** Do not take these medications if you are pregnant. **Caution:** Do not take these medicatopms if you have used an MAO inhibitor such as isocarboxazid (Marplan), phenelzine (Nardil), rasagiline (Azilect), selegiline (Eldepryl, Emsam), or tranylcypromine (Parnate) in the past 2 weeks. Life-threatening side effects can occur. Illegal laboratory conversion of pseudoephedrine into methamphetamine has become a major concern. As a result, drugs containing pseudoephedrine (e.g., Sudafed) are now offered "behind-the-counter" instead of over-the-counter.

Important Notice

- These OTC (over-the-counter) medications should not be recommended by the telephone triager unless this listing has been reviewed, amended as necessary, and approved by the supervising physician, office medical director, or call center medical director.
- Concise and limited information for these OTC medications is provided in these tables. The triager is strongly encouraged to read the *Physicians' Desk Reference for Nonprescription Drugs* or other trustworthy drug reference for all OTC medications that the triager recommends to patients. Extensive drug information is available at the National Library of Medicine drug information Web site (MedlinePlus).
- Patients should be instructed to read the package warnings and instructions on all OTC medications that they take.

Constipation

Adult OTC Drug Dosage Table

Treatment of Constipation

Medication	Dosage	Notes
Bulk Laxative Metamucil (psyllium fiber)	**Powder** 1 teaspoon or tablespoon (depending on the product) in an 4- to 8-oz (120- to 240-mL) glass of water once daily **Single-Dose Packet** 1 packet in an 8-oz (240-mL) glass of water once daily	Bulk-forming agents works like fiber to help soften the stools and improve your intestinal function. Long-term use of this type of laxative is generally safe. **Side Effects:** Mild gas or a bloating sensation may occur.
Osmotic Laxative Miralax (polyethylene glycol 3350)	**Powder** 1 heaping tablespoon (17 g) in an 8-oz (240-mL) glass of water once daily	Miralax is an "osmotic" agent, which means that it binds water and causes water to be retained within the stool. You can use this laxative to treat occasional constipation. Do not use for more than 2 weeks without approval from your doctor. Generally, Miralax produces a bowel movement in 1 to 3 days. **Side Effects:** Diarrhea (especially at higher doses). **Pregnancy:** Discuss with your doctor before using. **Available in the United States:** Approved for OTC use by the FDA in December 2006.
Milk of Magnesia (magnesium hydroxide) is a mild stimulant laxative.	**Liquid** 1-2 tablespoons (15-30 cc) by mouth once or twice daily	This is a mild and generally safe laxative. You can use milk of magnesia for short-term treatment of constipation. (Research suggests that Miralax may be more effective.) **Pregnancy:** Discuss with your doctor before using. **Caution:** Do not use if you have kidney disease.
Stool Softener Docusate sodium Colace	100 mg capsule 100 mg BID	

Important Notice

- These OTC (over-the-counter) medications should not be recommended by the telephone triager unless t[illegible] listing has been reviewed, amended as necessary, and approved by the supervising physician, office med[illegible] director, or call center medical director.
- Concise and limited information for these OTC medications is provided in these tables. The triager is str[illegible] encouraged to read the *Physicians' Desk Reference for Nonprescription Drugs* or other trustworthy drug reference for all OTC medications that the triager recommends to patients. Extensive drug informatio[illegible] available at the National Library of Medicine drug information Web site (MedlinePlus).
- Patients should be instructed to read the package warnings and instructions on all OTC medications [illegible] they take.

Diarrhea

Adult OTC Drug Dosage Table

Treatment of Diarrhea

Medication	Dosage	Notes
Bismuth Subsalicylate Pepto-Bismol	**Liquid** 2 tablets or 2 tablespoons by mouth every hour (if diarrhea continues) Maximum of 8 doses in a 24-hour period	Helps reduce diarrhea. May cause some temporary darkening of your tongue and stools (black color). **Caution:** Do not use for more than 2 days.
Loperamide Imodium A-D	**Caplets or liquid** 2 caplets or 4 teaspoonfuls initially by mouth. May take an additional caplet or 2 teaspoonfuls with each subsequent loose BM. Maximum of 4 caplets or 8 teaspoonfuls each day.	Helps reduce diarrhea. **Caution:** Do not use if there is a fever greater than 100° F or if there is blood or mucus in the stools. **Caution:** Do not use for more than 2 days.

Important Notice

- These OTC (over-the-counter) medications should not be recommended by the telephone triager unless this listing has been reviewed, amended as necessary, and approved by the supervising physician, office medical director, or call center medical director.
- Concise and limited information for these OTC medications is provided in these tables. The triager is strongly encouraged to read the *Physicians' Desk Reference for Nonprescription Drugs* or other trustworthy drug reference for all OTC medications that the triager recommends to patients. Extensive drug information is available at the National Library of Medicine drug information Web site (MedlinePlus).
- Patients should be instructed to read the package warnings and instructions on all OTC medications that they take.

Dry Skin

Adult OTC Drug Dosage Table

Treatment of Dry Skin

Medication	Dosage	Notes
Lotion Eucerin Lotion Lubriderm Lotion Vaseline Intensive Care Lotion **Cream** Eucerin Creme **Ointment** Vaseline petroleum jelly		Best time to apply is right after a bath or shower when the skin is moist. Vaseline is inexpensive. It has the drawback of feeling somewhat greasy; this can be lessened by using only small amounts and rubbing it in thoroughly. Eucerin Creme is especially helpful for dry/chapped hands. Avoid using products with any fragrance.

Important Notice

- These OTC (over-the-counter) medications should not be recommended by the telephone triager unless this listing has been reviewed, amended as necessary, and approved by the supervising physician, office medical director, or call center medical director.
- Concise and limited information for these OTC medications is provided in these tables. The triager is strongly encouraged to read the *Physicians' Desk Reference for Nonprescription Drugs* or other trustworthy drug reference for all OTC medications that the triager recommends to patients. Extensive drug information is available at the National Library of Medicine drug information Web site (MedlinePlus).
- Patients should be instructed to read the package warnings and instructions on all OTC medications that they take.

Earwax

Adult OTC Drug Dosage Table

Earwax Removal

Medication	Dosage	Notes
Debrox Drops Murine Drops	**Ear Drops** Tilt head to side and place 5-10 drops in ear canal. Keep head tilted for 2-3 minutes. Use twice daily for up to 4 days.	These ear drops help soften and remove excessive wax. **Caution:** Do not use if you have any earache, ear discharge, redness. **Caution:** Do not use if you have a perforation (hole) in your eardrum.

Important Notice

- These OTC (over-the-counter) medications should not be recommended by the telephone triager unless this listing has been reviewed, amended as necessary, and approved by the supervising physician, office medical director, or call center medical director.
- Concise and limited information for these OTC medications is provided in these tables. The triager is strongly encouraged to read the *Physicians' Desk Reference for Nonprescription Drugs* or other trustworthy drug reference for all OTC medications that the triager recommends to patients. Extensive drug information is available at the National Library of Medicine drug information Web site (MedlinePlus).
- Patients should be instructed to read the package warnings and instructions on all OTC medications that they take.

Fever

Adult OTC Drug Dosage Table

Treatment of Fever

Medication	Dosage	Notes
Acetaminophen Tylenol Regular Strength Tylenol Extra Strength Tylenol Adult Liquid Pain Reliever Tylenol Arthritis Extended Relief	325-mg regular strength tablets or caplets: 650 mg (2 pills) every 4-6 hours 500-mg extra strength gelcaps, caplets, or tablets: 1,000 mg (2 pills) every 8 hours 500-mg liquid per tablespoon: 1,000 mg (2 tablespoons or 30 cc) every 8 hours	**Treatment of Fever:** Drink cold fluids orally to prevent dehydration. Good hydration replaces sweat and improves heat loss via skin. Adults should drink 6-8 glasses of water daily. Dress in one layer of lightweight clothing and sleep with one light blanket. **Acetaminophen for Fever:** For fevers 100-101° F (37.8-38.3° C), fever medicine is generally not needed. For fevers above 101° F (38.3° C) you can take acetaminophen. The goal of fever therapy is to bring the fever down to a comfortable level. Remember that fever medicine usually lowers fever 2 degrees F (1 - 1½ degrees C). **Instructions for Taking Acetaminophen:** Take 650 mg by mouth every 4-6 hours. Each Regular Strength Tylenol pill has 325 mg of acetaminophen. Another choice is to take 1,000 mg every 8 hours. Each Extra Strength Tylenol pill has 500 mg of acetaminophen. The most you should take each day is 3,000 mg. **Extra Notes:** Acetaminophen is in many OTC and prescription medicines. It might be in more than one medicine that you are taking. You need to be careful and not take an overdose. An acetaminophen overdose can hurt the liver. **Caution:** Do not take acetaminophen if you have liver disease. ***Before taking any medicine, read all the instructions on the package.***

Fever *(continued)*

Adult OTC Drug Dosage Table

Treatment of Fever *(continued)*

Medication	Dosage	Notes
Ibuprofen Advil Motrin Nuprin	200-mg caplets or tablets: 200-400 mg every 6 hours	**Treatment of Fever:** Drink cold fluids orally to prevent dehydration. Good hydration replaces sweat and improves heat loss via skin. Adults should drink 6-8 glasses of water daily. Dress in one layer of lightweight clothing and sleep with one light blanket. **Ibuprofen for Fever:** For fevers 100-101° F (37.8-38.3° C), fever medicine is generally not needed. For fevers above 101° F (38.3° C) you can take ibuprofen. The goal of fever therapy is to bring the fever down to a comfortable level. Remember that fever medicine usually lowers fever 2 degrees F (1 - 1½ degrees C). **Instructions for Taking Ibuprofen:** Take 400 mg by mouth every 6 hours. Another choice is to take 600 mg by mouth every 8 hours. Use the lowest amount that makes your pain feel better. **Extra Notes:** Acetaminophen is thought to be safer than ibuprofen in people over 65 years old. **Caution:** Do not take ibuprofen if you have stomach problems, kidney disease, are pregnant, or have been told by your doctor to avoid this type of anti-inflammatory drug. Do not take ibuprofen for more than 7 days without consulting your doctor. ***Before taking any medicine, read all the instructions on the package.***

Important Notice

- These OTC (over-the-counter) medications should not be recommended by the telephone triager unless this listing has been reviewed, amended as necessary, and approved by the supervising physician, office medical director, or call center medical director.
- Concise and limited information for these OTC medications is provided in these tables. The triager is strongly encouraged to read the *Physicians' Desk Reference for Nonprescription Drugs* or other trustworthy drug reference for all OTC medications that the triager recommends to patients. Extensive drug information is available at the National Library of Medicine drug information Web site (MedlinePlus).
- Patients should be instructed to read the package warnings and instructions on all OTC medications that they take.

Gastroesophageal Reflux Disease (GERD) (Reflux, Heartburn)

Adult OTC Drug Dosage Table

Treatment of Gastroesophageal Reflux (GER)

Medication	Dosage	Notes
Antacids Maalox Mylanta Rolaids Tums	**Liquid and Tablets** Read package instructions.	**Caution:** There are other serious causes of epigastric discomfort, including: myocardial infarction and gallstones.
H_2 Blocker—Ranitidine Zantac	75-mg tablets 75 mg once or twice daily	**Caution:** There are other serious causes of epigastric discomfort, including: myocardial infarction and gallstones.

Important Notice

- These OTC (over-the-counter) medications should not be recommended by the telephone triager unless this listing has been reviewed, amended as necessary, and approved by the supervising physician, office medical director, or call center medical director.
- Concise and limited information for these OTC medications is provided in these tables. The triager is strongly encouraged to read the *Physicians' Desk Reference for Nonprescription Drugs* or other trustworthy drug reference for all OTC medications that the triager recommends to patients. Extensive drug information is available at the National Library of Medicine drug information Web site (MedlinePlus).
- Patients should be instructed to read the package warnings and instructions on all OTC medications that they take.

Hay Fever (Nasal Allergies)

Adult OTC Drug Dosage Table

Treatment of Hay Fever (Nasal Allergies)

Medication	Dosage	Notes
Cetirizine Zyrtec	10-mg cetirizine tablets 10 mg every day	**Caution:** Antihistamines may cause sleepiness. Do not drink, drive, or operate dangerous machinery while taking antihistamines. Cetirizine is a newer (second-generation) antihistamine and it causes less sedation than diphenhydramine. It has the added advantage of being long-acting (lasts up to 24 hours).
Diphenhydramine Benadryl	25-mg diphenhydramine tablets 25-50 mg every 6 hours	**Caution:** Antihistamines may cause sleepiness. Do not drink, drive, or operate dangerous machinery while taking antihistamines.
Loratadine Claritin Alavert	10-mg loratadine tablets 10 mg every day	**Caution:** Antihistamines may cause sleepiness. Do not drink, drive, or operate dangerous machinery while taking antihistamines. Loratidine is a newer (second-generation) antihistamine and it causes less sedation than diphenhydramine. It has the added advantage of being long-acting (lasts up to 24 hours).

Important Notice

- These OTC (over-the-counter) medications should not be recommended by the telephone triager unless this listing has been reviewed, amended as necessary, and approved by the supervising physician, office medical director, or call center medical director.
- Concise and limited information for these OTC medications is provided in these tables. The triager is strongly encouraged to read the *Physicians' Desk Reference for Nonprescription Drugs* or other trustworthy drug reference for all OTC medications that the triager recommends to patients. Extensive drug information is available at the National Library of Medicine drug information Web site (MedlinePlus).
- Patients should be instructed to read the package warnings and instructions on all OTC medications that they take.

Headache

Adult OTC Drug Dosage Table

Treatment of Headache Pain

Medication	Dosage	Notes
Acetaminophen Tylenol Regular Strength Tylenol Extra Strength Tylenol Adult Liquid Pain Reliever Tylenol Arthritis Extended Relief	325-mg regular strength tablets or caplets: 650 mg (2 pills) every 4-6 hours 500-mg extra strength gelcaps, caplets, or tablets: 1,000 mg (2 pills) every 8 hours 500-mg liquid per tablespoon: 1,000 mg (2 tablespoons or 30 cc) every 8 hours	For relief of headache pain you can take acetaminophen. Take 650 mg by mouth every 4-6 hours. Each Regular Strength Tylenol pill has 325 mg of acetaminophen. Another choice is to take 1,000 mg every 8 hours. Each Extra Strength Tylenol pill has 500 mg of acetaminophen. The most you should take each day is 3,000 mg. **Extra Notes:** Acetaminophen is in many OTC and prescription medicines. It might be in more than one medicine that you are taking. You need to be careful and not take an overdose. An acetaminophen overdose can hurt the liver. **Caution:** Do not take acetaminophen if you have liver disease. ***Before taking any medicine, read all the instructions on the package.***
Ibuprofen Advil Motrin Nuprin	200-mg caplets or tablets: 200-400 mg every 6 hours	For relief of headache pain you can take ibuprofen. Take 400 mg by mouth every 6 hours. Another choice is to take 600 mg by mouth every 8 hours. Use the lowest amount that makes your pain feel better. **Extra Notes:** Acetaminophen is thought to be safer than ibuprofen in people over 65 years old. **Caution:** Do not take ibuprofen if you have stomach problems, kidney disease, are pregnant, or have been told by your doctor to avoid this type of anti-inflammatory drug. Do not take ibuprofen for more than 7 days without consulting your doctor. ***Before taking any medicine, read all the instructions on the package.***

Important Notice

- These OTC (over-the-counter) medications should not be recommended by the telephone triager unless this listing has been reviewed, amended as necessary, and approved by the supervising physician, office medical director, or call center medical director.
- Concise and limited information for these OTC medications is provided in these tables. The triager is strongly encouraged to read the *Physicians' Desk Reference for Nonprescription Drugs* or other trustworthy drug reference for all OTC medications that the triager recommends to patients. Extensive drug information is available at the National Library of Medicine drug information Web site (MedlinePlus).
- Patients should be instructed to read the package warnings and instructions on all OTC medications that they take.

Hemorrhoid Pain and Irritation

Adult OTC Drug Dosage Table

Treatment of Rectal Pain and Irritation From Hemorrhoids

Medication	Dosage	Notes
Hydrocortisone Cream 1% Anusol HC Preparation H Hydrocortisone Analpram HC	After sitz bath and drying rectal area, apply 1% hydrocortisone ointment bid.	A stool softener may help reduce pain during bowel movements.

Important Notice

- These OTC (over-the-counter) medications should not be recommended by the telephone triager unless this listing has been reviewed, amended as necessary, and approved by the supervising physician, office medical director, or call center medical director.
- Concise and limited information for these OTC medications is provided in these tables. The triager is strongly encouraged to read the *Physicians' Desk Reference for Nonprescription Drugs* or other trustworthy drug reference for all OTC medications that the triager recommends to patients. Extensive drug information is available at the National Library of Medicine drug information Web site (MedlinePlus).
- Patients should be instructed to read the package warnings and instructions on all OTC medications that they take.

Hives (Urticaria)

Adult OTC Drug Dosage Table

Treatment of Hives (Urticaria)

Medication	Dosage	Notes
Cetirizine Zyrtec	10-mg cetirizine tablets 10 mg every day	**Caution:** Antihistamines may cause sleepiness. Do not drink, drive, or operate dangerous machinery while taking antihistamines. Cetirizine is a newer (second-generation) antihistamine and it causes less sedation than diphenhydramine. It has the added advantage of being long-acting (lasts up to 24 hours).
Diphenhydramine Benadryl	25-mg diphenhydramine tablets 25-50 mg every 6 hours	**Caution:** Antihistamines may cause sleepiness. Do not drink, drive, or operate dangerous machinery while taking antihistamines.
Loratadine Claritin Alavert	10-mg loratadine tablets 10 mg every day	**Caution:** Antihistamines may cause sleepiness. Do not drink, drive, or operate dangerous machinery while taking antihistamines. Loratidine is a newer (second-generation) antihistamine and it causes less sedation than diphenhydramine. It has the added advantage of being long-acting (lasts up to 24 hours).

Important Notice

- These OTC (over-the-counter) medications should not be recommended by the telephone triager unless this listing has been reviewed, amended as necessary, and approved by the supervising physician, office medical director, or call center medical director.
- Concise and limited information for these OTC medications is provided in these tables. The triager is strongly encouraged to read the *Physicians' Desk Reference for Nonprescription Drugs* or other trustworthy drug reference for all OTC medications that the triager recommends to patients. Extensive drug information is available at the National Library of Medicine drug information Web site (MedlinePlus).
- Patients should be instructed to read the package warnings and instructions on all OTC medications that they take.

Jock Itch

Adult OTC Drug Dosage Table

Treatment of Jock Itch (Tinea Cruris)

Medication	Dosage	Notes
Antifungal Cream—Clotrimazole Lotrimin **Antifungal Cream—Miconazole** Lotrimin AF Micatin Monistat-Derm	Apply antifungal cream 2 times per day to the area of itching and rash. Apply it to the rash and 1 inch beyond its borders. Continue the cream for at least 7 days after the rash is cleared.	Keep your penis and scrotal area clean. Wash once daily with unscented soap and water. Keep your penis and scrotal area dry. Wear cotton underwear (Reason: breathes and keeps area drier). Avoid nylon or tight-fitting underwear. **Expected Course:** The rash should clear up completely in 2-3 weeks.

Important Notice

- These OTC (over-the-counter) medications should not be recommended by the telephone triager unless this listing has been reviewed, amended as necessary, and approved by the supervising physician, office medical director, or call center medical director.
- Concise and limited information for these OTC medications is provided in these tables. The triager is strongly encouraged to read the *Physicians' Desk Reference for Nonprescription Drugs* or other trustworthy drug reference for all OTC medications that the triager recommends to patients. Extensive drug information is available at the National Library of Medicine drug information Web site (MedlinePlus).
- Patients should be instructed to read the package warnings and instructions on all OTC medications that they take.

Menstrual Cramps

Adult OTC Drug Dosage Table

Treatment of Menstrual Cramp Pain

Medication	Dosage	Notes
Ibuprofen Advil Medipren Motrin Nuprin	200-mg caplets or tablets The first dosage should be either 400 or 600 mg. Take 200-400 mg every 6 hours. Take with food.	For pain relief you can take ibuprofen. Take 400 mg by mouth every 6 hours. Another choice is to take 600 mg by mouth every 8 hours. Use the lowest amount that makes your pain feel better. **Extra Notes:** **Caution**: Do not take ibuprofen if you have stomach problems, kidney disease, are pregnant, or have been told by your doctor to avoid this type of anti-inflammatory drug. Do not take ibuprofen for more than 7 days without consulting your doctor. ***Before taking any medicine, read all the instructions on the package.***
Naproxen Aleve Anaprox	220-mg tablet The first dosage should be 2 tablets (440 mg). Take 220 mg (1 tablet) every 8 hours for 2 or 3 days. Take with food.	For pain relief you can take naproxen. Take 250-500 mg by mouth every 12 hours. Use the lowest amount that makes your pain feel better. **Extra Notes:** **Caution:** Do not take naproxen if you have stomach problems, kidney disease, are pregnant, or have been told by your doctor to avoid this type of anti-inflammatory drug. Do not take naproxen for more than 7 days without consulting your doctor. Naproxen is not available OTC in Canada. ***Before taking any medicine, read all the instructions on the package.***

Important Notice

- These OTC (over-the-counter) medications should not be recommended by the telephone triager unless this listing has been reviewed, amended as necessary, and approved by the supervising physician, office medical director, or call center medical director.
- Concise and limited information for these OTC medications is provided in these tables. The triager is strongly encouraged to read the *Physicians' Desk Reference for Nonprescription Drugs* or other trustworthy drug reference for all OTC medications that the triager recommends to patients. Extensive drug information is available at the National Library of Medicine drug information Web site (MedlinePlus).
- Patients should be instructed to read the package warnings and instructions on all OTC medications that they take.

Pain

Adult OTC Drug Dosage Table

Treatment of Pain

Medication	Dosage	Notes
Acetaminophen Tylenol Regular Strength Tylenol Extra Strength Tylenol Adult Liquid Pain Reliever Tylenol Arthritis Extended Relief	325-mg regular strength tablets or caplets: 650 mg (2 pills) every 4-6 hours 500-mg extra strength gelcaps, caplets, or tablets: 1,000 mg (2 pills) every 8 hours 500-mg liquid per tablespoon: 1,000 mg (2 tablespoons or 30 cc) every 8 hours	For pain relief you can take acetaminophen. Take 650 mg by mouth every 4-6 hours. Each Regular Strength Tylenol pill has 325 mg of acetaminophen. Another choice is to take 1,000 mg every 8 hours. Each Extra Strength Tylenol pill has 500 mg of acetaminophen. The most you should take each day is 3,000 mg. **Extra Notes:** Acetaminophen is in many OTC and prescription medicines. It might be in more than one medicine that you are taking. You need to be careful and not take an overdose. An acetaminophen overdose can hurt the liver. **Caution:** Do not take acetaminophen if you have liver disease. ***Before taking any medicine, read all the instructions on the package.***
Ibuprofen Advil Motrin Nuprin	200-mg caplets or tablets: 400 mg every 6 hours	For pain relief you can take ibuprofen. Take 400 mg by mouth every 6 hours. Another choice is to take 600 mg by mouth every 8 hours. Use the lowest amount that makes your pain feel better. **Extra Notes:** Acetaminophen is thought to be safer than ibuprofen in people over 65 years old. **Caution:** Do not take ibuprofen if you have stomach problems, kidney disease, are pregnant, or have been told by your doctor to avoid this type of anti-inflammatory drug. Do not take ibuprofen for more than 7 days without consulting your doctor. ***Before taking any medicine, read all the instructions on the package.***

Important Notice

- These OTC (over-the-counter) medications should not be recommended by the telephone triager unless this listing has been reviewed, amended as necessary, and approved by the supervising physician, office medical director, or call center medical director.
- Concise and limited information for these OTC medications is provided in these tables. The triager is strongly encouraged to read the *Physicians' Desk Reference for Nonprescription Drugs* or other trustworthy drug reference for all OTC medications that the triager recommends to patients. Extensive drug information is available at the National Library of Medicine drug information Web site (MedlinePlus).
- Patients should be instructed to read the package warnings and instructions on all OTC medications that they take.

Poison Ivy

Adult OTC Drug Dosage Table

Poison Ivy

Medication	Dosage	Notes
Prevention With IvyBlock Cream	Use it prior to possible exposure (e.g., planned hike in woods).	It works on the skin as an active barrier that blocks the allergenic oil (urushiol) of the poison ivy/oak plant. This cream has been approved by the FDA; it has been shown to prevent a skin reaction (Marks 1995).
Reducing the Itch of Poison Ivy Calamine lotion	Apply to affected area of the skin 3-4 times daily.	
Reducing the Itch of Poison Ivy Aveeno (oatmeal) bath for itching	Sprinkle contents of 1 packet under running faucet with comfortably warm water. Bathe for 15-20 minutes, 1-2 times daily.	After using Aveeno bath, pat the skin dry using towel; do not rub. You can also dry the area by using a blow dryer set on the cool setting.

Important Notice

- These OTC (over-the-counter) medications should not be recommended by the telephone triager unless this listing has been reviewed, amended as necessary, and approved by the supervising physician, office medical director, or call center medical director.
- Concise and limited information for these OTC medications is provided in these tables. The triager is strongly encouraged to read the *Physicians' Desk Reference for Nonprescription Drugs* or other trustworthy drug reference for all OTC medications that the triager recommends to patients. Extensive drug information is available at the National Library of Medicine drug information Web site (MedlinePlus).
- Patients should be instructed to read the package warnings and instructions on all OTC medications that they take.

Pubic Lice

Adult OTC Drug Dosage Table

Treatment of Pubic Lice

Medication	Dosage	Notes
1% Permethrin Nix	Pour about 2 ounces of the creme into previously washed and towel-dried pubic hair. Add a little warm water to work up a lather. Leave the Nix on for a full 20 minutes. Then rinse the hair thoroughly and dry it with a towel. Repeat the Nix treatment in 1 week to kill any nits that were missed.	**Dead Nits:** Wait 3 or more hours after Nix treatment is completed before removing the dead nits (Reason: let Nix permeate the nits). The nits can be loosened using a mixture of half vinegar and half warm water. After wetting the hair with this solution, cover the hair with a towel for 30 minutes. Then remove the dead nits by back-combing with a special nit comb or pull them out individually. **Pregnancy and Breastfeeding:** According to the Centers for Disease Control and Prevention, women who are pregnant or who are breastfeeding can be treated with products containing permethrin (e.g., Nix).

Important Notice

- These OTC (over-the-counter) medications should not be recommended by the telephone triager unless this listing has been reviewed, amended as necessary, and approved by the supervising physician, office medical director, or call center medical director.
- Concise and limited information for these OTC medications is provided in these tables. The triager is strongly encouraged to read the *Physicians' Desk Reference for Nonprescription Drugs* or other trustworthy drug reference for all OTC medications that the triager recommends to patients. Extensive drug information is available at the National Library of Medicine drug information Web site (MedlinePlus).
- Patients should be instructed to read the package warnings and instructions on all OTC medications that they take.

Ringworm

Adult OTC Drug Dosage Table

Treatment of Ringworm (Tinea Corporis)

Medication	Dosage	Notes
Antifungal Cream—Clotrimazole Lotrimin **Antifungal Cream—Miconazole** Lotrimin AF Micatin Monistat-Derm	Use it prior to possible exposure (e.g., planned hike in woods).	Apply antifungal cream 2 times per day to the area of itching and rash. Apply it to the rash and 1 inch beyond its borders. Continue the cream for at least 7 days after the rash is cleared. **Expected Course:** The rash should clear up completely in 2-4 weeks.

Important Notice

- These OTC (over-the-counter) medications should not be recommended by the telephone triager unless this listing has been reviewed, amended as necessary, and approved by the supervising physician, office medical director, or call center medical director.
- Concise and limited information for these OTC medications is provided in these tables. The triager is strongly encouraged to read the *Physicians' Desk Reference for Nonprescription Drugs* or other trustworthy drug reference for all OTC medications that the triager recommends to patients. Extensive drug information is available at the National Library of Medicine drug information Web site (MedlinePlus).
- Patients should be instructed to read the package warnings and instructions on all OTC medications that they take.

Sunburn

Adult OTC Drug Dosage Table

Treatment of Sunburn Pain

Medication	Dosage	Notes
Acetaminophen Tylenol Regular Strength Tylenol Extra Strength Tylenol Adult Liquid Pain Reliever Tylenol Arthritis Extended Relief	325-mg regular strength tablets or caplets: 650 mg (2 pills) every 4-6 hours 500-mg extra strength gelcaps, caplets, or tablets: 1,000 mg (2 pills) every 8 hours 500-mg liquid per tablespoon: 1,000 mg (2 tablespoons or 30 cc) every 8 hours	For pain relief you can take acetaminophen. Take 650 mg by mouth every 4-6 hours. Each Regular Strength Tylenol pill has 325 mg of acetaminophen. Another choice is to take 1,000 mg every 8 hours. Each Extra Strength Tylenol pill has 500 mg of acetaminophen. The most you should take each day is 3,000 mg. **Extra Notes:** Acetaminophen is in many OTC and prescription medicines. It might be in more than one medicine that you are taking. You need to be careful and not take an overdose. An acetaminophen overdose can hurt the liver. **Caution:** Do not take acetaminophen if you have liver disease. ***Before taking any medicine, read all the instructions on the package.***
Ibuprofen Advil Motrin Nuprin	200-mg caplets or tablets: 400 mg every 6 hours	For pain relief you can take ibuprofen. Take 400 mg by mouth every 6 hours. Another choice is to take 600 mg by mouth every 8 hours. Use the lowest amount that makes your pain feel better. **Extra Notes:** Acetaminophen is thought to be safer than ibuprofen in people over 65 years old. **Caution:** Do not take ibuprofen if you have stomach problems, kidney disease, are pregnant, or have been told by your doctor to avoid this type of anti-inflammatory drug. Do not take ibuprofen for more than 7 days without consulting your doctor. ***Before taking any medicine, read all the instructions on the package.***

Sunburn *(continued)*

Adult OTC Drug Dosage Table

Preventing Sunburn

Any sunscreen lotion with a rating of SPF 30 may be used. Sunscreens with ratings higher than 30 provide minimal additional protection.	Apply sunscreen to areas that can't be protected by clothing. Generally, an adult needs about 1 oz of sunscreen lotion to cover the entire body. Reapply every 2-4 hours and after swimming. You should also reapply after swimming, exercising, or sweating.	Sunscreens help prevent sunburn but do not completely prevent skin damage. Thus, sun exposure can still increase your risk of skin aging and skin cancer. Try to avoid all sun exposure between 10:00 am and 3:00 pm. Also, use a hat with a wide brim and cotton clothing with long sleeves when outdoors.

Important Notice

- These OTC (over-the-counter) medications should not be recommended by the telephone triager unless this listing has been reviewed, amended as necessary, and approved by the supervising physician, office medical director, or call center medical director.
- Concise and limited information for these OTC medications is provided in these tables. The triager is strongly encouraged to read the *Physicians' Desk Reference for Nonprescription Drugs* or other trustworthy drug reference for all OTC medications that the triager recommends to patients. Extensive drug information is available at the National Library of Medicine drug information Web site (MedlinePlus).
- Patients should be instructed to read the package warnings and instructions on all OTC medications that they take.

Superficial Skin Infection

Adult OTC Drug Dosage Table

Treatment of Superficial Skin Infection and Impetigo

Medication	Dosage	Notes
Antibiotic Ointment Bacitracin Neosporin Polysporin (bacitracin and polymyxin B) Triple Antibiotic (bacitracin, neomycin, and polymixin B)	Use after cleaning and drying the wound. Apply ointment BID-TID.	**Caution:** Stop ointment if a rash or allergic reaction occurs.

Important Notice

- These OTC (over-the-counter) medications should not be recommended by the telephone triager unless this listing has been reviewed, amended as necessary, and approved by the supervising physician, office medical director, or call center medical director.
- Concise and limited information for these OTC medications is provided in these tables. The triager is strongly encouraged to read the *Physicians' Desk Reference for Nonprescription Drugs* or other trustworthy drug reference for all OTC medications that the triager recommends to patients. Extensive drug information is available at the National Library of Medicine drug information Web site (MedlinePlus).
- Patients should be instructed to read the package warnings and instructions on all OTC medications that they take.

Vaginal Dryness

Adult OTC Drug Dosage Table

Treatment of Vaginal Dryness During Sexual Intercourse

Medication	Dosage	Notes
Vaginal Lubricant Astroglide K-Y Liquid KY Silk-E		

Important Notice

- These OTC (over-the-counter) medications should not be recommended by the telephone triager unless this listing has been reviewed, amended as necessary, and approved by the supervising physician, office medical director, or call center medical director.
- Concise and limited information for these OTC medications is provided in these tables. The triager is strongly encouraged to read the *Physicians' Desk Reference for Nonprescription Drugs* or other trustworthy drug reference for all OTC medications that the triager recommends to patients. Extensive drug information is available at the National Library of Medicine drug information Web site (MedlinePlus).
- Patients should be instructed to read the package warnings and instructions on all OTC medications that they take.

Vaginal Yeast Infection

Adult OTC Drug Dosage Table

Treatment of Vaginal Yeast Infection (Candidal Vaginitis)

Medication	Dosage	Notes
Butoconazole Femstat 3 **Clotrimazole** Gyne-Lotrimin 3 Mycelex-7 **Miconazole** Monistat 3 or 7	Read and follow the package instructions closely.	There are a number of OTC medications for treatment of vaginal yeast infections. If no improvement within 3 days, you will need to be examined by a physician. Do not use the yeast medication during the 24 hours prior to your appointment (Reason: interferes with examination). If you are pregnant, you will need to speak with your doctor before using.

Important Notice

- These OTC (over-the-counter) medications should not be recommended by the telephone triager unless this listing has been reviewed, amended as necessary, and approved by the supervising physician, office medical director, or call center medical director.
- Concise and limited information for these OTC medications is provided in these tables. The triager is strongly encouraged to read the *Physicians' Desk Reference for Nonprescription Drugs* or other trustworthy drug reference for all OTC medications that the triager recommends to patients. Extensive drug information is available at the National Library of Medicine drug information Web site (MedlinePlus).
- Patients should be instructed to read the package warnings and instructions on all OTC medications that they take.

Index

Q

R

S